Michael Schwartz
5535

Neurology

Neurology

Mark Mumenthaler

Translated by Edmund H. Burrows

Third, revised edition

1990
Georg Thieme Verlag Stuttgart · New York
Thieme Medical Publishers, Inc., New York

Mark Mumenthaler M. D.,
Professor of Neurology, Head of the
Department of Neurology,
Berne University, Inselspital,
CH-3010 Berne, Switzerland

Dr. E. H. Burrows
Brackendale, Hadrian Way, Chilworth
Southampton SO1 7HX, England

Library of Congress Cataloging-in-Publication
Data
Mumenthaler, Mark, 1925–
  Neurology.

  Translation of: Neurologie.
  Bibliography: p.   Includes index.
  1. Nervous system–Diseases. I. Title.
  [DNLM: 1. Nervous System Diseases.
  WL 100 M962n]
  RC346.M8213   1989   612.8   89-4512

1st German edition 1967
2nd German edition 1969
3rd German edition 1970
4th German edition 1973
5th German edition 1976
6th German edition 1979
7th German edition 1982
8th German edition 1986
9th German edition 1990
1st English edition 1977
2nd English edition 1983

1st French edition 1974
1st Greek edition 1990
1st Italian edition 1975
2nd Italian edition 1984
1st Japanese edition 1983
1st Polish edition 1972
2nd Polish edition 1979
1st Portuguese edition 1977
1st Spanish edition 1976
2nd Spanish edition 1982
1st Turkish edition 1984

Important Note: Medicine is an ever-changing science. Research and clinical experience are continually broadening our knowledge, in particular our knowledge of proper treatment and drug therapy. Insofar as this book mentions any dosage or application, readers may rest assured that the authors, editors and publishers have made every effort to ensure that such references are strictly in accordance with the **state of knowledge at the time of production of the book. Nevertheless, every user is requested** to carefully examine the manufacturer's leaflets accompanying each drug to check on his own responsibility whether the dosage schedules recommended therein or the contraindications stated by the manufacturers differ from the statements made in the present book. Such examination is particularly important with drugs that are either rarely used or have been newly released on the market.

Cover design by Dominique Loenicker

This book is an authorized and revised translation from the 9th German edition, published and copyrighted 1990 by Georg Thieme Verlag, Stuttgart, Germany. Title of the German edition: Neurologie.

© 1977, 1990 Georg Thieme Verlag, Rüdigerstraße 14, D-7000 Stuttgart 30, Germany
Thieme Medical Publishers, Inc., 381 Park Avenue South, New York, N.Y.10016

Printed in Germany by Clausen & Bosse, Leck

Typesetting (Digiset 40T30) by Appl, Wemding

ISBN 3-13-523903-9 (Georg Thieme Verlag, Stuttgart)
ISBN 0-86577-317-3 (Thieme Medical Publishers, Inc., New York)

1 2 3 4 5 6

Dedicated to the memory
of my American teacher in neurology

G. Milton Shy

and to my many friends in the UK and USA

Preface

In the beginning, the German and French schools shaped the face of neurology. During the course of this century, and particularly since World War II, significant impulses for the development of the specialty have come from English-speaking countries, especially Britain and the USA. I myself completed part of my training in the USA, and I am very pleased that the present text is now appearing in its third English edition.

Since the first (1977) and second (1983) editions were published, a further seven years have gone by. It was therefore necessary to prepare a completely new translation. This was undertaken energetically and expertly by Ted Burrows, M.D., Wessex Neurological Center, Southampton, Great Britain. I wish to express my gratitude also to David Goldblatt, M.D. at the University of Rochester Medical Center, New York. He reviewed the manuscript with patience, care, and constructive criticism. He recommended many changes and more precise formulations, and adapted the language of the text for the American reader. Thanks to the enthusiasm of all my collaborators, and especially to the cooperation of Mrs. Hadler, who is in charge of the English editing at the publishing company, this third English edition is identical to the 9th German edition, and is appearing simultaneously with it. I wish to express my gratitude to all those who contributed, and to those at the publishing company responsible for the production of the text.

The book is an attempt to present the basic knowledge required for the practice of neurology in a clear, instructive manner. The personal views, specific experience and special interests of the author have had their effect on the text. The author is fully aware that this book is an anachronism in itself: any attempt by a single individual to present the entire specialty of neurology is presumptuous, considering the ever increasing degree of subspecialization within the field. The advantage of single authorship lies in the fact that I have been able to make every effort to present, in a concise fashion, what in my view are the salient aspects of current knowledge. I have tried to act as a generalist of neurology. The fact that the book has been published in ten languages, and is being translated into a further two, seems to justify my efforts. The reader, however, must be the final judge of the acceptability of this method; I shall be very grateful for all suggestions and criticisms.

Berne, Switzerland   Fall 1989
MARK MUMENTHALER

Contents

1. Diseases Affecting Mainly the Brain and its Coverings

Intracranial diseases may be characterized by:

– **General symptoms and signs,**
  • headache,
  • disturbances of consciousness,
  • (generalized) epileptic seizures,
  • an organic mental syndrome,
  • meningism,
  • signs of raised intracranial pressure (vomiting, slow pulse).

– **Localizing signs,**
  • focal neurologic deficits,
  • neuropsychologic features,
  • disturbances of vision,
  • cranial nerve palsies,
  • focal epileptic seizures.

None of these features is necessary for diagnosis, and they are encountered in various combinations and degrees of severity.

Congenital and Perinatally Acquired Lesions of the Brain

Cerebral Palsy (Cerebral Movement Disturbances, Psychomotor Retardation)

Definition: By this term is understood, irrespective of etiologic considerations, a retardation of motor and usually mental development which is usually evident in the 1st year of life.

Pathogenesis: Disturbances occurring during pregnancy, premature birth, abnormal delivery, birth weight below 2,000 g or above 4,000 g, etc. deprive the brain of oxygen and commonly lead to cerebral movement disturbances. The Apgar scale provides a method of evaluating vital signs at birth: heart rate, respiration, muscle tone, reflex response to foot-sole stimulation, and skin color is each scored from 0 to 2 points. The highest score is 10 points, i.e., 5×2 points. The Apgar scale is determined at 1, 5, and 10 min after birth. Malformations (p. 3), intrauterine infections (p. 12), and icterus gravis (p. 14) are additional causes of cerebral palsy.

Clinical picture: *Warning signs* include, in addition to the above-mentioned features at birth, cyanosis, delayed first cry, feeding problems, hypotonia or by contrast a fixed arched position, a tendency to opisthotonus and spasticity giving rise to difficulties in changing diapers. Strabismus and lefthandedness are also frequently found.

Abnormalities in the *reflex responses* (213) may manifest early: no head-raising at 3 months in the prone position, abnormally strong grasp reflex, increased tonic labyrinthine reflexes, increased neck reflex, rotation en bloc response of the body to testing of the positional reflex. At the end of the 4th month the infant should be able to control his head in the sitting position, lift his head when placed prone, and use both hands together during play. The Moro reflex is fading, the Landau and parachute reflexes are appearing. Pathologic phenomena as described above. At the end of the 6th month the presence of the following features raises the strong suspicion or certainty (when dominant) of retarded development: retained tonic and Moro reflexes, absent Landau, labyrinthine positional, and parachute reflexes. The child should be able to raise his head from the supine position, turn himself on his stomach, utter spontaneous sounds, and use the whole hand including the thumb. Sits with support. At the end of

the 9th month a cerebral movement disturbance should be suspected if, in addition to the abnormal reflexes already mentioned, the following are shown: absence of supporting and "limping" reaction, i.e., the presence of a trunk postural reflex.

The infant should be able to sit unaided, and lumbar kyphosis becomes less pronounced. The *normal motor development of infants and small children* is given in Fig.1.1, the *normal reflexes* in Table 1.1.

Physical findings: For several weeks up to 6 months, hypotonia ("floppy infant") may be present. For several further months the child may exhibit a dystonia alternating with an increase in muscle tone depending upon posture and various other stimuli, leading finally to true spasticity. Some infants (with or without spasticity) develop involuntary movements (athetosis, chorea, choreo-

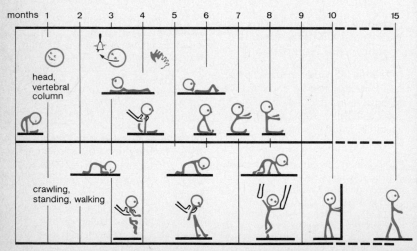

Fig.1.1   Motor development during infancy and early childhood

athetosis, torsion dystonia, tremor), ataxia, and rigidity. Sometimes epileptic seizures also supervene. Mental development is affected to a greater or lesser degree of severity. The term oligophrenia encompasses cases of reduced mental function, in which the cause is definitely congenital or acquired early in life. In some children varying degrees of agnosia and/or apraxia may produce *disturbances of fine motor control,* such as drawing and spatial appreciation. These children are often awkward as well as restless and even hyperkinetic. Choreiform movements may be present, which can usually be suppressed at will or by voluntary movements. In such cases one speaks of "the clumsy child." The higher level of verbal intelligence contrasts with poor performance of manual and other motor activities. Complex relationships exist with the congenital form of alexia, which presents as a difficulty in learning to read at school but is not identical with acquired alexia. Neurologic examination reveals no abnormality but the EEG often shows diffuse abnormalities. This symptom complex is invariably caused by mild or minimal brain damage, secondary to either intrauterine causis or birth trauma. Individual signs and symptoms may be attributed to an inherited disturbance of cerebral organization. Table 1.2 reviews the most important movement disturbances of cerebral origin.

Early detection: This is possible by establishing the presence of retarded development and specific abnormal findings in the infant in the course of neurologic examination. About 25% of patients improve spontaneously; however, 50% can be rehabilitated by prompt early treatment to a greater or lesser degree. For this reason, early recognition is essential. Much can be achieved nowadays in the brain-damaged child by appropriate therapy (136); 25% of the children remain severely damaged.

Malformation of the Brain Due to Developmental Disturbances

Most of the lesions in this group of diseases are present at birth or manifest immediately afterward, although in a few the signs become apparent only in the course of the first few years of life. Disturbed psychomotor development with defective intelligence is usually present. Epileptiform seizures and focal cerebral or cerebellar signs may occur. Individual entities are listed in Table 1.3.

Absence or Defective Development of Individual Parts of the Brain

The commonest defect is a *micropolygyria,* in which numerous narrow convolutions are present within a circumscribed area of the neocortex or over a more widespread area. The secondary convolutions may be reduced in number *(pachygyria)* or entirely absent *(agyria* or *lissencephaly).* In arhinencephaly the olfactory nerves and tracts are absent, in some cases the corpus callosum is absent as well *(agenesis of the corpus callosum),* the hemispheres then being rudimentary and fused. Occasionally a *cyclops* may occur. *Holotelencephaly* (a solitary ventricle in the rostral forebrain) combines microcephaly,

Table 1.1   Reflexes in infants and children

Description	Mode of Testing and Effect	Time	In Cerebral Palsy	Remarks
Positional tests / Postural reflexes				
Doll's eyes phenomenon	Awake recumbent infant, passive turning of the head to the side. Gaze remains in original direction	Birth to 10th day	Persistent	
Step reflex	Child held up passively by examiner's hands under axillae with soles of feet lightly touching the ground. Step movements executed, with the examiner supporting the child's weight	First week of life		
Crossed stretch reflex	Maximal passive flexion of hip and knee joints with child supine: extension of the opposite leg and foot	Always normal	Foot tone to be noted	Spinal reflex
Crossed flexion reflex	Maximal passive flexion of hip and knee with child supine: flexion of opposite leg as well	Birth to 7th–12th months	Abnormal after 1st year	Differential diagnosis: additional movements with hip joint contracture due to other causes
Supporting reflex	Legs: child lifted onto his legs or normal pressure on the soles of the feet by the examiner's hands stimulates extension. Arms: extension on pressure	Increasingly after birth to 4th–6th months	Excessive, persistent	Physiologic inability to stand in 2nd–3rd months
Foot position reflex	Child held up by examiner's hands under axillae so that the dorsa of feet lightly touch the edge of a flat surface. Leg will be actively raised and placed on the table top	Only in the first weeks of life		

Grasp reflex	Touching the palm of the hand with a finger; fist is clenched	Birth to 3 months	Increased after 3 months	Suspicious after 3 months, abnormal after 6 months
Toe reflex	Touching the sole of the foot causes clawing of toes	Birth to 12th month	Absent in neonates, later increasing	If marked, to clawing, which later interferes with walking
Spine reflex	Stroking the skin of the back with the child prone; flexion to same side, extension of ipsilateral leg and flexion of contralateral one	In first months of life	Increased	Usually only vaguely present
Neck reflex, asymmetric	Supine (or prone) position. If the head is turned slowly and passively, a change occurs in posture or tone. The arm and the leg on the side to which face is turned are extended and the opposite arm as well as the leg are flexed	Birth to 5th–6th months. Not during sleep	Increased after the 6th month during sleep as well	Occasionally spontaneous
Neck reflex, symmetric	Supine position, head flexed: both arms flexed, and the legs extended at the hips and sometimes at other joints as well	Birth to 5th–6th months. Not during sleep	Increased after the 6th month during sleep as well	
Tonic reflex	Supine position, passive flexion of head: head and shoulders retract actively, trunk and hip extensors contract, mouth opens	Never pure	Increased	Spastic subjects are unwilling to lie supine
	Prone position, backward movement of the head: head bends forward, arms and legs flex and adduct	Rarely pure	Increased	

Postural reflexes

Positional tests

Table 1.1 (Continued)

Description	Mode of Testing and Effect	Time	In Cerebral Palsy	Remarks
Labyrinthine postural reflex (head)	Child prone: retracts head. In hanging position suspended by the feet: head retracts as well	Starts in 2nd month	Absent	
	Child seated, trunk flexed to one side: head in vertical position	From 3rd–4th month to 6th month	Delayed	Sometimes asymmetric (in hemisyndromes)
Landau reflex	Child held horizontal in abdominal suspension: head retracted, trunk and legs extended. Passive flexion of head: all joints flexed	4th–18th month	Absent, delayed, sometimes prolonged	
Head-on-trunk reflex	Supine position, head turned passively and rapidly to one side: after ⅓ rotation, the trunk follows in torsion movement	Birth, fades by 12th month	Delayed, protracted, rotation en bloc	En bloc rotational movement requires treatment
Trunk postural reflex	Supine position, rotation of shoulder (or pelvic) girdle: in 1st stage, trunk follows en bloc. In 2nd stage, trunk follows in torsion movement	Birth to 4th–6th month	Increased, sometimes prolonged	Negative if pelvis begins to rotate after 80°
	Supine position, hips flexed to right angle, rotation of trunk by lateral inclination	4th–6th to 14th month. Birth to 6th month		

Movement reflexes

Movement reflexes

Moro's reflex	Supine position. Sudden blow on the bed, or horizontally suspending the patient's head and trunk and suddenly dropping the head, causes arms to move sideways and then forward in a clenching movement, hands outstretched	Birth to 4th–7th month	Positive for longer period	Absent in the first few months in severe cerebral damage
Supporting reaction	Pushing the child from a particular direction into any body position stimulates contraction of the ipsilateral muscles	Seated, from 7th month onward	Delayed or absent (deficient)	
Limping reaction	Pushing the child from a particular direction into any body position stimulates supporting reaction with the arms sometimes crossed to the opposite side	Seated, from 7th month onward	Delayed or absent (deficient)	
Parachute reflex	Child held in position of abdominal suspension or in upright kneeling position. When suddenly pushed forward the arms are extended, palms outstretched	From 6th–9th months onward	Absent, delayed, or incomplete	Abnormal, even if asymmetric or clenched hand outstretched. A statokinetic reaction

Balance tests

Table 1.2 Most important disturbances of movement of cerebral origin in infants

Description	Details	Pathologic Substrate	Causes
Infantile spastic diplegia (Little's disease)	Spasticity of the limbs more marked in the legs. Equinus. Scissor gait. Mentally often normal	Pachymicrogyria, lobar sclerosis	Perinatal damage (developmental disturbances, embryopathy, kernicterus)
Congenital cerebral monoparesis	Usually paralysis of the arm and face	Porencephaly, focal atrophy	Birth trauma (asphyxia, hemorrhage)
Congenital hemiparesis	Arm more severely involved than the leg. Epileptic attacks in about 50%. Usually mentally handicapped	Porencephaly	Birth trauma (asphyxia, hemorrhage)
Congenital tetraparesis (bilateral hemiplegia)	Arms more severely involved than the legs, sometimes bulbar signs. Epileptic attacks. A severe mental deficit	Porencephaly bilateral, often hydrocephalus	Birth trauma (asphyxia, hemorrhage). Additional prenatal damage
Congenital pseudobulbar palsy	Disturbance of deglutition causing difficulties with drinking. Speech difficulties. Mentally usually normal	Bilateral lesion of corticobulbar tracts	Prenatal damage or birth trauma. Malformation (syringobulbia)
Atonic astatic syndrome (Foerster)	Hypotonia and weakness of muscles. Inability to stand up. Incoordination. Severe mental deficit	Atrophy of frontal lobes? Cerebellar defects?	
Bilateral athetosis (athetose double) and congenital chorea (choreoathetosis)	Athetotic or other involuntary movements, often combined with spastic paralysis	Defects of basal ganglia. Status marmoratus (Vogt). Status dysmyelinatus if onset is late	Developmental disturbances, perinatal damage especially kernicterus
Congenital rigidity	Rigidity without involuntary movements. Postural anomalies. No pyramidal signs. Severe mental deficit. Epileptic attacks	Status marmoratus	Developmental disturbances, perinatal damage particularly kernicterus
Congenital cerebellar ataxia	Ataxia, intention tremor, and disturbances of coordinated movement. Retardation of motor development. Speech disturbances. May be combined with other motor syndromes	Malformation of cerebellum	Disturbances of cerebellar development

Table 1.3 Most important malformations and genetically determined growth abnormalities of the brain

1. *Absence or malformation of individual parts of the brain*
   - Micropolygyria — Local increase in narrow convolutions
   - Pachygyria — Reduced number of secondary convolutions
   - Agyria — Absence of convolutions
   - Lissencephaly — See agyria
   - Arhinencephaly — absent olfactory nerves and tracts, absence of the corpus callosum, among other defects
   - Cyclops — Fusion of orbital anlage
   - Holotelencephaly — Single ventricle in rostral part of cerebrum
   - Dandy-Walker syndrome — Cystic enlargement of the 4th ventricle and hydrocephalus
   - Arnold-Chiari malformation — Caudad displacement of the medulla oblongata and tonguelike elongations of the cerebellar tonsils

2. *Microcephaly* — Small head and brain

3. *Meningoencephaloceles* — Incomplete closure of the neural tube
   - Spina bifida occulta
   - Meningocele
   - Myelomeningocele
   - Myelomeningocystocele
   - Open anencephaly

4. *Sinus pericranii* — Vascular malformation in communication with venous sinus, usually frontal

5. *Cranial dermal sinus* — Located in midline, usually occipital, and often associated with dermoid cyst

6. *Phakomatoses* — Multisystem malformation implicating the CNS
   - Tuberous sclerosis (Bourneville's disease)
   - Encephalofacial angiomatosis (Sturge-Weber disease)
   - Von Hippel-Lindau disease
   - Neurofibromatosis (von Recklinghausen's disease)

hypotelorism, and retarded development. Parts of the cerebellum may be absent or incompletely formed. The *Dandy-Walker syndrome* of children (1062) is characterized by the presence of an enormous cystic enlargement of the fourth ventricle, which sometimes herniates into the middle cranial fossa, accompanied by hydrocephalus and enlargement of the posterior cranial fossa. It is caused by an atresia of the foramina of Luschka and Magendie and is often accompanied by a dysgenesis of the vermis, agenesis of the corpus callosum, aqueductal stenosis, and lower cranial nerve palsies (787). In the *Arnold-Chiari malformation,* part of the medulla oblongata and a tonguelike process of the cerebellum are found below the level of the foramen magnum in the cervical spinal canal. This malformation may sometimes – but not invariably – be associated with spina bifida and hydrocephalus. Anomalies of the craniovertebral junction may also be present (p. 20).

Microcephaly

Various prenatal insults, especially from cytomegalovirus (p. 13) – and in 15% also genetic factors – may lead to *microcephaly* (626). This group also includes xeroderma pigmentosum. Its manifestations are skin changes caused by exposure to sunlight, as well as small stature, mental retardation, deafness, and spinocerebellar deficits (814). The small size of the facial skeleton is combined with prominent orbital ridges and a receding chin ("bird face"). Mental deficiency is the rule, with spastic weakness, athetosis, epileptic seizures, strabismus, nystagmus, and optic atrophy being common findings. The EEG in two-thirds of cases is abnormal; hydrocephalus or cerebral malformation is also common.

Meningoencephalocele

The neural tube, which starts to develop on the 19th day of embryonic life, is usually closed in both its cranial and spinal parts by the end of the 1st month. The surrounding covering layers and bones develop from mesenchyme. Disturbances in development may lead to various defects. By far the commonest site of these malformations is the occipital region.

Clinical forms: The *following defects* are encountered in the brain and spinal cord:

- Incomplete bone fusion: cranium bifidum occultum (spina bifida occulta).
- Herniation of meninges through the bone defect, covered by skin: meningocele.
- Presence of brain substance within the herniating meninges: encephalomeningocele (myelomeningocele).
- Presence of part of the ventricular system in addition to the herniating brain and meninges: encephalomeningocele (myelomeningocele).
- The neural tube remains open and the malformed cerebral anlage presents an uncovered neural plate: open anencephaly (complete rachischisis).

Treatment: As a rule, only meningoceles and encephalomeningoceles are operable. Any operation should be carried out in the first hours of life. Great care is required to achieve a worthwhile result, not only for the newborn but also for his family. Associated spinal malformations, hydrocephalus, the mental attitude of the infant's parents, etc. require careful review. Even more important, therefore, is the intrauterine evaluation of malformations of the brain and spinal cord, which is made possible by evaluation of the child's albumin level in the blood of the mother, the alpha-fetoprotein. Malformations occur in 1 in 15 pregnancies in women with high levels, but only 1 in 10,000 pregnancies in women with normal levels (454).

Differential diagnosis: A finding not to be confused with meningocele, *sinus pericranii* is a lesion usually in the frontal region but not always in the midline (897). This congenital vascular malformation, which often presents as a fluctuating soft tissue mass communicating with the intracranial venous sinuses, is usually asymptomatic and unaccompanied by other defects. *Cranial dermal sinus* (419) is another midline lesion usually found in the occipital region and associated with a local swelling. Roentgenograms almost always reveal a skull defect and most cases are associated with a dermoid cyst.

Phakomatoses

The malformations in this group (see Table 1.3) involve not only the brain but also the skin, peripheral nervous system, and internal organs (22).

Tuberous Sclerosis (Bourneville's Disease) (425, 912)

The **clinical features** of this syndrome are

- mental deficiency,
- epileptic seizures,
- adenoma sebaceum,
- intracranial calcifications,
  nodular tumors of the brain,
  kidneys, and retina.

While the *mental deficiency* is usually manifest within the first 2 years, only three-fourths show *nonpigmented patches* (white spots) by this age. More than five such patches should prompt suspicion of tuberous sclerosis. In the presence of a seizure disorder even less than five vitiliginous spots are suggestive of this condition. The *adenoma sebaceum* (Pringle's nevus) sometimes appears only in the course of the first few years, affecting characteristically the nose and forehead. The lesions may be discrete, resembling acne, or consist of wartlike nodules which may be disfiguring. *Intracranial calcifications* may be visible in the conventional roentgenograms only after the 2nd–4th year. The *epileptic seizures* almost always occur in the first 2 years, starting as salaam spasms (p.267). Nodular mesenchymal tumors, usually angiomyolipomas, occur on the surface or in the cortex of the *kidneys,* and rhabdomyomas occur in the heart. Ophthalmoscopic examination may reveal knotlike prominences in the *retina* resulting from glial proliferation. In the brain, similar warty swellings are found which distort the gyri and consist of large abnormal astrocytes. These abnormal cell collections may also be present in the white matter or within the cerebral ventricles. The disease is a dominant hereditary disorder with a high mutation rate. It exhibits changes compatible with a disordered histiogenesis. When the diagnosis is suspected, an attempt to demonstrate tubers in the brain by computerized tomography or magnetic resonance imaging should be made in early infancy (genetic counseling for the parents).

Encephalofacial Angiomatosis (Sturge-Weber Disease)

This phakomatosis has a sporadic incidence but appears to be inherited as a dominant trait with variable penetrance. **Clinically,** it is characterized by the combination of a facial nevus in the distribution of one or more divisions of a trigeminal nerve, (focal) epilepsy, mental deficiency, and sometimes a contralateral hemiparesis. **Roentgenograms** show "railroad track" calcification on the convexity of the affected part of the hemisphere, the deposits being within tortuous blood vessels, mostly capillaries and small veins of the meninges. The parieto-occipital convexity is most often involved.

Von Hippel-Lindau Disease

This disease, inherited as an autosomal dominant, is characterized **clinically** by retinal angiomatosis combined with one or sometimes more cerebellar angiomas. The intracranial lesion is usually situated in the wall of a cyst and causes cerebellar symptoms and signs of raised intracranial pressure to develop in adulthood. Occasionally angiomas of other organs may be present. **Treatment** consists in total removal of the mural nodule of this cerebellar angioma. Early diagnosis enhances the good prognosis of surgically treated cases.

Generalized Neurofibromatosis (von Recklinghausen's Disease) (992)

This phakomatosis is characterized by the presence of countless neurofibromata which develop from the connective tissue of the nerve sheaths. They involve the *peripheral nerves* (progressive peripheral palsies) as well as the *nerve roots* (radicular syndromes). In the latter instance, if within the spinal canal, they may give rise to spinal cord compression and paraplegia. Growth into an intervertebral foramen produces foraminal enlargement which may be visible on appropriate roentgenograms; if a tumor has both intraspinal and extraspinal extensions, the term "dumbbell" neurofibroma is used (see Fig. 1.**29**). *Intracranially,* the most

Table 1.**4**   Intrauterine lesions of the brain

- German measles embryopathy
- Congenital toxoplasmosis
- Neonatal cytomegalovirus encephalitis
- Congenital syphilis
- Alcohol embryopathy

frequent clinical site is the eighth cranial nerve, presenting as a cerebellopontine angle tumor, occasionally bilateral (p. 37). The optic nerve and retina may also be involved (visual disturbances) and occasionally the CNS itself (epilepsy and evidence of a space-occupying lesion). Neurofibromas may undergo malignant change. In such patients, meningiomas are not uncommon. *Skin* manifestations typical of the disease are neurofibromas and pigmented patches (gray-brown café au lait, freckles). Transmission is by autosomal dominant inheritance with about 90% exhibiting new mutations.

Ataxia telangiectasia may also belong to the phakomatoses. It is discussed on p. 134.

Intrauterine Affections Involving the Brain

Table 1.**4** lists diseases caused by an abnormal factor influencing the brain during fetal development.

Embryopathy Following German Measles

German measles in the mother during the first 3 months of pregnancy carries a 10% risk of fetal damage: the later in pregnancy that the illness occurs, the smaller the risk of damage to the fetus (377). The commonest lesions are:

- cataract,
- deafness (developmental damage to the cochlea),
- microcephaly, and
- cardiac defects.

Congenital Toxoplasmosis

During pregnancy, maternal infection with the protozoan organism *Toxoplasma* first spreads by the bloodstream and produces partial necrosis of the placenta. During the second half of pregnancy, a generalized infection of the fetus occurs, followed by a florid encephalitis with CSF changes, epileptic seizures, cerebral damage, and internal hydrocephalus. These stages of the infection are usually completed during pregnancy; therefore, most of the affected children are already in a stage of encephalitic damage at birth. They show:

- psychomotor retardation,
- epileptic seizures,
- progressive hydrocephalus,
- intracerebral calcifications on X-ray (15%), and
- chorioretinitis (15%).

Serologic diagnosis is mentioned in the section on postnatal toxoplasmosis (p. 53).

Congenital Cytomegaly

Cases of this disease exhibit:

- prematurity or abnormal birth history,
- microcephaly (the main sign),
- hydrocephalus,
- seizures,
- paralyses,
- intracerebral calcifications, the deposits particularly lining the ventricular walls,
- involvement of other organs
  - chorioretinitis,
  - interstitial pneumonias,
  - hepatitis,
  - anemia, and
  - skeletal changes.

The diagnosis in life depends upon cytologic examination of urinary sediment, demonstration of the cytomegalic inclusion body virus, and complement fixation tests in later infancy. Very few patients have been described who appeared to be normal at birth and in whom a progressive cerebral syndrome subsequently developed (164).

Congenital Syphilis

This form of syphilis with neurologic features is more likely to occur if the mother has been recently infected. Characteristic clinical signs include:

- general stigmata, such as
  - saddle nose,
  - rhinitis,
  - perioral fissures,
  - skin lesions,
  - hepatosplenomegaly,
  - periostitis,
  - (later) defective dental growth (Hutchinson's teeth),
  - interstitial keratitis, and
  - deafness,
- signs of CNS involvement,
- acute syphilitic leptomeningitis (within the first month of life),
- chronic meningovascular syphilis (later).

The serologic reactions for syphilis are usually positive in the blood and CSF. Chorioretinitis is not uncommon. After several years tertiary manifestations may appear, particularly general paralysis of the insane or tabes dorsalis (p. 57).

Alcoholic Embryopathy
(or Fetopathy)

This term describes the damage caused to the fetus through alcohol abuse by the mother during pregnancy (930, 1126, 1285). Apart from various structural malformations of the brain, the following features are prominent:

- small stature,
- psychomotor retardation,
- microcephaly, and
- facial dysmorphism (short nose, narrow lips, micrognathia).

Cerebral Disturbances due to Birth Trauma

Subdural Hematoma

This is the commonest hemorrhagic complication of birth. The source of the bleeding may be a torn venous sinus (tentorium) or lacerated cortical veins. Usually there is a history of difficult labor, sometimes forceps delivery. Clinical signs of cerebral damage are present, and aspiration of the subdural space yields frank blood or blood-stained fluid. Treatment consists of repeated aspirations, sometimes craniotomy.

Intracerebral and Intraventricular Hemorrhages

These conditions usually lead to death. Smaller simple hemorrhages and multiple small hemorrhagic contusions may produce a picture of cerebral palsy: the clinical signs cannot be distinguished from those following *birth asphyxia* with resulting cerebral softening. Such patients later present a variety of pathologic anatomic changes, namely thin sclerotic convolutions *(ulegyria),* large cystic spaces *(porencephaly),* and *status marmoratus* of the basal ganglia. This appearance is caused by an excess of myelinated fibers and is associated with athetosis or *athétose double* (p. 121).

Icterus Gravis Neonatorum

Definition: Rh incompatibility leads to a deposition of bilirubin in the brain, particularly in the basal gan-

glia, and consequent motor weakness, dystonic and athetotic movements, deafness, and intellectual deficit.

Pathophysiology and pathologic anatomy: If an Rh-negative mother who through previous pregnancy or transfusion of Rh-positive blood has formed anti-Rh agglutinins again carries a fetus with Rh-positive blood, the anti-Rh agglutinins cross the placenta and damage the Rh-positive erythrocytes of the fetus. This leads to so-called kernicterus with bilirubin deposition in different parts of the basal ganglia and brainstem. The yellow pigment permeates particularly the subthalamic nucleus, globus pallidus, dentate nucleus, and inferior olive. Apart from the high concentration of bilirubin in the blood, anoxia appears to play some part in the brain damage.

Clinical picture: The newborn infant exhibits edema, anemia, erythroblastosis, and, at birth or within the first few days of life, a rapidly progressive jaundice. In about 20% of the cases of erythroblastosis, a so-called kernicterus develops. Two to five days after the onset of jaundice, the child becomes apathetic, ceases to nurse, and develops convulsions, opisthotonus, and respiratory difficulties; in the most severe cases, the infant dies after 3–7 days. However, in most instances it survives and exhibits a picture similar to cerebral palsy, with motor disturbances, e.g., paralyses, involuntary dystonic and athetoid movements, and defects of hearing and intelligence.

Table 1.5   Terminology in various types of hydrocephalus

Internal hydrocephalus	Enlargement of the ventricles only
– Obstructive	With occlusion of the drainage channels and CSF stasis in the ventricular system (e.g., aqueductal stenosis)
– Communicating	With maintained CSF flow from the 4th ventricle
– Malabsorptive	With delayed CSF absorption (e.g., cisternal adhesions or impaired absorption in the pacchionian granulations)
External hydrocephalus	Enlargement of the external fluid compartments (over the cortex and/or in the cisterns)
External and internal hydrocephalus	Combination of above
Hydrocephalus ex vacuo	Internal and external hydrocephalus secondary to primary brain shrinkage

Diagnosis: Estimation of the bilirubin level.

Treatment: Phototherapy is applied in mild cases when the bilirubin level rises to exceed 10 mg/100 ml, and exchange transfusion is carried out if the level is above 20 mg.

Hydrocephalus (377)

Definition: Hydrocephalus is present if the internal and/or external CSF spaces are enlarged. Table 1.5 defines the various forms.

Pathophysiology: The CSF is manufactured in the choroid plexus of the lateral ventricles and the third and fourth ventricles of the brain. It gains exit from each lateral ventricle through a foramen of Monro (interventricular foramen) into the third ventricle, from here through the aqueduct of Sylvius into the fourth ventricle, and then through the foramen of Magendie (single opening of the fourth ventricle situated in the midline) and the foramina of Luschka (lateral openings of the fourth ventricle, paired structures) into the cisterna magna (cerebellomedullary cistern) and the lateral pontine cisterns (Fig. 1.2). About one-fifth passes into the perimedullary subarachnoid spaces, while four-fifths directly traverses the basal cisterns and enters the bloodstream via the pacchionian granulations of the superior sagittal sinus. It seems likely that CSF is also produced in the subarachnoid space.

Pathogenesis: Hydrocephalus develops if the flow of CSF is hindered at any point along the pathways described above. The development of hydrocephalus through overproduction of cerebrospinal fluid has been postulated as an intermittent process following infections or trauma. It occurs as a progressive condition

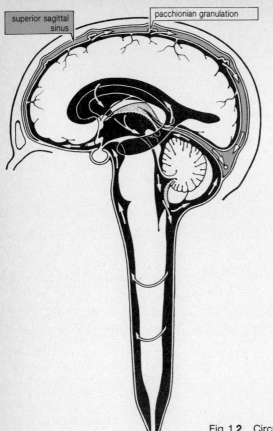

Fig. 1.2 Circulation of the cerebrospinal fluid (CSF)

in children due to plexus papilloma, which is surgically correctable. In individual cases, the following mechanisms are possible:

Obstructive Hydrocephalus:

- Tumor of the third ventricle (colloid cyst, etc.).
- Absence, gliosis, stenosis, or malformation of the aqueduct of Sylvius.
- Tumor of the posterior cranial fossa.
- Obstruction of the foramina of Luschka and Magendie.
- Malformations, particularly the Arnold-Chiari deformity (sometimes associated with meningocele).

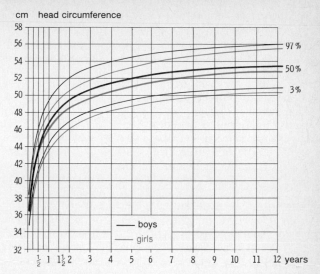

Fig. 1.3   Head circumference in children. The percentages indicate the statistical mean value, i.e., the proportion of children in whom the head circumference is smaller than the percentile value indicated

Communicating Hydrocephalus:

- Obliteration of the cistern by inflammatory adhesions (following meningitis).
- Obliteration of the subarachnoid pathways following hemorrhage.
- Subdural hematoma.
- CSF outflow hampered by venous sinus thrombosis (e.g., "otitic hydrocephalus," p.19).
- *Hydrocephalus ex vacuo* caused by loss of brain substance as in cerebral atrophy postnatally.

Hydrocephalus may develop in utero (unequivocal hydrocephalus is present in 0.2% of all births) and prevent spontaneous childbirth, or it may develop postnatally.

Clinical picture, diagnosis, and treatment: These aspects will be discussed separately in relation to the (etiologically different) forms of hydrocephalus.

Congenital or Infantile Hydrocephalus

Clinically, this form is characterized by an abnormally large and progressively increasing circumference of the head (Fig. 1.3). The fontanels are wide and may bulge. Percussion of the skull reveals a cracked-pot sound. Because of the bulging frontal bone and depression of the orbital plates, the eyes have a characteristic appearance: the upper halves of the sclerae are visible and the irises appear to have dipped toward the lower lids – the setting-sun sign. Diaphanoscopy is the technique whereby the brain is transilluminated in a dark room by means of a strong light and a cardboard tube held against the head. In the normal infant and in those in whom the cortical mantle is thicker than 1 cm, the rim of light around the edge of the tube has a diameter which never exceeds 1.5 cm. In hydrocephalics it is always larger. Premature infants may show a rim of light as large as 3.5 cm. The physical and mental development of hydrocephalic children is retarded, and without therapy or spontaneous remission the picture of increasing dementia, spasticity, and convulsive attacks leads eventually to death.

Ancillary investigations: If hydrocephalus is suspected and the fontanels are still open, ultrasound examination is performed. If the diagnosis is confirmed, a CT scan of the brain is carried out. If hydrocephalus is actively progressive, with evidence of transependymal leakage from the lateral ventricles, a ventriculoperitoneal shunt is immediately inserted. Under the same general anesthetic, preliminary pressure measurements are made, and a specimen of the CSF is obtained for laboratory exclusion of infective changes. In older infants and small children, in whom the hydrocephalus has been present for a longer period, initial pressure measurements are carried out under sedation following the CT scan, and prior to operation. In the course of normal basal pressure measurements, pressure monitoring for 24–48 h leads to the observation of peaks of pressure during sleep.

In nonprogressive or unexplained hydrocephalus, radioisotope cisternography is carried out, or exceptionally a small volume of contrast medium is injected into the ventricles. The only contraindication to the invasive treatment of hydrocephalus is a proven severe associated malformation of the brain.

Prognosis: Untreated hydrocephalus in childhood has a mortality of over 50%. Of the survivors, only very few develop normally without treatment. Shunt surgery has reduced the overall mortality during a 10-year period of observation to less than 10%, the operative mortality is less than 1%. More than two-thirds of the children with treated uncomplicated hydrocephalus (unaccompanied by malformation of the brain) are physically and mentally normal.

Differential diagnosis: A large head is encountered in familial macrocephaly. Infants with this condition are usually large and heavy but otherwise healthy, and they show normal psychomotor development. The setting-sun phenomenon is absent and the CT brain scan is normal. Follow-up observation reveals that their head circumference (already too large) continues to parallel the normal growth percentiles.

Treatment: Therapeutic management depends on the results of the ancillary investigations. Occasionally an obstructive lesion is operated upon directly (e.g., atresia of the foramina of Luschka and Magendie), but far more commonly shunt operations are performed. In obstructive hydrocephalus, ventriculocisternostomy (Torkildsen procedure, viz. short-circuiting an occipital horn to the cisterna magna by means of a subcutaneous catheter) is performed, while in communicating hydrocephalus a ventriculoperitoneal or ventriculovenous shunt operation is carried out, e. g., inserting a Spitz-Holter valve and a tube system which shunt the CSF from the lateral ventricle into the peritoneal space or a large vein, respectively (jugular or superior vena cava). The prognosis is poor if the residual cortical mantle is less than 1.5 cm thick.

Otitic Hydrocephalus

This term is used to denote a moderately raised intracranial pressure caused by thrombosis of a venous sinus, usually the transverse sinus. The syndrome is encountered more frequently after otitis media of the right ear, but also complicates primary lesions at other sites. The clinical picture includes headache, vomiting, papilledema, and often bilateral sixth nerve palsies. The patients are usually children. With appropriate treatment of the primary lesion, the prognosis is good.

Normal Pressure Hydrocephalus
(Nonresorptive Hydrocephalus, Malresorptive Hydrocephalus)

This is a lesion of adults which for didactic reasons is considered in this section.

Clinical features: These are: NPH

- progressive gait disturbances with
- spastic paraparesis,
- urinary incontinence,
- fluctuating mental changes,
- history of a previous event preventing normal CSF absorption,
  • subarachnoid hemorrhage,
  • craniocerebral trauma,
  • meningitis,
  • venous sinus thrombosis.

None of these elements is an essential criterion. The diagnosis is probably made too often (1294).

Ancillary investigations: CT scanning reveals symmetrical enlargement of the cerebral ventricles with the external CSF spaces normal or somewhat constricted in size. A characteristic feature is the dramatic improvement after lumbar puncture. Radioisotope cisternography shows that the labeled albumin diffuses into the ventricles against the normal CSF outflow, which is retarded (385). This test alone is an unreliable criterion for predicting the success of shunting. An important diagnostic aid is continuous monitoring of intraventricular pressure (260) or lumbar CSF pressure (488). A permanent or intermittent slight increase in pressure enables a nonresorptive hydrocephalus to be differentiated from an atrophic degenerative process. A test can be carried out by means of the continuous infusion of fluid into the CSF spaces, to show if the fluid is normally reabsorbed or raised CSF pressure results (749, 750).

Treatment: If the diagnosis is established, treatment consists of a ventriculoatrial shunt operation (see above). The patients who benefit are those with a clear-cut history of a preexisting causative event (1156) and who show the complete neurologic and mental syndrome (see above) (947). Only about one-third to two-thirds of patients benefit from the operation (435). In those in whom only an unexplained progressive organic mental syndrome and/or spastic syndrome is present, despite an abnormal radioisotope cisternogram, operative measures are not justified (980).

Craniostenosis (274, 363, 377)

Premature synostosis of the cranial sutures upsets the harmonious arrangement between the enlarging cranium and the growing brain. The following **clinical types** of craniostenosis are distinguished:

- *Scaphocephaly* (= dolichocephaly) due to synostosis of the sagittal suture (commonest form).
- *Oxycephaly* due to synostosis of at least the sagittal and coronal sutures. There is pressure in the direction of the anterior fontanel, giving rise to a high pointed cranium (second commonest form).
- *Brachycephaly* due to synostosis of the coronal and lambdoid sutures.
- *Plagiocephaly* due to unilateral or partial synostosis of one suture and resulting in asymmetric cranial growth (this deformity is more commonly found in children with cerebral palsy and asymmetric muscular tone).
- *Crouzon's disease* due to synostosis of the cranial and facial bones, particularly the coronal suture and maxillary sutures. The face and skull are broad, the eyes wide apart, and the chin protrudes.

These various patterns of synostosis alter the proportions of the growing skull, leading in many cases to later disturbances of mental development, convulsive seizures, and signs of raised intracranial pressure. **Treatment** should be instituted early, preferably before the fourth month of life. It consists of excision of a strip of bone parallel to and on either side of the synostosed suture (760).

Anomalies of the Craniovertebral Junction (297)

Classification: The following *malformations* are encountered, sometimes combined together:

- atlanto-occipital assimilation,
- os odontoideum,
- atlantoaxial instability,
- occipital vertebra,
- spina bifida of the atlas,
- platybasia, and
- basilar impression.

In the lateral *skull roentgenogram* of a case of basilar impression, the tip of the odontoid process does not lie above Chamberlain's line (connecting the posterior rim of the hard palate to the posterior edge of the foramen magnum), or more than 5 mm above McGregor's line (posterior rim of the hard palate to the lowest part of the occipital bone). Block vertebrae (Klippel-Feil deformity) may distort the cervical vertebral column. Occasionally malformations of the central nervous organs may accompany these skeletal deformities, particularly the Arnold-Chiari malformation (p.9).

Clinically, the patient has a short neck and a low hairline. Slowly progressive neurologic signs and symptoms as a rule appear only in adults. The typical clinical picture is a combination of lower cranial nerve palsies, brainstem signs (nystagmus), and long tract signs (usually bilateral pyramidal signs and sensory disturbances which are sometimes dissociated). A misdiagnosis of multiple sclerosis is often made. The optimal form of **treatment** has yet to be defined; it is by no means certain that wide decompression or shunting is beneficial. When a surgical decompression is performed – also in the case of an associated Arnold-Chiari malformation – the operation should include a duraplasty, and retroflexion of the head during anesthesia should be avoided (271).

Craniocerebral Trauma (253)

The **incidence** of craniocerebral trauma rises steadily, particularly following automobile accidents. In industrialized countries traffic accidents account for 8,000 cases per million inhabitants each year, of which 50% are admitted to a hospital. About 2.5-5% of the injured later require rehabilitation.

Depending on the degree of severity of the trauma, the *following* **types** are distinguished:

- *Scalp contusion* without damage to the brain and no evidence of concussion. This condition will not be further discussed.
- *Cerebral concussion* (with or without skull fracture).
- *Cerebral contusion* (not always a fracture and only exceptionally unaccompanied by concussion) due to an indirect traumatic mechanism.
- *Cerebral laceration:* direct brain damage, always with skull fracture.
- Posttraumatic early and late complications, perhaps with *cerebral compression*.

The boundaries between simple scalp trauma and concussion, as well as those between concussion and contusion of the brain, may be difficult to determine. The presence or absence of a skull fracture is no indication of the severity of the brain damage. Craniocerebral trauma may have a legacy of severe *permanent effects*.

Case History and Physical Findings in the Head Injured

Accident history from patient and witnesses: The following points should be noted:

- specific time and nature of the accident, including the direction of the blow,
- nature of head covering, if any,
- degree of unresponsiveness,
- patterns of motor activity,
- respiratory pattern,
- memory of the accident or retrograde amnesia for the period immediately preceding it,
- duration of the anterograde amnesia following the accident, and
- vomiting.

Examination: The following points should be noted in a recently injured subject:

- respiration,
- state of consciousness,
- visible external injuries, particularly scalp injuries,
- bleeding from the nose or ears or in the throat,
- periorbital and retroauricular hematoma,
- general condition, especially circulatory state (shock!),
- neurologic status (pupils, visual function, nystagmus, hearing, weakness, and pyramidal tract signs),
- skull roentgenograms, neuroradiologic, and if necessary EEG examination.

Expert opinion: In the subsequent evaluation of a head injury, the following should be noted:

- the *accident history* (see above),
- the injured person's *complaints* as well as their nature and intensity, namely headaches, dizziness, uncertainty in standing and walking, memory defects, irritability, fatigability, disturbances of behavior, CSF fistula,
- posttraumatic *complications* that can be directly related to the history: disturbances of smell, vision, and hearing, and epileptic seizures,
- abnormal *physical findings:* anosmia, vestibular disturbances, hearing and visual disturbances, paralyses, and pyramidal tract signs, a global or focal organic mental syndrome, EEG, and roentgenologic findings. A skull fracture in childhood tends to disappear rapidly, but occasionally a "growing fracture" is encountered. In adults the fracture line remains visible for 2–3 years, occasionally even longer,
- subsequent CT scanning commonly shows normal appearances, even if a cerebral contusion had been present initially.

Cerebral Concussion

Definition: The entity of cerebral concussion, concussion of the brain, is not accompanied by any macroscopic brain lesion. Consequently it is not followed either by late sequelae or by clinically detectable neurologic deficits. The clinical picture is characterized by brief loss of consciousness, retrograde amnesia, and often vomiting and postconcussional headaches, dizziness, and transiently reduced mental performance. Apart from slight scalp injury, all head injuries are accompanied by cerebral concussion.

Clinical picture: The typical feature is a *disturbance of the level of consciousness* (1040) which may, however, be brief. It may go unobserved by the bystander (particularly if the injured subject stands up immediately after the accident), although for the head-injured patient it is a tangible amnestic experience. Commonly, although not necessarily, this *amnesia* is *retrograde* so that episodes preceding the accident cannot be remembered. *Anterograde amnesia* from the time of the accident to the return of complete recall of events does not represent unconsciousness, but rather a *posttraumatic twilight state.* As a rule, the unconsciousness of simple cerebral concussion does not last more than

15 min, and that of the twilight state (delirium) less than 1 h. If the former exceeds 1 h and the latter 24 h, a cerebral contusion (see below) is undoubtedly present. *Vomiting* occurs regularly in concussion.

Examination: Physical examination as well as lumbar puncture and EEG always yield normal findings.

Postconcussional complaints: As a rule these complaints arise immediately after the injury and cease gradually after a variable interval. *Headaches* are prominent, usually diffuse, and develop under tension in the course of the day; only occasionally are they continuous from morning awakening. They are regularly aggravated by exposure to the sun or alcohol intake, perhaps also by frequent bending and standing up. *Dizziness* is often present and takes the form of a nonspecific staggering gait with uncertainty upon rapid movements and upward and downward gaze (walking upstairs). Occasionally a more localized, intense boring type of headache is present, which prompts suspicion of a meningeal scar. Head-injured subjects complain of a general *reduced mental performance*, including defective memory (for names), difficulty with concentration, rapid fatigability, and irritability. These complaints may last for months and should be evaluated in relation to the severity of the injury as well as to the personality and situation of each particular patient. While the incidence of accident neurosis is undoubtedly not rare in persons carrying accident insurance, genuine complaints may last for months or years. However, this situation is by no means identical with unfitness for work and compensation liability.

Treatment: Bed rest for at least a few days, then medical treatment to stabilize the autonomic nervous system, as well as a confident attitude of the physician.

Cerebral Contusion and Penetrating Brain Injuries

Definition: The cerebral contusion represents morphologically tangible evidence of damage to the brain substance. The unconsciousness and posttraumatic twilight state (1040) as a rule last longer than in cerebral concussion. However, occasionally a contusion may occur without concussion, particularly as a result of a direct blow to a small localized area of the brain.

Findings: Usually neurologic signs are present from the start as evidence of a focal brain lesion. The presence of traumatic anosmia (p. 328) in practice always indicates the presence of a cerebral contusion, even in the absence of other neurologic findings.

Disturbances of cardiac rhythm are common in contusional head injuries (1225), a finding that has been confirmed experimentally (345). Lumbar puncture may reveal blood-tinged or xanthochromic CSF, and prompt CT scanning usually reveals focal damage, such as hematoma. However, after weeks or months it may no longer show any abnormality.

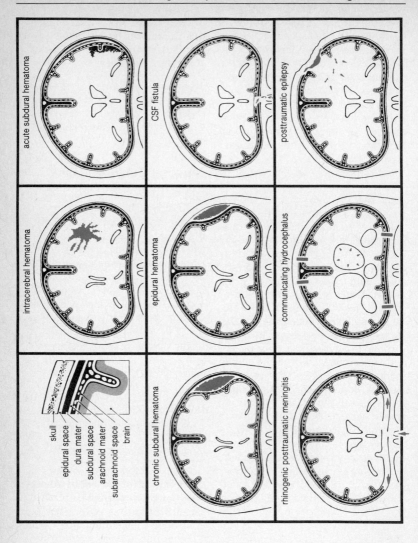

Fig. 1.4
Complications
of cranial trauma

Posttraumatic complaints: Epileptic seizures are always signs of an established cerebral contusion (see below). The head-injured subject's complaints after a cerebral contusion correspond to those after concussion but they are frequently, although not necessarily, more severe. Clinical evidence is also present of the local cerebral lesion, e.g., paralyses and disturbances of gait, speech, and vision. In many cases, a posttraumatic encephalopathy is present (see below).

Posttraumatic Complications and Late Effects

Classification: The following may be present:

- epidural hematoma,
- subdural hematoma,
- intracerebral hematoma,
- cranial nerve palsies,
- focal neurologic deficits,
- CSF fistula,
- with secondary meningitis or brain abscess,
- nonresorptive hydrocephalus, and
- posttraumatic encephalopathy with an accompanying psycho-organic syndrome.

The complications of craniocerebral trauma are illustrated in Fig. 1.4.

Intracranial Hematoma

An intracranial hematoma may be an early or late complication. Careful supervision of the acutely head-injured patient is necessary because of the risk of secondary cerebral compression from a hematoma. CT scanning and exceptionally angiography (645) contribute materially to the diagnosis.

Epidural Hematoma

Epidural hematoma usually results from rupture of a meningeal artery, causing blood to accumulate between the dura and the cranial vault, thereby leading to cerebral compression. If the initial injury was severe, the patient may not recover consciousness or may be conscious for only a short interval (absent or brief lucid interval). On the other hand, an epidural hematoma may follow a slight injury or even an incident unaccompanied by brain damage so that an unequivocal lucid interval may be present. In the presence of deep coma and accompanying additional brain damage, it is sometimes difficult to lateralize the hematoma; an ipsilateral dilated pupil or a fracture may localize it. *Immediate* evacuation, not necessarily within a neurosurgical center, is essential for complete recovery.

Acute Subdural Hematoma

This condition usually appears after a severe head injury, such as contusional bleeding, and may therefore occur without a lucid interval immediately following the initial loss of consciousness. Differentiation from an epidural hematoma is often impossible clinically. In acute subdural hematoma the CSF is always bloody, but this is also a sign of a simple cerebral contusion or a contusion and epidural hematoma. Deterioration in the level of consciousness following a lucid interval, or an unusually prolonged period before the patient wakes up, are signs meriting suspicion of a space-occupying hematoma. In such cases, CT scanning is essential or, if not available, exploratory burr holes are required. For subdural hematoma in arachnoid cysts, see p. 38.

Chronic Subdural Hematoma (209)

Only the posttraumatic variety will be referred to here, although the nontraumatic form, so-called *pachymeningosis haemorrhagica interna,* is clinically indistinguishable. Neurosurgeons question the existence of this entity, spontaneous subdural hematoma without preceding head injury. A history of injury, occasionally slight, is present in about three-fourths of cases. In patients receiving anticoagulant treatment who complain of headache, the possibility should always be remembered of *(bilateral) chronic subdural hematomas.*

Clinically, signs and symptoms of the subdural hematoma may appear some weeks after a slight injury or after a symptomless interval. They usually reach their maximum in 2–3 months. The patients are usually elderly men. Headache is a prominent symptom. A progressive fluctuating disturbance of consciousness is typical, leading eventually to a deep somnolence with few, if any, neurologic signs. Xanthochromic CSF, often with a low pressure, is a confirmatory finding. CT scanning confirms the diagnosis, the lesion being shown as a biconvex hypodense zone displacing the surface of the brain from the cranium (Fig. 1.5). A stage occurs during

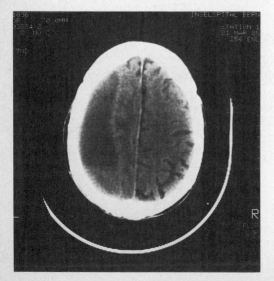

Fig. 1.5 Left-sided chronic subdural hematoma shown by computed tomography (CT). The surface of the hemisphere is displaced from the inner table of the skull. The patient is examined in a supine position, and the denser part of the hematoma fluid sinks toward the occiput (layer effect)

which the hematoma is isodense with the brain substance and therefore invisible. **Treatment** consists in surgical evacuation, either through burr holes or following an osteoplastic craniotomy. With small hematomas, the signs and symptoms may remit spontaneously.

Subdural Hygroma

In adults this condition is a collection of fluid over a cerebral hemisphere, occurring without evidence of trauma and occasionally accompanied by a low pressure syndrome (p.458). The clinical signs and symptoms and treatment are the same as those of subdural hematoma, provided a sufficient volume of fluid is present. In infants and small children, bilateral subdural hygromas are often observed days or weeks after meningitis. An unsatisfactory course of a meningitic infection in small children always merits exploratory aspiration for subdural hygroma, and repeated aspiration or surgical evacuation if one is found.

Intracerebral Hematoma

The intracerebral hematoma is a space-occupying lesion and provokes collateral edema. Apart from a loss of consciousness, the condition is characterized by neurologic deficits, blood-stained CSF, and abnormal CT scan findings.

Cranial Nerve Palsies

An example is anosmia, which is permanent in two-thirds of cases (735). Optic nerve lesions are as a rule permanent, while external ocular palsies show a tendency to regress after 3–4 months. Nonspecific visual disturbances, caused by decompensation of a heterophoria due to the head injury, may disappear. An actual lesion of the visual apparatus can be excluded by demonstrating that the visual evoked potentials are normal (355). For traumatic arteriovenous fistula in the cavernous sinus, see p.97. For posttraumatic facial palsy, see p.359. Traumatic disturbances of hearing following fractures of the skull base may be the result of inner ear damage, but more commonly they indicate a lesion of the statoacoustic nerve. The latter lesion is not amenable to operative treatment and therefore carries a more severe prognosis. In fractures of the skull base extending into a jugular foramen, the cranial nerves traversing it (glossopharyngeal, vagus, and accessory) may be damaged. This produces the Siebenmann syndrome of palatal paralysis, disturbances of swallowing, dysphagia, and paralysis of the sternomastoid and upper part of the trapezius muscles.

Focal Damage to Individual Brain Regions

The following may be produced: hemipareses, sensory disturbances, visual field defects, speech disturbances, and neuropsychologic deficits. Pseudobulbar signs are rare. After severe trauma, frequently including fracture of the base of the skull, the patient may develop diabetes insipidus (specific gravity or urine under 1.005) a few days later; in the survivors this sign usually disappears. In such cases, it is necessary to exclude polyuria with high specific gravity in the Schwartz-Bartter syndrome. A CT scan may reveal focal brain atrophy.

Lhermitte's Sign

This sign (p. 246) may appear weeks or even months after craniocerebral trauma. It usually disappears in several months if neurologic examination is normal and cervical roentgenograms, including lateral views made with the neck in flexion and extension, show no abnormality (35).

Cerebral Fat Embolism

In this complication, which most often accompanies fractures of a long bone, clinical manifestations of fat embolism occur in 1-5% of the cases, 80% of which show neurological symptoms (549). They appear twelve hours to three days following the injury, and are characterized by a picture of diffuse brain damage, which may be continuous with the initial signs and symptoms of head trauma. The diagnosis is confirmed by the appearance of the chest roentgenogram and the finding of petechiae in the skin and fat emboli in the retinal vessels.

CSF Fistula, Meningitis, Brain Abscess

A *CSF fistula* may occur following a fracture of the base of the skull with rupture of the dura, usually into the paranasal sinuses. The diagnosis is confirmed by laboratory examination of the fluid (glucose content). The abnormal flow may be aggravated by an increase in the jugular venous pressure. Dye injections made for diagnostic purposes are not without danger: the use of methylene blue for this purpose is contraindicated and has been superseded by radioisotopic cisternography. The most important complication of a CSF fistula is a *spreading purulent meningitis* which is usually recurrent and pneumococcal. Many years may elapse between the fracture and the onset of the meningitis. A *brain abscess* may be produced in the same way, or as the result of a penetrating injury. While the majority of cases of CSF rhinorrhea disappear spontaneously, persistence beyond 2-3 weeks is an indication for dural repair (covering the defect with fascia lata or a dura-periosteal flap).

Benign Posttraumatic Intracranial Hypertension

This condition, which follows a mild or moderately severe injury, is probably caused by thrombosis of a venous sinus which hinders normal CSF outflow and leads to signs of raised intracranial pressure. It manifests after an interval of days or months and is characterized by headache, nausea, swimming vision, and papilledema, but not by focal neurologic signs except sometimes an abducent palsy. The CSF pressure is raised. The signs and symptoms regress spontaneously.

Posttraumatic Encephalopathy

The possibility of permanent brain damage increases with the length of the initial period of unconsciousness (1040). Apart from the direct results of the injury, foci of necrosis, hemorrhage, and cerebral softening at a distance from the contusion appear to contribute to the picture. The condition manifests itself clinically as an organic mental syndrome in which disturbances of memory, behavior, and drive, as well as a marked personality change, may lead to severe disability. Several studies have confirmed that an accurate final evaluation of the permanent damage is only possible 2 or more years after the injury. Sometimes an apparently paradoxical progression of the signs and symptoms may be detected. It is possible that a progressive commu-nicating hydrocephalus resulting from disturbed CSF absorption (following subarachnoid hemorrhage) may play a part (p. 19). Socially, this condition is the most devastating complication of craniocerebral trauma.

Posttraumatic Epilepsy

This type of epilepsy, which occurs almost exclusively after a severe injury and commonly in the initial weeks or months following the injury, will be discussed on p. 275.

Raised Intracranial Pressure and Brain Tumors

Signs of Raised Intracranial Pressure and Benign Intracranial Hypertension

Signs of Raised Intracranial Pressure

Signs of raised intracranial pressure always prompt the suspicion of the presence of an intracranial space-occupying lesion – until the latter has been convincingly ruled out. Table 1.6 lists the main signs.

Causes of a raised *intracranial pressure* are:

- intracranial space-occupying lesion,
- encephalitis,
- meningitis,
- craniocerebral trauma,
- venous sinus thrombosis,
- CSF outflow obstruction due to
  • malformation at the cranio-vertebral angle,

- aqueductal stenosis,
- posthemorrhagic or postmeningitic arachnoid adhesions,
- markedly raised CSF protein in
  • polyradiculitis (663),
  • spinal tumor, especially neurofibroma (1212),
- drugs and toxic substances:
  • lead poisoning,
  • steroid medication,
  • ovulation inhibitors,
  • tetracycline medication,
  • insecticides,
  • neurobrucellosis (259 a),
- altitude sickness.

In altitude sickness during rapid ascent, cerebral edema represents one of the major signs, together with pulmonary edema, retinal hemorrhages, and coronary perfusional disturbances. Immediate return to a lower altitude and measures to reduce the intracranial pressure are essential (see below) (528).

Table 1.6   Signs of raised intracranial pressure

Subjective	Headaches (diffuse and constant, more severe in the morning), vomiting (fasting, projectile), apathy
Warning signs	Confusion, disturbances of respiration, bradycardia, hypertension, cerebellar fits (opisthotonus and extensor spasms of arms and legs), dilated pupils
Eye signs	Papilledema (may appear within hours), enlarged blind spot, attacks of amblyopia, oculomotor palsy, also 6th cranial nerve palsy
Skull roentgenograms	Increased digitate markings, abnormal pituitary fossa including demineralized dorsum sellae, diastasis of sutures in children
CT scanning	Reveals slitlike ventricles in brain swelling, periventricular lucencies, also sometimes the cause of the raised intracranial pressure as well
EEG	Diffuse nonspecific abnormalities
CSF	Pressure raised above 200 mm water (lumbar puncture theoretically contraindicated), pressure may be normal in obstructive lesions of the craniovertebral angle or spinal canal

Benign Intracranial Hypertension (Pseudotumor cerebri)

The cases remaining after exclusion of the entities listed above, i. e., the etiologically unexplained cases, are called *"benign intracranial hypertension"* (139, 198, 559). In these the neurologic and neuroradiologic findings are always normal with the exception of swollen optic disks, enlarged blind spots, and occasionally slitlike ventricles on neuroradiologic examination. The CSF shows increased pressure only and no abnormal values. The **clinical features** include the following:

- mostly young women,
- often obese,
- menstrual irregularity,
- relatively common during pregnancy (299),
- headache, usually diffuse,
- occasionally with vomiting,
- dizziness and tinnitus,
- occasionally nystagmus,
- double vision and other visual disturbances.

Etiology: Causative factors are found in only about three-fourths of cases (see above). In about one-fourth middle ear infection is responsible. Recovery is usually complete, relapses are rare. It must be stressed that in about 8% of patients the visual acuity remains permanently diminish because of papilledema (139). The risk of severely impaired vision is particularly great in patients with arterial hypertension (254). The increasing size of the blind spot on visual field testing is a particularly useful guide to dehydration therapy (559). **Treatment** of raised pressure is by repeated lumbar puncture, with dexamethasone 4 mg 4× daily i.v., later by mouth. Also recommended are urea solutions, mannitol or sorbitol. Furosemide 40 mg i.v. 2-3 × daily.

"Empty Sella" (374, 1258)

If, in addition to raised intracranial pressure, the presence of an inadequate diaphragma sellae permits herniation of the subarachnoid cisterns into the pituitary fossa, a so-called empty sella results. Appropriate CT slices reveal a fluid-filled pituitary fossa which is apparently empty. Patients with benign intracranial hypertension and empty sella usually exhibit visual disturbances.

Brain Tumors (442, 1038, 1315)

Incidence: One of 10,000-20,000 people will die of a brain tumor. In an additional 20% of patients the brain and its coverings will be invaded by a metastatic deposit from a tumor elsewhere, without the presence of clinical neurologic signs (968). In a series reported from a psychiatric hospital, the incidence of primary brain tumors was even higher and reported to be 1‰ (627).

Causes: Local factors are responsible for the origin of brain tumors apart from a general factor – the "humoral" anlage (1315). The former factor is linked to embryonal histiogenesis and is responsible for identical tumors occurring quite regularly at the same sites, particularly in those parts of the brain enveloping the neural groove. With very rare exceptions, trauma cannot be regarded as an etiologic factor (1315).

General Symptoms and Signs of Brain Tumors

General signs: Various tumors exhibit identical signs of raised intracranial pressure:

- steady progression of the clinical picture (however: progression also accompanies inflammatory and even vascular lesions. "Apoplectiform" events in tumors may be caused by hemorrhage into the tumor),
- frequently headaches (steady, diffuse, often nocturnal and improv-

Table 1.**7**   Incidence of various brain tumors in a pooled neurosurgical series (from Cushing 1932, Olivecrona 1967, and Zülch 1965; after Adams et al.)

	%
Glioma	
– Glioblastoma multiforme (astrocytoma IV)	20
– Astrocytoma I–III	10
– Ependymoma	6
– Medulloblastoma	4
– Oligodendroglioma	5
Meningioma	15
Pituitary adenoma	7
Neurinoma	7
Metastases	6
Craniopharyngioma, dermoid, epidermoid, teratoma	4
Angioma	4
Sarcoma	4
Not classified (mostly glioma)	5
Other (pinealoma, chondroma, granuloma, etc.)	3
	100

ing during the day), in about one-third of cases the presenting symptom,

- sometimes signs of raised intra-cranial pressure (see Table 1.6),
- mental changes (irritability, fatigability, memory loss, altered behavior),
- epileptic seizures (more often generalized than local), in about one-fourth of cases the presenting symptom.

Table 1.7 lists the commonest brain tumors and their incidence in a neurosurgical series. The *features of individual brain tumors* are further described below.

Focal clinical signs: Sooner or later these signs amplify the general signs and symptoms of brain tumors described above. To some extent they serve to localize the lesion. For example: a motor or sensory deficit may accompany a tumor of the contralateral cerebral hemisphere.

Localizing clinical features may be produced by the mass effect of the tumor.

- The contralateral cerebral peduncle may be compressed against the tentorial edge and cause homolateral pyramidal signs.
- Through constriction of the brainstem in the tentorial opening caused by herniation of the uncus, intra-axial hemorrhages arise which may produce bilateral pyramidal signs.
- Compression of the posterior cerebral arteries against the tentorial edge may lead to infarction of the visual cortex and various visual field deficits which may be bilateral.
- The occurrence of an oculomotor palsy (mydriasis and ptosis followed by disturbed eye movements) points

to compression of the third nerve against the petroclinoid ligament.
- Sixth nerve palsy is a nonspecific sign of raised intracranial pressure, without localizing value because of the unusually long intracranial course of this nerve.

Ancillary investigations: *CT scanning* (30, 864) is rapidly being replaced by MRI (magnetic resonance imaging) for many clinical indications. It must not be forgotten that a negative MR or CT scan by no means excludes a brain tumor, particularly slowly growing, infiltrating types such as low-grade astrocytomas. In all cases, if the signs and symptoms continue to increase, the clinician is obliged to repeat the examination. In the presence of MR and CT scanning, all other ancillary methods have receded into the background. *Angiography* remains a preoperative requirement in many patients to amplify the CT findings (655); *digital subtraction angiography* performed by intravenous injection of the contrast medium is a less invasive technique (666). In other patients, *stereotactic biopsy* is required to decide between operative and radiation treatment. The *EEG* often shows pathologic changes in tumors of the cerebral hemisphere, but it may be normal or show nonspecific changes in deep-seated tumors and lesions around the midline. Metastases are recognized only when their size reaches 2 cc. The CSF is either normal or, in the presence of tumors which are superficial or adjacent to the ventricles, shows a nonspecific increase in protein and cell content. Acoustic schwannomas always show a significantly high protein level. Malignant cells may be demonstrated by careful cytologic examination of the centrifuged specimen. *Skull roentgenograms* may reveal signs of raised intracranial pressure, including accentuated convolutional markings, an abnormal pituitary fossa with an osteoporotic dorsum sellae (differential diagnosis of intrasellar tumor!), separation of sutures in young subjects, or local posterior fossa changes in cerebellar tumors (deepened posterior fossa, thin occipital bone). The pineal calcification may be displaced from the midline. The cranial bones may show areas of sclerosis (meningioma) or destruction. In some meningiomas widened vascular channels may be visible in the vault. Some tumors may calcify (meningioma, oligodendroglioma, craniopharyngioma, choroid plexus papilloma, tuberculoma, lipoma of the corpus callosum). Giant aneurysms show curvilinear mural calcification. CT scans may be superior to MRI in revealing meningioma, since calcium is not detected by MRI.

Individual Brain Tumors

Glioma

Glioblastoma multiforme (astrocytoma grade 4): This tumor grows rapidly and is highly malignant. It is the commonest primary brain tumor, appearing mainly in subjects aged 40-60 years, and grows by infiltrating the brain. Usually the cerebral hemispheres are involved, occasionally bilaterally as a "butterfly" lesion in the corpus callosum, and it may also involve the basal ganglia. Glioblastomas account for 90% of gliomas of the cerebral hemispheres in adults. The case history is brief – weeks or months. Apart from the general tumor symptoms and signs, local features such as paralysis, speech disturbance, and other focal deficits are present. Postoperative survival is usually a few months and at most 2 years. Combined operative surgery, X-irradiation, and cytostatic chemotherapy do not significantly improve the prognosis (1097).

The low-grade *supratentorial astrocytoma* (grades 1 or 2) is usually encountered in patients in their 30s or 40s. This tumor usually grows slowly and appears sometimes to be well circumscribed, although it may infiltrate into the white matter of the frontal or temporal lobes. In these situations, over the course of years, the tumor may give rise to slowly progressive clinical signs. Most frequently these are mental changes, an increasingly severe hemiparesis, ataxia, papilledema, headache, or epileptic seizures; initially the tumor may not be demonstrable by neuroradiologic methods including CT scanning. Circumscribed fibrillary astrocytomas sometimes take many years to recur and cures have been reported following operative removal. In other cases, transformation into a glioblastoma multiforme occurs. Sometimes the tumor appears to sprout simultaneously in different places and shows different histologic degrees of malignancy. In such cases, one may speak of a gliomatosis of the brain (255).

Cerebellar astrocytoma (pilocytic astrocytoma of the cerebellum) (275, 1090): This variety is significantly more benign than the supratentorial astrocytoma. It is found commonly in young subjects between the ages of 5 and 15 years (25% of brain tumors of childhood and adolescence). The tumor is a well-differentiated, often cystic mass situated in the cerebellar hemisphere, the vermis, or the pons. It produces slowly progressive cerebellar signs such as ataxia, disturbances of balance, nystagmus, and later signs of raised intracranial pressure. A permanent cure can only be guaranteed if complete macroscopic removal is achieved (often impossible because of the site of the tumor).

Ependymoma (1038, 1090, 1315): These tumors are found mainly in children and young adults, seldom in later life. The comprise about 4% of all brain tumors (1315) and develop from displaced ependymal cells in the depths of cerebral tissues. The histologic picture of a periavascular pseudorosette arrangement of cells is characteristic. The tumor develops in the vicinity of the ventricular system, more often in the posterior fossa around the fourth ventricle than above the tentorium. Intraspinal ependymomas are usually found in the lumbar region. The infratentorial site of the tumor causes cerebellar signs and symptoms, frequently beginning only with CSF outflow obstruction and corresponding signs of raised intracranial pressure. Unusual (continuous) headaches in a child should always prompt the suspicion of an ependymoma. The tumor is relatively benign and patients may survive for many years – the survival time is longer, the older the child was at the time of onset of the first signs and symptoms (1107). When the tumor is located on the floor of the fourth ventricle, radical operation is impossible. Surgical removal should always be followed by X-irradiation, which must include the entire vertebral column. Combined operative and radiation treatment provides a 10-year survival of nearly 70% (1053).

Medulloblastoma: This malignant tumor of childhood and adolescence represents 20% of brain tumors in young subjects. Nine of ten cases are located in the inferior vermis (915), but a cerebellar hemisphere or the pons may be affected. The tumor infiltrates the fourth ventricle (thereby hindering CSF outflow) and releases metastatic seedlings into the CSF pathways. These seedings later cause spinal cord and cauda equina signs. Medulloblastomas produce the same signs as cerebellar astrocytomas (see above). Even after radical operative removal and irradiation – the tumor is radiosensitive (121) – recurrences are inevitable after months or years. The 5-year survival rate reaches 47%, the 10-year survival rate 42%, and these figures rise if the tumor is resected more radically (915).

Oligodendroglioma: This tumor is most common between the ages of 35 and 45 years. It may displace or infiltrate a cerebral hemisphere or the basal ganglia, particularly the thalamus, of young subjects. More than 50% of cases are located in the frontal lobes. Oligodendrogliomas grow very slowly and many years may separate the time of diagnosis from the first signs and symptoms. Apart from the presence of local tumor signs which develop in the course of months, epileptic seizures are particularly common, being the presenting symptom in 70% of cases and being present in about one-half of all the patients. Recurrences are almost invariable, even after "radical" surgical removal, but occasionally there is a 3- to 5-year interval. The average postoperative survival time of 5 years corresponds to that of supratentorial astrocytomas. After partial tumor resection subsequent radiotherapy increases the five year survival rate to 36% (706).

Brainstem glioma (474): This tumor is histologically indistinguishable from other types of glioma, but it gives rise to a typical clinical picture. Most cases occur before the age of 20 years. They manifest by progressive signs and symptoms of involvement of the pons and medulla oblongata, which may appear in the course of a few weeks or months:

- lower motor neuron cranial nerve palsies with
  - disturbances of swallowing,
  - fifth nerve involvement,
  - facial palsy,
- hemifacial spasm,
- disturbances of external ocular movement,
- signs of long tract involvement,
  - pyramidal tract signs,
  - paralyses of the extremities,
  - dissociated sensory disturbances.

The differential diagnosis from vascular malformations, brainstem encephalitis, or multiple sclerosis may be difficult. The tumor is inoperable. Ventricular atrial shunting may be required. Survival averages 1 year (474).

Glioma of the optic nerve and chiasm (1090, 1188): These tumors are encountered nearly exclusively in children and adolescents, being twice as common in girls. The following features are characteristic:

- disturbances of vision,
- visual field defects,
- proptosis,
- (later) brainstem signs,

- polyuria,
- obesity,
- infantilism, and
- disturbed sleep rhythm.

Generalized neurofibromatosis is present in 14% of cases (1188). Appropriate roentgenographic projections of the optic canals (Rhese) will show foraminal enlargement greater than 7 mm in diameter on the affected side. CT scanning is helpful. This finding excludes other entities considered in the differential diagnosis such as pituitary adenoma, intraorbital meningioma, medial sphenoidal wing meningioma, and Hand-Schüller-Christian disease. Combined operative and radiation treatment offers a long-term cure of 85% in gliomas of an optic nerve and of 50% in gliomas of the optic chiasm (1188).

Hypothalamic tumor: These tumors lie in the rostral floor of the third ventricle and are seen in children in the first 2 years of life. They are usually astrocytomas: progressive emaciation occurs, although the child does not refuse food and his normal behavior is not altered (Russell's syndrome). This picture must be differentiated from that of anorexia nervosa in older girls.

Meningioma

This is a benign neoplasm which arises from the meninges of the brain and grows slowly over the years, producing its symptoms and signs by compression. Malignant change is rare (1217). Occasionally it is encountered in the presence of another malignant neoplasm (104), such as breast cancer (806). Meningioma is the commonest intracranial tumor of mesodermal origin and occurs particularly in subjects aged 40–50 years. It is also a chance finding upon neuroradiologic investigation or autopsy.

The arachnoidal origin of meningioma dictates their intracranial *sites of predilection:*

- over the convexity,
- in the frontoparietal parasagittal region,
- in the Sylvian region,
- along the falx,
- in the olfactory groove,
- on a lesser sphenoidal wing,
- on the tuberculum sellae,
- on the (cerebellar) side of the tentorium,
- in the cerebellopontine angle,
- in the region of the foramen magnum,
- in the spinal canal.

The skull bone adjacent to the meningioma may be thickened and show radially arranged bony spicules. Exostoses may also be present. Meningiomas developing parallel to the bone, the so-called en plaque type, may distort the skeletal appearance and give rise to a picture resembling fibrous dysplasia of bone (287). Almost all supratentorial meningiomas cause epileptic seizures, which are often the presenting clinical event.

Olfactory meningiomas arise on the floor of the anterior cranial fossa. Often they cause only one neurologic sign, anosmia, but they may also cause headache and a frontal lobe syndrome. Epileptic seizures may be present. *Meningiomas of the lesser sphenoidal wing* tend to provoke a bony hyperostosis. More laterally situated meningiomas occupy the temporal fossa. Focal hemispheric signs and symptoms may be present, including optic atrophy and proptosis. *Meningiomas of the tuberculum sellae* produce a chiasmal syndrome. *Meningiomas of the superior sagittal sinus and falx* not infrequently cause pure motor paralysis of a lower limb. Sometimes this may be bilateral and thus give rise to spastic paraparesis, which has to be differentiated from spinal cord damage. *Meningiomas in the vicinity of the foramen magnum* may present a difficult diagnostic problem since the clinical picture is multifocal and resembles that of multiple sclerosis. *Intraventricular meningiomas* usually arise in the region of the trigone and may produce intermittent symptoms caused by obstruction of a foramen of Monro (attacks of severe headache and vomiting).

Pituitary Adenoma

Only about 10% show enlargement of the sella turcica and the signs of an intracranial space-occupying lesion. Adenomas occur commonly in subjects aged 30–50 years. Clinically, all cases exhibit *endocrine disturbances:* acromegaly accompanies eosinophilic adenoma (which is rarer). Signs of pituitary insufficiency such as thin wrinkled skin, and secondary endocrine deficiencies of the thyroid gland and gonads accompany *chromophobe adenoma.* In *prolactinomas,* prolactin levels in excess of 100 mg/ml, galactorrhea and usually secondary amenorrhea are present, with impotence in males. Larger pituitary adenomas cause *visual field defects* (usually bitemporal hemianopsia) and roentgenologic evidence of *sellar enlargement.* The visual field defect and visual disturbances of sellar and parasellar tumors are more likely to regress completely in those patients in whom residual function is present, the visual loss was brief and the tumor was slowly growing. *Basophil adenoma* (Cushing's disease) is caused by a tumor which seldom impinges on the brain, exerting its effect by increased ACTH production and thereby enhanced cortisone secretion from the adrenal cortex. The results are truncal obesity, hypertension, osteoporosis, and glycosuria, as well as abdominal striae, hirsutism, and amenorrhea.

Schwannoma (Neurilemmoma, Neurinoma)

The commonest variety of neurinoma is the one arising from the vestibulocochlear (statoacoustic) nerve. This tumor, the so-called *acoustic neuroma*, usually appears between the ages of 30 and 50 years and presents the clinical picture of a cerebellopontine angle tumor: progressive hearing loss, noises in the ear, vertigo, ipsilateral fifth and facial nerve lesions, and later signs of involvement of the cerebellum and pyramidal tracts and of raised intracranial pressure. Occasionally the stigmata of generalized neurofibromatosis (von Recklinghausen's disease, p. 12) may be present, not infrequently with bilateral tumors. Far more rarely, this syndrome is produced by a tumor of another histologic type, e.g., meningioma or epidermoid. Initially the patient complains of noise in the ear (tinnitus), increasing deafness, and vertigo. The retrolabyrinthine site of the lesion can be confirmed by absence of recruitment (p. 362). Later trigeminal nerve involvement with sensory disturbance of the face and keratitis neuroparalytica, as well as peripheral facial palsy, may supervene. The final picture comprises signs of cerebellar involvement, pressure effects on the brainstem, pyramidal tract signs, and papilledema. The CSF protein content is almost invariably increased. The diagnosis rests on the results of clinical and MR or CT examination. Very small tumors may require a roentgenographic technique involving demonstration of the internal auditory canal with gas or a positive contrast medium. Operative treatment using microsurgical technique usually allows the facial and trigeminal nerves to be spared.

Cerebral Metastases (968, 1267)

Brain metastases arise mostly from bronchogenic cancer (in men) and breast cancer (in women), then from melanomas and hypernephromas. By the time that the intracranial deposits are detectable clinically, three-fourths are multiple, especially melanoma metastases. The intracranial deposit is often the first symptom of the disease, particularly in lung cancer. According to statistics in the literature, metastatic deposits represent between 4% and 20% of all brain tumors. Of 122 patients from whom apparently solitary cerebral deposits were surgically removed, only 5% were alive 4 years later. Prognostically favorable factors include a supratentorial location, macroscopically complete resection, and advanced age; hypernephroma metastases were more often solitary than bronchial or melanoma metastases. Meningeal carcinomatosis see p. 203; paraneoplastic encephalopathy, see p. 156.

Teratomatous Tumors

The first of these is *craniopharyngioma*, which must be distinguished from a primary pituitary tumor. It arises most commonly in children and young adolescents, with the maximum incidence in the 2nd decade of life. However, clinical features may appear for the first time in older subjects (usually optic atrophy). Although pure suprasellar forms of the tumor occur, endocrine disturbances are invariably present. Craniopharyngioma is far more likely than a pituitary adenoma to invade the midbrain and third ventricle, producing corresponding clinical signs (hydrocephalus, disturbances of behavior and drive, diabetes insipidus, etc.). The tumor often calcifies. Craniopharyngiomas are not malignant tumors; however, they can sometimes only partly be removed for technical reasons. Another teratomatous tumor is the *epidermoid* (445), which shows a peak incidence between 25 and 45 years, in contrast to the *dermoid* which is a childhood tumor. Epidermoids are found at the base of the skull and in the cerebellopontine angle, as well as most frequently in the parapituitary, parapontine, and orbitomaxillary regions. The clinical picture depends on the site of the tumor – thus, chiasmal syndromes, lower cranial nerve palsies, brainstem compression, epileptic seizures, as well as mental symptoms and evidence of raised intracranial pressure. Occasionally these tumors, which grow extremely slowly and produce clinical signs by displacement, are found in the spinal canal. Radical removal carries an excellent prognosis.

Most cases of *pinealoma* appear to be teratomatous in composition. They compress the aqueduct and cause obstructive hydrocephalus. In addition, a paralysis of upward gaze is present (usually later) and there are widely dilated pupils which react to convergence but not to light (Parinaud's syndrome). Young males are most often affected.

Other Tumors

Several other tumors are mentioned only briefly due to their rarity: A malignant lymphoma can arise as a primary tumor affecting the cerebral hemispheres or cerebellum as a solitary or multilocular lesion, infiltrating the brain rapidly. They develop primarily in immune-compromised individuals. Therapy consists rarely in partial resection, but mainly in whole brain radiation and chemotherapy (549). Infrequently, a lymphoma of another organ metastasizes to the brain. A picture of intermittent CSF outflow obstruction prompts suspicion of an intraventricular tumor such as meningioma or *colloid cyst of the third ventricle* (711) (p. 458). *Choroid plexus papilloma* occurs most commonly in the first 10 years of life, particularly in the first 2 years. It arises most frequently in the fourth ventricle, grows slowly, may later calcify, and produces seedling metastases. Permanent cure can be achieved by radical removal. *Gumma and tuberculoma* are rarely seen in Western countries. Other evidence of the primary disease should be found. *Hydatid cysts* are also rare, while in endemic areas, cysticercosis of the central nervous system (738, 1066) occurs in up to 4% of individuals infected with *Taenia solium*. It manifests as a space-occupying lesion in 50% of the cases (1066). Angiomatous tumors of the brain, see p. 95.

Differential Diagnosis of Brain Tumors

Other space-occupying intracranial lesions must first be excluded, in particular

- chronic subdural hematoma (p. 26) (often history of trauma, fluctuating level of consciousness, relatively few neurologic symptoms and signs, xanthochromic CSF);

- brain abscess (p.60) (often rapidly progressive, initial fever and other signs of inflammation, raised ESR, obvious source of metastatic abscess, infective picture in CSF);
- arachnoid cysts (virtually confined to boys and nearly always on the left side, the cyst is associated with aplasia of the frontal and temporal operculum as well as marked cranial asymmetry); it is usually found when a subdural hematoma complicates a mild head injury (762);
- tuberculoma (calcification), gumma, and other granulomas such as sarcoidosis;
- parasites (echinococcus).

Certain *encephalitides* may resemble brain tumors:

- acute herpes encephalitis (p.49) (acute course, temporal lobe signs and symptoms, perhaps xanthochromic or inflammatory CSF findings);
- acute brainstem encephalitides (differentiate from brainstem glioma);
- multiple sclerosis may be difficult to distinguish clinically or roentgenologically from a brain tumor (1049).

Cerebrovascular disturbances may sometimes mimic a brain tumor:

- progressive ischemic softening without definite cerebral insult (in particular, unilateral or bilateral carotid artery thrombosis, see p.70);
- cerebral hemorrhage; although the diagnosis as a rule presents no difficulty, the space-occupying features of this condition may necessitate operation as if it were a neoplasm;
- arteriovenous malformation (p.95)

over a long period may produce only focal epileptic seizures, with or without apoplectiform features or other focal signs or symptoms.

Focal cerebral atrophy may also lead to confusion. Thus:

- Mills' unilateral progressive ascending paralysis, a slowly progressive hemiparesis sometimes with slight muscular atrophy as a result of local brain atrophy. However, this is a debatable entity, and may represent an atypical presentation of amyotrophic lateral sclerosis;
- some cases of Pick's disease (progressive focal neurologic signs and mental symptoms).

Signs of raised intracranial pressure in which a space-occupying lesion has been ruled out are usually referred to as *pseudotumor cerebri* (p.30).

Treatment of increased intracranial pressure: Treatment of increased intracranial pressure or brain edema is most effective in the presence of a brain tumor. It may also be used for pseudotumor cerebri (see p.31) after a stroke or head trauma. Foremost in the treatment is the administration of dexamethasone (Decadron), 4 mg every six hours intravenously, later by mouth. Water-soluble cortisone, 50–150 mg, may also be used. Treatment further includes the administration of urea, 200–500 ml of a solution of urea, 30 g in 70 ml of 10% dextrose in water, at 60 gtt/per minute. Mannitol as a 20% solution or sorbitol, 40% in a dose of 2.5–3.0 g/kg given over 30–60 minutes. In unconscious patients a Foley catheter should be inserted. Furosemide (Lasix), 40 mg intravenously as much as 2–3 times per day as a diuretic.

Inflammatory Diseases of the Brain and its Coverings

Inflammatory diseases of the central nervous system, particularly meningitis and encephalitis, may be primary or merely represent one aspect of generalized diseases involving the whole body. Consequently they occupy a boundary zone between neurology and internal medicine. This book will mainly deal with those aspects that confront the neurologist on his initial contact with the patient, namely, the clinical characteristics, practical approach, and differential diagnosis between individual types of encephalitis and meningitis. Table 1.**8** provides a systematic *review of the inflammatory diseases of the brain and its coverings*. Mention is made only of those entities which occur most commonly or which merit consideration for other reasons.

Meningitides

Introduction and classification: Various microorganisms may invade the meninges in a manner that varies to a greater or lesser degree in acuteness, intensity, duration, and exclusiveness. The particular clinical picture in an individual patient will depend on the type of microorganism, the number (concentration) of microorganisms, the general condition and notably the resistance of the patient, the presence of associated infections, and upon clinical management. Classification of the meningitides into purulent and aseptic, acute and chronic is not entirely satisfactory because overlapping situations occur, e.g., treated cases which were originally purulent, the leukocytic early stage of a subsequent lymphocytic virus meningitis, chronic meningitides with an initially acute course. On didactic grounds, the following classification can be justified:

- acute purulent (bacterial) meningitis,
- acute "aseptic" lymphocytic meningitis, and
- chronic meningitides.

General symptoms and signs: Most cases of meningitis exhibit the following features:

- headache, which is always present, sometimes very severe and diffuse and occasionally involving both sides of the occiput,
- backache is often present,
- fever is nearly always present, sometimes very high but may be absent, e.g., elderly patients,
- nausea and vomiting,
- sleepiness and dizziness,
- sometimes epileptic seizures,
- meningism (and positive Lasègue's sign) is nearly always present,
- abnormal CSF findings are invariably present, with
  - increased cell response (see individual forms below);
  - high protein level,
  - sometimes reduced glucose content (in purulent forms as well as in chronic bacterial, tuberculous, and fungal meningitides).

Table 1.8   Review of the major infective diseases of the brain and its coverings

Agent	Site (M = meninges, E = brain, SC = spinal cord, V = vertebrae)			Remarks
1. *Protozoa and parasites*				
Toxoplasmosis	M (+)	E +		Complement fixation test, dye test, see p.53
Trichinosis, cysticercosis, echinococcosis (738, 1066)		E +		Epileptic attacks, other organs involved, raised intracranial pressure, CSF pleocytosis and eosinophilia, blood eosinophilia
Schistosomiasis (1095)				
2. *Bacteria*				
Cocci	M + + +	E (+)		e.g., meningococcus, pneumococcus, *Hemophilus influenzae*, rarely *Staphylococcus aureus*, streptococci, klebsiellae, *Proteus*, *Pseudomonas*. Possible brain abscesses
Salmonellosis	M + +			
Brucellosis (295, 901)				Erythema, myalgia, lung infiltrates, conjunctivitis.
Leptospirosis	M +	E + +		Immunosuppressed or debilitated patients, complications such as brainstem involvement. Abscesses
Listeria monocytogenes				
Tularemia	M (+)	E + +	SC +	
Treponema pallidum		E (+)		Meningitis in early stage. General paresis. Tabes dorsalis
Mycobacterium tuberculosis	M + +		V +	Tbc in history, or in other organs or contacts. CSF glucose level markedly reduced – less than 1,000 cells. Monocytosis. Cranial nerve palsies
Shigella clostridium				
Neisseria gonorrhoeae				
Chlamydia trachomatis et psittaci				Ornithosis, lymphogranuloma inguinale

Table 1.8 (Continued)

Agent	Site (M = meninges, E = brain, SC = spinal cord, V = vertebrae)	Remarks
3. Fungi		
Blastomycosis	M ++ E ++	Enters body through lungs, skin involvement
Cryptococcus neoformans	M ++ E ++	Enters body through lungs or skin, chronic course, involves elderly and debilitated persons
Sporotrichosis	M + E +	
Actinomycosis	M (+)	Abscesses may form
Coccidioidomycosis	M + E +	Mimics tuberculous meningitis
Moniliasis	M (+) E ++	⎫ Debilitated persons, diabetics, alcoholics, drug addicts. Brain abscesses may develop
Mucormycosis	M (+) E ++	
Aspergillosis	M (+) E ++	
Nocardiosis	M (+) E ++	
Histoplasmosis	M +	⎭
4. Rickettsiae		
Q fever	M +	⎫ Headache, general debility, skin rashes
Typhus	E +	
Rocky Mountain spotted fever	E +	⎭
5. Viruses		
Poliomyelitis	M ++ E + SC ++	
Coxsackie	M ++ E + SC + V +	Neck and backache, two-peak, exanthemata, pleurodynia (Bornholm disease), neuritis and sometimes orchitis ⎫ epidemic affects children, usually in late summer
Echo	M ++ E + SC +	Skin rash ⎭

	M	E	SC	V	
Mumps	M +				Very high cell count, lifelong immunity. Affects males especially. Sometimes parotitis, pancreatitis, orchitis, oophoritis, deafness
Influenza					
Arboviruses					
– Spring meningoencephalitis	M (+)	E ++			Seasonal and geographic incidence
– Radiculomyoencephalitis	M +–	E +	SC +		
– Louping ill	M +	E +			
– E. & W. equine encephalitis (USA)					
– St. Louis encephalitis					
– Encephalitis japonica					
Encephalomyocarditis	M +	E +			Cardiac involvement. Rodent as host
Epidemic myalgic encephalomyelitis		E +			Muscle pains, attacks of disturbed mental function, neurasthenic picture
Herpes simplex	M (+)	E ++			Most severe, rapidly progressive encephalitis with grave prognosis
Herpes zoster	M (+)	E +	SC +	V +	Skin eruption. Usually lifelong immunity. In 5% associated neoplasm. In 1/3 pain persists
Lymphocytic choriomeningitis	M ++	E +	SC +		Domestic mouse as host. Pulmonary signs. Late spring/winter. Very high cell count. Possible brain or spinal cord bleeding
Epstein-Barr	M +				Infectious mononucleosis. Painful neck. Enlarged glands. Skin rash. Liver involvement
Uveomeningitic syndrome					Eye involvement
Rabies					Bite of an animal with rabies. Rarely dysphagia. Excitation situations. Throat spasms. Fatal

Acute Purulent Meningitis

Etiology: Bacterial invasion of the meninges occurs by the following routes:

- hematogenous,
- by continuity from the scalp, or
- by introducing the microorganism from outside, e.g.,
  - open craniocerebral trauma,
  - injections, or
  - shunt operations.

In adults the commonest microorganisms are the pneumococcus and meningococcus, in children *Hemophilus influenzae* (1091), the latter accounting for four-fifths of cases of childhood purulent meningitis. In infants the following must be included: *Escherichia coli,* group B streptococci, *Pseudomonas, Listeria,* and staphylococci.

Signs and symptoms: General, see p.40. In purulent meningitis the following features may be observed:

- signs and symptoms worsen within hours into a dramatically severe clinical picture;
- headaches (and backache) are unusually intense;
- temperature is very high (however, in elderly subjects with poor resistance and in infants high fever may be absent);
- meningism is massive, with positive Kernig sign (drawing up of legs) and Brudzinski sign (flexion of hip and knee upon testing for meningism); also here exceptions are found in elderly subjects and infants;
- very rapid onset of vomiting, confusion, drowsiness, and coma.

Diagnosis: *Lumbar puncture* is diagnostic. The CSF contains over 1,000 cells per ml, usually between 1,000 and 10,000, occasionally up to 100,000. Values over 50,000 prompt suspicion of a ruptured brain abscess; 80%–90% of the cells are polymorphonuclear leucocytes. Monocytic elements may predominate in chronic cases or in patients receiving treatment. The protein level is almost always raised, as is the CSF pressure. If the pressure exceeds 400 mm of water, the risk exists of herniation due to brain edema (or rupture of an abscess). The CSF glucose level is usually below 40% of the blood sugar. Direct Gram staining prior to treatment usually demonstrates the causative microorganism. Bacteriologic cultures must be made and are positive in about three-fourths of cases. Blood cultures should also be prepared since a positive result may be obtained even if the CSF cultures are negative, especially with the three commonest microorganisms.

Prognosis: This depends on the severity of the infection, associated diseases, the patient's resistance, and the treatment. The mortality rate of meningitis in neonates remains as high as 50%, that in children is between 10% and 20%. It is very high in meningococcal septicemia (Waterhouse-Friderichsen syndrome), in which adrenal failure causes vasomotor collapse. In pneumococcal meningitis it may reach 30%, in *Hemophilus influenzae* 15%. Permanent sequelae can be expected in about one-half of cases of infantile meningitis, e.g., deafness, malresorptive hydrocephalus, epilepsy, and defects of intelligence. These complications are much rarer in older individuals. Since the introduction of ampicillin in 1963, mortality from purulent meningitis has dropped, the level depending on the particular microorganism: for all microorganisms together, from 1,446 fatalities in 7,803 cases (18.53%) to 1,883 fatalities in 14,402 cases (13.07%) (191).

Treatment: Treatment should commence immediately after lumbar puncture. Adults should be treated with penicillin G (20 million units a day by intravenous infusion), ampicillin (2 g every 4 hours by intravenous injection), and gentamycin (80 mg every 8 hours by intramuscular injection). These antibiotics will combat not only the three commonest microorganisms mentioned above but also most Gram-negative microorganisms including *Pseudomonas* and the *Klebsiella-Aerobacter* group such as *Proteus*, and most staphylococci including those that are penicillinase resistant. If *Hemophilus influenzae* is suspected or observed (1091), chloramphenicol 100 mg/kg/day should be given for 3 days, then 50 mg/kg/day, in view of the increasing resistance to ampicillin. Treatment should be continued in reduced dose for 14 days. The treatment of neonates with meningitis is begun with ampicillin and aminoglycoside. As soon as a Gram-negative organism such as *E. coli* is isolated, a third-generation cephalosporin (e.g., ceftriaxone) is substituted. Similarly, a third-generation cephalosporin or cefuroxine is used as monotherapy in infants and children with meningitis caused by other microorganisms. Ampicillin is utilized in the presence of a *Hemophilus influenzae* infection, provided that no beta-lactamase producing organisms are present. Chloramphenicol, in view of its severe side effects in children, is held in reserve. Penicillin G is used if pneumococci or meningococci are isolated.

"Aseptic" or Lymphocytic (Serous) Meningitis

Etiology: Variable. The responsible microorganism may belong to the bacteria, protozoa, fungi, rickettsiae or – most commonly – the viruses.

Symptoms and signs: General, see p. 40. The following features are seen in the serosal form of the meningitis:

- headache is always present,
- temperature usually less raised than in the purulent meningitides,
- other organ involvement is common, e.g., lungs in tuberculous meningitis,
- course of illness has two peaks, especially in viral cases,
- commonly, there are signs of involvement of cranial nerves and their divisions, polyradiculitis, encephalitis, or myelitis.

Diagnosis: *Lumbar puncture* is essential for the diagnosis and to distinguish it from a purulent meningitis. It shows a cell count of less than 100–1,000 cells per ml. More than 1,000 cells are commonly found in lymphocytic choriomeningitis, mumps, and echo 9 infection. On

Table 1.9   Examination specimens and diagnostic methods in suspected viral infections of the CNS

	Early Stage (Always First Blood Test)	Late Stage (Always Second Blood Test)	Method of Choice
Meningitis			
Mumps virus	**CSF**, fauces, **feces**	(Urine)	IgM, G, T
Enteroviruses	CSF, fauces, **feces**	**Feces**	G
Herpes simplex type (1), 2	CSF, fauces, **blister**, heparinized blood		G, I, T
Varicella – zoster virus	CSF, fauces, **vesicle**		IgM, T
Epstein–Barr virus	CSF		IgM, G
Lymphocytic choriomeningitis			T, G
Arboviruses			IgM, T
Meningoencephalitis			
Herpes simplex type 1, 2	CSF, fauces, **skin eruption, heparinized blood** (brain)	(Brain)	I, G, T
Mumps virus	**CSF**, fauces, (urine)	(Urine)	IgM, G, T
German measles virus	CSF, fauces, urine		IgM, G, T
Measles virus	CSF, fauces	(Brain)	T, IgM, G
Arboviruses		(Brain)	IgM, T
Enteroviruses	**CSF**, fauces, **feces**	(Feces)	I
Adenoviruses	CSF, fauces, feces, urine		G, I, T
Cytomegalic inclusion virus	CSF, fauces, **urine, heparinized blood**	*Urine*	I, IgM, T
Varicella – zoster virus	CSF, **vesicle**		I, IgM, T
Epstein–Barr virus	Heparinized blood		IgM, I
Lymphocytic choriomeningitis	CSF		T, G
Rabies	CSF, brain		T, I
Spinal paralytic diseases			
Poliovirus 1, 2, 3	(CSF), **fauces, feces**	Feces	G, (T)
Other enteroviruses	**CSF, fauces, feces**	Feces	G
Mumps virus	**CSF**, fauces, feces	(Urine)	IgM, G
	CSF, fauces, urine	(Brain)	IgM, CFT
Guillain-Barré syndrome	After consultation with virologists (feces, in selected cases)		Special tests
Chronic CNS diseases			

G = growth   I = identification   T = rise of titer
(This table was compiled by Dr. *U. Schilt* of the Institute of Hygiene and Medical Microbiology, University of Berne. See also reference 1074)

the 1st day up to 50% of polymorphonuclear cells are present; thereafter, mononuclear and lymphocytic elements predominate. The protein level at most is slightly elevated; glucose in the viral forms is normal. If the glucose is reduced, a specific bacterial infection (tuberculosis) or a fungus should be suspected. Direct examination in viral meningitis reveals no microorganism, while fungi and individual bacterial types may be identified by the use of special stains. The diagnostic use of *cultures* and *serologic tests* is particularly important in this group for identifying the microorganism. Table 1.9 lists the body materials and the methods used for their examination in relation to the clinical stage of the illness.

Specific etiologic forms: The *viral meningitides* are numerically the main group. The commonest of these are the enteroviruses (echo, coxsackie, polio), followed by mumps, herpes II, lymphocytic choriomeningitis, and adenoviruses. Among the arboviruses is the tick-transmitted virus, spring meningoencephalitis. At least one-third of cases remain unidentified despite comprehensive virologic investigations. Leptospirosis (caused by a spirochete) produces similar signs and symptoms.

Mumps meningoencephalitis is diagnosed more often if a lumbar puncture is performed routinely in each case of mumps infection. Usually only trivial clinical signs of neurologic involvement are present, a mild meningitis. Disturbances of consciousness or neurologic deficits occur in a very small percentage. On the other hand, since only one of every two cases of mumps show noteworthy general clinical features and among these there is often no swelling of the parotid gland, the diagnosis of mumps should be pursued in all cases of serosal meningitis and meningoencephalitis by means of the complement fixation test. The prognosis is good in the meningitic form, and only one-third of the cases with encephalitis show late sequelae such as changes in behavior or seizures. Sudden deafness may occur in mumps, particularly in children.

Tuberculous meningitis has become rare and can now be cured. However, the prognosis is poor if treatment is delayed; therefore, the disease must be recognized early. The disease must be suspected in patients

- with a meningitic clinical picture which has progressed over the course of several weeks,
- with a lymphocytic cell count of fewer than 300 cells accompanied by a reduced glucose level,
- with lower cranial nerve palsies,
- with a past history or clinical evidence of tuberculosis of the lungs or other organs (although this is not necessary),
- with evidence of tuberculosis in the patient's community.

Focal clinical evidence of brain involvement may also be present. The CSF initially shows a polymorphonuclear picture but lymphocytes soon predominate. The CSF glucose is always markedly reduced (in contrast to viral meningitis). Direct identification with the Ziehl-Neelsen stain may involve a prolonged and careful search for the acid-fast microorganism. Laboratory culture requires a full 4 weeks. Patients in whom the disease is clinically suspected, even if the initial search for the tubercle bacillus proves negative, merit immediate treatment with the triple regime – isoniazid, ethambutol, and rifampicin, supplemented by prednisolone. Treatment must continue for 1–2 years. Sarcoidosis, see p.53.

Chronic Meningitis

This group includes infective meningitides as well as other processes causing meningeal reaction which run a chronic course. The CSF may show a cell count of 50–500 over several months, usually lymphocytes and large monocytes and reticulocytes. The protein content may be very high. The clinical picture may be mild: occasionally the patient is free from symptoms and completely ambulatory. The following diseases should be considered: treated tuberculous meningitis, *Borrelia burgdorferi* infection (Lyme disease), syphilis, fungal meningitides, toxoplasmosis, specific leptospiroses and brucelloses, recurrent meningitis (Mollaret), Hodgkin's disease, sarcomatosis and carcinomatosis of the meninges (1131), and sarcoidosis. Etiologically undetermined cases may run a course for months or years and then cure themselves spontaneously (520).

Important: parameningeal bacterial infections such as brain abscess may produce "aseptic" meningitis. If such a space-occupying lesion is suspected, CT or MR scanning should precede lumbar puncture. If an abscess is identified, lumbar puncture (which is hazardous and usually not diagnostically helpful) should not be performed.

Encephalitides

Involvement of the central nervous organs, i.e., by encephalitis or encephalomyelitis, accompanies many of the meningitides mentioned in the previous section. Nevertheless, it appears useful on didactic grounds to discuss the encephalitides as a separate clinical entity, including all infective illnesses which show a principal localization in the brain.

Etiology: The etiologic diagnosis is often difficult and involvement of other organs (e.g., embolic focal encephalitis, sarcoidosis) may be significant. The bacteriologic and serologic findings are usually diagnostic. In order to identify the causative microorganism (especially viruses) directly, specimens of stool, sputum, blood serum, and CSF must be obtained during the initial days of the illness. Serologic studies demand, in addition to serum taken at the start of the illness, further specimens 3–4 weeks later (presence of complement-fixing serum antibodies). A rise in titer is conclusive evidence and a fall from an abnormally high level after many months is similarly significant. Not infrequently the skin test becomes positive at a later stage. Further details are given in Table 1.9.

Diagnosis: The *most important features* of an encephalitis are the following:

- previous illness not involving the nervous system (particularly common in virus encephalitides) with signs and symptoms which may be either characteristic (e.g., typhus, measles) or nonspecific (e.g., influenza);
- headache, usually fronto-orbital, of varying degrees of severity;
- vomiting, photophobia, joint pains, neck- and backache;
- disturbances of the sleep rhythm;

- the patient appears critically ill;
- drowsiness or a deeper state of disturbed consciousness or confusion;
- pyrexia, which may not be obvious;
- cranial nerve palsies, focal neurologic deficits or papilledema;
- signs of cerebral irritation (epileptic seizures, myoclonus, choreiform disturbances of movement);
- generalized raised intracranial pressure;
- CSF shows increased cell count (rarely normal, usually up to 1,000) and increased protein content;
- EEG shows generalized changes of nonspecific nature;
- CT scanning may show parenchymal changes;
- other neuroradiologic examinations are usually normal, occasionally evidence is shown of a "space-occupying" lesion (e.g., hemorrhagic herpes encephalitis of the temporal lobe).

Viral Encephalitides

Only a few of the large group of virus encephalitides will be discussed. For additional information the reader is referred to Table 1.8 and to the literature (10, 1068).

Herpes Simplex Encephalitis (934)

This variety corresponds to the disease entity previously known as acute hemorrhagic encephalitis. The incidence may be as high as 10% of all encephalitides. The annual incidence in Sweden amounts to 2.3 cases per million inhabitants (1115). The clinical signs and symptoms begin after an influenza-like prodrome with a temperature above 38.5 °C. Next to appear are the nonspecific generalized signs of any encephalitis (see above). After several days specific signs of involvement of a temporal or frontal lobe appear, including hemispheric signs and other focal features, visual field disturbances, and epileptic seizures. A rapid course now develops of increasing mental changes, delirium, and drowsiness leading to coma. CT scanning may reveal a necrotic lesion in a temporal or frontal lobe; some of these later in the course of the disease will contain fresh blood. The *EEG* shows typical periodic sharp waves at 2- to 3-s intervals, later also a focal slowing (236). The *CSF* shows an increased lymphocytic cell count up to 700 cells and a slightly raised protein (50–200 mg %); the glucose is normal or slightly reduced. In 5%–10% of cases the CSF is normal. *Identification of the virus* in CSF or blood serum is virtually never possible. Observation of a rising titer of neutralizing antibodies in the serum over the course of weeks occurs too late to be useful in diagnosis during the early phase of the illness; moreover, it is not invariably present and also accompanies herpes labialis (698). In practical terms, only *brain biopsy* can confirm the diagnosis (91). Well-founded clinical suspicion is inadequate, and even in the hands of a highly experienced clinical group, it was confirmed in only 57% of 182 cases (1269, 1270). The **prognosis** depends on the treatment. Without treatment 70% are fatal and only 10% recover completely. In treated cases, the prognosis is better in younger patients and in those less deeply unconscious in the acute phase. None of the unconscious patients over 30 years recovered (1270). **Treatment** is with adenine arabinoside (1269), 10–20 mg/kg i.v. or with the less toxic substance acyclovir, 10–30 mg/kg i.v. Some authors advise, in view of the side effects of adenine arabinoside, that the diagnosis should first be established by brain biopsy (1270). Others commence treatment in those noncomatose younger patients in whom the clinical picture suggests a focal lesion and the CSF findings and the EEG and CAT appearances are compatible with the diagnosis. In a series of over 50 cases confirmed by biopsy, the action of acyclovir was superior (1115). Acyclovir administration is accompanied by measures to prevent epilepsy, gastric ulceration, and cerebral edema.

Arboviral Encephalitides

Insects serve as a reservoir for these viruses and transmit the microorganism by biting vertebrate animals including humans who are thus infected. Various forms of these encephalitides have individual regional distributions and a seasonal incidence, usually in spring through autumn. In the United States, *equine encephalitis, louping ill, and St. Louis encephalitis* is found, in Central and South America *Venezuelan equine encephalitis*, and in Central Europe *Russian spring-summer encephalitis* and the *Central European encephalitis* (tick encephalitis). The latter variety appears particularly in Czechoslovakia, Austria, and Yugoslavia and is carried by the tick *Ioxedes ricinus*. The incubation period is 10–16 days, and the course of the illness shows two peaks, the com-

monest clinical form is a meningitic one, showing an increased CSF cell count, usually polymorphonuclear. The prognosis is good. The diagnosis is confirmed when the complement fixation test becomes positive.

Rabies Encephalitis

Rabies results from the *bite of a rabid animal* after an incubation period lasting weeks or months. After a prodrome of fever and headache, mental **signs and symptoms** appear with irritability, anxiety, and episodes of agitation, accompanied by difficulty with swallowing, spasms of the facial and esophageal muscles as well as "hydrophobia." This picture is followed by atonia of the face, dysarthria, epileptic seizures, and psychotic episodes; actual paralysis is rare. Without treatment, death occurs in several days. **Treatment** consists in the prompt administration of immune serum to bitten persons and simultaneous passive immunization.

Encephalitis Lethargica ("Sleeping Sickness," von Economo's Encephalitis)

This disease occurred throughout the world between 1917 and 1925, and it is probably still encountered sporadically. Most patients show an uncharacteristic prodrome in which fever is either slight or absent and then exhibit a striking somnolence. Occasionally confusion is also present. Some patients show disturbances of external ocular movement and of pupillary function, others exhibit a striking hyperkinesia and hypersomnia, and yet others become stiff and show a paucity of movement. All these varieties carry a high mortality, about 40%, and most of the survivors are severely handicapped. However, numerous mild cases have been reported without manifest central nervous involvement, in which after a latent period of months or years, the typical features of postencephalitic parkinsonism appear (p. 108).

Several **other viral encephalitides** *and meningitides* are mentioned in Table 1.**8**. A variety of other affections which could be discussed in this chapter on encephalitis have been placed in other sections for various reasons: Creutzfeldt-Jakob disease (p. 169), kuru (p. 137), paraneoplastic progressive multifocal leukoencephalopathy (p. 156), herpes zoster (p. 385), and acute anterior poliomyelitis (p. 205).

Subacute Sclerosing Panencephalitis (SSPE)

Three main forms are considered under this title which were originally described separately but which now appear to be the same disease entity: *inclusion body encephalitis (Dawson),* panencephalitis (Pette-Döring), and *sclerosing leukoencephalitis (van Bogaert).* The **clinical signs and symptoms** begin furtively, usually in children of school age. First there are discrete and then definite mental changes (irritability, tiredness, loss of vitality). After several weeks speech disturbances and typical involuntary movements occur, the latter including myoclonic jerks and sudden movements evoked by noise and other stimuli. Choreiform and athetoid movements are also seen. The **prognosis** is poor: the characteristic changes worsen, speech dries up, autonomic disturbances appear, and the patient is finally left in a motionless state of increased extrapyramidal tone. The end result corresponds to decortica-

tion. The course extends over several months, rarely to 1 year. The *EEG* shows a pathognomonic appearance, namely periodic bursts of high slow waves at 3- to 4-s intervals in all leads, each periodic group identical with those in front and behind it. Invariably these electric phenomena synchronize with the myoclonic seizures. The *CSF* shows, in the presence of a normal cell count, one characteristic feature, a very high level of gamma globulins, and both the blood serum and CSF contain an increased titer of measles antibodies (174). The observation that many of these children suffered from measles early in life justifies the assumption that the measles infection occurred in the presence of passive maternal antibodies. An abnormal relationship exists between the measles virus and the immunologic reaction of the host. The high incidence of the disease in boys and in the rural population is compatible with an additional virus infection possessing an animal reservoir (174). **Treatment:** Isoprinosine (Inosiplex) (324) and amantadine appear to be effective (1005).

Epidemic Myalgic Encephalomyelopathy (Epidemic Neuromyasthenia) (543)

This curious disease usually occurs in isolated outbreaks or in house epidemics. The **etiology** is unknown, and a virus infection appears probable (543), – particularly infection with the Coxsackie B virus (101) – but the possibility of organic mercury poisoning has also been suggested. The **signs and symptoms** affect women more often. The disease runs a subacute course or develops furtively with muscular and nonspecific joint pains, paresthesias, muscular contractions, headache, generalized ill-health, and in about one-half of the cases pyrexia. The mental symptoms are important: the patient is irritable, ill-tempered, irascible, and often shows unreasonable and hysterical behavior. Physical examination shows the muscles, tendons, and periosteum to be markedly tender to pressure. The weakness often noted is actually a protective mechanism to pain. The tendon jerks are normal. Dysesthesia and hypesthesia are present and the gait is uncertain. The CSF is always normal. The **prognosis** is good and the patients usually recover after a few weeks. In individual cases, however, the disturbances may persist for months or years.

Radiculomyelomeningoencephalitis;
see under Berylliosis (204, 646)

One day up to 1 week after a tick bite, local **symptoms** appear, redness and swelling in the sense of an erythema migrans. However, the tick bite may have passed unobserved, and about 50% of cases show no skin changes. Days to weeks later, intense local (radicular) pains appear, leading to signs of polyradiculitis and myelitis: areflexia, weakness of other extremities, facial palsy, and sometimes of long tract involvement. Acute myelitic pictures are also described. The condition may be further associated with arthritis (411), myocarditis, liver involvement, and eye findings (including optic nerve). More and more, a chronic form is being reported which presents after one year or longer as a chronic myeloencephalitis with spasticity, weakness and personality changes. The CSF always shows an increased cell count, up to several hundred cells, as well

as an elevated protein content and an increase of immunoglobulins. In typical cases, the diagnosis is based on a history of a tick bite and the skin findings. In about 50% of the patients, however, one or both of these factors are absent. An elevated serum titer of borrelia-specific IgA of 1:124 is suggestive, of 1:1062 practically diagnostic of a borrelia infection. However, only an IgM titer indicates an acute infection with borrelia. In a recently acquired infection with borrelia with acute involvement of the central nervous system, the antibody titer in the cerebral spinal fluid exceeds that of the serum. The **prognosis** of the radiculomyelitic form is good, and both the pains and the other signs of illness disappear completely within weeks or months. **Treatment:** in view of the often very severe pain and the risk of developing a progressive chronic form, penicillin, 20 million units intravenously every day for two weeks, has to be administered. **Etiologically,** the responsible agent is *Borrelia burgdorferi,* a spirochete which is trasmitted by ticks, possibly also other insects. The incidence in the population is 10% in West Germany and in Switzerland.

Fungal Meningoencephalitides
Meningoencephalitis Caused by Cryptococcus neoformans (1119)

This saccharomycete involves exclusively the nervous system or, at least, neurologic **signs and symptoms** always dominate the clinical picture. Infestation is usually through the respiratory passages, sometimes through the skin. The disease is commoner in men.

Headache, vomiting, and disturbances of consciousness give way to focal neurologic deficits and cranial nerve palsies. A *CSF* pleocytosis (up to 400 lymphocytes) and a moderately increased protein level are present; the glucose content is usually low. The encapsulated bullet-shaped microorganism may be identified microscopically in an India ink preparation. At some stage in the course of the disease, the general condition of the patient will deteriorate markedly. The **prognosis** is poor. The majority of cases progress rapidly and die within a few months, although some may survive and remain capable of working, with the CSF showing a picture of chronic meningitis. Amphotericin B is given in treatment.

Blastomycosis

This condition, caused by the fungus *Blastomyces dermatitidis,* usually affects men working out of doors. The portal of entry is usually the lungs and all organs are eventually affected. About 50% of patients have lesions of the skin and lungs, 3%–10% in the CNS (384). This is due either to spread from skeletal foci or by contiguity or hematogenous dissemination into the brain parenchyma. Differential diagnosis includes tuberculous involvement of the nervous system and cryptococcosis.

Protozoal Brain Diseases

Toxoplasma Encephalitis

The congenital form has already been described on p. 13. A toxoplasma infestation with cerebrospinal manifestations may be acquired postnatally (1076). The **signs and symptoms** are usually those of an acute or subacute meningoencephalitis, meningomyelitis, or meningoradiculitis. Less often, signs and symptoms arising stepwise from separate locations may be present, giving a picture resembling multiple sclerosis. Earlier direct *identification of the microorganism* in CSF is possible by the immunofluorescence test, replacing the complement fixation and Sabin-Feldman tests. **Treatment** consists of combined administration of pyrimethamine (Daraprim) and an ultra long-acting sulfonamide (e.g., Fansidar) and spiramycin.

Sarcoidosis

It has not been established that sarcoidosis **etiologically** is an infectious disease. It is discussed here because it may involve the CNS, the clinical picture of a meningoencephalitis being most frequent. Neurologic **signs and symptoms** are present in about 5–10 1% of cases (1075, 1159, 1274), although in postmortem examinations this figure is far higher. The commonest is a brainstem picture, accompanied by diabetes insipidus and perhaps chiasmal involvement. Granulomata may be found, solitary or multiple, presenting as space-occupying lesions or as a picture of multifocal involvement of cranial nerves suggesting multiple sclerosis. Organic mental changes, even dementia, may occur. A transverse myelitis may be present if the spinal cord is involved. Rarely a peripheral neuropathy may occur (1274). The myopathy of sarcoidosis is described on p. 503. With CNS involvement, the *CSF* invariably shows an increased protein level and moderately increased cell count up to 200 cells. The **prognosis** is very serious: the disease runs a chronic course and is slowly progressive. **Therapeutically,** the patients respond variably to corticosteroids. Most cases respond well to treatment, provided the dose is appropriate and treatment is given early and consistently, with adjustment of the dose according to the clinical course (1159).

Bacterial Brain Diseases

Listeriosis (1111)

Listeria, a Gram-positive microorganism, is ubiquitous and may be transmitted to man. In listeriosis, in addition to various general and local symptoms, a meningoencephalitis may be present. **Clinically,** an acute cerebral picture is usually encountered with vomiting, headache, and high fever. The lesion, usually in the vicinity of the pons or medulla oblongata, causes corresponding local signs, e.g., paralysis of deglutition, and disturbances of vestibular function and external ocular movements. The microorganism may also affect neonates or adults whose resistance has been reduced by malignancy or immunosuppressive medication; such patients show an acute or chronic meningoencephalitis. Meningism may be absent, and a variable clouding of consciousness and epileptic seizures occur. The *CSF* shows a reduced sugar content and an increase in the cell count; the microorganism may be isolated from it. Without **treatment** (penicillin, tetracycline), death may occur within a few days.

Focal Embolic Encephalitis

Etiologically, this disease is a subacute bacterial endocarditis, in which dislodged (septic) thrombi from heart valves produce multiple cerebral emboli. The **signs and symptoms** correspond to these events, presenting either as a massive apoplectic insult with clinically detectable deficits such as hemiparesis or as a series of smaller insults. A long history of such episodes with micro-emboli in the smaller arterioles and capillaries is the characteristic feature of focal embolic encephalitis. The end result, in the absence of massive neurologic deficit, is a picture of mental disturbance, epileptic seizures, and personality changes. Pseudobulbar signs and symptoms may also appear, and more rarely a metastatic purulent meningitis. The multiple emboli may also produce mycotic aneurysms with subarachnoid hemorrhage, massive intracerebral hemorrhage, or brain abscesses. The *CSF* shows inflammatory changes. The correct diagnosis is usually made from the cardiac findings and other evidence of sepsis.

Rickettsial Diseases

Of these diseases, typhus and Q fever are the most important. They are transmitted to man from an animal reservoir by insects. General symptoms and signs are first present, such as fever, headache, a feeling of being gravely ill, and a skin rash (marked in Q fever). After a few days a steadily increasing encephalitic picture supervenes with confusion, coma, visual involvement, and focal neurologic deficits. Especially in Q fever, signs of meningitis may be present. The CSF is usually normal. Spontaneous recovery is possible. Treatment consists of chloramphenicol and tetracycline.

Encephalopathies Caused by Immune Reaction

Encephalopathies following infectious diseases or preventive inoculations (smallpox, measles, German measles, rabies) are not caused by microorganisms but result pathogenetically from an immune reaction. In addition to the conditions which will be described in more detail later, the neurological complications arising from a mycoplasm pneumonia infection should be mentioned. They occur in 5% of the cases, and consist of meningeal encephalitis, myelitis, or radiculitis (218, 965, 1259).

Measles Encephalitis (1, 407)

This complication may be expected in 1-5 of every 1,000 cases of measles. It is one of the parainfectious encephalitides, **etiologically** variable, which may complicate harmless infectious diseases (measles, German measles, chickenpox). A clinically similar picture may follow smallpox vaccination. The *histologic picture,* showing perivascular infiltration, is remarkably uniform, and this finding prompts the conclusion that this heterogeneous group possesses the same **pathogenetic** mechanisms, an antigen-antibody reaction. The measles virus does not appear to involve the brain directly (407). The clinical **signs and symptoms** of measles encephalitis appear on the 4th-6th day of the exanthem, when the fever is already subsiding. Within hours, headache, vomiting, confusion, and coma supervene. Epileptic seizures and focal cerebral and spinal neurologic deficits may also occur. *Lumbar puncture* reveals cell counts as high as 400 cells. The **prognosis** is poor: about 10% of cases die in the first few days. Practically all the survivors later have neurologic deficits, and about one-half exhibit severe mental defects.

Encephalitis After Smallpox Inoculation

This complication occurs on average in 1 in 100,000 injections, occasionally as often as 1 in 1,000. It is particularly likely to occur at the time of the first injection in an older child, but never under the age of 2 years and only rarely in subjects older than 30 years. **Clinically,** the encephalitic features appear after the 8th and before the 25th day (usually 9th-12th day) after vaccination. It starts acutely with headache, vomiting, fever, and seizures, as well as various neurologic deficits. The acute phase lasts 1-2 weeks. The CSF cell count is raised (up to 100) and the protein level is increased. The **prognosis** is poor, and the mortality is 10%-50%, death usually occurring between the 15th and 18th day of the illness. If a patient survives the critical phase, he may show a remarkable recovery, although residual paralyses and other disturbances may remain.

Syphilis of the Central Nervous System (1252)

General Aspects and Terminology of Neurosyphilis

About 10% of cases that are not cured by early treatment - including congenital syphilis - develop clinical signs of involvement of the nervous system. It may be affected in each of the three stages of the disease:

- If only the serologic reactions are positive, and there are neither clinical signs nor CSF evidence to indicate involvement of the nervous system, the term *seropositive latent syphilis* is used.

- The spirochetes may reach the nervous system before the exanthem appears, i.e., before the onset of generalized signs of the secondary stage 5–12 weeks after the infection. At least 10% of cases exhibit a lymphocytosis in the CSF during this stage. Such cases are termed *CSF-positive latent syphilis.*
- If clinical signs finally appear, true *neurosyphilis* is present. Neurosyphilis may be classified into three main types:
  - *cerebrospinal syphilis* in which inflammatory changes of the meninges and blood vessels are prominent, producing either an acute exudative or a more proliferative picture,
  - *tabes dorsalis,* affecting particularly the spinal cord, and
  - *general paresis,* in which the lesions are mainly localized to the brain. Tabes dorsalis and general paresis together comprise the *tertiary syphilitic diseases* (metasyphilitic diseases).

The incidence of cerebrospinal syphilis compared with that of tabes dorsalis and general paresis is 4:3:5.

Serologic Diagnosis of Syphilis

Blood serum reactions (357, 458) permit the diagnosis of syphilis. Of the nontreponema tests, purified cardiolipin with lecithin is used as the antigen to detect reagins. One such test is the VDRL test, which is negative in at least one-fourth or one-third of patients with primary syphilis as well as in advanced cases. Of the specific treponema tests,

the TPHA including the FTA (fluorescence treponema antibody absorption test) merit mention, since they are negative in only about 5% of advanced cases. The result can be evaluated quantitatively to permit conclusions concerning activity, reinfection, efficacy of treatment, and further therapeutic possibilities. The 19-S IgM (FTA) absorption titer is positive only if live treponema microorganisms are present in the body. Thus, it is a reliable indication of the possibilities of treatment, although it fails to implicate or exclude CNS involvement with certainty. By contrast, the *CSF tests* (458) yield definite results which permit confident conclusions. These tests include the ratio of the IgG concentrations in blood serum and CSF to each other, and other tests, especially cytology. For practical purposes, a positive VDRL reaction in the CSF indicates involvement of the central nervous system, and this test remains positive even in patients who have been successfully treated. On the other hand, this test may rarely be negative in patients with neurosyphilis. The activity of neurosyphilis is proved by an increased cell count or raised protein level (see treatment, p.59). Raised IgG levels in the CSF immunoelectrophoresis and raised IgM in the blood serum are other tests by which active neurosyphilis may be confirmed in a particular patient.

Cerebrospinal Syphilis

In the *secondary stage,* an acute and sometimes *fatal syphilitic meningoencephalitis* may occur, with cellular infiltration of the meninges, endarteritis of the meninges and cerebral blood vessels, cranial nerve palsies, upper motor neuron lesions, epileptic seizures, and coma. A very high cell count is found in the CSF. Occasionally polyneuropathies have been described in this stage.

In the *tertiary stage,* i.e., 2 or more years after the infection, *various manifestations of cerebrospinal syphilis* may be seen which reflect the vascular and perivascular inflammatory lesions causing <u>obliterative endarteritis.</u> This pathologic process leads to necrosis with caseation or to proliferative granulomatous changes (gumma).

- *Gummatous cerebral leptomeningitis* is a membranous thickening of the meninges which is mainly confined to the base of the brain. Clinical features include headaches, pupillary anomalies, cranial nerve palsies, signs of chiasmal compression, epileptic seizures, and mental symptoms.
- *Syphilitic cerebral arteritis* may lead to apoplexy with cerebral softening.
- *Cerebral gummas* are seldom large and may manifest clinically as space-occupying lesions. They are usually situated in the subcortical layer of a hemisphere.
- *Hypertrophic spinal pachymeningitis* may be associated with osteomyelitis of a vertebral body, most commonly in the cervical spine. The dura mater is thickened and fused to the arachnoid, and the blood vessels show inflammatory changes. The clinical picture consists of severe pains, muscular atrophy of the upper extremities, radicular sensory disturbances, and sometimes paraplegia (see below).
- *Syphilitic myelitis* and meningomyelitis are accompanied by changes in the meninges and blood vessels leading to superficial changes or softening of entire segments of the spinal cord. The clinical picture is that of girdle pain leading to a transverse lesion of the spinal cord after several weeks.
- In Erb's *syphilitic spinal paralysis* the clinical picture described above develops more slowly: it includes disturbances of bladder function, but no sensory changes occur.
- Muscular atrophy may be the most prominent feature of a syphilitic meningomyelitis - a *syphilitic amyotrophy.*
- The main signs of a *syphilitic radiculitis* are pain and sensory changes, sometimes accompanied by herpes zoster.
- *Optic atrophy* may be a feature of cerebrospinal syphilis, caused by either arteritis or arachnoiditis. Papilledema due to papillitis may be present, or it may be a sign of metasyphilitic disease.

Tabes Dorsalis

General: Tabes dorsalis is a manifestation of metasyphilitic involvement of the <u>nervous</u> system. It usually appears 8-12 years after the infection and is characterized by <u>bouts of lancinating pain, ataxia,</u> <u>absent tendon reflexes, and pupil-</u>lary abnormalities (reflexly unreactive (Argyll Robertson) pupil, pp. 350 and 351). Tabetics account for 30% of the patients with neurosyphilis; men are four times more often affected than women.

Subjective complaints: Typical attacks of *pain* herald the clinical picture. They appear suddenly, last seconds or minutes, and have a shooting or lancinating nature, affecting the legs or other parts of the body. Such painful *tabetic crises* may involve the epigastrium, rectum, penis, or bladder. *Paresthesias and sensory changes* ("walking on cotton wool") also occur commonly, as well as *ataxia* causing disturbance of gait. *Irreversible bladder disturbances* occur early, usually a giant, painless atonic bladder with a large residual volume but without pain. Impotence is another early feature.

Clinical examination: The *sensory changes* always appear first: initially they amount to diminution or absence of vibration sense, later affecting also positional sense. Sensitivity to pain is reduced, particularly in the deeper structures (absence of pain sensation on testicular or Achilles tendon pressure). The (perineal) pain sensation is usually delayed. In about one-third of cases, ataxia is present – partly as a result of this absence of deep sensation – which may lead to a severe disturbance of gait. This disturbance is worse in darkness or if the patient shuts his eyes; the Romberg test is abnormal and the patient cannot walk on a straight line. Involvement of afferent fiber from muscles in the posterior nerve roots may produce marked hypotonia with a hypermobility of joints. For the same reason, the *tendon jerks* are absent in more than one-half the patients, usually the ankle jerks and then the knee jerks. Less often, pyramidal signs are present. *Inequality of pupils* is eventually present in about 90% of patients with tabes dorsalis. The commonest finding is a uniformly contracted pupil that reacts poorly (or not at all) to light. All variations may be observed, the complete Argyll Robertson pupil is seen in about 20% of tabetics (pp. 350 and 351). About one patient in ten has *optic atrophy* which, despite energetic treatment, usually progresses to blindness. *Disturbances of ocular*

movement are less common. *Trophic changes* include chronic *perforating ulcer* of the foot or *tabetic arthropathy* with gross destruction of the joint surfaces (Charcot joint).

The *CSF* may contain up to 80 mononuclear cells. The protein level is either normal or slightly elevated. The colloidal gold curve is abnormal as a result of the increased gamma globulins. The Wassermann reaction is positive in about 70% of cases in blood, in 75% of cases in the CSF. In 5% it is positive only in blood and in about 10% only in CSF. Thus, in about one-fifth of all cases, the Wassermann reaction is negative in the blood as well as the CSF. In contrast, the specific tests (TPHA and FTA) are always positive.

Neuropathology: Shrinkage and fibrosis of the posterior columns of the spinal cord are visible upon naked-eye examination. Microscopic study shows degenerative changes in the afferent fibers in the posterior roots entering the spinal cord. The posterior column fibers show demyelination with axonal degeneration and glial proliferation.

General Paresis (1310)

General: This condition comprises about 45% of cases of neurosyphilis. Men are four times more often afflicted than women. The condition appears 10–15 years after the primary infection, occasionally much later: the older the patient at the time of the infection the earlier its appearance. The dominating feature is a progressive dementia, often accompanied by a facile and expansive expression, epileptic seizures, slurred speech, pupillary irregularities, and various neurologic deficits.

Symptoms: The clinical picture initially may be nonspecific: headaches, generalized lassitude, and sleep disturbances. About 10% of patients experience epileptic seizures. Individual patients show transient hemiparesis or other focal deficits (Lissauer type, epilepsy paralysis).

Clinical examination: Less than one-half the patients show pupillary anomalies of the type described in tabes dorsalis. A typical feature is the dysarthric "slurred" speech, which is particularly marked for certain test phrases (e.g., "around the rugged rocks the ragged rascal ran," "hopping hippototamus," "Methodist Episcopal"). Muscular jerks known as "sheet lightning" may be observed, particularly in the region of the mouth. The reflexes are often abnormally brisk, sometimes accompanied by pyramidal signs. Optic atrophy, or posterior column deficit, or other signs of tabes dorsalis may be present, so that the term "taboparesis" is used. An occasional finding is nonresorptive hydrocephalus, and in such cases shunting may improve that part of the clinical status produced by the hydrocephalus.

Mental picture: The mental symptoms sometimes overshadow the neurologic deficits, and the commonest is a slowly progressive dementia with memory loss, disturbance of affect, reduced discriminatory ability, and corresponding deterioration of moral and social behavior. Less frequently the disturbance is of the hyperreactive or expansive type in which the patient tries to perform bizarre exploits by overestimating his own ability (delusions of grandeur).

The *CSF findings* and the serologic reactions are almost invariably abnormal. The Wassermann reaction is positive in the blood serum as well as CSF, usually more frequently than in tabes.

Neuropathology: Macroscopic examination reveals the brain to be shrunken and hardened. The meninges are thickened and the convolutions atrophic, especially in the frontotemporal region. The ventricles are enlarged. Microscopically, the picture of a subacute encephalitis is present: loss of ganglion cells and an increase in astrocytes and microglia, particularly in the cerebral cortex, corpus striatum, and hypothalamus. The arterial vessels have thickened walls and contain a marked perivascular cellular infiltration. Abundant spirochetes may be identified in the cerebral tissue.

Prognosis: Without treatment, prognosis is poor and survival seldom exceeds 3 years. Spontaneous improvement is rare.

Treatment and therapeutic follow-up of neurosyphilis (206, 1015, 1166, 1252, 1310): The *indications* for treatment and the follow-up measures necessary in cases of neurosyphilis are signs of activity in the

CSF. The most important of these signs is an increased cell count, and it is the indication for *treatment with penicillin,* e. g., 15–20 million units in the course of 2–8 weeks. A combination of penicillin with some other form of treatment offers no advantage. In patients who show signs of recrudescence of the infection, despite a correctly administered course of intramuscular penicillin, the treatment should be carried out by the intravenous administration of soluble penicillin, 20 million units per day for 10 days.

CSF follow-up: Regular CSF examination is essential at 3-month interval in the 1st year of treatment, every 6th month in the 2nd and 3rd years, then annually until the 5th year. If treatment is successful, the cell count returns to normal within 6 months, and the protein content shows definite improvement. The only indication for *repeating the course of treatment* after 6 months or years later is a persistently high cell count – above 15/mm³. *Interval observation:* In some cases, the other CSF changes gradually return to normal in the course of 3 years: the protein content, the increased gamma globulin level, the abnormal colloidal gold curve, also the Wasserman reaction in both CSF and blood serum. In other cases, certain deviations from the normal remain present indefinitely, but they should not be viewed as signs of activity. The treponema immobilization test (Nelson) remains positive, always in the blood serum and nearly always in the CSF, following successful treatment of neurosyphilis. The test may be falsely positive in patients receiving antibiotic treatment. For tabetic crises, carbamazepine 400–800 mg/day is effective.

Brain Abscess (170)

Etiology: Cerebral abscesses are rarely the direct result of trauma, far more commonly they are metastatic. The commonest primary sources of infection in the body are a middle ear infection, sinusitis, bronchiectasis and other purulent pulmonary lesions, and endocarditis (particularly in congenital heart disease). In children more than 50% of brain abscesses are caused by congenital heart disease, and about 5% of such lesions are complicated sooner or later by a brain abscess. The antibiotic era has seen an ever-increasing proportion of cases – at present about 25% – in which the primary source remains unknown. The commonest microorganisms are the streptococcus and staphylococcus, less frequently pneumococcus and others. The interval elapsing between the primary purulent process and the first symptoms of cerebral involvement is less than 2 months in one-half the cases, in the remainder the interval varies from many months to years.

Localization: Abscesses are found significantly more frequently in the cerebral hemispheres than in the cerebellum (1103) and only a small percentage occur in the brainstem (1039). In the latter, the clinical picture mimics a low-grade brainstem glioma. Listeriosis is frequently localized in the brainstem (p. 54).

Clinical signs and symptoms: The clinical picture is only rarely multiphasic, in the context of focal embolic encephalitis (p.54). This may be the case, for example, when an abscess is superimposed on a hemorrhage or on an area of cerebral softening due to embolism or infarction. In the course of investigating such patients, microorganisms are usually identified without a source of infection being found (203). Far more commonly, progressive signs of an intracranial space-occupying lesion are present with focal signs such as epilepsy and raised intracranial pressure so that a brain tumor is suspected. The differential diagnosis is made more difficult by the fact that the majority of patients are afebrile. Most patients exhibit a leukocytosis and a raised ESR, but in at least one-fourth these values are normal. In one of three patients the CSF cell count is not increased. The rate of progression of the signs and symptoms corresponds to that of a glioblastoma or a cerebral metastasis. Under certain circumstances, the final differential diagnosis between neoplasm and brain abscess is possible only by means of neuroradiologic investigation, and sometimes only by biopsy. In enhanced CT scans, brain abscesses may image as solitary (or multiple) ring lesions.

Treatment: The success of treatment depends on the phase of the illness and the size and site of the abscess. Radical extirpation should be the aim: in early abscesses that are not yet encapsulated, treatment involves aspiration followed by drainage and an intensive course of locally applied and systemic antibiotics. A radical operation should then be carried out within 24 h (685). More and more, cerebral abscesses are being treated conservatively by a high-dose antibiotic regimen for 4–6 weeks. The mortality remains about one-third of cases.

Epidural Abscess and Subdural Empyema (127, 395)

Etiology: Extradural abscesses may arise either on the basis of a (traumatic) osteomyelitis or by contiguous spread; e.g., from a frontal sinusitis. Subdural empyema usually develops from an (acute) frontal or ethmoidal sinusitis, more rarely from an otitis media. About half the patients are under 20 years of age; most empyemas occur in men.

The **clinical picture,** which varies according to the underlying lesion, usually begins with the signs of osteomyelitis. However, focal signs and symptoms such as hemiparesis and epileptic seizures become rapidly superimposed upon the general features such as high fever, increasing headache, irritability, and confusion. An occasional complication is rupture into the subarachnoid spaces, leading to meningitis or brain abscess. If no rupture occurs, the CSF cell count may remain normal. Conventional skull roentgenograms may sometimes reveal the presence of osteomyelitis, and CT scanning will image the extracerebral space-occupying lesion.

A severe, so-called *otitis externa* may lead to osteomyelitis of the skull base, especially in diabetics. The *pathogenic organism* is *Pseudomonas aeruginosa.* The presenting picture is a clinical triad: granulomatous destruction of the external auditory canal, earache, and a yellowish-green discharge from the ear. *Cranial nerve palsies* may occur (348), especially paralysis of the facial nerve, associated with palsies of other cranial nerves (3rd–12th) in various combinations. Osteomyelitis of the cervical vertebrae is also known, complicated by involvement of the nerve roots and appropriate clinical signs. **Treatment** consists in evacuating the purulent focus. While antibiotic cover has revolutionized the prognosis for the better, in spite of this combined treatment the disease still carries a mortality of about 30%.

Circulatory Disturbances and Hemorrhages of the Brain and its Coverings

Physiologic and Anatomic Aspects of the Cerebral Circulation

Cerebral Metabolism

Glucose is virtually the only energy source of the cerebral metabolism, and a total of 115 g/day is utilized. The respiratory quotient is about 1. Approximately 15% of the cardiac output per minute enters the brain, although brain tissue accounts for only 2% of the total body weight. Ischemic symptoms appear clinically if the normal blood flow of 58 ml/100 g brain/min falls to 35–40 ml.

Regulatory Mechanisms

These mechanisms guarantee an adequate supply of oxygen to the brain. In the conscious subject, the fall in pressure leads first to compensatory dilatation of the cerebral vessels so that arterial perfusion remains at a constant level. Only if the systolic pressure falls below about 70 mm Hg in healthy subjects (or below 70% of the initial value in hypertensives) does cerebral perfusion clearly diminish (768). Occlusion of one carotid artery leads to a 70% hyperperfusion of the opposite side: the same may be observed following occlusion of a middle meningeal artery and cannot be explained merely by a rise in blood pressure. Cerebral perfusion diminishes in the presence of hyperventilation or raised intracranial pressure.

Total (Experimental) Cerebral Ischemia

In this situation, all the free oxygen is exhausted within 2–8 s. After 12 s unconsciousness occurs, and after 30–40 s a silent EEG tracing is obtained. After 3–4 min, histologically detectable irreversible foci of parenchymal necrosis are found. The subject cannot survive a total ischemia of more than 9 min (Fig. 1.**6**).

Intra- and Extracranial Collateral Circulation

This collateral flow is an important factor in understanding the mechanism of cerebrovascular accidents (1204). The brain is supplied mainly by the two internal carotid arteries and the two vertebral arteries. The most important intracranial collateral connection is the arterial circle of Willis, which joins together the four main arteries at the base of the brain. It ensures passage of blood from one side to the other, also from front (carotid territory) to back (vertebral territory), and vice versa. These channels are represented diagrammatically in Fig. 1.7. A number of factors determine the extent to which these channels play a part in individual cases of arterial occlusion, viz.:

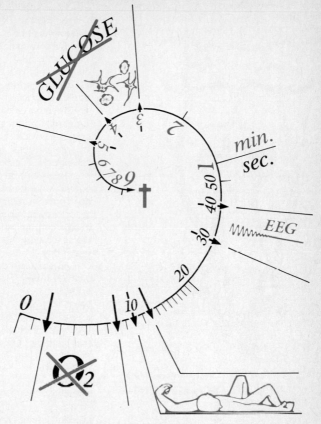

Fig. 1.6 Diagrammatic representation of the effect of total cerebral ischemia on tissue oxygenation, the level of consciousness, the EEG, the morphology of the cerebral nerve cells, and the glucose content

- size (diameter) of the anastomosis,
- state of the arterial wall and its ability to widen,
- local pressure changes, i.e., a fall in pressure in the bypass,
- systemic blood pressure and general circulatory state, and
- the speed with which an artery becomes occluded.

Ulcers and Platelet Thrombi

Platelets may aggregate on mural irregularities such as stenotic plaques or ulcers of the cervicocranial vessels supplying the brain – these lesions may be diagnosable by Doppler sonography or angiography as areas of stenosis or ulcers. Some of these aggregates become detached and are carried distally into the cerebral circulation, producing

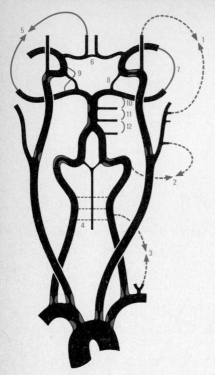

1 external carotid artery – facial artery – angular artery – ophthalmic artery – carotid siphon
2 external carotid artery – occipital artery – muscular branches – vertebral arteries
3 subclavian artery – thyrocervical trunk – occipital muscular branches – vertebral arteries
4 vertebral arteries – meningeal branches – spinal arteries
5 anterior cerebral artery – pericallosal artery – callosal branches – posterior cerebral artery
6 right anterior cerebral artery – anterior communicating artery – left anterior cerebral artery
7 middle cerebral artery – parieto-occipital branches – posterior cerebral artery
8 carotid siphon – posterior communicating artery – posterior cerebral artery
9 carotid siphon – anterior choroidal artery – posterior choroidal artery – posterior cerebral artery
10 posterior cerebral artery – cortical branches – superior cerebellar artery
11 superior cerebellar artery – cortical branches – anterior inferior cerebellar artery
12 anterior inferior cerebellar artery – cortical branches – posterior inferior cerebellar artery

Fig. 1.7 The most important collateral channels of the cervicobrachial arteries and their branches

signs and symptoms of a cerebral ischemic attack. This is likely to happen in atheromatous lesions of the internal carotid artery. On account of the laminar character of blood flow, emboli from a particular site in an arterial wall will repeatedly be delivered to the same intracranial arterial branch, sometimes resulting in recurrent monosymptomatic insults (see transient ischemic attacks, p. 70). The pathogenesis of a cerebral insult may be clarified considerably if microemboli (which consist partly of cholesterol crystals) are observed in the retinal vessels. In the individual case, it is always difficult to decide whether the damage is caused by microemboli or by the altered hemodynamic factors mentioned previously.

Localization

The concept should be abandoned that the site of the lesion in the cerebral parenchyma must always correspond topographically to the location of the pathologic lesion in the arterial system of supply. Localized ischemia of a specific zone within the brain is seldom caused solely by focal changes or a congenital anomaly in the feeding artery. Usually an additional factor is present, such as a generalized reduction in the supply of blood to the brain, e.g., hypotension, a reduction in the cardiac minute volume, or significant stenosis of an artery nearer to the heart.

Clinical and Etiologic Aspects of Cerebrovascular Accidents
(307, 399, 1204)

About 15% of all deaths are caused by cerebrovascular accidents. Of these, three-fourths are due to ischemic attacks. Men and women are affected equally.

Clinical features:

- most patients are elderly,
- exceptionally in young individuals
  - in the presence of high-risk factors (see below),
  - in arteritides,
  - in cardiac embolism or disturbances of rhythm in the context of cardiopathy,
  - in dissecting aneurysm of the carotid artery (p. 73),
- "stroke"-like onset of (central) neurologic symptoms and signs,
- progressive stroke (PS), i.e., a march of neurologic manifestations in the course of hours and, rarely, days,

- topographic localization to a particular site in
  - a cerebral hemisphere,
  - the brainstem and cerebellum (p. 73), and
- rarely heralded by a previous disturbance of consciousness.
- Causes may be obvious, e. g.,
  - fall of blood pressure (during sleep, postprandial, sudden orthostasis, cardiac infarction),
  - disturbances of cardiac rhythm.
- Presence of vascular risk factors (see below).
- Clinical or instrumental evidence of abnormality of cardiac function.
  - Cardiac infarction shown by ECG,
  - disturbances of cardiac rhythm,
  - cardiac lesion producing emboli,
  - bruits or murmurs over the great vessels or abnormal findings upon Doppler sonography.
- Clinical course
  - prompt and complete recovery (TIA = transient ischemic attack),
  - slower but complete recovery (PRIND = primary reversible ischemic neurologic deficit),
  - incomplete or absence of recovery with permanent deficits (CS = completed stroke),
  - PS = progressive stroke (see above).

Etiologic factors: The following are frequently present and should be sought in each case:

- Arteriosclerosis of the cervical and cerebral vessels. Search for
  - bruits or murmurs over the great vessels,
  - bruits or murmurs or absent pulses over other arterial territories of the body,
  - Doppler sonographic evidence of stenosis or occlusion of neck and large intracranial vessels (see Fig. 1.9),
- vascular risk factors
  - hypertension,
  - diabetes mellitus,
  - nicotine abuse,
  - obesity,
  - hyperlipidemia,
  - ovulation inhibitors,
  - polycythemia vera,
  - specific familial diseases such as Osler-Rendu syndrome (p. 164),
  - homocystinuria,
  - Fabry's disease,
  - progeria,
  - Ehlers-Danlos syndrome, and
  - pseudoxanthoma elasticum.
- Presence of a (generalized) arteriopathy and
- collagen diseases
  - amyloid angiopathy
  - livedo reticularis generalisata (Sneddon syndrome) (981, 1145),
  - cranial arteritis (very rarely intracranial),
  - fibromuscular dysplasia of the cerebral vessels (1121),
  - spontaneous or posttraumatic dissecting aneurysm of the internal carotid artery (p. 73).
- Sources of emboli
  - local plaques in the neck vessels as a source of platelet thrombi, usually at the carotid bifurcation,
  - cardiac lesions as a source of larger emboli,
    1. cardiac infarction with myocardial thrombus,
    2. auricular fibrillation with or without rheumatic valvular lesion (5- to 17-fold greater risk of emboli [1883]),
    3. endocarditis,
    4. mitral valve prolapse (click syndrome, with mesosystolic click and holosystolic murmur), which may be detectable only by echocardiography (84) and may be familial, and
    5. auricular myxoma.
- Sudden onset of (focal) vascular insufficiency as a cause of ischemia, due to a
  - fall of arterial blood pressure (sleep insult during the night with discovery of the paralysis upon awakening, stress insult, e.g., after heavy meal, relaxation insult following unusually severe physical demands),
  - acute blood loss, e.g., internal bleeding,
  - cardiac infarction,
  - subclavian steal syndrome (p. 80),
  - local arterial compression, e.g., one vertebral artery during rotation or therapeutic manipulation of the neck,
  - Coronary surgery (1104),
  - Heart transplant patient with an incidence of cerebral vascular complications of up to 60% (825).

Acute Disturbances of Perfusion of the Cerebral Hemispheres

Introduction: The classic stroke of the cerebral hemisphere (307, 399, 1204) is characterized – as the name implies – by focal neurologic deficit occurring out of the blue, often during sleep, in a patient otherwise in good health. Only occasionally does the patient experience premonitory signs of headache and a general feeling of malaise for several hours, rarely 1–2 days (progressive stroke). The case history and etiologic factors have already been summarized.

Clinical signs and symptoms: The clinical deficit is the same in the various etiologic types – hemodynamically induced insufficiency, arterial thrombosis, extracranial carotid stenosis, or embolism. Specific details about the last-named two groups of patients will be given below.

In the *acute stage,* physical examination should include assessment of the following: respiration, circulation, and level of consciousness. Lesions in the territory of supply of the middle cerebral artery produce a near total hemiplegia. Lesions of the *internal capsule* (which is supplied by the lenticulostriate branches of the middle cerebral artery) tend to be more severe clinically, on account of the tightly packed corticospinal, corticobulbar, thalamocortical, and optic tracts traversing this structure. Initially, tone is frequently diminished and the reflexes are normal or reduced, but the Babinski sign is usually present. Sensation is normal or only slightly affected. Cases of *pure motor hemiplegia* may follow softening of a small part of the internal capsule or the foot of the peduncle (238). Stimulation of the median nerve on the paralyzed side may show evidence of damaged sensory pathways in the tracings of the sensory-evoked potentials (237). *Hemianopsia* should be identified and *speech and communication disturbances* noted (p. 173). No meningism is present and the CSF is initially normal; the pleocytosis accompanying extensive areas of softening develops later. Secondary hemorrhagic infarction may produce xanthochromia of the spinal fluid.

In the *later stages,* after days or weeks, spasticity develops, producing a flexed position of the arm and an extended position of the leg. The head and eyes are now turned toward the side of the lesion (conjugate deviation), and the patient "looks to the side of the distaster." Recovery from the hemiplegia is usually faster in a lower limb than in an upper limb. The patient when walking circumducts the paralyzed leg but fails to swing the paralyzed arm, which he holds in a position of slight flexion (Wernicke-Mann) (Fig. 1.8). When the patient raises the affected arm to the horizontal position, the elbow and the finger joints tend to be slightly flexed, and there is a tendency for the little finger to be abducted – the digiti quinti sign (28).

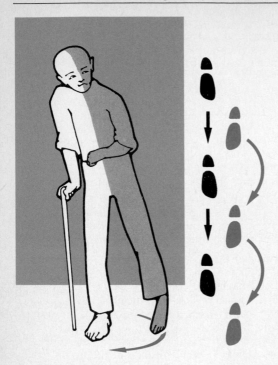

Fig. 1.8 Typical posture of the hemiplegic during walking. He circumducts the spastic paralyzed leg because of extensor dominance, and adducts and flexes the paralyzed arm because of flexor dominance

Features of a Cerebral Hemispheric Insult

Occlusion of a specific arterial trunk produces a specific pattern of signs and symptoms. Occlusion of the trunk of the *middle cerebral artery* leads to a more severe weakness of the arm and face with relative sparing of the leg, and homonymous hemianopsia. Occlusion of the *anterior cerebral artery* usually does not produce unconsciousness and presents as a purely motor spastic paralysis of the contralateral lower limb. A thalamic infarct (145, 408) can give rise to a variety of symptoms, depending on its localization, including visual field defects and memory impairment. This is particularly prominent, and may persist over years if the infarct is bilateral – when both thalami are supplied by brances from one medial arterial trunk (408). Lesions in the *vicinity of the thalamus* may produce a persistent, burning unilateral pain. Touch becomes unpleasant and this sensation is often delayed and prolonged. Temperature appreciation is also disturbed so that dissociated hemianesthesia may be present. Often, *Horner's syndrome* is present on the side of the lesion (p. 241), and also the thermoregulatory mechanism of *sweat secretion* may be reduced or abolished (1073). This can be attributed to a *subthalamic lesion* of the uncrossed descending central sympathetic tract. An oversensitivity to light stimulation is described (203). *Epileptic attacks* occur in about 10%-20% of patients with cerebral ischemia, most commonly at the onset of the attack and only rarely weeks or years later; they may be focal or generalized. More unusually, chronic epilepsy develops. Cases of bilateral perisylvian ischemia with localized softening of the anterior part of the operculum may cause an isolated apraxia of varying degree, affecting the mouth and throat muscles during voluntary movements only, the *Foix-Chavany-Marie syndrome* (761). *Aphemia* is recognized as a lesion of the pars opercularis, the inferior parietal gyrus, and the adjacent white matter beneath it giving rise to dysarthria and impaired speech production without aphasia (1070).

Examination of the Unconscious Patient

A special examination technique is required to attempt to demonstrate neurologic deficits. The unconscious patient immediately after the apoplectiform seizure turns his head and eyes away from the lesion. Even in unconscious patients, it is sometimes possible to elicit details of the neurologic deficit. A facial palsy may be demonstrated by asymmetry in the pain grimace in response to pain stimulation. Passive elevation of the upper eyelid is easier on the paralyzed side. The corneal reflex, if still present, is different on the two sides. With the patient supine, the lower limb on the paralyzed side is externally rotated (1093). Paralyzed extremities, when raised passively, fall more promptly and floppily to the bed clothes when released. Pain stimulation provokes a more prompt defense response on the healthy side. Finally, differences in the tendon reflexes or pyramidal signs may be observed.

Cerebral Embolism

This particular etiologic form of acute cerebral insult accounts for only about 10% of cases of apoplexy. At least one-half of these cases are caused by mitral stenosis with associated atrial fibrillation, one-third by myocardial infarction with mural thrombosis. Far less frequently the causes listed on p. 66 are present. The significance of a mitral valve prolapse is controversial (631). The incidence is 5-20% in young adults, but 40% in patients with a cerebral infarct. Its demonstration by echocardiography is not always easy and requires an experienced examiner. If the diagnosis is established, treatment with lung anticoagulants is justified. The diagnosis of a cerebral embolic event is justified if one of the above-mentioned cardiac lesions is present, if the neurologic deficit appeared suddenly without loss of consciousness, and if it was maximal at its onset. Emboli lodge more commonly in a cerebral vessel on the right side of the brain than on the left. Often the symptoms and signs regress rapidly. An unequivocal arterial occlusion often disappears upon follow-up angiography or may not be present at autopsy examination. There is no meningism and the CSF at least initially is normal.

Prognosis of Vascular Accidents in the Cerebral Hemispheres

About one-fifth of patients with brain softening die during the first attack, of the remainder about one-half die of a recurrence within 5 years. Patients with a preexisting arteriopathy and transient ischemic attacks are as likely to develop myocardial infarction as cerebral infarction (510). In the acute phase, advanced age, a complete hemiplegia of the extremities, impaired level of consciousness, and a combination of hemiplegia with hemianopia constitute poor prognostic signs (26). Arterial hypertension, which is present in about two-thirds of these patients, also affects the prognosis unfavorably and accelerates recurrent attacks. Possibly the significantly better prognosis of attacks in young persons can be explained by the absence of associated risk factors: of young persons, as high as 80% regain their work capacity partly or completely (514). Treatment, see p. 81.

Intermittent Disturbances of Perfusion of the Cerebral Hemispheres (Transient Ischemic Attacks)

Apart from the impressive attacks described above with their serious deficits which regress only slowly or remain permanently present, there is another clinical picture, which results from *intermittent cerebral vascular insufficiency* or *transient ischemic attacks*. The commonest cause appears to be platelet thrombi released from ulcerated plaques in the internal carotid artery. The layman speaks of a little stroke. In this condition, short-lasting cerebral disturbances of unspecified nature or focal neurologic deficits occur. The patient may briefly lose consciousness, then recover again without paralysis. For several hours he may be confused and disoriented, have difficulty in finding words, be dysarthric, or exhibit transient weakness of an arm or a leg. This type of attack may recur repeatedly in the course of months or years, discrete deficits sometimes remaining, and in at least one-half of the cases ending eventually in a completed stroke (984). About one-fifth of patients with a transient ischemic attack die within 3-5 years from myocardial infarction or they become incapacitated by permanent hemiplegia (600). Because of the frequency of these two complications, the physician is obliged at the time of the first episode of a transient ischemic attack to **search diligently or a (treatable) cause.** Lesions of both intracranial and extracranial branches of the arterial system may be responsible for intermittent disturbances of perfusion or for apoplexy with permanent deficit. While occlusion of the middle cerebral artery almost invariably leads to immediate and permanent deficit, transient clinical signs are commoner with lesions sited closer to the heart. More than 60% of patients with carotid artery occlusion have experienced transient signs and symptoms only once or twice before the onset of irreversible damage. Intermittent disturbances may either be caused by hemodynamic factors or by recurrent emboli consisting of cholesterol crystals and fragments of thrombi.

Lesions of the Cervical Portion of the Internal Carotid Artery

This is the commonest site of arterial stenosis in the neck (307, 1117, 1204).

Flow murmurs: Auscultation of the neck occasionally reveals a murmur of arterial stenosis synchronous with the pulse to be discovered. It can be intensified by compression of the opposite carotid artery (caution!). A flow murmur is not a very reliable clinical sign. Only rarely present with a complete occlusion, it is found relatively frequently on the side opposite to the occluded artery, it is absent in about three-fourths of cases of stenosis, and is audible over more than 10% of blood vessels without stenosis (1313). Not uncommonly cervical flow murmurs are encountered as chance findings in individuals without cerebral signs (498, 509). The risk of stroke increases, and in a series submitted to a 6-year period of observation in such individuals it reached about 14% (509), compared with 3.4% of similar subjects without flow murmurs. The risk of damage rises further if combined lesions of the carotid and vertebral arteries are present (498). Nevertheless, only a loose correlation can be shown between the site of the insult and the murmur, and between the subsequent clinical disease (myocardial infarction!) and the bruit in the neck. Many authorities have concluded that an asymptomatic flow murmur indicates a generalized arteriopathy and when present as the only sign does not justify invasive diagnostic tests or surgical arterial repair (509).

Abnormally marked coiling or kinking of the extracranial internal carotid artery is claimed to be responsible for cerebral circulatory disturbances, but the causal significance of these anatomic variants remains questionable.

Further findings: Occlusion of the internal carotid artery produces abnormally strong pulsations of collateral branches supplying the ophthalmic artery, which are palpable in the periorbital region (567). An EEG recording made with carotid compression provides information concerning the extent to which one hemisphere is dependent upon the blood flow from the contralateral carotid artery (and the vertebral arteries). Measurement of the retinal artery pressure may provide useful information, as may ophthalmodynamometry (1272). An ipsilateral reduction in visual evoked potentials is described following exposure to a very bright light source and is attributed to reduced regeneration of the visual pigment caused by inadequate retinal perfusion (305).

Doppler sonography (112, 578): This is the most important screening test. It rests on the fact that a signal is reflected from a moving surface – in this case the flow of blood in an artery – and thereby its frequency is modified. These frequency changes are proportional to the initial frequency and the flow velocity. Apart from simple acoustic evaluation, averaged recordings can be triggered by the ECG, processed by means of a computer, and displayed on a cathode ray oscillograph. This method enables the flow characteristics of blood vessels to be observed. Hemodynamically significant stenoses of the internal carotid artery may be observed with an accuracy of 90%, although without providing precise localization (609). Figure 1.9 provides an example. The Doppler technique is also useful in establishing vertebral artery occlusions (610) and even in recording the flow in intracranial branches (2) and in evaluating brain death.

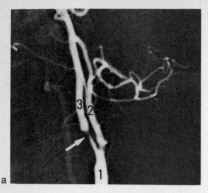

a

Fig. 1.9 Doppler sonographic examination in stenosis of the right internal carotid artery. Below are tracings of the electrocardiogram and of the Doppler signal showing (a) the flow component toward the probe and (b) away from the probe in the neck arteries. The tracings in the three arteries of a patient with stenosis (left side) are contrasted with those of a normal subject (right side). Stenosis of the internal carotid reduces flow in the common carotid artery as well as in the poststenotic part of the internal carotid, particularly the diastolic component. In stenosis the turbulence distorting physiologic laminar flow may be amplified acoustically and heard by means of earphones or a loudspeaker

	stenosis	**normal**
ECG		
common carotid artery 1	a b	
external carotid artery 2	a b	
internal carotid artery 3	a b	

b

Occlusion or Stenosis of the Intracranial Carotid Artery

Occasionally this lesion accompanies a stenosis of the basilar artery. It gives rise to a collateral circulation consisting of a network of delicate blood vessels in the basal ganglia, to which the name *moya moya* (Japanese: "a puff of smoke") is attached.

The condition is a cause of stroke in both young and old patients (894).

Stenotic Lesions of the Internal Carotid Artery Proximal to Its Ophthalmic Branch

Pathognomonic of this lesion is the combined association of a transient ipsilateral monocular visual loss *(amaurosis fugax)* and a contralateral hemiparesis. Abnormal (homolateral) visual evoked potentials in carotid stenosis have been mentioned above (305).

Dissecting Aneurysm of the Internal Carotid Artery (143, 820, 821, 1154, 1262)

This could be demonstrated as the cause of a first stroke in 2.5% of the cases (143). It may arise spontaneously or follow trauma, produces a characteristic clinical picture. It is heralded by intense homolateral hemicranial and hemifacial pains, and soon a Horner's syndrome appears. Rarely, an ipsilateral lesion of the hypoglossal nerve has been observed, with paralysis of the tongue (428). Only a minority of patients show contralateral neurologic deficits. A homolateral 12th nerve palsy has been described. The angiographic appearances are typical. A cystic median necrosis may underlie the spontaneous dissection (1262). The prognosis of the spontaneous cases is rather unfavorable, and more than 50% die or are left with severe sequelae (143). In the traumatic cases, the prognosis is reported by some authors as poor (1154), by others as good (818) – no doubt depending on the selection of the groups of patients reported on.

Acute Disturbances of Perfusion In the Brainstem and Cerebellar Region (Vertebrobasilar Territory) (114, 1204)

Anatomy

The vertebral arteries and the basilar artery, with their branches, supply blood to the upper cervical spinal cord, the medulla oblongata, the cerebellum, the pons, and most of the remaining mesencephalon. In three-fourths of cases both posterior cerebral arteries receive their main supply from the basilar artery so that large parts of both occipital lobes, particularly the visual cortex, are also dependent on the vertebrobasilar tree. The left and right vertebral arteries, which arise, respectively, from the left and right subclavian arteries, lie in close anatomic relationship to the uncovertebral joints of the cervical vertebrae in their courses through the costotransverse canals. Within these canals the arteries may be compressed by osteophytic overgrowth or by mechanical compression during neck movements. Extension and lateral flexion as a rule reduce perfusion through the contralateral vertebral artery.

Classic Brainstem Insult

Characteristic clinical features: About 15% of cerebral vascular accidents occur in the vertebrobasilar territory. Typical are:

- *stroke-like* onset,
- sometimes *triggered* by head movements,
- *without loss of consciousness* (with exception of actual basilar artery thrombosis which is rare),
- often intense *rotatory vertigo* and vomiting,
- *paralysis of deglutition* and *hoarseness,*
- and/or *visual disturbances,*
  - oscillopsia with nystagmus,
  - double vision,
  - visual field defects, cortical blindness,
- *cerebellar* (ataxic) signs develop,

Table 1.10 Brainstem syndromes (description of individual syndromes in the literature are not always similar)

Description	Site of Involvement	Ipsilateral Signs	Contralateral Signs	Special Features
Chiray-Foix-Nicolesco syndrome (upper red nucleus syndrome)	Midbrain, red nucleus	Oculomotor palsy	Hemiataxia sometimes develops, also intention tremor, hemiparesis (often without Babinski's sign), sensory disturbances	
Benedikt syndrome (upper red nucleus syndrome)	Midbrain, red nucleus	Oculomotor palsy, sometimes paralysis of ocular movement toward the affected side	Hemiataxia sometimes develops, also intention tremor, hemiparesis (often without Babinski's sign)	Staggering gait
Claude's syndrome (lower red nucleus syndrome)	Midbrain, red nucleus	Oculomotor palsy	Hemiataxia or hemi-incoordination, hemiparesis	No hyperkinesia
Weber's syndrome	Middle cerebellar peduncle	Oculomotor palsy	Hemiparesis	
Parinaud's syndrome	Region of the quadrigeminal bodies			Paralysis of upward gaze (superior quadrigeminal bodies). Paralysis of downward gaze (inferior quadrigeminal bodies)
Nothnagel's syndrome	Region of the quadrigeminal bodies	Oculomotor palsy	Hemiataxia	

Raymond-Céstan syndrome	Anterior tegmentum of the pons	Gaze paralysis to the side of the lesion	Sensory disturbance, sometimes including the trigeminal nerve, and hemiparesis	Nystagmus
Gasperini's syndrome	Posterior tegmentum of the pons	Paralysis of 5th, 6th, 7th, and 8th cranial nerves	Sensory disturbance	
Millard-Gubler syndrome	Posterior tegmentum of the pons	(Peripheral) facial palsy	Hemiparesis	
Brissaud's syndrome	Posterior tegmentum of the pons	Facial spasm	Hemiparesis	
Foville's syndrome	Posterior tegmentum of the pons	Sixth cranial nerve palsy, sometimes also a facial palsy	Hemiparesis	
Babinski-Nageotte syndrome	Posterolateral part of the pontobulbar junction	Cerebellar ataxia, Horner's syndrome	Hemiparesis, sensory disturbances	Nystagmus, lateropulsion (territory of posterior inferior cerebellar artery)
Wallenberg's syndrome	Posterolateral part of the medulla oblongata	Horner's syndrome, paralysis of the vocal cord, soft palate, and posterior wall of the pharynx, trigeminal nerve involvement, hemiataxia	Dissociated sensory disturbances	Nystagmus, involvement of posterior inferior cerebellar artery
Céstan-Chenais syndrome	Lateral part of the medulla oblongata	Horner's syndrome, paralysis of the vocal cord, soft palate, and posterior wall of the pharynx, hemiataxia	Hemiparesis, hemihypesthesia	
Avellis' syndrome	Lateral part of the medulla oblongata	Paralysis of the soft palate, posterior wall of the pharynx, and vocal cords	Hemiparesis, hemihypesthesia	

Table 1.10 (Continued)

Description	Site of Involvement	Ipsilateral Signs	Contralateral Signs	Special Features
Schmidt's syndrome	Lateral part of the medulla oblongata	Paralysis of the posterior pharyngeal wall, vocal cord, sternomastoid, and upper trapezius and tongue muscles	Hemiparesis, hemihypesthesia	
Tapia's syndrome	Lateral part of the medulla oblongata	Paralysis of the soft palate and posterior pharyngeal wall, vocal cord, and tongue	Hemiparesis, hemihypesthesia	
Vernet's syndrome	Lateral part of the medulla oblongata	Paralysis of the soft palate and posterior pharyngeal wall, sternomastoid paralysis, loss of taste sensation over posterior third of tongue, hemihypesthesia of the pharynx	Hemiparesis	
Jackson's syndrome	Inferior part of the medulla oblongata	Paralysis of tongue (lower motor neuron)	Hemiparesis	

- involvement of the cranial nerves and of the *contralateral* extremities
  - e.g., lower motor neurone facial paralysis with hemiparesis of the contralateral extremities (Millard-Gubler syndrome),
  - further details, see Table 1.**10**.

Causes: Softening in the vertebral territory may occur under similar circumstances to those in the carotid artery, i.e., following a drop in blood pressure, as upon morning rising. Often no particular cause can be found, and only rarely a mechanism leading to mechanical occlusion of the vertebral artery (see above), such as an onset associated with extreme head movements, e.g., hanging out the washing, shaving under the chin, reversing a car, washing the hair during bathing with the head thrown back, chiropractic maneuvers (317). The consequences of an actual thrombosis of the vertebral artery (665) are more serious the more distally it is located in the trunk of the artery. The overall mortality is 25%. A high lateral occlusion of the vertebral artery leads to brain stem symptoms in 60% of the cases, has a mortality of 4.5% per year, and carries a risk of stroke of 1.8% a year (144). The cerebellar and brain stem symptoms described above are frequently heralded or accompanied by occipital headaches.

Specific Syndromes

Brainstem ischemia gives rise to fairly characteristic clinical syndromes which depend on the site of the lesion. Table 1.**10** summarizes the eponymous brainstem syndromes, although it must be pointed out that none of these syndromes is frequently seen in a pure form.

The Wallenberg Syndrome

The Wallenberg syndrome (dorsolateral syndrome of the medulla oblongata) is one of the commonest (Fig. 1.**10**). *Subjectively,* it arises very suddenly with severe rotatory vertigo which may put the patient on the floor. There is no disturbance of consciousness. Vomiting and hoarseness (vagal nucleus ambiguus) may be present. *Clinical findings* include nystagmus (descending vestibular nucleus), ipsilateral Horner's syndrome (central sympathetic tract), ipsilateral trigeminal nerve involvement (descending tract of the trigeminal nerve), and ipsilateral disturbance of swallowing with paralysis of the palate and posterior pharyngeal wall (vagal and glossopharyngeal nuclei). The last of these leads upon gagging to distortion of the soft palate and sideways displacement of the posterior pharyngeal wall to the healthy side which remains innervated, the so-called stage curtain phenomenon (Fig. 1.**11**). Accompanying these features is an ipsilateral ataxia of the extremities (anterior spinocerebellar tract) and a crossed dissociated sensory disturbance of the extremities (lateral spinothalamic tract). Features usually absent are paralysis of the extremities, altered reflexes, and upper motor neuron signs. As a rule, the acute signs disappear within a week and most patients appear to recover satisfactorily. The syndrome

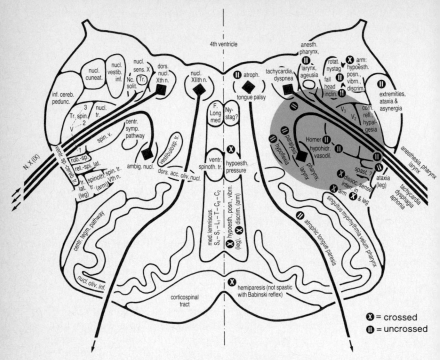

Fig. 1.10 Section through medulla oblongata. The colored zone is damaged in Wallenberg's syndrome (after *Hassler*)

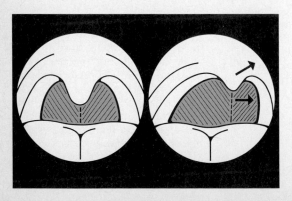

Fig. 1.11 Displacement of the soft palate (and posterior pharyngeal wall) during swallowing to the healthy left side in a case of paralysis of the right vagus nerve (stage curtain sign)

is the clinical manifestation of ischemia in the territory of the posterior inferior cerebellar artery and sometimes follows occlusion of a vertebral artery at the level of the atlas as it penetrates the dura mater. In young subjects, a "benign form" of the Wallenberg syndrome is described, which has an excellent prognosis (117).

Acute cerebellar infarct. In approximately 1 of 200 autopsies encephalomalacia of the cerebellum is found. A cerebellar infarct occurs more infrequently in men, and about 60% of the patients are hypertensive. Aside from headaches, the clinical findings (636, 1214) are usually ataxia, not infrequently disturbance of eye movements, alteration of consciousness, and increased intracranial pressure. This indicates a poor prognosis. Therapeutically, in the event of progressive symptoms the development of an acute posterior fossa syndrome has to be prevented by external ventricular drainage or possibly surgical evacuation – provided that the brain stem is not involved.

Specific forms of presentation and signs: Disturbances may occur which vary from *cortical visual field defects* to complete blindness, either isolated or combined with brainstem signs. The patient often sees only shades of gray or is blind, but denies it. The picture of bilateral blindness or other severe visual disturbance in an elderly patient with intact pupillary reflexes should always prompt suspicion of cortical blindness due to a vascular lesion. Transient cortical blindness has been described after vertebral angiography. Larger areas of softening of the medulla oblongata may produce *acute bulbar palsy,* with bilateral cranial nerve palsies, disturbances of swallowing, bulbar disorders of speech, and severe paralysis of the extremities. The pupils are contracted. Clonic convulsions may occur, sometimes decerebrate rigidity. The prognosis is very poor. Areas of softening in the pons occasionally present as an unusual disturbance of consciousness, so-called *coma vigile* (p.89), or as a locked-in syndrome. The *palatal nystagmus* accompanying brainstem lesions and occasionally associated with rhythmic vertical movements of the eyes (ocular bobbing) is attributable to damage of the central tegmental tract or the dentate nucleus.

Prognosis of established brainstem insult: This may be compared with insults in the cerebellar hemispheres (216) (p.68).

Intermittent Insufficiency of Vertebrobasilar Perfusion

This picture is characterized by the following *features:*

- recurrent signs and symptoms, usually identical, occurring over months or years,
- often triggered by rotation or other head movements,
- in particular
  - rotatory vertigo,
  - double vision,
  - paresthesias and sensory disturbances of the face,
  - transient cortical visual disturbances, and
  - paresthesias of the extremities.
- Bilateral signs and symptoms, or symptoms first on one side and then on the other,
- occipital headache, and
- drop attacks (p.287).

Predisposing factors of vertebrobasilar insufficiency include *generalized arteriosclerosis,* particularly in the context of diabetes mellitus. The condition may also be a complication of *atlantoaxial instability* in patients with rheumatoid arthritis (580). A further cause is the so-called *subclavian steal syndrome,* in which the vertebral arteries function as a collateral circulation and blood flows in a retrograde direction from within the cranium through the vertebral artery on the affected side into the subclavian artery distal to the site of obstruction. This lesion may lead to signs of vertebrobasilar insufficiency and vertigo on exercising the arm of the affected side.

Transient Global Amnesia

These episodes appear to reflect a disturbance of perfusion in the basilar territory, specifically a transient ischemia of the hippocampus on both sides. The term *ictus amnésique* is also used to describe an episode of transient global amnesia (373, 380, 852, 854, 1141, 1142). The *description of the episode* is characteristic: the patient loses his ability to fix new events in his memory and has forgotten events of the preceding days, weeks, or even months (retrograde amnesia). He manages to carry on his daily life satisfactorily, but exhibits anxiety since he vaguely realizes his predicament. He keeps on asking the same questions over and over, immediately forgetting the answers he obtains. Subjects in middle or advanced age are affected, and the disturbance usually lasts only for a few hours. *Physical examination* shows normal findings. First the capacity to recall new events returns, then within hours or days the retrograde amnesia clears up. Finally, only the memory gap for the actual period of

amnesia remains. *Recurrences* are rare. Similar manifestations have been observed personally in young subjects after the ingestion of *oxyquinoline derivatives* (853). It has been observed that the episode itself lasts slightly longer and a permanent residual retrograde amnesia remains. Amnestic episodes are rare in brain tumors. When accompanying epileptic seizures, the term *amnestic encephalitis* has been used. *Topographic amnesia* is another variety (827).

Criteria for further invasive investigation of cerebrovascular insults: These depend upon the following elements and should be investigated in the following way:

– only when the initial neurologic *deficits* have completely or largely *regressed;*
– only when *no indications of severe generalized arteriopathy* exist, or no other severe illness is present;
– a cardiac source of embolism is ruled out;
– *clinical* analysis by auscultation and palpation of the *cervicocranial* arteries, and
– a careful *Doppler sonographic examination* is carried out.
– When these examinations yield evidence of a hemodynamically significant stenosis or a mural plaque as a potential source of emboli
– and the whole situation indicates that vascular surgery offers a good prospect of success,
– then careful and complete arteriographic examination of both the extracranial and intracranial vessels is carried out.

Treatment of Disturbances of Cerebral Perfusion

Prevention: The disappointing results of treating established vascular accidents emphasize the importance of prophylaxis in stroke. Removal as well as prevention of the risk factors (see pp. 65–66) and precise early diagnosis in transient ischemic attacks are necessary if attempts are to be made to eliminate the cause.

Conservative treatment of cerebrovascular accidents (307, 1204): In the *treatment of the cardiovascular apparatus,* arterial hypertension should only be treated promptly if very high levels are found, in the context of a hypertensive encephalopathy (p. 84). More often the blood pressure should be restored to values which are normal for the patient – therefore sometimes even hypertensive values. For this purpose, the following may be used: ephedrine hydrochloride 7–10 mg, or norephedrine (Levophed) i.v., or an infusion of macromolecular solutions. In patients with cardiac failure, digitalis should be given and disturbances of cardiac rhythm corrected.

Measures for improving blood flow include the infusion of papaverine hydrochloride 200–500 mg in 1 liter over 8 h, but the benefit is questionable since such infusions dilate the blood vessels in undamaged regions of the brain. The author does not use them.

Cerebral edema is seen only exceptionally with large areas of softening (increasing drowsiness, Cheyne-Stokes breathing). As in brain tumors (p. 31), it is treated with corticosteroids and diuretics or with glycerine (43, 417).

In order to *reduce the viscosity of the blood,* dextran is prescribed (431), e.g., dextran 500 ml as a 40% solution, as Macrodex or Rheomacrodex for several days. The patient should be monitored for a sudden or significant rise in blood pressure, which calls for treatment with diuretics and perhaps antihypertensives.

Anticoagulants are justified only in cases of embolism from cardiac sources, e.g., mitral valve prolapse. They should not be given for the first 3 weeks after a severe insult (or only after extensive cerebral softening or cerebral hemorrhage has been excluded by CT scanning), in order to avoid provoking a hemorrhage into the softening. In cases of recurrent ischemic attacks caused by proven carotid stenosis, anticoagulant medication appears to have as beneficial an effect as endarterectomy (42). The significant reduction in the incidence of recurrence produced by anticoagulants is observed only during the 1st month after the initial insult. It does not influence the survival rate (1265). Careful evaluation of the literature fails to reveal any convincing evidence of a beneficial action of anticoagulants in cases of chronic intermittent insufficiency (188).

Treatment with *thrombolytics* cannot be recommended since no beneficial effects have been proved.

Aggregation inhibitors should be prescribed in all cases after

2–3 weeks (156, 211, 1059). An acetylsalicylic acid preparations, 1 g/d – one that is well tolerated by the stomach – may be used for as long as 1 year.

According to statistical data, medication is indicated only in males, but it appears to be absurd to exclude female patients from treatment (216). Patients unable to tolerate acetylsalicylic acid may be given sulfinpyrazone or a combination of acetylsalicylic acid and dipyridamol. This combination appears to be more beneficial in cases of carotid territory infarction than acetylsalicylic acid alone, but the same success has not been shown with infarcts in the vertebrobasilar territory (156).

Vascular surgery: The indications for arterial surgery have yet to be conclusively defined. In a 1978 study of 225 patients with transient ischemic attacks who were submitted to long-term follow-up, no prognostic difference could be detected between the conservatively treated patients and those undergoing arterial surgery (1203). Increased experience and improved operative techniques including the introduction of external-internal anastomoses (45) have widened the indications for operative treatment. Provided an excellent microsurgical technique can be guaranteed, indications may now be defined.

– Arterial surgery possesses prophylactic value, but it will not cure existing neurologic deficits.
– It may be utilized to treat isolated arterial lesions, but has no place in patients exhibiting marked generalized arteriosclerotic changes.
– Occlusion of a common carotid and subclavian artery is an indication for operation.
– In lesions at the carotid bifurcation in the neck, operation should be considered
  • in those patients with transient ischemic attacks in whom the signs have regressed completely and provided a stenosis is demonstrated (42, 361, 440). In such cases, it does not appear to be important whether the stenosis produces hemodynamic changes or not (440),
  • the presence of residual clinical deficit or a total occlusion of the artery tends to invalidate the indication for operation.
  • Endarterectomy of a stenotic carotid artery does not benefit the signs and symptoms of vertebrobasilar insufficiency (744).
– Indications for external-internal anastomosis – usually between the superficial temporal artery and a branch of the middle cerebral artery – may include the following (45, 288):
  • presence of an intracranial flow disturbance proximal to the origin of the middle cerebral artery,
  • transient ischemic attacks,
  • especially if the retinal artery pressure is too low (pressure to be measured with the patient erect), and
  • no collateral channels from other sources have opened to

irrigate the ischemic part of the brain beyond the site of obstruction.

The morbidity and mortality of the operation amount only to a small percentage. More than 90% of the surgical anastomoses remain open (689). More recently, as the result of a comparative study, the benefit of this bypass operation has been questioned (330).

Rehabilitation: Rehabilitation of the hemiplegic patient is crucially important. The program, managed by trained staff, must start on the 1st day and continue for an adequate period, even months. Optimally, rehabilitated patients regain a significantly improved functional ability compared with patients who are inadequately rehabilitated. By contrast, the effectiveness of speech therapy has been challenged (644).

Intracerebral Hemorrhage

Lesions in the Cerebral Hemispheres (247, 400, 502, 591, 1257)

Epidemiology: Cerebral hemorrhage accounts for about 10%–20% of all acute strokes. The introduction of CT scanning has seen a threefold increase in the number of cases diagnosed (400). Male patients predominate, and 80% are hypertensives. The average age is somewhat lower than the average for infarction but three-fourths of patients are over 50.

Clinical aspects: In two-thirds of cases the hematoma is situated in the basal ganglia. *Acute (juvenile)*

subcortical hemorrhage is a condition which is characterized – somewhat restrictively – by the onset of acute hemispheric signs usually accompanied by severe localized headache. In most cases, the lesion is caused by a small *arteriovenous malformation,* but hemorrhage into a neoplasm or tumor metastases must also be considered. The hematomas may be multiple (1257) and may rupture into the ventricular system (247). This picture may also follow secondary *hemorrhage into a cerebral infarct* caused by arterial occlusion (247). Therapeutic anticoagulation may lead to spontaneous intracerebral hematomas, or cause bleeding from arteriovenous malformations (502). While the onset is abrupt as a rule, usually during the day at work, about 10% arise gradually. Only slightly more than one-half of the patients are unconscious at the onset, presenting in deep coma with stertorous breathing and extensor spasms; in such patients, the prognosis is poor. In three-fourths of patients ventricular rupture occurs, in 15% the hematoma disrupts the cortex. Despite this, massive subarachnoid hemorrhage is seldom seen.

Ancillary investigations: The *CSF* is xanthochromic only if the hematoma is close to the surface or a ventricle and is blood-tinged when it perforates. In 15% of cases, the CSF is completely normal (502). *CT scanning* demonstrates the hematoma, which in two-thirds of cases exerts a space-occupying effect. Review of a large series of cases has permitted the retrospective conclusion that about one-fourth of intracerebral hematomas were misdiagnosed as cerebral softening in the pre-CT era (315). Initially the hematoma is uniformly hyperdense and shows a low-density rim. When exceptionally in the course of weeks it does not shrink and it exhibits its customary ringlike enhancement after the injection of contrast medium (up to 9 weeks), the differential diagnosis from secondary hemorrhage into a tumor may be difficult (502). As a rule, hematomas resorb completely within 6–8 weeks. Occasionally angiography is required to rule out an arteriovenous malformation.

Treatment: Since no effective conservative method of treatment is known, an attempt at surgical removal of the hematoma is justified in some cases. According to neurosurgical statistics (591), early operation and use of the dissecting microscope enable the majority of patients to be salvaged. However, from the neurologist's viewpoint, the result is not always satisfactory (400). Evaluation of the same patient by different specialists gives rise to marked divergence of approach to the planning of treatment (770).

Spontaneous Cerebellar Hemorrhage (Cerebellar Apoplexy) (166, 664, 800, 907)

This condition accounts for 10% of all brain hemorrhages. In more than one-half of cases, an arterial hypertension is present while other patients have received anticoagulant medication or are shown to harbor an arteriovenous malformation. Usually for no apparent reason, the first symptoms are intense headaches (mainly occipital), vertigo, and nausea.

Incoordination of movements and gait ataxia are the rule, as well as dysarthria and a paralysis of horizontal gaze or nystagmus in the direction of gaze. Meningism is found in 40%, the CSF is blood-stained in 80%–90% of cases. If untreated, two-thirds of patients lapse into coma within hours or days. CT scanning or vertebral angiography confirms the diagnosis. Spontaneous improvement is very rarely described (907); therefore, prompt operation is unavoidable despite the high surgical mortality (166).

Vascular Encephalopathies

Hypertensive Encephalopathy (234, 768)

The term hypertensive encephalopathy is used to describe the cerebral disturbances accompanying severe constant arterial hypertension – headache, confusion, drowsiness, and mental deterioration. Superimposed on this picture are crises of deterioration, mostly associated with a further rise in the level of the blood pressure. The most likely event is spasm of the smaller arteries occurring on the basis of the hypertensive attack, leading to a severe disturbance of consciousness with vomiting, papilledema and retinal hemorrhages, blindness, hemianopsia, epileptiform seizures, and a raised CSF pressure. Treatment should be energetic, aimed at achieving a fall in the blood pressure level by means of antihypertensive drugs and measures to reduce possible cerebral edema (p. 29).

Generalized Cerebral Arteriosclerosis

This leads to *arteriosclerotic dementia,* which is discussed on p. 168.

Subcortical Encephalopathy
(Binswanger's Disease)
(48, 212, 370)

The term subcortical encephalopathy is used to describe a chronic progressive vascular lesion of the cerebral hemispheres. The frequency is given as one to a few percent, depending on the population analyzed (370). It is characterized by fluctuations in mood and consciousness of the patient, sometimes signs of vascular accidents, later pseudobulbar symptoms and evidence of vascular insufficiency in other body regions. The patients are middle-aged, and practically all are hypertensives. The course of the disease may extend over 10 years. The vascular lesions are usually situated in the subcortical layers of the cerebral hemispheres and show marked thickening of the walls of the smaller blood vessels with foci of softening and gliosis. A generalized hydrocephalus is invariably present. The EEG reveals a diffuse change combined with local changes in various sites. The CT scan (720) shows a characteristic appearance, a diffuse thinning of the white matter, global cerebral atrophy, and sometimes multiple infarcts.

Thromboangiitis Obliterans
(Buerger's Disease)

Epidemiology: This disease may be confined to the blood vessels of the brain. Males are more commonly affected than females, young adults as well as the elderly.

Pathoanatomically, large areas of softening or small cortical foci (granular atrophy) may be present. The characteristic feature of the disease, viz. changes in the walls of the blood vessels, can always be demonstrated in the superficial temporal artery by histochemical methods (elastica stain).

Clinical features: The clinical picture is identical to that of cerebral arteriosclerosis so that a presumptive clinical diagnosis is possible only in those patients in whom the disease presents early in adult life or in whom signs of arterial involvement are present elsewhere in the body (intermittent claudication, anginal pain). The serum contains antielastic antibodies and increased IgE levels, and these are diagnostic pointers which differentiate the disease from ordinary arteriosclerosis. The ESR may be increased and the rheumatoid factors abnormal. The CSF may reveal inflammatory changes. The prognosis is poor.

Multi-Infarct Dementia

This condition is described as a separate entity (667). It is the result of a summation of numerous vascular insults which lead to progressive dementia rather than neurologic deficits.

Pseudobulbar Palsy

Pathogenesis: This condition usually arises on the basis of cerebral arteriosclerosis, sometimes accompanied by hypertension. The anatomic substrate comprises several ischemic lesions *bilaterally* in the region of the corticobulbar tracts. The bilateral nature of the lesions is essential to explain the pseudobulbar signs because of the bilateral corticobulbar control of the lower cranial nerves.

Clinical signs: A typical case is the patient in whom signs of an earlier apoplectic insult causing hemispheric signs had completely disappeared by the time that a later, fresh insult took place. Only this latter lesion was accompanied by definite pseudobulbar signs *(acute pseudobulbar palsy)*. The same signs may develop on the basis of a series of relatively small insults, instead of one large insult, as *status lacunaris*. The clinical signs may be described as an <u>upper motor neuron lesion</u>, a spastic <u>paralysis of the mouth</u> and throat muscles.

Features:

- Speech is poorly articulated, dysarthric (p. 173), in extreme cases it is not possible (anarthria).
- The tongue cannot be fully protruded and shows clumsy movements.
- Absence of atrophy or fasciculation of the tongue.
- Deglutition is severely upset, food remains in the mouth for a long time.
- Reflexes of the facial muscles are increased, including the masseter and perioral reflexes.
- Extremities may show signs of pyramidal tract involvement.
- Marked lability and (apparent) incontinence of affect, with uncontrollable bouts of crying and laughing.

Differential diagnosis: Nonvascular intrapontine lesions as well as extra-axial mass lesions may produce a pseudobulbar picture, particularly incontinent laughing and crying. In true bulbar palsy (p. 223), fasciculation and atrophy of the tongue are invariably present, although initially signs due to upper motor neuron in-

volvement may be prominent, and differentiation from pseudobulbar palsy may then be difficult.

Coma and Other Effects of Acute Anoxic Cerebral Damage

Pathogenesis: An acute (diffuse) deficient supply of oxygen to the brain may follow cardiac failure, shock, respiratory difficulty, CO intoxication, head injury with traumatic brain swelling, or other causes. The partial anoxia leads first to *coma* (958). Diffuse bilateral lesions of the cerebral hemispheres, as well as a more localized lesion at the diencephalic level, may cause coma.

Clinical aspects: Despite the strongest stimuli, the patient is unable to perform any voluntary act, i.e., any act consciously willed. However, unconscious reflex responses can be elicited, and the autonomic functions may remain intact despite the patient's comatose condition. It is important to establish the level of coma according to a graduated system of severity. This level allows conclusions to be drawn concerning the prognosis and the evaluation of improvement or worsening of the disturbance of consciousness. One should not speak simply of coma without always specifying its depth.

Coma stages:
- responds to painful stimuli by specific defense movements;
- reacts in a diffuse way to painful stimuli without exhibiting purposeful defense movements;
- exhibits no reaction even to the most painful stimuli, but retains reflexes

(pupillary light reflex, corneal, swallowing, and tendon reflexes);

- exhibits no reaction to severe painful stimuli and all or some of the named reflexes are absent, with retained spontaneous respiration, circulatory regulation, and cardiac action;

- fails to react, fails to show reflex response to stimulation, and has ceased to breathe spontaneously, but the heart continues to beat. The patient who requires artificial respiration and whose circulation needs to be supported is on the threshold of cerebral death.

The patient's posture: The posture of comatose patients may provide useful clues to the site of the causative lesion. Patients with a diffuse (anoxic) lesion

of both cerebral hemispheres assume a position with flexed arms and extended legs, called *decorticate rigidity.* By contrast, the *decerebrate posture* includes overextension of the arms with adduction and medial rotation and flexion of the hands and fingers, with extensor spasms of the legs and sometimes opisthotonus (Fig. 1.12). This posture usually accompanies bilateral deep diencephalic lesions of the rostral midbrain, but it may also follow bilateral hemispheric damage. Either of these coma positions may be modified by additional hemispheric lesions or upon stimulation, and they may alternate.

Respiratory anomalies in coma are defined and their topographic significance is outlined in Table 1.11.

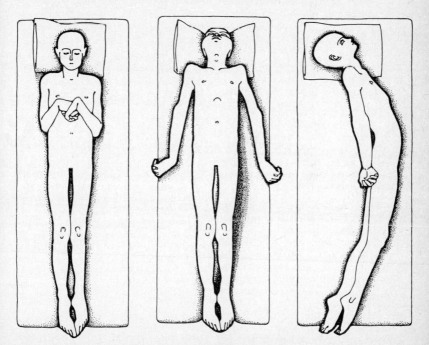

Fig. 1.**12**   Posture of decorticate patient (left) contrasted with that of the decerebrate patient (middle and right) (from *Mumenthaler* [845])

Table 1.11   Respiratory disorders of cerebral origin

Condition	Definition	Site, Localization	Remarks
Cheyne-Stokes respiration (periodic breathing)	Alternating hyperpnea and apnea	Diffuse deep-seated hemisphere damage or midbrain lesion	Aggravated by pulmonary congestion and prolonged circulation time
Central reflex hyperventilation	Persistent hyperventilation with hypocapnia	Posterior brainstem and tegmentum: rostral reticular formation	Rare
Apneustic breathing	Brief respiratory spasm in full inspiration. Variants: brief cessation of respiration during inspiration	Medial or caudal aspect of pons or dorsal tegmentum	e.g., infarction following vertebrobasilar occlusion
Ataxic breathing (Biot's breathing)	Irregular exchange of superficial and deeper respiration with irregular pauses	Dorsomedial aspect of medulla oblongata	Posterior fossa lesions, meningitis, etc.
Temporary failure of automatic respiration (Ondine's curse)	Normal ability to breathe while awake, but ceases during sleep or distraction	Lesion in the reticulospinal projections of the respiratory center in the medulla oblongata	Acute lesions of the medulla oblongata. Differential diagnosis: upper respiratory tract obstruction with sleep apnea

Pupillary anomalies in comatose patients also possess topographic significance:

- pupils equal, small, and reacting to light: thalamic lesions and metabolic disturbances;
- pupils unequal, one dilated and reacting neither directly nor consensully to light: oculomotor lesion, e.g., homolateral supratentorial space-occupying lesion (rarely a contralateral hemisyndrome);
- pupils equal and of average size, not reacting: midbrain lesion;
- pupils equal but widely dilated and not reacting, sometimes with tremor of the iris or hippus (rhythmic spontaneous intermittent enlargement): lesions of the roof of the midbrain;
- pinpoint pupil: lesion of the pons.

Ancillary investigations: The results of specific ancillary investigations in comatose patients may assist in localizing and defining the extent of the damage. The somatosensory and auditory evoked potentials (1244) are particularly useful.

Prognosis of comatose patients: This depends on the degree of brain damage suffered by the patients. Of a large series of resuscitated patients, only 30% exhibited no significant neurologic deficit (84). The group with the more favorable prognosis are those patients in whom the coma is less severe initially and who regain consciousness within 24 h after the initial episode (1120). Investigation of the evoked potentials in comatose patients, e.g., following craniocerebral trauma, provides a reliable method of predicting the patient's chances of recovery (33). Modern resuscitation measures permit patients to survive a coma (coma dépassé).

When spontaneous respiration and normal circulatory function return, a variety of clinical deficits may remain.

Brain Death

In brain death the arterial blood pressure falls without support and the body temperature sinks below 35 °C. Spinal reflexes remain or may reappear (1003), but the brainstem reflexes disappear. This can be documented by the absence of a response from the orbicularis oculi muscle upon electric stimulation of the supraorbital nerve (787).

The oculocephalic reflex also is absent: sudden passive rotation of the head fails to evoke the vestibular reflex that would normally maintain the position of the eyeballs in their original direction of vision; instead, they remain fixed within the orbits and go en bloc with the head. The EEG shows no cerebral electric activity ("silent EEG"), and cerebral arteriography shows a failure of contrast medium to enter the intracranial vessels (circulatory arrest).

The Apallic Syndrome

This characteristic picture may develop after an apparently good initial recovery with a free interval of several days. The patient lies passively without moving, or he makes a few sparse spontaneous movements. Protective or defense responses are absent. He tends to remain motionless in any passive position in which he is placed. Primitive reflexes such as sucking and grasping are prominent; groping and reaching after seen or felt objects can be described as grasping. Rigidity and extrapyramidal hyperkinesia may develop. Initially extensor spasms and mass movements may be present. Since the patient lies with his eyes open but is unable to respond appropriately to commands or other stimuli, the condition is called coma vigile.

Akinetic Mutism

This title describes a condition arising either after cerebral hypoxia with diffuse white matter lesions or after midbrain lesions causing damage to the reticular formation. It is also observed after bilateral anterior cerebral artery occlusion (383). In this condition, the patient is able to move and - in contrast to the above description - even to speak, but he cannot be prompted to do so.

Locked-In Syndrome (885)

This syndrome must be distinguished from akinetic mutism. Patients with the locked-in syndrome are, for practical purposes, mute and akinetic. A lesion of the pons at the level of the abducent nucleus interrupts the corticobulbar and corticospinal tracts and produces a quadriplegia. The patient retains only eyelid and vertical eye movements, which the patient uses to make himself understood. In most cases, the syndrome is caused by hemorrhage or infarction, and only rarely is a tumor responsible.

Alpha Coma (1263)

Brainstem infarction or anoxia may provoke an actual deep coma with a virtually normal alpha rhythm in the EEG. This condition must be differentiated from psychogenic coma and from *coma dépassé*.

Klüver-Bucy Syndrome (21)

Damage to the limbic system, particularly bilateral lesions of the mediobasal temporal lobes, may lead in humans to the Klüver-Bucy syndrome demonstrated in animal experiments. In this syndrome, all objects are placed in the mouth and an oral automatism arises. The patient exhibits a general disinhibition, an increased sexual appetite, a loss of restraint, and occasionally euphoria and a gluttonous desire for food. This picture is also seen in the posttraumatic apallic syndrome (410).

Acute Subarachnoid Hemorrhage (SAH)

Introduction
The following features may be defined:

- *stroke-like* onset within the space of a minute, followed by
- *very intense headache,*
- without any *specific warning beforehand* and with a history in only one-third of cases of unusual physical exertion (weight lifting, straining at stool, coitus), about one-third of patients become *unconscious,* a further one-third are confused, and
- *nausea* or vomiting may occur.
- The *headache* is usually diffuse,

occasionally occipital in distribution.
- *Clinical examination* reveals
  • meningism (and Kernig's sign) is invariably present, but may not be elicited in the most deeply unconscious,
  • up to about one-half of patients exhibit an extensor plantar reaction, in the remainder neurologic examination reveals no abnormality (exceptions, see below),
  • one-tenth of cases show a sub-hyaloid fundal hemorrhage, usually situated close to the optic papilla. As a late sequela occasionally one finds a conical membrane at the posterior pole of the vitreous, called Terson's Syndrome (1256).
- Specific and essential for the diagnosis is *blood-tinged CSF* obtained by lumbar puncture. Only 8 h after the hemorrhage does, it becomes xanthochromic after centrifugation.
- *Ancillary investigations,* see below.

This clinical picture is found irrespective of whether the source of bleeding is a basal saccular aneurysm or an arteriovenous malformation. If the source of bleeding is located in the spine, the acute pain not infrequently occurs first in the back and later (in the recumbent patient) in the head. Specific questioning reveals that about one-fifth of patients – commoner with malformations than aneurysms – experience brief uncharacteristic episodes (attacks of headache and nausea) for several days and up to 3 weeks before the hemorrhage (1209).

The *degree of severity of SAH* with respect to the operative risk was classified by Botterell (155) into 5 grades:

1. Conscious, with or without blood in the CSF.
2. Confused, without significant neurologic deficit.
3. Confused, with neurologic deficit and probable intracerebral hematoma.
4. Marked neurologic deficit with tendency to worsen, either as a result of a large intracerebral hematoma or, in elderly subjects, with less severe deficits of degenerative cerebrovascular disease.
5. Moribund or nearly moribund, vital functions failing, and extensor spasms present.

Aneurysms of (Basal) Cerebral Arteries

The commonest cause of the SAH described above is an arterial aneurysm (berry aneurysm) at the base of the brain. Aneurysms develop during young adult life at specific sites which are vulnerable because of weakness of the internal elastic membrane of the artery, particularly in the bifurcations of cerebral arteries.

The *commonest sites* are shown in Fig. 1.13; about 50% of aneurysms are located on the anterior communicating artery. A roughly similar number (each about 10%) are found elsewhere – intracranial internal carotid artery, posterior communicating artery, and middle cerebral artery. Other sites and multiple aneurysms are much less common. Other intracranial sources of hemorrhage – also without demonstrable focal signs – are small arteriovenous malformations on the surfaces of the cerebral or cerebellar hemispheres and traumatic aneurysms of the middle meningeal artery. Review of a large autopsy material has shown that, in the presence of an arterial aneurysm, about 50% showed evidence of rupture. This applies particularly to aneurysms of the anterior communicating artery, and especially those in subjects under 65 years (1010). Cigarette smoking and simultaneous use of ovulation inhibitors significantly increase the risk of SAH in women (940).

Clinical picture: This corresponds to the above-mentioned generalized syndrome of acute SAH. ECG changes including T-wave reversal and ST flattening are common findings in cases of SAH – and occasionally also in other vascular intracranial lesions (apoplexy, venous sinus thrombosis); the picture may prompt suspicion of myocardial infarction. Aortic stenosis giving rise to secondary hypertension in the cervicobrachial arterial branches of the arch must also be excluded, particularly in a child or adolescent with acute SAH.

In individual cases, **details of the clinical picture** may permit conclusions about the site and nature of the source of the hemorrhage:

– Aneurysm of the *anterior communicating artery* may upon rupture produce a large hematoma in the base of the frontal lobe and cause focal hemispheric signs. As a rule, a severe disturbance of consciousness is present, and deep coma follows rupture into the lateral ventricle.
– Intracranial aneurysms of the internal carotid artery may be *supraclinoid,*

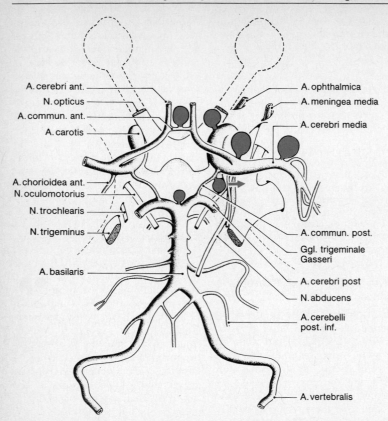

Fig. 1.**13**   Commonest sites of intracranial aneurysms and their relations to cranial nerves (after *Krayenbühl* and *Yasargil*)

i.e., situated within the subarachnoid space, or *infraclinoid,* i.e., situated extradurally. Rupture of the latter aneurysm does not cause SAH. Carotid artery aneurysms often cause weakness of the external ocular muscles, which may appear suddenly or show a slowly progressive course. Fairly often they are accompanied by optic nerve or chiasmal involvement, exophthalmos, trigeminal nerve signs (first division), and a hemisyndrome.

Individual cases of internal carotid aneurysm may mimic a pituitary tumor clinically (visual field defects, endocrine disturbances) and radiologically (sellar enlargement). Angiographic demonstration of the aneurysm may be prevented by thrombosis of its sac. A segment of curvilinear calcification demonstrable in the parasellar region on conventional skull roentgenograms may indicate the diagnosis.

- Aneurysms at the mouth of a *posterior communicating artery* may occasionally manifest without SAH, giving rise to third nerve palsy or migrainous pains in the first division of the trigeminal nerve (commonest cause of so-called ophthalmoplegic migraine). Occasionally the aneurysm may produce a contralateral hemiplegia by pressure on the cerebral peduncle.
- Aneurysm of the *middle cerebral artery* is usually found at the sylvian trifurcation. In about one-fourth of patients this aneurysm produces a contralateral hemiparesis and sometimes other focal features (epileptic attacks, aphasia) due to hemispheric damage.
- Aneurysms of the intracranial *vertebral arteries* and *basilar artery* may produce signs of bulbar and cerebellar involvement, a cerebellopontine angle syndrome, or lower cranial nerve palsies. Since SAH is not an invariable accompaniment, the distinction between aneurysm and tumor can be made only by CT scanning or vertebral angiography. MRI is more likely to show the aneurysm itself than CT scanning is.

Subarachnoid hemorrhage from a spinal source of bleeding (arteriovenous malformation), see p. 212; intracranial arteriovenous malformations, see p. 95.

Practical approach: In any clinically typical acute SAH from an intracranial source of bleeding, the following measures should be taken:
- urgent admission to a hospital with neurosurgical facilities;
- immediate *CT scanning,* since the examination frequently indicates the site of the aneurysm or reveals another source of hemorrhage, as well as the displacement produced by an associated hematoma. CT examination on the day of the hemorrhage provides evidence of fresh blood in 96% of cases, but only in 74% on the 3rd day (8).
- The CT demonstration of fresh blood makes *lumbar puncture* superfluous. However, this examination should be carried out (in order to observe xanthochromia, compare with a test tube of water), even before CT examination, if there is doubt about the diagnosis (see postcoital headache, p. 455) or if no CT is available.
- Careful *arteriographic investigation* is indicated
  • after verified SAH
  • or if a confident clinical diagnosis is possible,
  • provided that the patient is a candidate for operation
  • and consents to operation,
  • if CT scanning reveals an intracerebral hematoma.

In principle, both carotid arteries should always be injected and, where necessary, one vertebral artery.

In at least 10% of cases detailed angiographic examination will reveal no source of hemorrhage, and this result is a good prognostic sign. In a large series of cases, only 8.7% suffered a recurrent hemorrhage, which was significantly more frequent in hypertensives (20%) than in normotensives (3%) (1106). Survival of these patients for 6 months reduces their relapse risk to 0.86% a year (884). The presence of intracranial arterial spasm, a factor which influences the surgeon's approach, may be demonstrated by a special Doppler sonographic technique (2).

Spontaneous course: The natural history of the disease is typical in that at least 30%-45% of patients die from the first hemorrhage or within a few weeks of bleeding. Of the survivors, about one-half die within a few years from a further hemorrhage. In a retrospective study of patients over a period of 2-21 years, recurrent hemorrhage occurred at the rate of 3.5% a year in the first 10 years in patients who had survived the initial hemorrhage for 6 months. The average mortality from this recurrence was 67%, irrespective of the age of the patient, but the prognosis was worse in hypertensives and in women if the aneurysm was situated on the posterior communicating artery (861). A further study of 568 cases treated conservatively revealed that 40% suffered a recurrent hemorrhage within 6 months. In the 1st decade, an annual recurrence rate of 2.2%, and in the 2nd decade of 0.86%, must be expected; 78% of all recurrent hemorrhages were fatal (883). Prognostically unfavorable signs include deep coma, paralysis of extraocular muscles, and focal neurologic signs (see below). The presence of angiographically demonstrable arterial spasm, which is also claimed to be unfavorable, does not appear to bear any direct clinical relationship to mortality or to the subsequent course in patients managed surgically or conservatively (566).

Surgical treatment: The poor prognosis of medically managed spontaneous SAH makes it clear that in the majority of cases surgical treatment is indicated, utilizing the microsurgical technique. Exceptions are unusually severe hemorrhages with deep coma and specific locations of the aneurysm. The chances of survival of patients who survive the first episode of hemorrhage are doubled by successful operation. Patients in good general condition who possess no abnormal neurologic signs and in whom meningeal irritation has faded are suitable for immediate operation. Care is required in patients who are shown, by one or other investigative methods, e.g., transcranial Doppler sonography (3), to have arterial spasm.

During the past 20 years, no statistically significant effect of operation, including the important surgical risks, has been confirmed. In individual cases, the outcome depends on many factors which are statistically difficult to assess. For example, operative treatment of middle cerebral artery aneurysms seems to be indicated only in males. Carotid ligation appears to be superior to conservative treatment in aneurysms of the posterior communicating artery, while direct attack carries a high operative risk. A statistical analysis of all series of cases published in the literature before 1972 compared the outcome of medically and surgically treated patients and failed to show that operation significantly improved the prognosis (29). This controversial subject has been transformed in recent years by the introduction of the operating microscope and its increasing use by neurosurgeons in treating diseases of the cerebral arteries (1300, 1301). Microsurgery represents a distinct advance, having already produced a fall in operative mortality and complications. It is now accepted that aneurysm surgery, with the exceptions mentioned above, is the field of the experienced neurosurgeon using microsurgical techniques.

Conservative treatment with antifibrinolytic substances, especially in anticipation of surgical management, has proved ineffectual (1300). Calcium-channel blockers diminish the risk of vasospasm.

Late effects of subarachnoid hemorrhage: The late complications include nonresorptive communicating hydrocephalus (1302). It occurs more frequently if the hemorrhage was severe, and particularly if arterial spasm was present. In about one-third of patients, the ventricles become enlarged in a few weeks and then progress in size over months or years. Ventriculoatrial shunting is indicated. Mental symptoms, behavioral disturbances, spasticity, and epileptic attacks may occur and surprisingly often - arterial hypertension.

Arteriovenous Malformations

Anatomy: The arteriovenous malformation (angioma racemosum arteriosum) - sometimes called arteriovenous aneurysm or angioma - is a congenital lesion. It is made up of hypertrophied feeding arteries and draining vessels which are separated by a knot of capillaries. In addition, arteriovenous shunts are present. The individual components of the lesion can be demonstrated histologically or angiographically; they are microscopically abnormal structures. Most arteriovenous malfor-

mations occupy superficial situations in relation to the meninges and penetrate to a varying degree into the brain substance; only rarely are they purely subcortical or intraventricular. By far the commonest localization is the supratentorial chamber, and they are most often irrigated by the middle cerebral artery. The right and the left cerebral hemispheres are equally involved. Infratentorial and extracranial sites (external carotid artery and muscular branches of the vertebral artery) are rare. *Arteriovenous malformations of the brainstem* (162) may manifest clinically only in the 3rd–5th decades of life, producing a picture of cranial nerve, cerebellar, and pyramidal tract involvement which runs a particularly protracted course, up to 10 years or more. A special variety of this lesion is the orbital arteriovenous malformation which may give rise to unilateral pulsating exophthalmos that is worse when the head is lowered.

Clinical signs and symptoms (936) may be completely absent. However, in typical cases, combinations of the following signs appear in varying degrees of severity, usually manifesting for the first time in 10- to 30-year olds. All ages and both sexes are equally affected:

- Subarachnoid (or intracerebral) hemorrhage is the commonest manifestation, occurring in over 50% of cases (1314), recurring after variable intervals in one-fourth, and causing death in about 20% fatal (Cooperative Study, 66). The probability of a recurrence of a hemorrhage is 2–3% per year (180, 552), and the size of the angioma or the presence of arterial hypertension do not influence the prognosis. Over 20 years, in a population of over 200 cases which were treated conservatively, the risk of hemorrhage was 32%, of epilepsy 18%, and of neurologic deficits 27%. The risk of a fatal autcome was 29% (257).

– Epileptic attacks, usually but not always focal, appear in about 40% of patients with arteriovenous malformations (1314). In about one-fourth, an epileptic attack rather than intracranial hemorrhage is the presenting clinical feature (162).

– Headaches, present in at least 50% of patients, may possess many features of migraine, e.g., fortification spectra. A monotonous repetition of attacks with similar signs and symptoms should raise suspicion of an arteriovenous malformation.

– Neurologic signs in the context of an intracranial hemorrhage, of which acute (juvenile) subcortical hemorrhage (p.85) is an example.

– In about one-fourth of cases a pulse-synchronous intracranial murmur is audible, most easily heard over the eyeball or the mastoid.

– CT scanning, even without tissue enhancement, provides a pathognomic appearance in most cases of arteriovenous malformation.

Treatment: This depends on the symptomatology, the extent, and the location of the arteriovenous malformation. Antiepileptic medication may be adequate if the clinical features are confined to seizures and if extirpation appears to be technically difficult. An angioma which has not ruptured should not be treated surgically (32), but rather be embolized by an experienced neuroradiologist (see below). However, if hemorrhage occurs and/or permanent neurologic signs develop, the possibility must be considered of operative excision, utilizing careful angiographic investigation and a microsurgical technique (731). Operation should always be considered in those malformations best suited to excision, i.e., the localized variety situated on the surface of a cerebral hemisphere. In larger and more unfavorably situated lesions, the average operative risk, particularly in patients over 50 years of age, is higher than the risk of conservative management. An exception is justified if the surgeon is a particularly skilled operater. About two-thirds of intracranial arteriovenous malformations are potentially operable. The very extensive and diffuse variety of the lesion is surgically untreatable: direct attack is not feasible, and the well-developed collateral channels render carotid ligation valueless. Therapeutic embolization of the feeding vessels is replacing surgical intervention more and more. This form of interventional neuroradiology, in the hands of an experienced radiologist who is equipped with the appropriate catheters, is the method of choice for the treatment of cerebral and particularly intraspinal arteriovenous angiomas. Stereotactically applied radiotherapy may be used for smaller angiomas of special localization.

Arteriovenous Fistula of the Cavernous Sinus

Arteriovenous fistulous connections of the cavernous sinus are almost invariably traumatic in origin. They present clinically as cases of pulsating exophthalmos with pain, engorgement of the conjunctival and retinal vessels, external ocular palsies, visual disturbances, and vascular murmurs. The latter, which synchronize with the pulse, are always audible upon auscultation and the patient may be aware of their presence. Surgical occlusion is successful in only about one-third of cases, and the particular technical procedure undertaken (embolization with muscle fragments, extracranial ligation of vessels, intracranial ligation of vessels) must be planned from case to case upon the basis of the angiographic findings (162).

Cavernomas (Cavernous Angiomas)
(1036, 1110, 1155)

This rare vascular malformation, in terms of its pathological anatomy, consists of the well circumscribed conglomerate of vessels without nervous tissue inbetween them. They can occur anywhere in the brain or even in the brain stem and not infrequently they are multiple. Their clinical manifestations are seizures and/or hemorrhage. Radiographically they appear on CT scan as a hyperdense area with positive contrast enhancement. Small calcifications, which are often present, can also be visualized. On MRI the

hemosiderin deposits, which are also common, can be shown. Treatment consists of microsurgical resection.

Cerebral Venous Thrombosis

Epidemiology: Cerebral venous thrombosis (536) may be septic or bland and most cases arise from a primary focus elsewhere in the body. The most frequent form is thrombosis of the superior sagittal sinus and the superficial cortical veins. Women are more often affected than men.

Clinical features: These comprise the following:

- sometimes evidence of a thrombus-forming generalized *preceding illness* or local lesion,
  • thrombophlebitis migrans,
  • hypercoagulable state, e.g., puerperium (one-fourth of cases) or after operation,
  • administration of ovulation inhibitors (1030),
  • blood dyscrasias,
  • infectious illness, especially focal infections of the head such as sinusitis or otitis media,
  • cranial trauma
- Often, but not always, an attack is preceded by malaise lasting hours or days with headache and nausea.
- Usually the onset of neurologic signs is acute, with
  • sudden severe headache,
  • retching or vomiting,
  • focal epileptic attacks,
  • disturbances of consciousness, even coma.

- Meningism may be present.
- Focal neurologic deficits, particularly hemisyndromes; and
- less frequently, papilledema, disturbances of external ocular movement, dyskinesias (1129), venous engorgement of the head and face.
- Occasionally generalized features such as fever, raised ESR, and leukocytosis.
- In about one-half of cases, the CSF is blood-tinged or xanthochromic.
- Unilateral otogenic thrombosis of the transverse sinus may be recognized by a diagnostically valuable sign: when Queckenstedt's test is performed on the affected side, the CSF fails to rise. However, this can only be considered to be abnormal, if compression of both sides fails to elevate the CSF more than isolated compression of the opposite side.

Ancillary investigations: CT scanning may confirm the clinical suspicion. Angiography will reveal the site of the venous occlusion.

Prognosis: The prognosis is poor. At least one-half of the patients die, although more children survive. Some patients recover completely but others exhibit severe residual symptoms such as hemiplegia, mental syndromes, or epileptic seizures. In children the picture of *otitic hydrocephalus* usually appears 1–2 weeks after an apparently healed otitis media caused by thrombosis of a sigmoid or transverse sinus (p. 19). Puerperal cerebral venous thrombosis is likely to recur in about one-third of women during further pregnancies.

Treatment: Clinically mild cases are given appropriate medication to prevent infection, edema, and convulsions. The author in common with others (412) does not agree with anticoagulation because the pathoanatomic lesions include venous infarction of the cerebral parenchyma as well as subarachnoid hemorrhages. However, some authors recommend anticoagulation treatment, believing that the risk of thrombotic spread with secondary venous infarction is the greater hazard. Of course, the CSF must not contain blood.

Extrapyramidal Syndromes

Anatomy: The extrapyramidal system is a functional unit comprising:

- corpus striatum (caudate nucleus and putamen),
- lentiform nucleus (putamen and globus pallidus),
- corpus Luysi (subthalamic nucleus),
- substantia nigra, and
- red nucleus.

These structures are interconnected by ascending and descending tracts, as well as with the thalamus, cerebral cortex, and midbrain structures. These connections are illustrated in Fig. 1.14

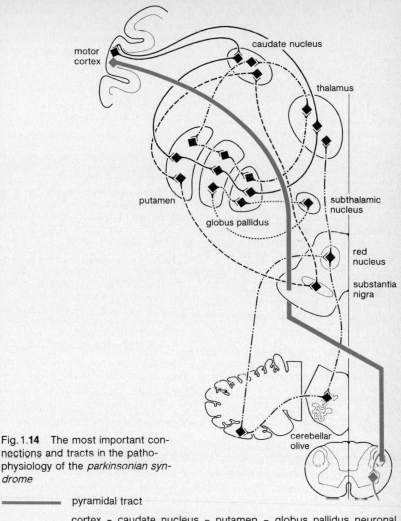

motor cortex

caudate nucleus

thalamus

putamen

globus pallidus

subthalamic nucleus

red nucleus

substantia nigra

cerebellar olive

Fig. 1.14 The most important connections and tracts in the pathophysiology of the *parkinsonian syndrome*

pyramidal tract

cortex – caudate nucleus – putamen – globus pallidus neuronal system – ventral thalamic nuclei – motor cortex neuronal system

pallidosubthalamic – pallidal neuronal system

pallidothalamostriatal neuronal system

striatonigrostriatal neuronal system

rubro-olivocerebellorubral neuronal system

in relation to the parkinsonian syndromes.

Pathophysiology: The ganglionic areas mentioned above are linked together to form a complex *neuronal system*. In healthy subjects these relays serve to control tone and to harmonize muscular activity. A lesion in any one of the relay systems results either in the transmission of uncontrolled impulses (e.g., tremor or dystonic movements) or in abnormally persistent muscular contractions (e.g., rigidity and akinesia). In general, nerve impulses are damped by the putamen, caudate nucleus, and substantia nigra, and stimulated by the globus pallidus. However, the pattern of pathologic changes does not invariably correspond with the clinical picture. The theory concerning the origin of tremor (346) serves as an example: In lesions of the substantia nigra with functional depression caused by the nigrostriatal tracts, the globus pallidus overstimulates the ventrolateral thalamic nucleus. This in turn reacts with rhythmic discharges in response to cerebellar afferents. The latter for their part receive afferent impulses through the ventral spinocerebellar tract from deeper motor centers. These impulses may arise from the motor cortex as well as by a reflex mechanism from the periphery.

Biochemistry of the transmitted impulse: This is essential for an understanding of the extrapyramidal diseases. Dopamine is the transmitter substance of the nigrostriatal neuron, which exerts a damping effect on the cholinergic interneuron of the corpus striatum. Gamma-aminobutyric acid (GABA) is the transmitter substance of the inhibitory striopallidal and strionigral tracts. About 80% of the cerebral dopamine in healthy human subjects is contained in the corpus striatum and in the pars compacta of the substantia nigra, which is severely reduced in Parkinson's disease (for further details, see p. 110).

Classification of Extrapyramidal Syndromes

Two distinct pictures are differentiated:

- *Akinetic-rigidity syndrome* with
  - reduction of spontaneous activity and associated movements,
  - with an increase in muscle tone and involuntary movements;
  (the parkinsonian syndrome is the clinical manifestation of this combination of signs).

- *Hyperkinetic-hypotonic syndrome* producing
  - involuntary and irregular movements of variable localization,
  - interval of reduced resting muscle tone (represented by the following: chorea, athetosis, ballismus, and dystonias).

Table 1.**12** provides a review of the most important extrapyramidal syndromes.

The Parkinsonian Syndrome
(725, 726, 766, 805)

Epidemiology: It is estimated that 1‰–2‰ of the total population suffers from a parkinsonian syndrome (657), and 1% of subjects over the age of 60 years (598). The annual incidence (in Japan) is given as 10.2 per 100,000 population (475).

Clinical symptomatology: This is headlined in Table 1.**13**. None of the signs, and especially the tremor, is essential for the diagnosis, which

Table 1.12 The commonest extrapyramidal syndromes

Disease	Clinical Features	Pathologic Features	Etiology
Parkinsonian syndrome	Akinesia. Rigidity, rhythmic, alternating resting tremor of 4–8/s	Cell degeneration of the substantia nigra and other melanin-containing nuclei, as well as the globus pallidus and corpus striatum	Genetically determined. Encephalitis lethargica. Toxic or drug causes. (Vascular). Unknown
Chorea	Involuntary, irregular, rapid asymmetric, short-lasting movements of the extremities	Cellular degeneration of the small cells in the caudate nucleus and putamen	Genetically determined. Infectious. Postapoplectic
Athetosis	Involuntary, irregular, slow movements of the extremities, varying in location. Exaggerated postures of the limbs	Putamen, caudate nucleus, and external part of globus pallidus	Birth damage (especially kernicterus). Genetically determined. Space-occupying lesions. Postapoplectic
(Hemi)ballismus	Frequent, involuntary, irregular, lightning-like, copious, centrifugal movements involving various muscle groups	Subthalamic nucleus of Luys	Cerebral softening. Tumors
Dystonic syndromes – Spastic torticollis – Torsion dystonia – Localized dystonias	Involuntary, prolonged, tonic contractions of individual muscles or muscle groups (against resistance of the antagonists)	Putamen, thalamus	Genetically determined. Birth damage (particularly kernicterus)
Hepatolenticular degeneration (Wilson's disease)	Progressive tremor "wing-beating," rigidity, dysarthria, mental changes, liver symptoms, Kayser-Fleischer rings	Putamen	Genetically determined. Disturbance of copper metabolism
Myorhythmias	Involuntary, rhythmic jerks involving the same muscle groups, 1–3/s	Central tegmental tract in "palatal myoclonus"	Birth damage, vascular, encephalitis
Myoclonias	Involuntary, irregular, frequent, brief jerks of individual muscles or muscle groups	Dentate nucleus, inferior olive, red nucleus, perhaps also peripheral nervous system?	Birth damage, vascular, toxic

Table 1.13 Symptomatology of the Parkinsonian Syndrome

1. *Effect on primary automatic movements*
   Akinesia
   Absent accessory movements
   Pro- und retropulsion

2. *Increased extrapyramidal tone*
   Rigidity
   Increase in tone of resting muscles
   Increase in tone of antagonist muscles
   Cogwheel phenomenon
   Specific postural features

3. *Tremor*

4. *Other physical symptoms*
   Micrographia
   Speech disturbances
   Breathing difficulties
   Motor "weakness"
   Accentuated nasopalpebral reflex
   Autonomic symptoms ("postencephalitic" seborrhea, drooling, sweating attacks)
   Oculogyric crises and other disturbances of eye movement
   Dystonic movements

5. *Mental symptoms*
   Prolongation of the thought process
   Lability of mood
   Disturbance of affect
   Dementia

6. *Late effects, e.g., results of L-dopa treatment*
   On-off phenomenon
   Drug-induced dystonia
   Hallucinations and psychoses

will be discussed in greater detail below.

The most impressive manifestation of the *inhibition of primary automatic movements* is the generalized poverty of movement, or *akinesia*. This feature includes the expressionless face (masked facies). The patient seldom blinks; the head is turned in company with the shoulders and trunk in an en bloc movement, the tempo of all movements is slow and viscous. Thus, the patient to some extent resembles a wooden doll. The small handwriting, the *micrographia* of the parkinsonian subject, is an expression of this poverty of movement. It is often altered by the tremor. The *absence of associated movements* may be observed particularly in the lack of armswing on walking and in specific tests for this phenomenon, e.g., if the patient is seated on a chair which is suddenly tipped backward, he retains his stiff seated posture, failing to bend his trunk forward and flex his knees, as does a normal subject. The phenomenon of *propulsion* (or retropulsion) is characterized by the fact that the standing patient, if pushed forward (or backward), is able to regain his balance slowly by small and slow steps – or fails to do so altogether and falls over. This phenomenon also occurs during walking or, for example, upon pushing open a door which suddenly yields. Propulsion is an unfavorable sign since the patient usually fails to respond to treatment after it has appeared. The term *paradoxical kinesia* is used to describe the fact that the parkinsonian patient may, under the influence of intense emotion, be able suddenly to walk or speak fluently and in a lively fashion, in contrast to the usual restriction of all his movements.

The *increase in extrapyramidal muscle tone* is reflected clinically as *ri-*

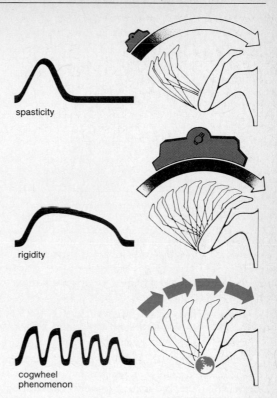

spasticity

rigidity

Fig. 1.15 Diagrammatic representation of the various forms of increased tone

cogwheel phenomenon

gidity. It is observed as increased, waxlike or viscous resistance of a limb during the whole range of a passive movement. This is compared in Fig. 1.15 to (pyramidal) spasticity, in which the increased muscle tone is demonstrable only in the early phase of the passive movement. Rigidity is best demonstrated by passive and irregular flexion and extension movements of the elbow joint. It may also be shown at the wrist by shaking the forearm. Apart from rigidity during movement, the muscles exhibit an *increase in resting tone*. Parkinsonian patients, at the end of any passive movement, exhibit an abnormally strong fixation in the new position. For example, the tibialis anterior muscle contracts actively if the patient's foot is passively dorsiflexed (fixation reflex). The *increase in antagonist tone* is shown by the fact that if resistance to a contracted muscle is suddenly removed, the movement is immediately braked by the antagonist muscle(s) which is also abnormally contracted. This is the opposite of the so-called positive rebound phenom-

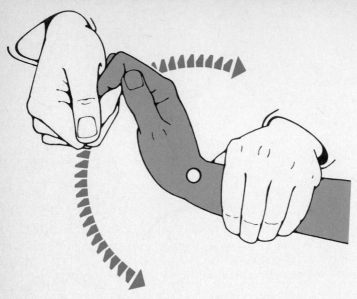

Fig. 1.**16** Testing for the cogwheel phenomenon. The examiner grasps the patient's fingers and tests mobility at the wrist joint

enon demonstrable in cerebellar lesions. The increased antagonist tone is best demonstrated by the "head dropping test": if the head of the recumbent patient is held in the examiner's hands and then suddenly released, it does not drop passively downward but sinks slowly onto the pillow or remains suspended for some time. Sometimes the patient lies recumbent on the bed with his head suspended in midair, as if an invisible pillow were there *("oreiller psychique")*. When testing muscle tone, the most striking feature found, apart from rigidity, may be the *cogwheel phenomenon*. If a joint is flexed and extended rapidly through its range of motion, the im-

pression is gained of a joint surface consisting of two cogwheels moving stepwise in relation to each other (see Fig. 1.15). This phenomenon is often particularly obvious at the wrist joint (Fig. 1.16).

Tremor as an involuntary movement is particularly common in patients with Parkinson's disease, although it need not necessarily be present (so-called akinetic parkinsonian syndrome). It takes the form of a rhythmic, regular tremor more marked at rest, which diminishes or disappears upon active movements. It has a frequency of 4-8/s and varies in intensity. The fingers often perform characteristic rhythmic movements described as "pill rolling" or "counting money." The tremor is increased by emotion, and abolished in sleep. It is reduced during concentration and deliberate movements, and also in extreme positions of the limbs.

The altered *posture* of the parkinsonian patient upon standing and walking should also be noted. He stands bent slightly forward, with knees and elbows flexed, and maintains this posture when walking (Fig. 1.17).

Apart from the main features of the disease mentioned above, a number of *other somatic signs and symptoms* may be present. An occasional early feature, resulting from the loss of the postural reflexes, which protect normal subjects from falling, is a reduced postural stability, the patient *falling forward* in an uncontrolled fashion (623, 845). This phenomenon must be differentiated from the drop attacks of vertebrobasilar insufficiency (p.73). *Speech* is soft, monotonous, and poorly articulated. In postencephalitic parkinsonism it may also be staccato in type and possess reiterative features such as palilalia (involuntary repetition of sentences or phrases with increasing rapidity). Occasionally an actual akinetic mutism is present in this syndrome, which may be possible to overcome only by emotional stimulation. Special technique will reveal the presence of disturbances of *respiration* (irregular frequency and depth). Sometimes the impression of *motor weakness* is gained, although the muscles can be shown to possess their normal power. This was first suggested by James Parkinson who

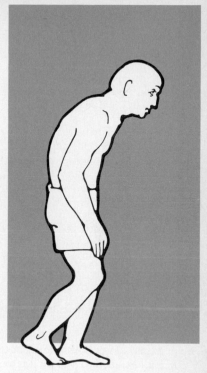

Fig 1.17 Typical posture of parkinsonian patient when walking

in 1817 described the syndrome as "the shaking palsy." The tendon reflexes are present and normal. Signs of pyramidal tract involvement are usually absent in uncomplicated cases of the parkinsonian syndrome but there are countless exceptions to this rule. A constant feature is *accentuation of the nasopalpebral and other reflexes* of the facial muscles. Pain is perceived by many patients as tenderness of the muscles and bones. They are to be distinguished from equally painful dystonias as they occur as a side effect of L-dopa therapy (727). Signs of *autonomic involvement* in the parkinsonian syndrome, particularly in the postencephalitic form, may be impressive (increased salivation, excess of sweating, hot flushes, abnormally increased sebaceous secretion amounting to seborrhea). Exclusively found in the postencephalitic form and in dyskinesias occurring following phenothiazine ingestion are the so-called *oculogyric crises:* the patient's vision is fixed upward for minutes or hours, and occasionally his head is tilted back. *Blepharospasm* in patients with postencephalitic parkinsonism may lead to convulsive closure of the eyelids for varying intervals. Occasionally disturbances of convergence and accommodation may accompany the oculogyric crises (progressive supranuclear palsy, see p. 109). *Dystonic features* may be present in addition to the parkinsonian signs and symptoms. A rare occurrence – occasionally in association with L-dopa treatment – is a *parkinsonian crisis,* a condition of extreme akinesia, severe rigidity, hyperpyrexia due to disturbed regulation of body temperature, and profuse sweating.

Mental symptoms are nearly always present but they vary greatly in intensity. The patient is often emotionally labile and hypersensitive. Mental processes are slowed to the same extent as the patient's physical activity; to a certain extent, he must force himself to think. In addition to cases of the hereditary parkinsonism-dementia complex (p. 108), at least one-third of parkinsonian patients show an organic mental syndrome of varying severity. The patients belonging to this group appear on average to be older, parkinsonian signs develop later and are more rapidly progressive, and L-dopa is less effective (499).

Individual parkinsonian signs and symptoms may be evaluated separately and *quantitatively defined.* This approach affords a yardstick for measuring progression of the disease and the efficacy of a treatment. The rating scale suggested by Webster in 1968 (1251) is reproduced in Table 1.**14**.

Specific Etiologic Forms

The clinical symptomatology is usually similar in the various etiologic forms. However, particular features may be accentuated in specific etiologic entities (see below). Table 1.**15** lists the main etiologic forms of the disease.

True Parkinson's disease:

This term, or paralysis agitans, is applied to the familial autosomal dominant disease which only rarely assumes a recessive or sporadic form. Males are more often affected, usually aged 50–60 years. The degree of involvement varies greatly and only about 60% of carriers of the defect are symptomatic. In most patients the prominent features are diminished movements and a fine tremor. True Parkinson's disease belongs to the group of heredodegenerative diseases (p. 164). Familial cases of combined *parkinsonism with dementia* which are observed in natives of Guam Island in the Pacific Ocean, some of whom simultaneously exhibit amyotrophic lateral sclerosis have been similarly classified, but have recently been considered to be of toxic origin (cycad

Table 1.14 Simplified rating scale for evaluating the severity of individual parkinsonian signs (after *Webster* 1968)

1. *Bradykinesia of the hands, including writing*
   0 = normal
   1 = appears slightly slowed
   2 = moderately slowed, writing markedly affected
   3 = severely slowed

2. *Rigidity*
   0 = normal
   1 = detectable
   2 = moderate
   3 = severe, demonstrable despite medication

3. *Posture*
   0 = normal
   1 = slight forward stoop commencing arm flexion
   2 = beginning arm flexion
   3 = severe forward stoop, flexion of arms and hands, and knees

4. *Upper extremities swing*
   0 = both sides normal
   1 = one arm reduced
   2 = one arm not swinging at all
   3 = both arms not swinging

5. *Gait*
   0 = normal, turns about without trouble
   1 = shortened steps, slow turns
   2 = more severely reduced steps, stamps both heels on the ground
   3 = shuffling gait, gait occasionally blocked, turns around very slowly

6. *Tremor*
   0 = none
   1 = as small as 2.5 cm deflection
   2 = over 10 cm, tremor severe but not constant
   3 = constantly over 10 cm, feeding and writing impossible

7. *Facies*
   0 = normal
   1 = loss of expression apparent
   2 = definite poverty of expression, lips parted, sometimes excessive salivation
   3 = masklike face, mouth open, marked salivation (drooling)

8. *Seborrhea*
   0 = none
   1 = increased perspiration
   2 = greasy skin
   3 = marked secretion in face

9. *Speech*
   0 = normal
   1 = reduced modulation, normal speech volume
   2 = monotonous, no longer modulated, commencing dysarthria, difficult to understand
   3 = marked harshness and weakness, very difficult to understand

10. *Self-care*
    0 = no impairment
    1 = slight difficulty in dressing
    2 = requires help in critical situations, all acts take much longer
    3 = unable to dress or feed himself, or to walk unaided

Table 1.**15** Etiology of the parkinsonian syndrome

1. *Hereditary forms*
   Parkinsonism-disease (paralysis agitans)
   Parkinsonian – dementia complex (Guam)
2. *Parkinsonism in other degenerative (heredofamilial) disorders*
3. *Postencephalitic parkinsonism*
4. *Arteriosclerotic parkinsonism*
5. *Rarer causes*
   Trauma (single; in boxers)
   Carbon monoxide poisoning
   Manganese poisoning
   Other intoxications
   Drugs (phenothiazine, rauwolfia)
   Tumors
   Polycythemia
6. *"Idiopathic"*

nut). In this disease, also, males are more commonly affected than females; it appears between the ages of 30 and 60 years. The clinical picture is dominated by rigidity and absence of movement; there may be no tremor. In this particular group, the parkinsonian syndrome is always associated with a marked degree of dementia.

Postencephalitic parkinsonism:
This postinfectious form may appear during the course of an encephalitis or after a latent period that may extend from months up to 30 years after the acute illness. The most celebrated cases are those who survived the epidemic of encephalitis lethargica of the 1920s (p.50). However, typical cases of the parkinsonian syndrome continue to occur in association with recent and isolated episodes of encephalitis, which do not possess the features of the von Economo form. Clinically, severe auto-

nomic features dominate the picture of postencephalitic parkinsonism. Oculogyric crises, dystonic movement disturbances, and palilalia are pathognomonic features. The assumption that many present-day parkinsonian cases may have been caused by (clinically silent) infection with the virus of encephalitis lethargica (179) is no longer accepted.

Drug-induced parkinsonian syndromes:
These are most likely to follow treatment with phenothiazine and less likely after tricyclic antidepressants and rauwolfia alkaloids. Poverty of movement and rigidity are more striking features than tremor. For other side effects of chlorpromazine, see p. 149.

Parkinsonism due to MPTP:
MPTP, developed as a "Design-Drug" (1-methyl-4-phenyl-1, 2, 3, 6-Tetrahydropyridin) causes a Parkinson syndrome after oral ingestion, injection or even inhalation (74). In terms of the pathological anatomy one finds an almost selective loss of melanin-containing ganglion cells in the pars compacta of the substantia nigra. The same clinical picture is produced in primates, so that a model for the study of Parkinsonism is available. It is not completely apparent yet if the loss of cells continues progressively after discontinuation of the exposure.

Arteriosclerotic parkinsonism:
This etiologic entity is probably too often diagnosed. The presence initially of unilateral signs is no valid basis for diagnosis; indeed, unilateral signs are not an unusual finding in the parkinsonian syndrome. Other signs of cerebral arteriosclerosis must be present, e.g., mental changes, pseudobulbar palsy, or focal neurologic signs. The course in the arteriosclerotic form of the disease is often rapidly progressive. The tremor is less marked than in the postencephalit-

ic forms. The patients are usually over 60 years of age. Many contradictory statements occur in textbooks about arteriosclerotic parkinsonism so that the concept of this form as a separate entity has fallen into disuse.

Idiopathic forms:

In very many patients with the parkinsonian syndrome no specific cause can be determined, and they are designated as examples of the idiopathic form of the disease. Not infrequently unilateral involvement is the presenting feature, which is progressive. Males, usually aged 50-60 years are more often affected than females. The importance of heredity in such patients is difficult to determine (638). The probability that children of parkinsonian parents will inherit the disease is said to be 19%; therefore, a single dominant or recessive pattern is unlikely. A multifactorial pathogenesis must be assumed.

Degenerative (familial) disorders:

Parkinsonian features may also appear in other specific degenerative conditions such as Friedreich ataxia, olivopontocerebellar atrophy, orthostatic hypotension, and the Creutzfeldt-Jakob disease. Striatonigral degeneration (809) is caused by a lesion of the putamen and substantia nigra which occasionally also involves the olives, pons, and cerebellum. The signs are those of parkinsonism, and occasionally pyramidal tract involvement and cerebellar signs are prominent. The response to antiparkinsonian treatment is usually unsatisfactory.

Progressive supranuclear palsy

(steele-richardson-olszewski syndrome) (300, 1151): This entity is by no means rare. It is characterized by akinetic parkinsonian signs and paralysis of ocular movements. The disease is sporadic and only exceptionally familial, affecting mostly males between 50 and 70 years of age. As a rule, a slowly progressive reduction in movements sets in, which over the course of one or more years develops into a true akinesia. **Clinically,** the patients mimic the picture of Parkinson's disease. The limitation of ocular movement, which is a diagnostically important feature, may not be noticed initially by the patient, although it leads eventually to complete external ophthalmoplegia. While voluntary and following movements of the eyes are more or less abolished, the doll's eyes phenomenon (p. 339) can be demonstrated and Bell's phenomenon is retained – therefore, a nuclear or peripheral ophthalmoplegia can be excluded. The condition leads gradually to a dementia which shows specific characteristics known as "subcortical dementia." Features are present which correspond to the psychopathologic picture associated with a lesion of both frontal lobes, viz. prolongation of thought processes, apathy, and occasional outbursts of irritability, as well as difficulty in applying knowledge. The dementia may be the presenting symptom and the eye movement disturbance may appear late or not at all (278). About one-half of the cases exhibit pyramidal tract involvement, fewer show cerebellar signs. The **prognosis** is poor, and death usually occurs within a few years. Individual cases of this syndrome fulfill the clinical and roentgenologic criteria of normal-pressure hydrocephalus (p 19). **Treatment** consists of ventricular shunting which may have a favorable effect on the mental symptoms, urinary incontinence, and ataxia, but it does not abolish the paralysis of vertical eye movements or the parkinsonian symptoms and signs (826).

Rarer causes of a parkinsonian syndrome:

A *traumatic parkinsonian syndrome* should be diagnosed only in the presence of proof of severe cerebral concussion or contusion with identifiable evidence of permanent brain damage; the parkinsonian signs should either have appeared immediately in association with the episode, or within days or weeks of it. The *parkinsonian syndrome in boxers* is attributed to the countless episodes of cerebral concussion and knockout blows experienced by these athletes, and it is sometimes accompanied by a dementia (dementia pugilistica, "punchdrunk state"). The *parkinsonian syndrome following carbon monoxide intoxication* presents after a shorter latent period – at most, several weeks after the acute episode – and bilateral signs are present. The parkinsonian syndrome following *chronic manganese intoxication* (1019) is encountered in miners extracting manganese, as well as factory workers in this industry. The clinical signs and symptoms usually present only after exposure for many years, and comprise memory disturbances, disorientation, hyperexcitability, and hallucinations. Asthenia and poverty of movement lead to rigidity, fixed facial expression, cogwheel phenomena, and resting tremor. Occasionally an intention tremor also may be present. Individual cases are described following *other intoxications,* methyl alcohol, certain sedatives, carbon disulfide, carbon dioxide, and thallium. In elderly subjects with an autosomally inherited disease comprising initial depression, a disturbed sleep rhythm, and finally parkinsonian features, *taurine deficiency* (937) has been demonstrated in the blood and CSF and in the brain at autopsy. Individual cases of the parkinsonian syndrome may follow electric injury, chronic subdural hematoma, brain tumors (especially meningiomas), and polycythemia vera.

Pathologic Anatomy
(436, 1217, 1298)

Changes are always present in the substantia nigra in the parkinsonian syndrome. They include degeneration of the melanin-containing ganglion cells and neuroglial proliferation. These changes were first observed in cases of postencephalitic parkinsonism. The other melanin-containing basal nuclei, the globus pallidus, corpus striatum, the reticular formation of the brainstem, the dentate nucleus, and the thalamus, are less constantly affected. The only essential diagnostic changes are those present in the substantia nigra. The cytoplasm of the diseased ganglion cells contains bullet-shaped hyaline Lewy bodies in which tyrosine is present. Other pathoanatomic features may be present, depending on the etiologic agent, e.g., Alzheimer's neurofibrils which are found in postencephalitic parkinsonism and in the parkinsonism-dementia complex. Immunofluorescence studies enable the reduced dopamine content of the substantia nigra and corpus striatum to be observed histologically.

Pathophysiology and Pathochemistry (205, 725, 766)

The signs and symptoms of the parkinsonian syndrome can be explained by an anatomic or functional failure of one of the components of the complex neuronal system illustrated in Fig. 1.**14**. In particular, the following tracts and neuronal system should be noted: efferent fibers from the substantia nigra to the anterior horn cells of the spinal cord; the substantia nigra receives numerous activating stimuli from various parts of the cerebral cortex, as well as inhibitor stimuli from the corpus striatum; efferent fibers pass from the anterior part of the substantia nigra to the medial part of the globus pallidus, whence the stimuli are transmitted as impulses to the premotor cortex (6A, 4S) via the ansa lenticularis and various thalamic nuclei. The clinical feature of akinesia may be explained by the fact that the stimuli regulating the involuntary automatic movements no longer reach the anterior horn cells in the normal way from the substantia nigra, the latter being diseased. The clinical feature of rigidity is the result of increased alpha activity. This induces the so-called plastic appearance of the muscles, which gives rise to viscous movements.

Biochemically, a deficiency of dopamine has been observed in the caudate nucleus, putamen, and substantia nigra in parkinsonian patients – nuclei which are otherwise rich in dopamine. Thus, an imbalance is produced which causes predominance of the cholinergically transmitted impulses within the complex neuronal system. *Acetylcholine* exerts an excitatory effect on most neurons of the caudate nucleus. Electrical stimulation of the anterior ventral nucleus of the thalamus enables excessive acetylcholine to be isolated from the corpus striatum. Cholinergic substances provoke or aggravate the parkinsonian signs and symptoms. Under normal conditions, there is a greatly increased concentration of dopamine in the caudate nucleus and putamen compared with other parts of the brain. Histochemically, it is found particularly in the nigrostriatal system, and in parkinsonian patients the dopamine content of this zone is reduced markedly below normal levels. Pharmacologic agents such as rauwolfia alkaloid and chlorpromazine derivatives, which interfere with catecholamine metabolism in the brain, provoke parkinsonian features. Thus, acetylcholine and dopamine represent the two specific transmitter substances which act like reins upon the neural system of the brainstem. Parkinsonism appears to be associated with a defect of the dopaminergic system. It may be caused by infectious, mechanical, vascular, toxic, or drug-induced damage to the system at one of the following levels: morbid-anatomic, histologic, ultramicroscopic, or molecular (enzymatic). In this way, an imbalance is produced which causes predominance of the cholinergic system. The resulting clinical picture depends on the extent and site of the underlying lesion. The various motor signs and symptoms may vary from a simple absence of automatic movements to tremor and dystonia.

Treatment

Rational treatment depends on confirming involvement of the dopaminergic nigrostriatal tracts and observing a deficiency of dopamine in the region of the substantia nigra and corpus striatum. This basis, together with the pathophysiologic data described above, suggests the following treatment options:

- substitution therapy with dopamine,
- treatment with dopamine agonists,
- administration of anticholinergics (to restore the balance between damaged dopaminergic and overacting cholinergic systems),
- influencing the release (catabolism) of dopamine in the nigrostriatal neurons, and
- influencing the neuronal system by stereotactic operations.

Medical treatment: The patient should be prescribed drugs when his signs and symptoms interfere with his daily life. In common with other authors, we tend to favor an early start of treatment (764, 836). The treatment of choice nowadays is synthetic dopamine (82, 206, 725). Since dopamine itself does not penetrate the CNS from the bloodstream, a precursor is used which is pharmacologically decarboxylated in the presynaptic nerve endings to dopamine. This precursor is administered in the form of L-dopa. It is decarboxylated in the CNS to dopamine, acts particularly on the akinesia and to a lesser extent also on the other parkinsonian features. Its effect in 50%-80% of patients is excellent or satisfactory. The pure substance is rarely prescribed, particularly since it is poorly tolerated, and L-dopa combined with a decarboxylase inhibitor (Sinemet, Madopar, etc.) allows the dose to be reduced. Treatment is started with a low dose, 62.5-125 mg/day, which is increased within a few weeks to a final dose of about 500-750 mg/day. Gastric side effects may be lessened

by the administration of domperidone. Psychotic episodes may follow too swift an increase in dose or prolonged medication. In more than one-half of the patients, these episodes consist of agitated confusion, in about 10% a dementia is present (82). These complications may perhaps represent a drug-induced long-term evolution of the disease. Anticholinergic drugs also may significantly increase the incidence of confusional states in mentally disturbed parkinsonian patients (290).

Bromocriptine (which also acts as a dopaminergic drug) is an ergotamine derivative which exerts antiparkinsonian effects roughly similar to those of L-dopa (207, 422, 703). Treatment starts with 1.25 mg/day, followed after 1 week by 1.25 twice daily, and then each further week or every 2-4 weeks (1093) rising by 2.5 mg to a total dose of 15-30 mg/day. Nowadays smaller daily doses, as low as 5-20 mg, have replaced the higher doses previously used (861). The use of bromocriptine should be restricted to those patients in whom L-dopa proves unsatisfactory or an increase of the dose produces such ill effects (see below) that the L-dopa treatment cannot be continued. When combined with L-dopa, it serves to reduce the side effects of bromocriptine (861). The milder forms of the syndrome may be treated first with *parasympatholytic drugs and amantadine* (916), which have few side effects. Apart from extracts of belladonna, wide use is now made of substances such as synthetic parasympatholytics (glaucoma is a contraindication). A combination of L-dopa with amantadine 200 mg/day may sometimes improve the results of treatment. The beneficial effect of beta-blocking agents previously postulated in parkinsonian patients has not been substantiated (767).

Side effects of L-dopa (and bromocriptine) treatment: Apart from the psychotic episodes referred to above, about three-fourths of patients under treatment experience very marked *dyskinesias*. These are involuntary movements affecting the muscles of the mouth and face as well as the extremities. They are confined to either side or to the area in which the patient's parkinsonian features first began. Sometimes they disturb others more than the patient but they may prevent him from walking, eating, or speaking correctly. Sometimes the involuntary movements assume a prolonged dystonic character and appear to be painful; however, myoclonus is rare. Severe hemiballistic movement disturbances may be associated with increased tremor and last 30–60 min. The phrase "on/off phenomenon" is applied to the sudden change from a satisfactory state, mostly accompanied by orofacial dyskinesias, to an acute state of akinetic rigidity lasting from minutes to hours (82). All these phenomena become more frequent as treatment is prolonged. Their occurrence is sometimes, but not always, related to the timing of individual drug doses. Additional *psychopathologic phenomena* such as hallucinations, confusion, and psychotic states occur in about three-fourths of the patients treated for a longer period (1086). It is by no means certain and no proof has been adduced that these phenomena are a direct side effect of the treatment. A more likely explanation is an abnormality of synthesis of metabolism of endogenous dopamine, which occurs in 50% of patients undergoing years of treatment (766). This complication is the main argument used by those authors who recommend that the start of treatment should be delayed as long as possible (350). Moreover, the fact should not be concealed that the efficacy of a specific dose unquestionably declines as treatment continues.

Stereotactic operations: These are nowadays only rarely undertaken as an alternative to medical treatment. They are performed through burr holes, using roentgenographic methods to verify the position of a special head frame for stereotactic surgery. These operations are intended to produce mechanical, chemical, electric, or cryogenic lesions within the globus pallidus (to diminish the patient's rigidity) or within the lateral ventral nucleus of the thalamus (to reduce tremor). The operative mortality is less than 1%. The best results abolish the rigidity, and slightly less successful operations reduce the tremor; but the akinesia can seldom be influenced. Slowly progressive cases respond more favorably than those which are rapidly progressive. Stereotactic operations are particularly indicated in unilateral cases (hemiparkinsonism), while bilateral cases may sometimes benefit from unilateral operation. It is also justified in patients who, despite correct medical treatment, are significantly restricted in their work capacity or social adaptability in daily life, provided there is no contraindication. The latter include previous apoplectic attacks, marked mental deterioration, and severe hypertension. Over the age of 65 years the operative risk is greater, although advanced age is no absolute contraindication.

Prognosis

The parkinsonian syndrome in its various etiologic forms is – with the exception of the drug-induced forms, which are almost all completely reversible – by definition a progressive disease. Within a few years the patient becomes an invalid. Even the most successful therapy available at present, L-dopa, does not delay the fatal outcome of the disease beyond a few years (131, 728). This pattern suggests a neuropathologic lesion rather than a biochemical defect as the primary etiologic factor (131).

In a group of 36 patients with Parkinson's disease who had been treated with L-dopa and who subsequently died, no changes were found in the brain at autopsy, other than those which may be expected in any untreated parkinsonian patient. In particular, the presence of varying degrees of neuronal degeneration in the substantia nigra indicated that the disease had continued to advance despite the L-dopa medication. Moreover, the efficacy of treatment bore no relation to the extent of these pathologic lesions. No unusual changes were observed in the basal ganglia of any of the patients who had experienced involuntary movements during treatment (1298). In a recent series reported from Japan, the average duration of the illness was 7.4 years. Most died

at about the age of 70 years from heart disease or pneumonia (475).

Chorea (11, 253, 766)

Clinical features: Chorea is one of the hyperkinetic-hypotonic extrapyramidal syndromes. The individual case, irrespective of its etiology, presents with irregular and asymmetric *involuntary movements* of sudden onset and short duration affecting the distal extremities. They may be so slight as to be viewed merely as "fidgety" movements, and their organic basis may initially go unrecognized. On the other hand, they may be severe, aimless, and extremely disturbing to the patient. In the face they may take the form of grimaces or lip-smacking movements. These involuntary movements interfere with the execution of voluntary actions and tend to upset the patient's daily life and to prevent adequate rest; sometimes they lead to total exhaustion. Sleep may be prevented. Additional athetoid components (p. 120) are not uncommon. An example of senile hemichorea exhibiting this picture in a motion picture recording is shown in Fig. 1.18. Neurologic examination reveals – apart from the involuntary movements described above – only a severely reduced muscle tone. The rest of the nervous system is normal. Examination of the knee jerk with the patient seated and his feet off the ground may reveal an abnormally prolonged relaxation following the contraction (Gordon's knee phenomenon; hung-up knee jerks) or provoke an additional extensor movement. Both responses are ex-

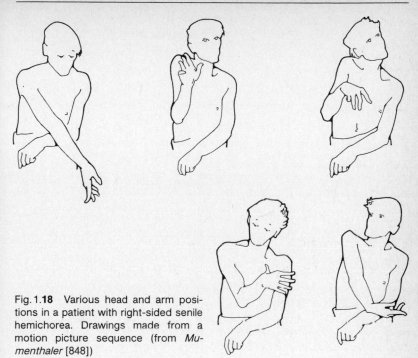

Fig. 1.**18** Various head and arm positions in a patient with right-sided senile hemichorea. Drawings made from a motion picture sequence (from *Mumenthaler* [848])

amples of an involuntary movement interfering with the reflex arc. Sometimes the abdominal musculature is drawn inward upon inspiration, as in paralysis of the diaphragm.

Table 1.**16** provides an overview of the hyperkinetic extrapyramidal syndromes and lists the various **etiologic types** of chorea which will now be discussed.

Chorea Minor

This is the commonest childhood type. It was described by Sydenham in 1686 *(chorea rheumatica, chorea*

infectiosa). It affects particularly *school-age* girls chiefly between the ages of 6 and 13 years and is rarely seen up to the age of 40 years. There is a striking association in childhood with infectious illnesses, particularly *rheumatic fever.* In about two-thirds of cases a relevant history of preceding disease is present, such as rheumatic joint involvement, sore throat, or endocarditis, which is followed within a few weeks by the choreiform signs. Evidence should be sought of a family predisposition to chorea and other neurologic diseases. The **signs and symptoms** develop within weeks or days and are

Table 1.16 Diagnosis of the Hyperkinetic Extrapyramidal Syndromes

Name	Description	Etiology	Details
Chorea			
Chorea minor	Sudden, usually frequent movements which are distal and brief, irregular and involuntary. Hypotonia	Immunologic and streptococcal infection	Common after angina. Especially young girls. Greatest incidence between 6 and 13 years
Chorea mollis		Immunologic and streptococcal infection	Hypotonia a prominent feature
Chorea gravidarum		During 3rd–5th months of pregnancy	Especially during first pregnancy. Often a history of chorea minor
Chorea after ovulation inhibitors			Rare. Reversible upon withdrawal of ovulation inhibitors
Huntington's chorea		Inherited autosomal dominant	Usually manifests between ages of 30 and 50 years. Associated with progressive dementia
Benign familial chorea		Inherited autosomal dominant	Starts during childhood. Later no longer progressive. No dementia
Choreoacanthocytosis		Autosomal recessive	Orofacial involvement. Tongue-biting, increased creatine kinase. Reflexes diminished. Acanthocytosis
Postapoplectic chorea		Vascular	Sudden hemichorea and hemiparesis, often combined with hemiballismus
Senile chorea		Vascular and degenerative	Presenile precursor, associated with dementia, often unilateral manifestation
Rarer forms			See p.119

Athetoses

Status marmoratus	Prolonged and exaggerated movements executed against resistance of antagonists. Distal involvement, movements tortuous and cramped	Perinatal asphyxia	Soon after birth, increasingly severe athetotic hyperkinesia. Often mental deficiency. Later spasticity develops as well
Status dysmyelinisatus		Icterus gravis neonatorum	Starts soon after birth, often with other signs of perinatal brain damage. Later progressive
Hallervorden-Spatz disease	Leads to exaggerated position of the joints (see Fig. 1.19)	Autosomal recessive disturbance of pigment metabolism	Starts between ages of 5 and 15 years, choreoathetotic movements, rigidity, dementia, and in 1/3 retinitis pigmentosa. Progressive. Fatal by 30 years
Hemiathetosis		Focal lesion of globus pallidus and corpus striatum	Unilateral. May appear following latent interval after the lesion
Ballismus (and hemiballismus)	Unilateral, severe and instantaneous throwing movements affecting severe limb segments	Lesion of the subthalamic corpus Luysix – usually an ischemic lesion caused by a vascular insult	Sudden onset. Most patients are also hemiparetic

Dystonic Syndromes

Torsion dystonia	Short or long-lasting, slow and tonic contractions of muscles or muscle groups, usually executed against the resistance of the antagonists	Familial forms	Often Jewish families. Commences in 1st or 2nd decades. Frequently just with local dystonia. Later rotating movements of the head and trunk as well as the extremities, and athetotic movements of the fingers
Spasmodic torticollis	Slow contractions of the neck muscles with rotatory movements of the head executed against the resistance of the antagonists	Idiopathic, sometimes following neck injury but also a variety of other causes	1/3 recover, 1/3 remain unchanged, 1/3 develop into a tonic dystonia
Localized dystonias	See p 125		e.g., writer's cramp, faciobuccolingual dystonias, oromandibular dystonias

usually heralded by nonspecific complaints such as tiredness, mental lability, and irritability. These general features are followed by the movement disturbances already described which, as stated above, may initially be dismissed as "fidgeting" or "embarrassment" movements. However, within weeks a typical picture of chorea develops. Exceptionally the movement disturbance is unilateral, initially or permanently. Fever is present only initially. The CSF is invariably normal. Occasionally a mental disorder including an actual psychosis may dominate the picture. If the reduced tone and weakness of the muscles is very marked and involuntary movements are virtually impossible, the term *chorea mollis* is used. The **prognosis** of chorea minor is good, and the signs and symptoms can be expected to regress within a few weeks or at most months. However, there is a significant tendency to recurrence, and about one-third of patients exhibit residual features (fidgetiness when excited, anxiety, tics). **Treatment** consists chiefly in salicylate medication, antihistaminics, cortisone, pyridoxine, and long-term penicillin.

Chorea Gravidarum

Typically this type is encountered in the 2nd trimester of a first pregnancy. The associated circumstances, signs and symptoms, and prognosis do not differ from those of chorea minor. With surprising frequency the pregnant patient will give a history of chorea minor in childhood. This type of chorea has also been observed to complicate the adminis-

tration of *oral contraceptives*. The signs and symptoms disappear if the drug is withdrawn (873).

Huntington's Chorea

Chronic progressive chorea, usually associated with the name of Huntington, is transmitted as an autosomal dominant. A polymorphic DNA marker is genetically linked with this type of chorea (452) so that in the near future it will be possible to predict the pattern of the disease in the descendants of patients with chorea. However, early diagnosis remains questionable. Lymphocytic cell cultures taken from established cases appear to be particularly sensitive to X-irradiation (832). The more florid and prolonged the signs and symptoms in established cases, the more abnormal will be their visual evoked potential (VEP). However, clinically asymptomatic descendants have normal VEPs, utilizing present-day laboratory techniques. The **clinical signs and symptoms** usually manifest at the age of 30–50 years. The hyperkinetic features develop very slowly and the movements are seldom as rapid as those of chorea minor. In addition, more associated athetoid movements are present. The gait is often markedly abnormal. Mental disturbances are a feature of the typical picture of Huntington's chorea, but they do not parallel the severity of the movement disturbances and may precede or follow them after a long interval. They include disturbances of affect, apathy, delusions, and paranoid delusions which lead eventually to dementia. The average age of onset appears to rise above

50 in those cases in which the abnormal gene is carried by the mother, compared to patients with paternal inheritance (860). Cases starting in childhood (214) may show initial signs of generalized rigidity and spasticity, cerebellar and pyramidal involvement, epileptic attacks, and a rapidly progressive dementia. Only later do the choreiform movements appear, and they then progress with particular rapidity. The **prognosis** is very poor, and the disease progresses steadily to a fatal outcome, usually within 10–15 years. No effective **treatment** exists (control of choreiform movements, see below).

Benign Familial Chorea

Apart from the progressive (Huntington) type of chorea, a benign, apparently autosomal dominant form of the disease exists without dementia (99). It commences in childhood but may later run a static course in some siblings.

Rarer Etiologic Types of Chorea

Another familial form which is transmitted as an autosomal recessive gene is so-called *choreoacanthocytosis* (1052). It appears in the 2nd decade of life, usually as orofacial dyskinesias with tongue biting, and later in a discrete form with choreiform movements of the extremities. The tendon reflexes are reduced or absent, the creatine kinase is increased, and an acanthocytosis with normal beta-lipoprotein is present. The patients are not demented.

Postapoplectic hemichorea is rare, even in the presence of softening of the putamen. Chorea following hemiplegia is not accompanied merely by the paretic signs of hemispheric involvement but by hemiballistic movement disturbances. *Hemichorea accompanying tumors* or other space-occupying intracra-

nial lesions is rare. Similarly, chorea seldom follows *viral encephalitis*. Senile *nonhereditary chorea* is part of the picture of senile dementia and rarely accompanies the presenile form. Choreiform attacks have been described in *lupus erythematosus* (303), *acute exanthemata, Hallervorden-Spatz disease, hepatolenticular degeneration, ataxiatelangiectasia, Creutzfeldt-Jakob disease, polycythemia vera* (331), *thyrotoxicosis* (360), hypernatriemia (1133), *hyperparathyroidism* (1124), and *after intoxication with CO, manganese, carbon disulfide, phenytoin,* and *chlorpromazine poisoning.* The chorea following icterus gravis neonatorum is usually associated with athetosis and other signs of kernicterus (p. 14). Exceptionally chorea may complicate *hypoxic encephalopathy* of childbirth. Choreoathetosis may rarely accompany portocaval encephalopathy. Another condition, called the *Lesch-Nyhan syndrome* (240, 817), is caused by an X-chromosomal, recessive disturbance of purine metabolism with very high serum uric acid levels in the first days or weeks of life, and it may be accompanied by choreoathetotic or dystonic signs. Other features are retarded psychomotor development and self-mutilation. The absence of hypoxanthine guanidine phosphoryboxyl transferase in the tissues has been confirmed at autopsy (817). Conventional gout medication does not prevent neurologic signs, and L-5-hydroxytryptophan to prevent self-mutilation in children (817) has not remained unchallenged (36). *Glutaric acidemia* and *aciduria* is a rare, genetically determined metabolic disturbance resulting from defective glutaryl-CoA-dehydrogenase activity. The disease, which appears in the first years of life and usually shows a progressive course (692), is characterized by choreiform, choreoathetotic or dystonic movements, spasticity, and dementia. Some cases may show an intermittent course (663). *Progressive pallidal atrophy* (Hunt), a sporadic hereditary disease, may present as choreoathetotic and dystonic movement disturbances which in the course of years are followed by tremor, rigidity, and akinesia. The disease usually affects children aged 5–15 years and is progressive into middle age. For paroxysmal choreoathetosis, see p. 276.

Pathologic Anatomy and Pathophysiology of Chorea

Pathoanatomically (436, 1217), a lesion of the small ganglion cells of the corpus striatum, especially the putamen and caudate nucleus is present. This produces obvious flattening of the medial wall of the lateral ventricle. A well-circumscribed lesion, e.g., a tumor metastasis, only very exceptionally produces chorea. More often there is diffuse damage involving the entire system.

Pathophysiologically, interruption of the striatonigral pathway abolishes the control exerted by the substantia nigra over associated movements and muscle tone. As a result, the substantia nigra transmits the impulses it receives from the premotor cortex in an irregular fashion to the anterior horn cells. Since the striatal fibers to the outer globus pallidus are also interrupted, this inhibition affects the pallidoreticular fibers as well as those linking the inner globus pallidus, the ventral nuclei of the thalamus, and areas 6A and 4S of the premotor cortex. The efferent impulses arising in the latter areas are therefore deprived of their physiologic control and exert an uninhibited action on the reticular inhibitory system, the substantia nigra, and the anterior horn apparatus.

Treatment

Drugs such as perphenazine in doses commencing with 4 mg and increased until effective are useful in controlling the involuntary movements of various types of chorea (576). Drugs such as haloperidol which may produce tardive dyskinesia should be avoided if possible.

Athetoses (11, 766)

Clinical features: Athetosis is characterized by slow, involuntary and irregular movements exaggerated particularly in the extremities, the movements appearing to be tormented and cramplike. They often cause hyperflexion or hyperextension of joints. Intense antagonist traction is a striking feature, resulting in bizarre postures in which the joints remain fixed for several seconds: the position of the hands is particularly striking (Fig. 1.**19**) and in the course of time may lead to subluxation of the digits ("bayonet finger"). All voluntary movements are affected by this strong abnormal accessory innervation as well as the execution of automatic movements such as gait. Not infrequently the athetotic picture described above is masked by choreiform movements. In uncomplicated cases, no abnormal *neurologic findings* are present. The tendon reflexes are brisk. A dystonic postural disturbance of the great toe results in dorsiflexion which may be interpreted as a "pseudo-Babinski" sign. Dorsiflexion and supination of the foot and toes whenever the patient is required to flex the knee and hip against resistance (Strümpell phe-

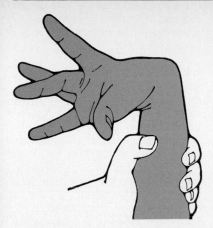

Fig.1.19 Typical position of the hand in athetosis with outstretched digits (thalamic hand) (after *Hassler*)

nomenon) may occasionally be observed. In individual patients other neurologic manifestations, depending on the primary pathologic process, may overshadow the athetotic picture.

Etiologic types: *Status marmoratus* is the commonest cause of the so-called *athetose double*, a form of infantile cerebral palsy. Usually it follows perinatal damage (asphyxia), the putamen and caudate nucleus showing microscopic evidence of neuronal damage and foci of hypermyelination. Clinical features are generally present shortly after birth or within the first few years of life, and seldom appear later. Apart from bilateral athetotic and hyperkinetic movements affecting particularly the arms, about one-half of the patients are mentally deficient. Other organic signs of cerebral damage may also be present, e.g., spastic diplegia or pyramidal signs (rare). The disease becomes stationary.

Status dysmyelinisatus consists of a demyelination of the fibers of the globus pallidus and degeneration of the myelinated fibers in the subthalamic nucleus. The pallidal cells are severely reduced in number and the pallidal nuclei appear to be shrunken. The pathogenesis of this disease picture is unclear, several different lesions seem to be capable of producing it. Apart from birth trauma and asphyxia, Rh incompatibility with *icterus gravis neonatorum* (p.14) may be responsible. In such cases, the athetotic disturbances of movement begin immediately after birth, or within the 1st year of life. They are often accompanied by other signs of cerebral damage.

The *Hallervorden-Spatz syndrome* is a familial disease, probably transmitted as an autosomal recessive gene, appearing in the first or early years of the 2nd decade of life It is characterized by progressive rigidity of the extremities, choreoathetotic movements, a dementia which is often progressive, and epileptic attacks. In one-third of patients retinitis pigmentosa is present, exceptionally the onset of the disease is delayed to adulthood. It runs a rapidly progressive course and patients seldom survive beyond 30 years. The substrate is a disturbance of pigment metabolism which can probably be explained on the basis of a genetically determined enzyme defect. The globus pallidus and reticular zone of the substantia nigra appear to be stained by intracellular and extracellular lipoid pigment

Hemiathetoses may be caused by *focal lesions* and are encountered in children as well as adults; they follow birth trauma, encephalitis, and - particularly in adults - stroke. It the last-mentioned condition, a symptom-free interval of weeks or months may elapse between the cerebrovascular accident and the onset of the hemiathetosis. However, the spastic hemiparesis remains constantly present.

Pathologic anatomy and pathophysiology of athetoses: Athetotic disturbances of movement accompany *macroscopic* lesions of the corpus striatum, globus pallidus, and rarely the thalamus and red nucleus. Pathophysiologically, the impulses from the inner globus pallidus to the thalamic nuclei are interrupted. The latter then fail to relay impulses to the extrapyramidal areas of the premotor cortex, which in turn transmits uncontrolled stimuli to the deeper centers and the spinal cord. Likewise, the rubroreticular system is deprived of its physiologic drive from the globus pallidus and is exposed to unregulated stimuli from the premotor cortex.

Treatment: See dystonic syndromes, p. 125.

Hemiballismus and Ballismus
(11, 766)

Clinical features: The typical clinical picture of these conditions is the occurrence of unilateral and sudden, throwing and spreading *movements,* which involve several parts of several limbs simultaneously. The impression may be gained of a coordinated movement which, however, is exaggerated and goes beyond the subject's intentions. The excursions of each limb movement are wide, and the arm or leg may be driven with force against an object or the whole body swung around. Injuries are not uncommon. While these hyperkinetic movements cease during sleep, in acute cases they may occur virtually continuously throughout the day, and they are aggravated by external stimuli. *Physical examination* usually reveals the presence of a hemiparesis.

Causes: The commonest cause is a *vascular accident* with softening in the vicinity of the subthalamic nucleus. In such cases, a contralateral hemiballismus occurs immediately. Another cause is a *local space-occupying lesion* which also provokes hyperkinetic movements. Bilateral heredodegenerative ballismus is a rare cause.

Pathologic anatomy and pathophysiology: *Pathoanatomically,* hemiballismus is usually caused by a primary lesion of the contralateral subthalamic nucleus, and less often by secondary changes in this nucleus resulting from damage to structure to which it is connected, the corpus striatum and the globus pallidus. *Pathophysiologically,* such lesions abolish the regulating effect which the subthalamic nucleus exerts on the red nucleus. Consequently, uncontrolled impulses are transmitted in the rubrospinal tract to the anterior horn cells, producing a clinical picture of hemiballismus.

Treatment: Reserpine may be effective (895).

Dystonic Syndromes (11, 766, 1051)

Clinical picture: This group of diseases includes a number of *disturbances of movement,* in which individual muscles or muscle groups exhibit involuntary tonic contractions of variable duration. The disturbed timing of contraction and relaxation of the agonist and antagonist muscles, respectively, is a characteristic feature. These disturbances may

- either affect one muscle group only, over and over again, e.g., spastic torticollis or writer's cramp
- or exhibit a somewhat wider involvement, e.g., torsion dystonia (see also Table 1.**16**).

Physical findings: These are
- clearly involuntary movements, otherwise normal neurologic findings, or
- evidence of the underlying cause of the dystonia.

An attempt has been made in Table 1.**16** to define *individual forms of dystonia* from the etiologic viewpoint, and these forms will now be discussed.

Torsion Dystonias

Clinical findings: The clearly generalized form (11, 767) is characterized by prolonged and powerful, mainly rotatory movements of the head, trunk, and pelvic girdle. These are accompanied by movements of the extremities, particularly athetotic finger movements. The affected muscles give the appearance of being permanently contracted to overcome the resistance of the antagonists and to be causing the patient painful discomfort. The postures adopted, even if unusual and uncomfortable, are often maintained for a long time. Torsion dystonia is triggered by voluntary movements

and emotional factors and abolished by sleep. Muscle tone is often reduced and the joints are often overdistended. The patient gradually assumes a permanent dystonic posture which may be striking, e.g., an exaggerated lumbar lordosis with flexion of the hips and medial rotation of the arms and legs. The fingers are typically spread, the metacarpophalangeal joints being hyperextended and the interphalangeal joints being flexed (thalamic hand, see Fig. 1.**19**).

The *myostatic form of torsion dystonia* denotes those patients in whom no hyperkinesia remains but in whom an abnormal dystonic posture and markedly increased muscular tone are present.

Hereditary idiopathic torsion dystonias occur commonly in Jewish families, being inherited as an autosomal recessive disease. However, familial cases in non-Jews are also described, in which the inheritance is an autosomal dominant (11). The *initial clinical signs* usually appear in the 1st or 2nd decade, in two thirds of patients before the 15th year (767). At first only mild local movement disturbances are present (spastic torticollis, writer's cramp), but later the complete picture of torsion dystonia develops. When the disease begins in childhood, the first sign is usually a disturbance of gait, which may be difficult to interpret. Within 5–10 years, the picture progresses to an impressive generalized dystonia in three of four patients. If the disease begins in adulthood, the initial signs are often limited to the trunk and upper extremities; only about one-third develop the generalized form (767). A raised serum dopamine-beta-hydroxylase level has been described in familial cases (329). **Pathoanatomically,** changes are found in the putamen and other basal ganglia, in which the large ganglion cells are more severely damaged than the small cells.

Symptomatic torsion dystonias may be the clinical manifestation of an early Wilson's disease, Huntington's chorea, Hallervorden-Spatz disease, brain tumor, previous encephalitis, and especially epidemic encephalitis (p.50). A progressive dyskinesia may follow cerebral venous thrombosis (1129). A juvenile progressive dystonia has been described in a case of GM_2 gangliosidosis (786).

Progressive dystonia with marked daily variations has been described as a hereditary disease (908, 1096), which commences in childhood as a variable localized dystonia. While the signs vary widely from day to day, they intensify in the course of years. The disease responds well to L-dopa treatment.

Spastic Torticollis

Clinically, this is the commonest hyperkinetic extrapyramidal disease entity among the dystonias, being characterized by focal hyperactivity of the throat and neck muscles. Prolonged and apparently distressing movements occur, in which the head is slowly but powerfully rotated to one side in the course of several seconds, and simultaneously tilted to the same or the opposite side. Since the antagonist muscles are also contracted, the impression is clearly gained of two forces opposing one another, with the one slowly overcoming the other. The muscles mainly involved are the sternomastoid and the upper part of the trapezius (innervated by the 11th cranial nerve), and to a lesser extent other throat and neck muscles. Spastic torticollis affects men as frequently as women and may appear at any age, usually in mid-adulthood. If the activity is symmetric, the head may be tilted strongly backward (retrocollis). The commonest variety of the disease is *mobile torticollis,* but a permanent dystonic posture may be encountered, so-called *fixed torticollis,* which must be differentiated from congenital shortening of the neck muscles. Voluntary movements and emotion reduce the muscular hyperactivity, which may be abolished during sleep. Certain small maneuvers such as light pressure which the patient exerts on his chin may also suppress them. If blepharospasm and contracted facial muscles accompany the torticollis, Meige's syndrome may arise, see below. An unusually large proportion of patients with spastic torticollis have abnormal personalities.

Etiology: This is variable. Apart from the hereditary factor, a history of encephalitis is not infrequently present. Sometimes a spastic torticollis may be the presenting feature of a torsion, dystonia, Wilson's disease, or Huntington's chorea. It is a strikingly frequent complication of craniocerebral or neck trauma.

Pathologic anatomy: Spastic torticollis is always caused by a lesion of the corpus striatum, but the nature of the lesion varies.

Course: In about one-third of cases, the signs are intermittent, and in the remaining two-thirds either stationary or progressive, i.e., they alter in the direction of a torsion dystonia.

Differential diagnosis: Many cases turn out to be psychogenic tics. A stiff neck may mimic spastic torticollis, especially the fixed type. It may be due to congenital anomalies of the craniovertebral angle, contralateral trochlear palsy, syringomyelia or a high spinal tumor (621), or a cervical disk lesion.

Treatment: This is correspondingly difficult. If the spastic torticollis is neither a progressive nor a spontaneously regressive type, bilateral intraspinal rhizotomy of the sensory and motor roots of Cl-4 and the spinal accessory nerve is indicated. However, this procedure carries the risk of instability of head control. Success with stereotactic operations has been reported. Haloperidol treatment, see below. First results with a biofeedback treatment seem to be promising: the auditory and visual signals of the abnormal activity of the neck muscles provided by the EMG enable the patient to acquire voluntary control over his muscular activity (183). In localized forms, the injection of botulin toxin into the muscle involved may have a temporary effect (434, 531).

Localized Dystonic Syndromes

General observations: This term describes those cases in which the dystonic movements are restricted to one part of the body. Often they are missed because their dystonic nature is not recognized. Individual muscle groups may exhibit a tendency to ever-recurring tonic contractions which disturb normal voluntary movements and result in abnormal postures. Various parts of the body may be affected, particularly the shoulders, and the feet or legs during walking, or the hands during the execution of specific movements.

Writer's cramp is the commonest localized dystonia, the hand muscles being affected only when the patient tries to write (1105). It has recently been claimed that dystonic writer's cramp is caused by a chronic lesion of the median nerve as it traverses the fascia beneath the pronator teres muscle (634).

Dystonic movements of the mouth and tongue, usually transient, occur as side effects of various drugs, particularly the phenothiazine derivatives, see p.150. They may occur as a dramatic acute effect of the first dose, as well as oculogyric crises. So-called *faciobuccolingual dystonias* (or dyskinesias) occur in older subjects and may rarely indicate a midline lesion of the cerebellum. One such *oromandibular dystonic syndrome* (dystonic jaw and lip movements with forced opening and closing of the mouth and concomitant tongue movements) may be combined with **blepharospasm** (389a) and is described as **Brueghel's syndrome** (765) or *Meige's syndrome,* which may be familial (890). Not infrequently it is combined with a cervical dystonia (551). In these patients, usually elderly subjects, the picture may broaden into a true torsion dystonia. Exceptional cases of buccofacial dystonia may be associated with dental malocclusion, which requires odontologic treatment (1173). The differential diagnosis from spasmus nutans is discussed on p.367. Sandifer's syndrome (1261), a disease of infants including gastroesophageal reflux, sometimes manifests by dystonic movements such as torticollis.

Treatment of dystonic syndromes: Dystonias as well as choreoathetotic disturbances in rare cases may be abolished by stereotactic operation. The most useful drugs (1178) are those which produce as a side effect the parkinsonian syndrome (767), e.g., haloperidol (3-5 mg/day) or reserpine (0.5-3 mg t.i.d.). Buccolingual dystonias respond to tetrabenazine (25-200 mg/day). For the myostatic forms, treatment with L-dopa is advised (1282). The dystonias also respond to diazepam (1311) and high doses of bromocriptine (1143). Blepharospasm may respond to clonazepam, and also to local injection of botulin toxin into the orbicularis oculi muscle (531, 1094).

Other Extrapyramidal Diseases

Essential Tremor

Clinical aspects: Essential tremor does not differ in its mode of presentation from *familial tremor,* which is an inherited autosomal dominant disease. The incidence in a population group in the United States was 414 per 100000 (456). Always present is a tremor of the hands, occasionally also of the legs. Sometimes there is also pain in the legs, dyskinesia, and ataxia (259). In such combined forms and especially if these are progressive, other causes of the tremor should be considered, e.g., hepatolenticular degeneration (p.145). The tremor of the hands is present at rest and has a frequency of 5-9/s, and it is aggravated by excitement or attempts to maintain a particular position (e.g., holding a full glass in the hand). It usually starts early, often in the 1st decade of life (923). Often it is diminished by alcohol intake. Rarely the tremor may be unilateral. The cause is a loss of the small cells of the corpus striatum. A tremor similar to the idiopathic form appears to be common in men with extra X chromosomes

(94). In children who will later develop a familial tremor, *attacks of shivering* lasting only a few seconds occur early in life and may recur, but usually disappear during the 1st decade (1229). An increasing incidence of Parkinson's disease in patients, with essential or familial tremor was not observed by several authors (727, 1182) while others only found a clearly increased incidence of Parkinson in patients with essential tremor (409). Less commonly a (familial) nonprogressive *intention tremor* may be found without other signs of disease. In neonates, a *low serum magnesium level* may provoke attacks of tremor and epileptiform seizures. *Senile tremor* has a frequency of 4-5/s and appears at rest, involving the head and mandible as well as the hands.

Differential diagnosis of tremor: The distal rhythmic tremor of the parkinsonian syndrome must be considered, as well as toxic tremor forms such as alcoholic tremor (p.151) and other addictions, the fine-movement tremor of hyperthyroidism, the irregular gross tremor of liver disease including outstretched arms ("flapping tremor"; asterixis), etc.

Treatment of these tremors, particularly the essential and familial forms, involves the use of beta-receptor agents such as propranolol 20 mg, 3-6 × /day (1189), also pyridoxine 900-1200 mg i.m. (566), and primidone 750 mg or more/day.

Organic Tics

Organic tics may sometimes be difficult to differentiate from psychogenic tics, and their cause is poorly understood. Most cases of *blepharospasm* (p.124) are cases of organic tics, as well as other repetitive, nonrhythmic movements which are confined to specific muscle groups. The organic tic disease, *Gilles de la Tourette's syndrome* (now usually called Tourette syndrome) (387, 416, 690, 874), is a complicated psychomotor disturbance characterized by tic-like jerks affecting particularly the face and neck combined with compulsive acts, vocal tics, coprolalia, and the use of indecent language; the sufferers frequently are left-handed and show motor asymmetry. The syndrome has been described as a transient phenomenon following neuroleptic medication (1112). Another similar condition is the inherited disease described as the *"jumping Frenchman of Maine,"* in wich the patient executes sudden jumping movements when given a fright as well as echolalia and compulsive automatisms. Another familial condition is startle disease *(hyperexplexia),* which should not be confused with the noninherited disease of childhood discussed later. In this condition, the hyperexplexia is inherited as an autosomal dominant. Unexpected external stimulation in such patients provokes a severe generalized jerking or occasionally collapse to the ground without loss of consciousness. Children with the condition may show hypertonicity and hypokinesia. It is possible that this condition is related to the so-called *jerking stiff man syndrome* (23).

Electrophysiologically, testing of the somatosensory evoked potentials shows a marked C response 60–70 ms after peripheral nerve stimulation (763). *Jactatio capitis* (377), a rhythmic to-and-fro movement of the head, is a condition usually found in children and occurring only rarely in adults. It is seen most commonly when the child lies in the supine position. The cause is usually to be found in environmental influences, and psychotherapy is indicated.

Myoclonias

This term is used to describe nonrhythmic jerking movements of one or several muscles. The source is not necessarily to be found in the extrapyramidal system. The movements are particularly prone to occur in the overlap period between sleeping and waking, but also in the early phase of sleep, as harmless *sleeping jerks.* The myoclonia accompanying voluntary movements *(action myoclonus)* may be caused by an anoxic lesion (Lance-Adams syndrome); it is usually accompanied by cerebellar signs. Treatment with the following drugs is recommended: nitrazepam, primidone, or chlorpromazine, as well as L-5-hydroxytryptophan up to 750 mg combined with a decarboxylase inhibitor (1227). Valproate is also useful (1009).

Myorhythmias (772)

Myorhythmias are rhythmic, jerking movements always affecting the same muscle or group of muscles with the same frequency (1–3/s). They affect particularly the face (platysma, orbicularis oculi) and the throat muscles (rhythmic protrusion of the tongue). If the diaphragm is affected, hiccup may be persistent and troublesome *(hoquet diabolique)* in encephalitis, multiple sclerosis (741), after anesthesia or surgery, or even spontaneously. The condition is treated with methylphenidate (Ritalin) 20 mg i.v. (734) or isometheptene 100–200 mg slowly i.v. (819). Myorhythmias of the palate and palatal nystagmus, see p.79.

Other Forms

In the *myokymias,* the individual fibers of the muscle or muscle groups are involved in successive waves of contraction (e. g., facial myokymia, p. 360). Myokymias may follow gold therapy (816). Treatment is with phenytoin. *Paramyoclonus multiplex* is a condition of spontaneous irregular muscular contractions involving especially the shoulder muscles. *Myoclonic epilepsy* and *myoclonus epilepsy,* see p. 267–8. *Myoclonus multiplex fibrillare* or *chorea fibrillare* (Morvan's syndrome) (282) is the term used to describe irregularly timed, partial muscular contractions accompanied by pain, autonomic disturbances, and mental changes. Sometimes hallucinations, a troublesome insomnia, and occasionally excessive sweating may occur. It appears that the toxic effects of mercury salts probably play an etiologic role. Pathophysiologically, the condition appears to be caused by an inhibition of tryptophan hydroxylase. The condition usually regresses within months. *Infantile polymyoclonus* (323) consists of irregular dancing eye movements, myoclonus, ataxia, and irritability, which commence in childhood. The illness runs a steplike protracted course. It is caused by an anomaly of the IgG system and a CSF plasmacytosis is always present.

Cerebellar Syndromes

Cerebellar function: *The cerebellum*

- coordinates the action of individual muscle groups so that
- agonists, accessory muscles, and antagonists act in a fluent and precise way, and
- carry out purposeful, economic, and appropriate movements.

For this purpose, certain *anatomic and pathophysiologic preconditions* must be fulfilled.

- The cerebellum must receive constant "feedback" information about movements going on, and about movements intended.
- It must be able to effect corrections and modifications during each individual movement.

The cerebellum should also be viewed as a stabilizing control system, which

- receives forewarning of each motor impulse,
- evaluates each impulse in the light of the sensory "feedback" mechanism, and
- modifies or corrects this impulse.

Information about the position of the extremities and the activity of muscle groups is transmitted

- by the spinocerebellar tracts through the restiform body (inferior cerebellar peduncle) and partly
- through the brachium conjunctivum.
- Likewise, stimuli reach the cerebellum via the restiform body from the vestibular nuclei.
- The brachium pontis (middle cerebellar peduncle) transmits impulses from the cerebral cortex.

Efferent fibers pass

- along the brachium conjunctivum (superior cerebellar peduncle) from the cerebellar nuclei to the globus pallidus and ventrolateral nuclei of the thalamus on the opposite side.
- Other fibers pass to the red nucleus and then turn to the thalamus and pass via the rubrospinal tract caudally to the brainstem and spinal cord.

Symptomatology of cerebellar disorders: The clinical features of cerebellar diseases comprise a disturbance of the harmonious execution of voluntary movements including their normal tempo. The automatic coordination of the movement is disturbed. The principal signs and symptoms are named and defined below.

- *Dyssynergia:* Defective coordination of the various muscles and muscle groups participating in a movement (extending the trunk backward without simultaneous flexion of the knees, thus endangering balance; when the subject is on all fours, the limbs are not used in the regular crossed order).
- *Dysmetria:* Absence of the appropriate amplitude and tempo for an intended movement (exaggerated splaying of the fingers to grasp small objects; the leg is lifted too high when the patient, with his eyes shut, attempts to put his foot on a chair).
- *Ataxia:* Muscle groups no longer contract harmoniously to execute a movement (finger to nose and heel to shin tests carried out with

to-and-fro deviation of the limb from the ideal course).

- *Intention tremor:* Increasing deviation from the ideal pathway as the patient tries to carry out a particular movement. This is the case when the dentate nucleus or its efferent fibers are involved (observed in finger-nose test, see Fig. 1.20, heel to shin test, or finger-finger test).
- *Pathologic rebound phenomenon:* The antagonists fail to counter overshoot movements promptly, i.e., the flexor muscles of the elbow when contracted against the resistance of the examiner's hand continue to contract if the hand is suddenly removed. An example is shown in Fig. 1.21.
- *Impairment of rapid alternating movements:* Rapid alternation of the action of agonist and antagonist muscles can no longer be promptly and fluently carried out: rapid pronation and supination of the forearm (Fig. 1.22), rapid tapping of the thigh alternately with the palm and the back of the hand (dysdiadochokinesia).
- *Hypotonia:* During passive movements (passive shaking of an extremity; excessive arm swing if the erect patient is shaken by the shoulders or rotated back and forth on his own axis).
- *Fall-away in positional testing:* The patient's muscular tone is inadequate to maintain the appropriate posture and, when the eyes are shut, the outstretched arm on the side of the lesion falls away slowly.
- *Deviation in Bárány's pointing test:* When the arm is raised, a

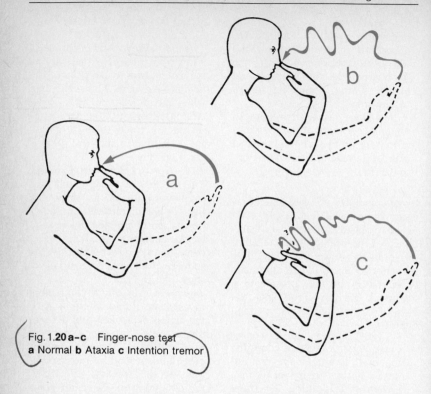

Fig. 1.**20 a–c**   Finger-nose test
a Normal **b** Ataxia **c** Intention tremor

finger is aimed at a point in front of the patient, and the arm on the side of the lesion is then lowered with the eyes closed, it tends to drop away to the side of the lesion.

- *Unsteady posture* (in Romberg test).
- *Truncal ataxia* when seated.
- *Unsteady, broad-based gait,* described by the patient as "dizziness" but not representing a true rotatory vertigo.
- *Nystagmus:* In cerebellar lesions a coarse nystagmus is present toward the side of the lesion, which increases when gaze is directed toward this side and diminishes when the eyes are closed.
- *Speech disturbance:* Staccato explosive speech.

There is a topical representation of individual body parts in the cerebellum. Specific cerebellar regions possess specific functions. Thus, individual signs may possess a **localizing significance:**

- in basal and midline lesions: a disturbance of truncal posture and equilibrium, especially when the patient is seated;

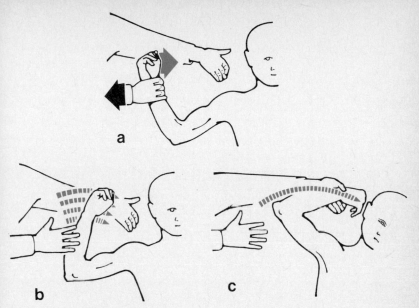

Fig. 1.**21 a–c**   Testing the rebound phenomenon in cerebellar disorders. **a** Technique of examination **b** Normal reaction with prompt control upon release **c** Abnormal rebound phenomenon with insufficient control in ipsilateral cerebellar lesions

- in lesions of the rostral part of the midline: disturbances of coordination involving stance and gait;
- in lateral lesions (cerebellar hemispheres): incoordination and lack of dexterity of movement of the ipsilateral extremities.

CT and MR scanning enable focal cerebellar lesions including infratentorial atrophic processes to be visualized.

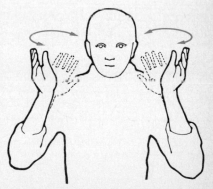

Fig. 1.**22**   The test for diadochokinesis. This sign is elicited by rapid pronation and supination of the hands

Table 1.17 Diseases with Predominantly Cerebellar Symptomatology

Onset	Disease	Age of Patient	Details
Hours	Psychogenic ataxia	Teenagers and young adults	Identifiable signs elicited by their various examination tests
Hours	Acute cerebellar hematoma	Any age	Especially hypertensives. Intense headache, increasing drowsiness and signs of raised intracranial pressure
Days	Acute cerebellar ataxia of childhood	1st decade of life	After nonspecific prodromal illness. Prognosis usually favorable
Days	Miller Fisher syndrome	Any age	Mostly young adults, especially men. Abnormal eye movements and absent reflexes. A good prognosis invariable
Days	Multiple sclerosis	Young adults	A history of other preceding bouts of illness is usually present, only rarely are they the first signs of MS. Tendency to regress
Days	Poisoning	Any age	e.g., DDT, diphenylhydantoin, organic mercury salts, piparazine, 5-fluorouracil
Hours to days (intermittent)	Hartnup disease, pyruvate dehydrogenase deficiency	Early childhood	Autosomal recessive. Additional choreoathetotic signs
Hours to days (intermittent)	Familial episodic ataxia	Any age	Usually autosomal dominant. Ataxia, dysarthria, nystagmus. Responds to acetazolamide
Hours to days (intermittent)	Multiple sclerosis	Young adults	Attacks of dysarthria, tonic brainstem attacks. Responds to carbamazepine
Months	Symptomatic progressive cerebellar atrophy	Any age	e.g., paraneoplastic disease

Months	Myxedema	Any age	Other signs of severe thyroid deficiency are invariably present
Weeks	Cerebellar tumor	Especially children	Raised intracranial pressure
Weeks	Encephalopathia myoclonica infantilis	First years of life	Rapidly progressive ataxia with myoclonic signs and opsoclonus. Seen in neuroblastomas. May regress
Months to years	Hereditary cerebellar ataxia	Any age	Family history. Gradual progression. Often other progressive neurologic signs are present, e.g., nystagmus, spasticity, optic atrophy
Months to years	Atrophie cérébelleuse tardive à prédominance corticale	4th and 5th decades of life	Increasingly severe uncertainty of gait, and less frequently nystagmus. Truncal ataxia. No hereditary factor
Months to years	Olivopontocerebellar atrophy	3rd to 5th decades of life	Ataxia, tremor, parkinsonian signs, and urinary incontinence leading to dementia. ½ are familial

Clinical Aspects of Some Cerebellar Disorders

General: In individual cases of cerebellar disorder, the clinical classification – and sometimes also etiologic classification – is based on the speed of appearance of the cerebellar signs and symptoms, upon details concerning them, and upon associated neurologic deficits. A classification based on such criteria is given in Table 1.17. The most important cerebellar affections will be described below, while other disease entities exhibiting cerebellar signs and symptoms included in Table 1.17 will be specified in other sections.

Acute Cerebellar Ataxia of Childhood (377)

About one-half of these cases follow a nonspecific preceding illness. Children aged 2–5 years are most commonly affected. The condition has a subacute onset, with a course of increasingly ataxic gait, tremor, nystagmus, and disturbances of external ocular movement. About two-thirds of cases recover completely within weeks or months. A small proportion may continue to show unsteady gait and ataxia for many years. It is not known if the condition is a simple encephalitis. The transient ataxia encountered in Fisher's syndrome is discussed on p. 298.

Intoxications with Cerebellar Signs

Several poisonous substances may within days produce a cerebellar syndrome which is, as a rule, completely reversible. They include DDT, organic mercury, piperazine, the mitotic inhibitor 5-fluorouracil, and phenytoin. However, the last-named drug may cause persisting cerebellar signs (73), commonly in female patients and in individuals with preexisting cerebellar lesions (p. 149).

Cerebellar Heredoataxias of Known Etiopathogenesis (105, 479, 1016)

A variety of systemic degenerations show a predilection to involve the cerebellum (105, 436, 476, 479). In several of these, the pathologic mechanism is known. The best known of these are *α-betalipoproteinemia* (Bassen-Kornzweig syndrome) (p. 140), *hexosaminidase deficiency, glutamate dehydrogenase deficiency* (663, 954, 955), and *pyruvate dehydrogenase deficiency* (599).

Disturbance of the mechanism of DNA synthesis underlies *xeroderma pigmentosum* (1002), which tends to be heralded by cerebellar signs, and *Cockayne's syndrome* (398, 1125), in which hearing difficulty may predominate. *Ataxia telangiectasia* (Louis-Bar syndrome) (1043), a recessive hereditary lesion, presents as a cerebellar ataxia in children and is slowly progressive so that the patient is disabled before he reaches adolescence. Choreoathetotic disturbances are sometimes present. The telangiectatic lesions usually appear later, first in the conjunctiva and then in other parts of the body, especially the skin folds. Pulmonary and upper respiratory infections are common; the eye movements are strikingly slowed. Histopathologic study shows lesions to be present in Purkinje's and granular cells, but no vascular anomalies are described in the cerebellum. A defect of the IgA system is present, the disease belongs to the group of syndromes with increased chromosomal fragility and higher neoplastic potential (137). The *Rett syndrome* comprises a progressive ataxia found only in girls, associated with autism, dementia, and loss of purposeful use of their hands (457).

Several hereditary cerebellar ataxias with known etiopathogenesis present with **signs of intermittent ataxia.** They include *Hartnup disease, pyruvate dehydrogenase deficiency* (599), and other syndromes. Included in this group is a *familial periodic ataxia* of which the pathologic mechanism has not yet been clarified (304, 437, 1287). The sufferers from childhood experience episodes of ataxia lasting hours or days which may recur at about weekly intervals. The attacks consist of ataxia, dysarthria, nystagmus, and vertigo. Between attacks, only the mildest of cerebellar signs and symptoms may be present. Most cases are inherited as autosomal dominants (1287). Acetazolamide prevents the attacks.

Cerebellar Heredoataxias of Unknown Etiopathogenesis
(105, 479)

In most of the heredoataxias in this group, a disturbance of amino-acid metabolism is the most likely cause (1016). Reports in the literature describing individual *families* differ in specific detail from each other so that no uniform clinical picture can be defined. Those cases in whom the ataxia commences in the 1st or 2nd years of life show an autosomal recessive pattern of inheritance, while those with a later onset (up to the 7th decade) are usually autosomal dominants. The clinical picture is characterized mainly by a progressive ataxia. Later on, muscular hypertonicity, paralysis, and atrophy may develop, as well as pyramidal signs, disturbances of external ocular mobility, nystagmus, optic atrophy, and dementia. The disease has a slowly progressive course, extreme cases surviving for several decades. Histopathologic examination shows degeneration of various cerebellar nuclei and cortex, as well as atrophy of the long spinal tracts. The *Marinesco-Sjögren syndrome* consists of cerebellar ataxia, congenital cataract, and mental deficiency.

Olivopontocerebellar atrophy (110, 436, 1248) is a disease which appears as commonly in a familial form as sporadically. Usually it manifests in middle age; only occasionally does it present earlier and may be fatal in 1–4 years. Ataxia, tremor, and disturbances of speech and gait are prominent features, as well as the characteristic parkinsonian signs of rigidity and akinesia, and often a disturbance of urination. Occasionally the patient may be demented. Histopathologic study shows destruction of the cells of the cerebellar cortex and nuclei, and atrophy involving the ganglia of the pons and the olives. Cellular degeneration of the substantia nigra and locus ceruleus may also be found. In individual cases, glutamate dehydrogenase deficiency has been demonstrated (955, 1016). The Menzel type is an autosomal dominant form which on the average has its onset at the age of 35 years (14–73), and has a duration of 12.5 years (519). In this type occasionally also additional symptoms such as chorea retinopathy, and optic atrophy occur. The Dejerine-Thomas type is sporadic, possibly autosomal dominant, has a later onset, age 50 years (17–65), and is more rapidly progressive over 6.5 years (1–18). Disturbance of autonomic regulation, orthostatic hypotonia, impotence, and a supranuclear gaze paresis may be additional findings.

Cerebello-olivary atrophy of the Holmes type is usually autosomal dominantly inherited, starts on the average at age 46 years (10–70), and has a duration of 17 years. Spasticity, dementia, and urinary incontinence may be part of the clinical presentation. *Dyssynergia cerebellaris progressiva (Ramsay-Hunt syndrome)* is difficult to differentiate clearly from myoclonus epilepsy (p. 268). The syndrome is characterized by myoclonic jerks which are aggravated by intention movements, typical cerebellar signs (indicating involvement of a cerebellar hemisphere), occasionally cerebellospinal signs such as absent reflexes, and epileptic attacks. However, in contrast to myoclonic epilepsy, there is no dementia. The disease is progressive over the course of years, not infrequently it is familial. The pathologic appearances vary greatly – the lesions resemble those of Friedreich's ataxia, involving especially the dentate nucleus, superior cerebellar peduncles, and the red nucleus, as well as sometimes the cerebellar cortex.

Systemic Nonheritable Cerebellar Affections

Late onset cerebellar cortical atrophy, or *„atrophie cérébelleuse tardive à prédominance corticale"* as the condition was described by Marie, Foix, and Alajouanine, is a nonheritable cerebellar disease involving the paleocerebellum symmetrically; the vermis shows more marked changes than the hemispheres. The histologic picture shows a marked reduction in the number of Purkinje's cells, as well as the granule cells. The primary degenerative form commences in middle age (average age, 47 years); the onset is usually rapid and the course is slowly progressive. Initially, the most striking features are the insecurity of gait, truncal ataxia upon walking or sitting, and uncertainty in the use of the hands. Rarely, nystagmus is found, sometimes muscular hypotonia, and pyramidal signs. The patient's mental state is usually unaffected and his life expectancy is not shortened. Primary degenerative forms exist which are due to focal process of premature aging (476).

Diffuse cerebellar atrophy may be the symptomatic reflection of quite different etiologic diseases. Initially, a picture similar to that of the late onset cerebellar cortical atrophy described above may be found; only the course of the disease gives rise to suspicion regarding the primary cause. For example, the late *cerebellar atrophy of chronic alcoholism* (p. 151) may resemble closely the picture of late onset cerebellar cortical atrophy. *Subacute cerebellar cortical atrophy as a paraneoplastic manifestation* will be described later (p.156). *Encephalopathia myoclonica infantilis* (Kinsbourne) is viewed as a separate syndrome, in which about 50% of cases is a paraneoplastic manifestation due to neuroblastoma in children (163). At the age of a few months or within the first few years of life, the picture appears of myoclonic contractions of varying severity, irregular eyeball dyskinesia, and opsoclonus (p.343). The child is often irritable, later he may become demented. The EEG shows no epileptic discharges. After treatment of the neuroblastoma or after ACTH administration in nontumor cases, the signs and symptoms may disappear completely.

Kuru is a disease found in New Guinea, more often in young women, who present a picture of ataxic gait, shivering, other cerebellar signs, and dementia, which ends fatally within months or years. The disease appears to be caused by a slow virus transmitted by cannibalism.

Other Cerebellar Syndromes

One of the cerebellar syndromes caused by *infectious diseases* is that found in infectious mononucleosis (465). *Macroglobulinemia* may present, in addition to polyneuropathy (p.314), as progressive cerebellar ataxia, which disappears with successful treatment of the primary disease (1130). *Myxedema* may commence with various neurologic symptoms including cerebellar signs (470). *Adult sprue,* although more commonly accompanied by polyneuropathies and spinal cord degeneration (p.317), may show a cerebellar picture including palatal nystagmus (363), sometimes before the intestinal symptoms become manifest. *Heat stroke* may cause irreversible cerebellar signs. *Cerebellar tumors* (p.33), which are diagnosed by their focal signs and symptoms and evidence of raised intracranial pressure, will not be discussed further in this section.

A condition not to be confused with cerebellar disease is so-called *bedrest ataxia,* a condition of unsteadiness and insecurity of movements encountered in persons who have been bedridden for a long time. *Optic ataxia* describes a severe degree of clumsiness in grasping or holding objects which is part of the picture of a bilateral lesion severing the connections between the visual cortex and the motor cortex (147).

Metabolic Disorders Involving the Brain

Biochemical progress has revealed an increasingly large number of brain diseases caused by metabolic anomalies. The majority are inherited enzyme defects (11, 943, 1016). For example, these defects may result in storage of metabolic by-products in the CNS as well as elsewhere in the body. Concerning the cerebral metabolism of the commonest early-life brain affections, the situation may be simplified by stating that wherever phospholipids and gangliosides are accumulated, these substances are laid down in the cell bodies and the synapses. This produces *neuronal disturbances* which soon provoke dementia, convulsions, and visual abnormalities. Later on, spasticity and ataxia may appear. By contrast, whenever sulfatides or cerebrosides are accumulated, the picture of a *disturbance of myelination* appears (see below), in which pyramidal signs such as spasticity and ataxia are initally present; only later do dementia and convulsions occur. Only the commonest and most fundamental metabolic disturbances have been chosen for discussion below. These diseases may be classified according to metabolic defect (943) or clinical age of onset (11).

Disturbances of Lipid Metabolism
(11, 558, 943, 949, 1016)

Gaucher's Disease

This is one of the glucoceramidoses, caused by a defect of glucocerebroside beta-glucosidase. It results in the accumulation of cerebrosides, in which the galactose part of the kerasin is replaced by glucose in the cells of the reticulohistocytic system (Gaucher's cells). The disease is transmitted as an autosomal recessive. The adult forms are characterized by hepatosplenomegaly and deposits in the bones; however, evidence of CNS involvement (extrapyramidal signs and mental disturbances) is exceptional. In the infantile forms, the above-mentioned features are accompanied by a progressive spasticity of all limbs, bulbar signs, external ocular palsies, and mental retardation. Gaucher's cells are found in different parts of the body, including the brain. Involvement of the peripheral nervous system in the form of a polyneuropathy may be demonstrated by electronmicroscopic examination of sural nerve biopsy material and electrophysiologic analysis.

Angiokeratoma Corporis Diffusum

This X-chromosomal inherited anomaly, Fabry's disease (569, 871, 1016), is another glucoceramidosis, based on a defect of ceramide trihexosidase which leads to deposition of the glycolipids, di- and trihexoglyceramide, in various bodily cells and tissues. The deposits are prominent in the skin, autonomic ganglia, brainstem, posterior root ganglia, hypophysis, smooth muscles of blood vessels, myocardium, renal tubules, and glomeruli. The clinical symptoms and signs are caused either by the deposits in the cells or their effect on the vascular system. Burning pains in the limbs are nearly always present early in adolescence, as well as absent sweat secretion. Patients respond to phenytoin (713). Cerebrovascular accidents are frequent. The striking histologic abnormality is a loss of unmyelinated and thinly myelinated nerve fibers (1109). Occasionally heterozygous carriers may exhibit clinical signs, e.g., ataxia, tinnitus, pyramidal signs, and bladder disturbances (130). The diagnosis is made by examination of urinary glycolipid or estimation of the alpha-galactosidase in white cells.

Gangliosidoses

An additional glucoceramidosis was originally designated *amaurotic familial idiocy* (Tay-Sachs disease). It is caused, depending on the type, by a defect of the beta-galactosidase (GM_1 gangliosidosis) or the hexosaminidase A (GM_2 gangliosidosis).

The disease is characterized by a deposition of gangliosides exclusively within the nervous system. The ganglion cells become ballooned, the glial cells proliferate and have a foamy cytoplasm, and the myelin sheaths are partially destroyed. Ganglioside deposition in the retina imparts a whitish tint which makes the normal fovea appear as a cherry red spot. The absence of hexosaminidase can be confirmed by examination of the hair roots (524). A rare *congenital form* is known. The *infantile form* presents in the 1st year of life as apathy, hypotonia, and lack of normal movements. An initial absence of reflexes gives way to generalized spasticity with increased reflexes, gradual blindness, dementia, marasmus, and death within 2–3 years. The *late infantile form* commences at 2–4 years of age and lasts 3–4 years. The *juvenile form* appears between the 5th and 10th years and also leads to death, usually before the age of 20. Speech disturbances, visual defects including blindness, increasing apathy, extrapyramidal signs and athetotic movements, cerebellar signs, pyramidal signs, and convulsive attacks may occur. This form of disease affects non-Jewish children. The *late form* begins after puberty. In beta-hexosaminidase A deficiency — occurring mainly in Jewish families – a GM_2 gangliosidosis predominates, presenting with progressive **spinocerebellar signs and symptoms** which may be difficult to differentiate from Friedreich's ataxia (1278).

Niemann-Pick Disease

This disease belongs to the phosphoryl-ceramidoses caused by sphingomyelinase deficiency. An excessive accumulation of sphingomyelin occurs, but it is not yet clear which is responsible – excessive production, faulty breakdown, or a stereochemical anomaly of the type of sphingomyelin produced. The disease is usually inherited as a recessive, commonly in patients of Jewish extraction. All tissues may store the substance. Neurologic signs occur only in the infantile form. The child exhibits a progressive mental retardation, and an initial spasticity is followed by hypotonia and absent reflexes. Later, there is blindness (in about one-fourth a cherry red macular spot occurs as in amaurotic idiocy), as well as deafness. The children die from cachexia between the age of 6 months and 3 years.

Heredopathia Atactica Polyneuritiformis (Refsum's Disease) (601, 983)

This is a congenital defect of lipid metabolism inherited as an autosomal recessive anomaly. The formation of phytanic acid is prevented by a defect of alpha-oxidation (phytanic acid alpha-hydroxylase deficiency), resulting in the deposition of tetramethylhexadecanoic acid. Symptoms and signs of the disease appear in the 1st and 2nd decades of life. Apart from skeletal anomalies, ichthyosis of the skin, and cardiac signs, retinitis pigmentosa, progressive hearing loss, polyneuropathy and cerebellar signs, especially ataxia, may be found. The albumin content of the CSF is always increased. Appropriate dietary measures including the omission of fruit, vegetables, and butter from the diet, and the reduction in the intake of animal fats, reduce the levels of phytanic acid and CSF albumin and may abolish some of the clinical signs and symptoms (983).

A-Lipoproteinemias

The first of these diseases is α-β-lipoproteinemia, the *Bassen-Kornzweig syndrome*. It is associated with acanthocytosis and may be accompanied by progressive CNS symptomatology such as ataxia and absent reflexes, occasionally with pyramidal signs (31); differentiation from Friedreich's ataxia or even multiple sclerosis may be difficult. Another entity belonging to this group is a *hypo-β-lipoproteinemia,* an atactic syndrome with signs of a polyneuropathy but without acanthocytosis (17). A third entity, *acanthocytosis with normal serum β-lipoprotein levels,* may be inherited as an autosomal recessive disease which is characterized by biting of the tongue, signs of polyneuropathy, choreiform disturbances of movement, and raised serum creatine kinase levels. The disease picture is also known as choreoacanthocytosis (1052). The an-α-lipoproteinemia, *Tangier disease* (enormous speckled tonsils, splenic tumor, and foam cells), is only rarely accompanied by a polyneuropathy.

Disturbances of Protein and Urea Metabolism

These enzyme abnormalities lead to an accumulation of amino acids.

Pyruvic Acid (Phenylpyruvic) Oligophrenia (11)

This recessive hereditary disease is caused by defective oxidation of phenylalanine to tyrosine. Since the latter substance is the precursor of melanin, the patient has blond hair and shows a partial absence of skin pigmentation. The breakdown of excessive phenylalanine to pyruvic acid leads to the excretion of the latter in the urine: its presence may be demonstrated by the ferric chloride test. The main clinical feature of the disease is progressive dementia, which is accompanied by increased muscular tone and epileptiform attacks. The brain damage occurs in the 1st year of life and appears to cease after brain maturation is complete. For this reason, early treatment with a phenylalanine-poor diet is vitally important.

Maple Syrup Urine Disease

This disease, a disturbance of valine, leucine, and isoleucine metabolism, also presents as an increasingly severe dementia. It is caused by a defect of branched chain keto acid decarboxylase. The patient's urine has a characteristic smell.

Hartnup Disease (11, 1183)

This disease, apparently inherited as an autosomal recessive anomaly, is a disturbance of tubular resorption and intestinal transport of amino acids, although the precise enzyme abnormality is not clear. An amino aciduria is present, particularly for alanine, tryptophan, and histidine. The clinical picture consists of attacks of pellagra-like dermatosis accompanied by episodes of ataxia, gait disturbance, and nystagmus, as well as a progressive dementia and spasticity. Histologic study shows a destruction of cortical ganglion cells and Purkinje's cells.

Encephalopathy with Fatty Infiltration of Viscera
(Reye's Syndrome)

This disease is **etiologically** unclear (39, 226, 229, 261). In certain cases, a deficiency of ornithine transcarbamylase is present (1094); in others, a carnitine deficiency plays a part (226). The cause of the syndrome appears to be multifactorial, and animal experiments point to a combined effect of viruses and insecticides (261). **Clinically,** children aged between a few months and 8 years are affected. After nonspecific prodromal signs, an acute picture appears consisting of vomiting, delirium, and coma, sometimes with convulsions. Pyramidal signs are present, later a picture of decortication. The liver is enlarged and hard to palpation. Frequently hypoglycemia and increased serum transaminase and ammonia levels are present. There may be a terminal jaundice. The CSF is normal or shows a diminished glucose content, but the liver function tests are abnormal with increased urea levels. **Pathoanatomic** study reveals neuronal degeneration but no evidence of inflammation. The enlarged, yellowish liver shows periportal infiltration with lipids, mainly triglycerides, and the renal tubules and heart are similarly infiltrated. Glycogen is virtually absent, and this finding prompts the possibility of **treatment** with ornithine or arginine (1194).

Disturbances of Carbohydrate Metabolism

Gargoyle Group

Dysostosis multiplex (Hurler's disease) (11) is mentioned to represent this group. It is characterized by a deposition of mucopolysaccharides in the connective tissues, periosteum, cartilaginous tissues, and walls of blood vessels, as well as of hexosamine-free ganglioside in the brain. The disease has an autosomal and occasionally a recessive autosomal pattern of transmission. The clinical picture manifests early, usually in the 1st or 2nd years of life, as dwarfism with various skeletal anomalies and grotesque deformity of the facial skeleton. Mental retardation progresses to dementia. Occasionally extrapyramidal abnormalities are present, as well as disturbances of hearing and vision.

Glycogenoses

In *Pompe's disease* (p. 495), cerebral involvement may be present. In *myoclonic epilepsy* (Unverricht-Lundborg), there is an abnormal accumulation of mucopolysaccharides, especially in the brain (p. 268). *Subacute necrotizing encephalomyelopathy* (Leigh) exhibits a progressive dementia, rolling eye movements, and cachexia, and leads to death. In the more frequent familial infantile form of the disease (probably autosomal recessive), the blood pyruvate and lactate levels are elevated. The less common, sporadic form which affects adolescents and adults, shows a subacute development with focal features including brainstem signs. Histologic study shows multiple foci of necrosis and glial proliferation in the basal ganglia, hypothalamus, brainstem, cerebellum, and spinal cord (1114).

Intermittent Disturbances of Glucose Metabolism

Clinical aspects of hypoglycemic states (186, 754): The symptomatology does not vary among the different etiologic forms: *disturbances of consciousness* (coma with sweating, pyramidal signs) lasting from 30 min to hours, *focal neurologic signs* with upper motor neuron weakness persisting after the coma, double vision, unsteady gait, and *epileptic attacks*. Apart from grand mal seizures, dreamy states and periods or agitation are particularly common, and may last for several days. Simple and complex myoclonias including jacksonian attacks have been described (186). These attacks tend to occur during those periods of the day when the blood sugar level is lowest, but they may be provoked by food intake itself and therefore manifest postprandially, especially in children. The EEG not infrequently shows, apart from a diffuse generalized disturbance, an abnormal focus which is usually in the temporal lobe and persists after the attacks. The most important diagnostic test is estimation of the blood sugar level during an attack and provocation of an attack by means of food deprivation. In addition to the transient clinical attacks, permanent neurologic deficits occur, particularly mono- or hemiplegias, hemianopsias, rigidity, progressive muscular atrophies which clinically may resemble amyotrophic lateral sclerosis, and finally dementia.

Causes of hypoglycemia: The following should be mentioned: *transient hypoglycemia of the neonate* (diabetic mother, hypothermia, after respiratory distress). Isolated attacks may be provoked by *leucine,* an additive to nutritive protein. Similarly, enzymopathies may lead to hypoglycemic attacks (glycogenoses, galactosemia, fructose intolerance, disturbed glycogenesis). *Specific drugs* may induce a hypoglycemic state (salicylate, paracetamol, antihistaminics), and especially the use of insulin and sulfonylurea. Under certain circumstances *glucose* may provoke hypoglycemia, as in the late dumping syndrome and in the early phase of adult diabetes. *Islet cell adenoma* may lead to severe hypoglycemia, simply as a result of beta-cell hyperplasia, but in a small percentage as a result of pancreatic adenocarcinoma (186). *Other endocrine diseases* occasionally lead to hypoglycemia (adrenal insufficiency, anterior pituitary insufficiency, and hypothyroidism). Poorly nourished *alcoholics* may become hypoglycemic 3-12 h after alcohol intake. Specific *liver diseases* and rarely also large *retroperitoneal tumors* (neurofibromatosis) may occasionally be accompanied by hypoglycemia. Rare causes are fasting, malignancy, enteritis, or myxedema. Diabetes mellitus (insulin), alcoholism or sepsis are responsible in 90% of the cases (754).

Treatment is surgical if an insulinoma is present; otherwise, frequent carbohydrate meals and sometimes corticosteroids are advised, in addition to preventive measures in the case of the exogenous causes and treatment of the underlying diseases mentioned above.

Leukodystrophies, Including Those Still Unexplained, and Other Metabolic Diseases

General remarks: The demyelinating diseases (leukodystrophies, lipodystrophies of the myelin sheaths) (11, 558, 949, 1016, 1216) have only been partly explained with regard to their biochemistry. Clinical suspicion should always be aroused by the combination of an increasing disturbance of motor development, progressive spasticity, visual disturbances, and a slowly progressive mental retardation. The diagnosis depends upon biochemical tests, including the identification both of products of myelin breakdown and of the enzyme defect (932). CT and MR scanning may provide useful clues to type diagnosis (1260).

Metachromatic Leukodystrophy

This disease is caused by the deposition of sulfatides in the CNS and peripheral nerves, as well as elsewhere and especially the kidneys. The diagnosis is reached by measuring the conduction velocity in a peripheral nerve by nerve biopsy and by demonstrating metachromatic substances and a reduced arylsulfatase A level in the urine. Infantile, juvenile, and adult forms are recognized. The disease, which is inherited as a recessive, may be heralded by pes cavus and muscular hypotonia. Later on, spastic quadriparesis with pyramidal signs develops. The CSF protein level is raised early. The disease runs a fatal course within a few years.

Alexander's Disease
(384, 865, 1243)

The cause of this early childhood disease is poorly understood. It presents as a loss of acquired motor development,

mental deterioration, epileptic attacks, and macrocephaly. Histologic study reveals a characteristic picture of destruction of the cerebral white matter, especially in the frontal lobes, and the presence of Rosenthal fibers which are by-products of glial cell destruction (384). Only rarely does the disease present in adulthood (1243).

Globoid Cell Leukodystrophy
(Krabbe's Disease)

Further examples of glucoceramidoses are cerebroside sulfatidosis (Scholz's disease with arylsulfatase A deficiency) and galactocerebrosidosis. The latter disease appears usually in the 1st and sometimes in the 2nd year of life and runs a rapidly fatal course. The initial picture of spastic paralysis with pyramidal signs and rigidity gives way to pseudobulbar signs, ataxia, increasing dementia, and finally a decerebrate picture. Histologic study reveals the abnormal substances, cerebrosides, deposited in the CNS, being particularly abundant in multinucleated giant cells (globoid cells) in the demyelinated areas.

Degenerative Diffuse Sclerosis of the Neutral Fat Type (1058)

This entity is so similar clinically to metachromatic leukodystrophy that the diagnosis can only be made histochemically by the demonstration of sudanophilic lipids and the absence of metachromasia in the white matter. The disease is inherited as a sex-linked recessive abnormality and progresses to death within months or years with increasing mental deterioration, neurologic deficit, and epileptic attacks.

Pelizaeus-Merzbacher Disease
(Chronic Infantile Cerebral Sclerosis)

This disease, inherited as an autosomal recessive abnormality, appears to be caused by a disturbance of glyceryl phosphatide metabolism in the myelin sheaths (1216). It manifests in the 1st year of life, with the picture of tremor, cerebellar ataxia, nystagmus, and visual disturbances. Later, an increasing spastic paraparesis develops, as well as disturbances of speech and dementia. The disease usually runs a fatal course within a few years; rarely, it may extend over several decades.

Batten-Kufs Disease (215)

This name is given to a group of genetically determined metabolic disorders. Their common feature is the deposition of histochemically and ultrastructurally characteristic abnormal autofluorescent material in the cell bodies of ganglion cells, as well as in cells of the skin, muscles, and gastric mucous membrane. The specific properties of the biochemical substance have not yet been clearly defined, but they resemble the pigments of age; therefore, the title *ceroid lipofuscinosis* has been suggested. The infantile and late infantile forms (Jansky-Bielschowsky) usually become manifest between the ages of 1 and 3½ years, with epileptic attacks, retinal degeneration, and psychomotor deterioration; death follows within a few years. Occasionally the onset may be delayed to adolescence (Spielmeyer-Vogt) or adulthood (Kufs). Hallervorden-Spatz disease, see p.121.

Adrenoleukodystrophy (831)

This is a sex-linked, recessively inherited abnormality which affects boys in the first 2 decades of life. Usually it presents as a picture of mental changes, disturbance of gait, visual loss, dysarthria, and an increasing spastic quadriparesis. While the young patients exhibit only mild evidence of adrenal insufficiency, adults may present as cases of adrenal insufficiency accompanied by mild spastic paraparesis (195, 449). The clinical picture includes epileptic attacks, personality change, and paraparesis. Histologic evidence can be shown of demyelination of the corticospinal and spinocerebellar tracts. A diet low in long-chain fatty acids slows progression of the condition.

Diffuse Cerebral Sclerosis (Schilder) (Diffuse Periaxial Encephalitis)

Several of the conditions described above and a few mentioned elsewhere were previously grouped under this term. However, very few genuine cases are encountered which correspond to Schilder's original description of a disease commencing in childhood or adolescence and possessing a progressive or episodic course, characterized by dementia, hemi- or tetraplegia, pseudobulbar signs, cortical blindness, and deafness. The CSF shows changes similar to multiple sclerosis. Focal areas of demyelination are found which sometimes involve an entire lobe and show secondary proliferation of glial fibers and corresponding tissue sclerosis. Perhaps Balò's sclerosis (p.253) belongs to this entity. Death supervenes within months or years.

Disturbances of Copper Metabolism

Normally copper is absorbed from the intestine in minute quantities, 98% of the serum copper being bound to an alpha-2-globulin, ceruloplasmin (normal 200–350 mg/l). A small proportion is bound to serum albumin and represents the active transport fraction in tissue metabolism. A disturbance may theoretically occur in the event of inadequate intake of copper, disturbed absorption from the intestine or, most likely, reduced availability of the copper-transporting protein ceruloplasmin.

Hepatolenticular Degeneration
(Wilson's Disease,
Westphal-Strümpell
Pseudosclerosis) (11, 301)

This disease is the most important disturbance of copper metabolism. **Clinically,** it is characterized by increasing tremor of the hands, commonly a truncal tremor, and shaking of the head. The tremor of the arms is the principal sign: commencing either as a resting tremor or as an intention tremor, it increases if the arms are outstretched sideways and may then assume a characteristic appearance. This picture of a distally accentuated irregular retention of resting muscular tone leads to a movement of the arms which is described as akathisia, "wing-beating" or "flapping tremor." This sign may be encountered in other afflictions, e.g., portocaval encephalopathy (see p. 162), focal thalamic or parietal lesions (358). These shaking movements are also responsible for the title "pseudosclerosis," to differentiate it from true multiple sclerosis. In many patients an increasing rigidity develops, as well as dysarthria, dysphagia, a grimacing (dystonic) smile torsion movements, epileptic attacks, and spasticity. Occasionally severe behavioral disturbances supervene which may be interpreted as a schizophrenic psychosis. The hepatic changes correspond to a typical *multilobular cirrhosis* and are present in 25% of cases of Wilson's disease; especially in children and young subjects, neurologic signs may be absent. The deposition of brown pigmented granules in Descemet's membrane in the vicinity of the limbus of the cornea gives rise to the pathognomonic clinical feature of the disease – the yellow-brown *Kayser-Fleischer ring.* These rings are present in virtually all cases exhibiting neurologic signs (1271), although they may be detectable only with the slit lamp; in the presence of purely hepatic involvement, the rings may be absent. Renal symptoms and osteomalacia are less specific signs. The diagnosis is clinically based on the combination of progressive neurological symptoms, primarily the trauma and psychiatric changes with a Kaiser-Fleischer ring of the cornea and signs of liver cirrhosis. Diagnostic laboratory data include a low ceruloplasmin level of less than 200 mg/l, and an increase of the free copper in the serum and of the excreted copper in the urine (more than 0.6 μmol/24 h. The diagnosis can be confirmed with a radioisotope copper test and the determination of the copper content in a liver biopsy. *CT scanning* reveals hypodense zones in the brain substance, especially the basal ganglia and occasionally the cerebellar nuclei, thereby confirming brain involvement in many patients (484). CT changes occurring in the course of treatment may likewise be observed (484, 1277), although these changes do not always correlate with the clinical picture. An MRI study regularly shows signal changes in the caudate, the putamen, in the white matter, but also in the palms and the midbrain (1147), on T_2-weighted images in the presence of neurological symptoms.

The disease is **inherited** as an autosomal recessive anomaly, but isolated cases may occur. The presence of the abnormal gene is 1:140-1:200, and the incidence is 1:250000 to 1:1 million. The onset is usually between the ages of 10 and 40 years. The average duration is 4-5 years, but it may be shorter, or indeed, more prolonged - cases have been recorded with a 40-year clinical duration. The **pathophysiology** of the disease is well known. The ceruloplasmin level is markedly reduced, but the free copper content of the serum is increased. Thus, more copper is excreted in the urine and more copper is deposited in the copper-containing tissues such as the brain, especially its basal ganglia, and the liver. This can be demonstrated in 2 mg of liver tissue by atomic absorption spectrophotometry.

Treatment consists of D-penicillamine (not the L-isomer, D-L-penicillamine, which is neurotoxic), given in an average daily dose of 1000 mg in equally divided doses before meals. A low copper diet should be prescribed. In order to prevent copper absorption from the intestine, potassium sulfide in gelatin capsules 3×20 mg is given. Regular evaluation of copper balance may indicate the need for higher doses. As a rule, a daily urinary excretion of over 1 mg of copper is sufficient to maintain a negative copper balance. Because of the possible side effects of penicillamine (causing myasthenia or lupus erythematosus), treatment with zinc sulfate is recommended (518).

Other Hereditary Disturbances of Copper Metabolism (1280)

Another hereditary disturbance, *not identical to Wilson's disease,* is characterized by a progressive dementia, spastic dysarthria, paralysis of vertical gaze, gait disturbance, and splenomegaly. Neither sensory disturbances nor pyramidal tract signs are present, and there are no Kayser-Fleischer rings. The disease begins before puberty and progresses slowly over the course of many years. The ceruloplasmin level may initially be normal, but later it falls; however, it is never as severely reduced as in Wilson's disease. The copper metabolism in these patients is similar to the picture shown in carriers of Wilson's disease.

Menkes' disease (kinky hair disease) (270, 388), which is transmitted as an X-chromosomal recessive disease, presents in the first months of life with epileptic attacks, mental deterioration, blindness, hyperthermia, skeletal abnormalities, and abnormal wiry hair. The ceruloplasmin and serum copper levels are diminished due to reduced intestinal absorption of copper.

Other Generalized Diseases with Neurologic Symptomatology

Almost all systemic disease processes exhibit evidence of involving the nervous system. The following list includes only those diseases in which neurologic signs and symptoms may predominate or contribute to establishing the diagnosis. The chapter headings which list the main categories provide a classification.

Intoxications With Central Nervous Symptomatology

Metals

Poisoning with metallic mercury (1237) or with inorganic mercury salts causes a fine tremor upon movement of the hands and later of the head, tongue, and legs. No sensory changes occur, and the tendon jerks remain normal. Speech is occasionally difficult to understand. Other features include stomatitis, excessive salivation, cataract, and mental changes in the sense of a neurasthenic syndrome, depression, or lack of self-confidence. *Organic mercury salts* such as insecticides cause dermatoses, cataract, diarrhea, and nausea. Neurologic findings include paresthesias and a feeling of numbness of the fingers, and sometimes tremor and ataxia. Usually the patient shows slurred speech, dysphasia, and occasional pyramidal tract signs. Pathologic lesions may be found in the cerebral hemispheres and the cerebellum. In the context of the poisoning of fish by industrial waste products, organic mercurials may cause severe or fatal poisoning (Minamata disease) in humans who eat the fish. Such cases have very occasionally been reported to exhibited signs of muscular atrophy, fasciculation, and pyramidal tract signs which are indistinguishable from amyotrophic lateral sclerosis. Inorganic mercury salts may produce signs and symptoms similar to intoxication with organic mercury compounds (1237).

In summary, **mercury intoxication** produces the following *main signs:*

- tremor,
- slurred speech,
- stomatitis,
- neurasthenic features,
- paresthesias, and
- sometimes features similar to amyotrophic lateral sclerosis.

Lead intoxication more commonly produces severe and intense signs in *children* than in adults: headache, vomiting, convulsions, papilledema, abducent palsy, and optic atrophy. Because of the life-threatening rise in intracranial pressure, immediate operative decompression may be required. In *adults,* general symptoms such as irritability, headache, tremor, nausea, vomiting, colic, etc. may slowly make their appearance. Delirium and coma may supervene. Up to about 30% of these patients die. Physical examination should include a search for the lead line on the gums, basophilic stippling of erythrocytes, and elevated pressure and increased protein content of the

CSF. Treatment with chelating substances such as versene is advised. Reference should be made here to *lead neuropathy,* which usually manifests itself as a wrist drop due to paralysis of the radial nerve. This complication presents over days or weeks as an increasing weakness of the long extensor muscles of the fingers and spreads to involve the extensors of the wrists. Occasionally other peripheral nerves are also involved. Sensation usually remains intact. Workers in factories producing car batteries and paint are most commonly affected. It appears that the encephalopathy that follows the prolonged inhalation of gasoline – both the acute (reversible) variety and the rarer progressive and persistent variety – can be attributed to the lead content of this substance (1223).

In summary, a case of **lead intoxication** produces the following *main signs:*

- signs of raised intracranial pressure, especially headache,
- optic atrophy,
- epileptic attacks,
- delirium,
- peripheral neuropathy, especially radial palsy, and
- colic.

Bismuth salts: Prolonged ingestion of these insoluble salts may produce an *encephalopathy.* The drug is usually taken for chronic constipation (196), although in other cases the patient's condition following colectomy for carcinoma was the reason for taking the medication (200). Therapeutic doses taken over the course of months or years may pro-

voke progressive fatigue, change of mood, headache, and tremor. The serum bismuth level is 10- to 100-fold higher than in patients without complications (718). A rare cause of bismuth poisoning is repeated application of a bismuth-containing suntan lotion (647). Over the course of weeks the patient becomes increasingly tired, ill-tempered, and complains of headache and shivering. Then rapidly in 1 or 2 days he becomes disoriented and develops myoclonic contractions, disturbances of gait, ataxia, and dysarthria. Examination reveals cerebellar signs and muscular hypotonicity, sometimes pyramidal signs, and increased facial reflexes. Epileptic attacks are rare, but typical EEG changes are always present (1171). The CSF is normal. CT scanning reveals abnormal hyperdense deposits of bismuth in the basal ganglia, an appearance which is not modified by contrast enhancement (807). Withdrawal of the bismuth-containing drug usually leads to complete regression of the signs and symptoms. However, fatal cases have been described (718).

In summary, **bismuth intoxication** produces the following *main signs:*

- confusional states,
- gait disturbances,
- ataxia,
- dysarthria, and
- myoclonic contractions.

Arsenical and thallium intoxication: Poisoning with these heavy metals is most commonly complicated by a polyneuropathy (p.318). In addition, poisoning provokes a subacute myelopathy with involvement of the optic nerve, similar in appearances to SMON (p. 253) (98).

Organic Solvents and Other Industrial Products

Chronic trichlorethylene poisoning presents as a neurasthenic syndrome with alcohol intolerance, as a toxic encephalopathy with an organic mental syndrome, as retrobulbar neuritis, and as peripheral polyneuropathy. The last of these is also a prominent feature in poisoning with carbon disulfide and industrial *n*-hexane (p. 320). Toluene, however, more commonly causes organic mental changes, even dementia, and pyramidal tract signs, cerebellar and brainstem symptoms, and cranial nerve deficits (522).

Triarylphosphate poisoning is discussed in detail on p. 319. The clinical picture is dominated by polyneuropathy, often accompanied by CNS signs which worsen in the course of years into a picture of spasticity and pyramidal tract involvement. Acute *carbon monoxide poisoning* may cause a parkinsonian syndrome (p. 110), apart from acute disturbances of consciousness.

Drugs

Table 1.**18** lists various drugs which are often observed by the neurologist to be responsible for side effects.

Phenytoin intoxication: This condition may appear even after normal doses of this antiepileptic drug. It is

Table 1.**18**   Drugs and their actions: most common neurologic effects

Drug	Principal Neurologic Signs	Remarks
Chlorpromazine derivatives (and other neuroleptics)	Hypokinetic parkinsonian signs, oral dyskinesias, malignant neuroleptic syndrome: pyrexia, rigidity, stuporous state	Rarely permanent signs. Akathisia, see p. 150
Phenytoin	Ataxia, nystagmus, dysarthrias, rarely myasthenia	Rarely permanent cerebellar signs
Lithium salts	Tremor, ataxia, polyneuropathies, rigidity, cramps, coma	Rarely permanent signs
Oxyquinoline derivatives	Polyneuropathies, myelopathies with spasticity, optic neuropathy (SMON), acute global amnesia	An association is probable but the mechanisms are complex
Penicillin	Myoclonias, epileptic attacks, disturbances of consciousness	Occur with 200 million units a day and above
Bismuth salts	Encephalopathy: confusion, tremor, ataxia, and gait disorders	CT shows hyperdense foci in brainstem, see p. 152

characterized by hypertrophy of the gums, cerebellar ataxia, nystagmus, and slurred speech. Ballismus, choreoathetotic movements, or paroxysmal dyskinesias are less frequent (314, 967). Myasthenia or an external (supranuclear) ophthalmoplegia is rare (1137). The author has encountered hiccups. The CSF protein may be raised. While these signs are usually reversible, permanent cerebellar damage may occasionally occur (1099). The vermis is preferentially involved. Women appear to be more at risk, and also patients with existing brain damage (73). The polyneuropathies are usually subclinical (967). In *mesantoin intoxication* a facial chloasma may appear.

In summary, phenytoin intoxication produces the following *main signs:*

- ataxia,
- nystagmus,
- gait disturbances,
- dysarthric speech, and
- hypertrophy of the gums.

Penicillin encephalopathy: This condition presents occasionally as a neurotoxic syndrome produced by high-dose penicillin treatment (20 million units/day or more). About 24–48 h after the start of treatment, myoclonic spasms, epileptic convulsions, and increasingly severe disturbances of consciousness occur, which lead eventually to coma. These signs appear if the CSF concentration of penicillin exceeds 10 units/ml.

Neuroleptics: These drugs and especially (chronic) *chlorpromazine med-*

ication produce several delayed side effects apart from akinetic parkinsonism (p. 108) and choreoathetotic disturbances of movement. These include *oral dystonic phenomena* with abnormal tongue and lip movements, disturbances of respiration and phonation, and dystonic movements of the head and trunk. These side effects may be partly abolished by simultaneous administration of antiparkinsonian drugs, and they almost always disappear after the neuroleptic medication is withdrawn. Very marked tongue and mouth dyskinetic movements may be an acute side effect of single-dose treatment with specific phenothiazine derivatives (e.g., trifluoroperazine, p. 125). Exceptionally, dystonic movement disturbances of the tongue and mouth may appear after the end of a long course of treatment, and they may then persist (88), being then called *tardive dystonias* or *dyskinesias*. An occasional lasting feature is an *akathisia,* a permanent restlessness of the muscles of the face and limbs. This usually commences only after drug medication has been withdrawn or the dose markedly reduced. The serum iron is decreased in these patients, and the iron-binding capacity is increased (180), as is also the case in the restless leg syndrome (p. 464–5). A Gilles de la Tourette's syndrome has also been described. During the early stages following the withdrawal of certain neuroleptic drugs, a so-called *malignant neuroleptic syndrome* may appear, consisting of fever, muscular rigidity, and unconsciousness (49, 828, 951). Premonitory signs such as sweating, tachycardia, and hypotension may occasionally occur. The creatine kinase level is increased. Dopamine receptor blockade in the basal ganglia and hypothalamus is believed to be responsible. About one-third of cases have a fatal outcome. A specific relationship exists to malignant hyperthermia (p.497). Treatment comprises L-dopa preparations, amantadine hydrochloride, and bromocriptine, as well as dantrolene 100 mg/day by mouth. A similar clinical syndrome may be observed after withdrawal of L-dopa treatment in parkinsonian patients.

Lithium salts: Lithium treatment in about two-thirds of patients produces mild side effects such as tremor, rigidity, and the cogwheel phenomenon. Diabetes insipidus and weight increase are common. On the other hand, severe and acute side effects are uncommon; these include rigidity, hypokinesia, mutism, convulsions, and coma (302), also a polyneuropathy (911). Prolonged attacks are exceptional (302). Myeloneuropathies have been described following *nitrous oxide (laughing gas) exposure* (682).

Table 1.**19**   Results of chronic alcoholic abuse on the nervous system

1. *Acute effect of alcohol intake*
   - Acute intoxication
   - Pathologic intoxication (drunkenness)
   - Alcoholic poisoning
   - Dipsomania

2. *Psychopathology of chronic alcoholic abuse*
   - Predelirium
   - Delirium tremens
   - Alcoholic hallucinations
   - Alcoholic Korsakoff's syndrome
   - Jealousy
   - Development of paranoia
   - Hepatic encephalopathy (portocaval encephalopathy)
   - Alcoholic dementia
   - Personality change of chronic alcoholic abuse
   - Alcohol-mediated hypoglycemia

3. *Alcoholic epilepsy*
   - Preexisting tendency triggered by alcohol
   - As forerunner of delirium tremens
   - Rum fits

4. *Alcoholic encephalopathy*
   - Encephalopathia haemorrhagica superior (Wernicke)
   - Marchiafava-Bignami disease
   - Central pontine myelinolysis
   - Cerebellar atrophy (p.136)
   - Lead encephalopathy in moonshine drinkers

5. *Alcoholic myelopathy*
   - In portocaval syndrome
   - In funicular spinal disease of malnutrition

6. *Tobacco-alcohol amblyopia*

7. *Alcoholic polyneuropathy*

8. *Alcoholic myopathy*
   - Acute with rhabdomyolysis
   - Chronic, sometimes with cardiomyopathy
   - Combined proximal myopathy and neuropathy
   - Subclinical forms

9. *Pachymeningosis haemorrhagica interna*

10. *Alcoholic embryopathy (fetal alcohol syndrome)*

An encephalopathy has been described during treatment with *interferon* (1174).

Alcohol

Table 1.**19** lists the neurologic syndromes of chronic alcoholism (461, 495). The commonest is *polyneuropathy* (see p.317).

Psychopathologic Disturbances

In addition to *alcoholic dementia,* the patient may present a true *Korsakoff's psychosis* or *delirium tremens.* The latter condition commonly occurs after (enforced) alcohol abstinence for 2–4 days and is characterized by restlessness, shivering, sleeplessness, confusion, and hallucinations.

Epileptic Attacks

These attacks in 10% of cases lead to or accompany delirium tremens. They are nearly always generalized. They are significantly commoner in drinkers of concentrated alcohol ("rum fits") and recur only with renewed delirium. True epilepsy occurs significantly less frequently in the elderly chronic alcoholic.

Wernicke's Encephalopathy, (Encephalopathia Haemorrhagica Superior) (485)

This encephalopathy, which may occur also in hemodialysis, is characterized by the presence of bilateral ocular signs such as bilateral abducens nerve palsy, visual failure, internuclear ophthalmoplegia (1072), as well as nystagmus and pupillary anomalies. Disorientation, confusion, and inability to concentrate are frequent findings; apathy and somnolence are sometimes present. The patient may eventually present a true Korsakoff's psychosis or delirium tremens. An associated polyneuropathy is a frequent finding and occasionally an ataxia. Autopsy examination of the brain reveals foci of hemorrhagic parenchymal necrosis and vascular changes extending from the paraventricular parts of the thalamus to the region of the third ventricle, aqueduct and fourth ventricle, and the mammillary bodies. The mortality rate is about 10%. Treatment consists of the immediate intravenous administration of thiamine, 100 mg 3–4×/d or more.

Marchiafava-Bignami Disease

This is an acute demyelinating lesion involving the corpus callosum as well as sometimes a large part of the central white matter (219). It occurs particularly in subjects who drink red wine and is characterized clinically by epileptic attacks, confusion, spasticity, and pyramidal signs and leads to terminal coma.

Central Pontine Myelinolysis (804)

This is a rare lesion which is usually fatal. The patient exhibits external ocular palsies, speech disturbances, difficulty in swallowing, and mental changes, and terminally a locked-in syndrome may be present. Alcoholic nutritional deficiency is the main causative factor, and there is a relationship with pellagra. In this connection, the fact should be mentioned that a simple failure to take nourishment may produce a similar picture, in addition to the hepatic disorders. Too rapid rehydration of a patient with hyponatriemia is another cause (804). MR scanning shows the lesion and allows its course to be observed (294).

Myopathies

Three types of myopathy are encountered in chronic alcoholics, namely an acute form with rhabdomyolysis, a chronic form which sometimes includes cardiomyopathy, and a combination of proximal myopathy with neuropathy. Subclinical forms are also found.

Other Addictions

Heroin: In this condition, which is aggravated by the foreign substances usually injected with the drug, neurologic signs may complicate the abnormal psychosocial picture. These include disturbances of coordination and sensation, tremor, and nystagmus. In other patients, ataxia, parkinsonian features, toxic amblyopias, transverse myelitis, neuritides, myopathies, and rhabdomyolysis may be found (108). Dementia is described in cases of chronic *hashish* addiction.

The encephalopathy of *gasoline inhalers* is well known (p.151).

The polyneuropathy found in *glue sniffers* is mentioned on p.320.

Parkinsonism after *MPTP consumption* in addicts was mentioned on p.108.

Nerve Poisons

Pathophysiology: These substances block acetylcholinesterase, the enzyme responsible for the degradation of acetylcholine, the substance which transmits neural stimuli in the peripheral and CNS. They include organic phosphorus derivatives, which are used as insecticides (1238), and from which the principal substances for chemical warfare are derived. These alkylphosphates phosphorylate cholinesterase and thereby block its action. Although the process remains reversible for a period of minutes to hours, the combination of enzyme with nerve poison undergoes an "aging" process which converts it into an insoluble complex. Once this chemical process is complete, the acetylcholine can no longer be broken down. This acetylcholine poisoning leads to depolarization blockage of the synapses.

Clinical features: The efferent nerve endings of *the parasympathetic system* are subjected to a muscarinic effect, producing prolonged contraction of the *smooth musculature* which results in various effects, e.g., bronchospasm with asthmatic respiratory disturbances; pupillary contraction with forced accommodation for near vision; intestinal colic with diarrhea; involuntary incontinence of urine; and an orthostatic fall of the arterial blood pressure. The pulse rate is slowed. Mucus and lacrimal and bronchial secretions are increased. The motor end plates of *the striated musculature* and the autonomic ganglia are subjected to a nicotinic effect, which produces a depolarization blockage with fasciculation and motor paralysis and a rise of the arterial blood pressure. *The synapses of the CNS* are directly affected by acetylcholine poisoning, producing feelings of anxiety, excitation states, and finally convulsions or central respiratory arrest.

Treatment (521): This must always be carried out in an intensive care unit. During the early stages, treatment consists of administering oxygen and very high doses of atropine (up to several 100 mg), as well as respiratory support.

Endocrine Disturbances with Neurologic Signs and Symptoms

Hypothyroidism (1177)

Usually as part of severe myxedema, the following **neurologic signs and symptoms** may occur:

Cerebellar signs with disturbances of balance and movement, ataxia, and occasionally dysarthria and nystagmus (470).

Involvement of the peripheral nervous system with paresthesias (in 80% of hypothyroid patients), disturbances of sensation, and a carpal tunnel syndrome.

Delayed relaxation time upon eliciting reflex (ankle jerk) may be observed in about one-fourth of patients with hypothyroidism. Myoedema (local swelling) may be visible upon tapping a muscle. Muscular weakness and spasms (p. 501) are the expression of *involvement of the musculature* itself. Muscular hyperplasia in myxedematous athleticism, see p. 502.

Cranial nerve palsies: Impaired hearing and tinnitus are common. The following are rare: ataxia, ptosis, hoarseness (mucopolysaccharide infiltration of the vocal cords), pain of the face and head.

Mental changes are a classic component of congenital hypothyroidism (cretinism) and also occur in a proportion of the advanced cases of the acquired type in adults. These changes include apathy, memory defects, dementia, and psychoses with hallucinations. Epileptic attacks may occur and lead to a terminal myxedematous coma.

CSF: The protein level is usually elevated.

All the clinical features can be reversed by medical correction of the hypothyroidism.

Hyperthyroidism (1177)

The commonest cause is a diffuse goiter (with exophthalmos), and less frequently a toxic thyroid adenoma, thyroiditis, or a TSH-secreting pituitary tumor. In all of these conditions, the following **neurologic signs and symptoms** may appear:

Involvement of muscles: Thyrotoxic myopathy (p. 501). Thyrotoxic *periodic paralysis* with attacks of localized or generalized muscular weakness lasting from minutes to several days. The onset and clinical findings are similar to familial paroxysmal paralysis (p. 501). Hyperthyroidism may be combined with *myasthenia gravis,* the severity of which is aggravated by hyperthyroid decompensation.

Polyneuropathy: Very rare.

CNS signs and symptoms: Spasticity with pyramidal signs is a rare complication, which is reversible.

Tremor is frequent; *chorea* is rare and reversible, being produced by overactivity of the dopamine receptors in hyperthyroidism.

Ocular signs: The most frequently encountered signs are exophthalmos, which occasionally is unilateral, lid retraction (von Graefe's sign) and abnormalities of convergence

(Möbius's sign). *Ophthalmoplegia* and *optic neuropathy* also occur.

Hypoparathyroidism

Clinically, the postoperative as well as the idiopathic form of this condition may be accompanied by a variety of neurologic signs and symptoms (421):

- tetany (numbness of the extremities, carpopedal spasm, Trousseau's sign, stridor, see also p. 291),
- epileptic attacks (rarely initially as hemitetany),
- headache and papilledema,
- signs of basal ganglia involvement, e.g., choreoathetotic movements (1124),
- muscular weakness and jerking movements,
- abnormal lassitude, apathy, confusion, hallucinations, and actual toxic psychosis,
- abdominal pain, nausea, and vomiting, and
- brisk tendon jerks, both Chvostek's and Trousseau's signs may be present.

Some of these symptoms disappear if the hypocalcemia is corrected (525).

Laboratory findings include increased serum phosphorus and reduced serum calcium levels. The urine shows hypocalciuria in an acidotic metabolic milieu, which eventually becomes a hypercalciuria. The CSF pressure is often raised; ophthalmologic examination may confirm the presence of a punctate cataract.

Roentgenologic examination reveals deposits of perivascular calcification in the basal ganglia and deep layers of the cerebral and cerebellar cortex. Similar radiologic findings may be present after encephalitis lethargica, CO poisoning, postanoxic state, tuberous sclerosis, toxoplasmosis, and hypothyroidism. They are also found in Fahr's disease, a progressive abnormality with a familial incidence.

Pseudohypoparathyroidism

In this syndrome, which forms part of the hereditary osteodystrophy of Albright, there is no absence of parathormone – indeed, it is present in excess, but it fails to influence the renal tubules to reduce the absorption of phosphorus. Thus, although the same biochemical situation is present as in hypoparathyroidism, patients with this syndrome fail to respond to treatment with parathormone.

Pseudopseudohypoparathyroidism

In this condition, a normal calcium-phosphorus ratio remains in the serum, although the clinical features of pseudohypoparathyroidism are present (with the exception of tetany and intracranial calcification). These features are: small stature, saddle nose, brachydactyly, exostoses, thick cranial vault, soft-tissue calcification, dental anomalies, cataract, epileptic attacks, and mental retardation. Both conditions can probably be attributed to an anomaly of the renal tubular epithelium or a disturbance of parathormone function localized to the renal tubules.

Hyperparathyroidism (920)

Clinically, the following signs and symptoms are present:

- depression, confusional states, lability of mood, restlessness, lassitude, sleeplessness,
- motor retardation and terminal dementia (although other causes of hypercalcemia may be responsible for dementia, 467),
- motor weakness,
- ataxia, spasticity, and disturbances of ocular movement,
- epileptic attacks,
- infrequently, cerebral ischemic insults resulting from vasospasm,
- diminished muscular reflexes and reduced response to sensory stimulation,
- swallowing disturbances and constipation,
- myopathic features and muscular atrophy, and
- fasciculation.

Malignancy: Remote Effects on the Nervous System

Malignant tumors involve the nervous system, not only by direct invasion but also through remote effects. These *paraneoplastic neurologic manifestations* (500, 886) are grouped together in Table 1.**20**.

Subacute Cerebellar Cortical Atrophy

This is the commonest paraneoplastic manifestation of CNS involvement. Men and women are equally affected. Although the primary tumor is most commonly a bronchial or ovarian carcinoma, other malignant lesions such as Hodgkin's disease should not be ignored. Frequently the neurologic signs and symptoms precede clinical evidence of the tumor. The onset is usually

Table 1.**20** Paraneoplastic manifestations involving the brain and muscles

1. *Encephalopathies*
   - Multifocal leukoencephalopathy
   - Diffuse polioencephalopathies with mental disturbances (limbic encephalitis)
   - Subacute atrophy of the cerebellar cortex
   - Brainstem encephalitis
   - Central pontine myelinolysis
   - Cerebellar encephalitis
   - Myelitis
   - Encephalopathy in active endocrine tumors
     • Hyperparathyroidism
     • Adrenal cortical tumors
     • Insulinoma
   - Encephalopathy in the paraproteinemias
   - Opsoclonus (especially in neuroblastomas)

2. *Subacute cerebellar cortical atrophy*

3. *Chronic myelopathy*

4. *Peripheral neuropathies*
   - Sensory neuropathy with posterior column involvement
   - Mixed peripheral neuropathy
   - Mononeuritis multiplex (vasculitis)

5. *Myopathies*
   - Polymyositis
   - Dermatomyositis
   - Eaton-Lambert syndrome
   - Myopathies in active endocrine tumors

subacute, with disturbances of gait and coordination and sometimes speech. Often a combination is present of cerebellar signs and evidence of involvement of other areas of the brain, e.g., double vision, pyramidal signs, posterior column signs, polyneuropathy, or dementia. The CSF frequently shows a raised protein level while the cell count remains normal. The course may be fatal within months, or the disease may be slowly progressive over several years. Histologic examination reveals diffuse involvement of the cerebellar cortex with widespread damage of Purkinje cells – in contrast to the localized picture found with alcohol-induced cerebellar atrophy.

Progressive Multifocal Leukoencephalopathy (500)

Pathologically, this syndrome may appear in carcinoma, but mainly in leukemia and diseases of the reticuloendothelial system (leukemia, lymphosarcoma, Hodgkin's disease, sarcoidosis) and also after anoxia. Diffuse plaques of demyelination, in which the axons remain intact, are found in the white matter of the brain, less frequently also in the spinal cord. The astrocytes are markedly enlarged, inflammatory cells may be present. **Clinically,** this syndrome is encountered – corresponding to the age of predilection for the primary disease – in middle-aged or elderly subjects. The onset is rapid and the course is usually fatal within a few months. The clinical picture consists of weakness, occasionally amounting to quadriplegia, visual field defects, cerebellar signs, confusion, dementia, and coma. The CSF is normal, the EEG shows nonspecific changes. CT scanning may occasionally reveal foci of demyelination, which are always visible with MR imaging. **Etiologically,** the possibility is discussed that the lesion

may be caused by reduced immunologic resistance (severely debilitated patients, or patients who are X-irradiated or treated with corticosteroids or immunosuppressant drugs) with a secondary viral infestation of the brain.

Multifocal Vascular Lesions

Intravascular coagulation may give rise to thrombi composed of fibrin, particularly in patients with lymphoma or leukemia, which lead to multifocal brain lesions, causing mental symptoms and multiple neurologic deficits (249).
Further paraneoplastic syndromes: opsoclonus, see p.343; polyneuropathies, see p.322; myopathies, see p.493.

Collagen Diseases and Immunologic Disorders with Nervous System Manifestations

Polyarteritis Nodosa

CNS complications are encountered in this disease, as well as the more common polyneuropathy (p.316). *Subjectively,* the patient complains of headache, visual disturbances, dizziness, and seizures. *Objectively,* an organic mental syndrome is found, as well as hemipareses, papilledema, and a retinopathy. Occasionally the CSF is abnormal, and not infrequently the EEG. Cogan's syndrome (p.363) is now considered to be a variant of this disease.

Lupus Erythematosus

In about 25% of cases, the nervous system is involved. **Clinically,** the *neurologic manifestations* occur most commonly on the basis of a vasculopathy (303, 582, 648, 1009): hemipareses, extrapyramidal disturbances of movement especially choreiform disturbances (303), epileptic attacks, and paraplegia. Less common are *retrobulbar neuritides* (410), *psychotic episodes, polyneuropathies* (p. 315), and (vacuolated) *myopathies* (p. 502).

These multifocal symptoms give rise to a diagnostic picture which must be differentiated from encephalomyelitis, a demyelinating disorder and a space-occupying lesion and also a distinction from secondary effects of the lupus involvement of other organs on the nervous system and from side effects of the lupus therapy (582).

Sjögren's Syndrome

Pathogenetically, the neurologic signs appear to be associated with a vasculitis which correlates with the presence of cytoplasmic antibodies. **Clinically,** the picture consists of focal cerebral disturbances, transverse myelitides, chronic myelopathies, optic nerve involvement, and aseptic meningoencephalitides. Not infrequently, an associated polyneuropathy is also present.

Granulomatous Angiitis of the CNS (418)

This is a giant-cell arteritis of unknown etiology. The condition is confined to the CNS and causes headaches, mental confusion, and focal neurologic deficits. It leads to death within weeks. Corticosteroids may occasionally be beneficial.

Thrombotic Microangiopathy
(Thrombotic thrombocytopenic Purpura of Moschcowitz)

In this disease, platelet thrombi cause multiple small vessel occlusions and lead to hemolytic anemia with jaundice, thrombocytopenia, cutaneous hemorrhage, and signs of damage to the kidneys and other internal organs. Sometimes neurologic signs appear, such as focal or generalized CNS deficits or a polyneuropathy (p. 317).

Malignant Atrophic Papulosis
(Köhlmeier-Degos) (739)

This is a microangiopathy caused by hyaline thrombi, in which the skin changes are characteristic. They are accompanied by gastrointestinal symptoms as well as neurologic signs which include the following: focal CNS deficits, spinal cord involvement, polyneuropathy, cranial nerve palsies.

Wegener's Granulomatosis

This is a condition in which granulomatous changes and focal arterial abnormalities are found in the respiratory organs, kidneys, and other parts of the body, including the nervous system at times. A nasal granuloma may penetrate by local destruction through the base of the skull and produce focal cranial nerve deficits, especially involving eye movement and the optic nerve. In other patients, a vasculitis may cause clinical signs similar to those encountered in periarteritis nodosa in the central and peripheral nervous system.

Acquired Immune Deficiency Syndrome (AIDS), HIV Infection

Pathogenetically, this syndrome is an infection with the HIV virus which is always transmitted by sexual intercourse or direct contact with infected body fluids. By the end of 1987, 50000 cases had been observed in the USA alone, and it was estimated that there were 150,000 cases worldwide. While earlier patients were almost exclusively homosexuals, those with a high level of promiscuity, or addicts dependent upon intravenous drugs. Presently individuals who do not belong to a high-risk group and also children of HIV-positive mothers are being infected with increasing frequency. The patients belong to the young and middle adult age group. Pediatric cases occur in children born to drug-addicted mothers harboring the virus. Their cell-bound immunity system has been breached, and consequently their resistance to infections and certain neoplasms is reduced. **Clinically**, the commonest mode of presentation is *Pneumocystis carinii* pneumonia or Kaposi's sarcoma (551). However, countless other opportunistic infections and other tumors, especially lymphomas, are encountered. **Neurologic signs and symptoms** occur in 30–40% or more of AIDS patients (368, 615, 1118). They may develop in patients who have recovered from a *Pneumocystis* pneumonia. The most important are encephalitic illnesses, which are characterized by progressive neuropsychologic manifestations, sometimes dementia, a lack of well-being, and development of psychotic symptoms. As the AIDS dementia complex, they represent an increasingly frequent cause of dementia in young adults. The cause is probably in most cases a direct infection of the brain with the HIV virus or infection with the cytomegalovirus. In other cases, the following have been observed: toxoplasma abscess, meningitic infections caused by *Cryptococcus*, *Candida*, and *Mycobacterium*, CNS lymphoma, and myelopathies with secondary CNS vascular complications caused by emboli or brain hemorrhage. The commonest peripheral neuropathies, which are symmetrical in distribution, are demyelinating lesions often accompanied by painful dysesthesias. **Treatment** is directed at eliminating the infection or the tumor. The chances of recovery are slight since the immune deficiency persists and most patients succumb again to recurrent or fresh infections.

Treatment with azidothymidine has recently been tried experimentally.

Renal Insufficiency and the Nervous System

Pathogenesis

In patients with renal insufficiency (971), the neurologic signs and symptoms are caused by abnormal concentrations of electrolytes and other substances in the CSF and serum. The signs depend on the relationship of these substances to each other, and upon the speed with which the concentrations alter. See also p. 160.

Acute Renal Insufficiency

This condition is accompanied by psychotic episodes. In addition, fleeting double vision and transient blindness may occur, as well as constriction and inequality of the pupils. Hemiplegic and hemianopsic deficits may indicate a vascular lesion. Muscular weakness is common. The tendon jerks are brisk or increased or reduced or absent (especially in hyponatremia). Pyramidal signs are not invariably present. Extrapyramidal signs such as myoclonus may sometimes be observed, occasionally there is a asterixis or fasciculation of the muscles.

Chronic Renal Insufficiency

Signs and symptoms similar to those of acute renal disease may be seen. However, the picture may be that of chronic encephalopathy, the patient experiencing variations in mood, neurasthenic irritability, reduced activity, and sleeplessness. Neurologic examination and the EEG tracing may be normal. If the patient's condition worsens, fasciculation, myoclonus, and muscular weakness become prominent. The muscular weakness may be the manifestation of a secondary hyperparathyroidism (with renal osteodystrophy) and may disappear after subtotal parathyroidectomy (683). Other features may be the signs of renal hypertension which is associated with vascular accidents and hypertensive crises. If a renal polyneuropathy (see p. 312) is present as well, the patient's clinical picture may mimic that of amyotrophic lateral sclerosis – a combination of atrophic muscles and absent reflexes in the lower extremities with increased reflexes and fasciculation in the upper extremities. While there is no direct parallel between the severity of the neurologic signs and the extent of renal insufficiency, the former seldom develop before the serum creatinine level has risen to values between 6 and 10 mg/100 ml. Convulsions occur in the end stages of the disease only, when the greatly restricted glomerular filtration rate has led to severe overhydration (water retention).

Cerebral Dysequilibrium Syndrome

This syndrome may be caused by dialysis, particularly after *rapidly executed extracorporeal hemodialysis*. The clinical picture consists of disturbances of consciousness and other features of a progressive encephalopathy, including convulsive attacks. A preexisting polyneuropathy can usually be observed to worsen as soon as dialysis is commenced. The cerebral signs are caused by delayed clearance or urea from the CSF in the presence of a rapidly falling plasma urea level and a corresponding (osmoregulatory) flow of water into the CNS. Signs and symptoms may also appear which are characteristic of Wernicke's encephalopathy (see p. 152) and central pontine myelinolysis (see p. 152).

Dialysis Encephalopathy (1279)

This denotes a severe progressive neurologic complication of *prolonged hemodialysis*. It starts as a disturbance of speech, with stuttering and myoclonic contractions and goes on to mental changes and a fatal outcome. The EEG changes are characteristic: bilaterally synchronous discharges of slow groups of spike and sharp waves, similar to what is seen in nephrosis, intoxications, and uremia. Treatment with diazepam restores the EEG tracing to normal and improves the clinical picture (688, 863).

Electrolyte Disturbances with Cerebral Signs and Symptoms (56, 780, 870)

Disturbances of Sodium Concentration (56)

Pathophysiology

The osmolarity of the extracellular fluid, which is largely responsible for the sodium ion concentration, is regulated by mechanisms which determine the intake and excretion of water from the body. These mechanisms include thirst, antidiuretic hormone, and renal function. Water retention leads – provided the amount of sodium in the body remains constant – to hypo-osmolarity, and increased excretion to hyperosmolarity. The amount of sodium also may alter. In normally regulated osmolarity, the sodium content determines the extracellular fluid volume of the body, recognizable by circulatory signs and symptoms. The osmolarity, not the amount of sodium, is responsible for neurologic symptomatology. Changes in the blood osmolarity within a few hours affect the CSF and the extracellular fluid content of the brain. Hypo-osmolarity of the blood, i.e., a level below 260 mOsm/l, leads to cerebral edema through a transfer of water into the intracellular compartment. Hyperosmolarity, levels above 330 mOsm/l, leads to tissue dehydration through a transfer of water into the extracellular compartment. A significant factor is the speed with which changes in osmolarity take place.

Hypernatremia

This condition and the consequent hyperosmolar syndrome is **caused by** water deficiency relative to sodium, sodium transfer relative to water, or a disturbance of normal osmoregulation. Water deficiency occurs if the patient's thirst, normal or abnormal, is not quenched. Salt treatment in infants and small children, inadequate infusion therapy, or the instillation of hypertonic saline solutions into body cavities, e.g., criminal abortion, leads to sodium excess. The usual body response is a feeling of thirst, with water intake, which prevents the development of a hyperosmolar state. If adequate water intake is impossible, if thirst is absent due to hypothalamic disturbance, or if diabetes insipidus decompensates, an acute or chronic hypernatremic syndrome develops. Very high blood sugar levels in nonacidotic diabetic coma may be associated with hyperosmolarity and corresponding clinical signs and symptoms, without hypernatremia necessarily being present. The **signs and symptoms** correspond to those of a metabolic encephalopathy. They consist of changes in the level of consciousness with irritability, agitation, disorientation, reduced awareness and ability to

concentrate, and sometimes delirium. The terminal picture is one of somnolence and coma. Muscular tone is usually increased, the reflexes are abnormally brisk, myoclonic contractions may occur, and less often epileptic attacks (especially at the start of treatment). Neurologic signs and symptoms appear at a level of 150 mval/l if this level is rapidly reached. In chronic lesions they appear at 160 mval/l. The CSF has a normal cell count with an increased protein content. The EEG is abnormal only in the sense of showing a slowed background activity. The **prognosis** is poor: according to various sources, between 10% and 70% of patients die, and about 10% exhibit permanent neurologic damage. At **autopsy,** multiple petechiae are found in the cortex and subcortical white matter, as well as thrombi in the intracranial capillaries, veins and sinuses. **Treatment** consists of slowly correcting the hypo-osmolarity. Normalization should be accomplished in the course of 48 h. It is achieved in the hypovolemic form by oral or parenteral administration of salt and water, in the isovolemic form by carbohydrate solutions, in the hypervolemic form by the additional use of diuretics. Hypernatremia of acute onset can and must be more promptly corrected than hypernatremia of chronic onset.

Hyponatremia

This situation indicates an excess of water in relation to the sodium content. Hyponatremia is **caused by** an excess of water which exceeds the sodium loss, or by a sodium deficiency which exceeds a simultaneously occurring water deficiency. Hyponatremia may also be the manifestation of a disturbed osmoregulation. The commonest causes of abnormal water retention are the edema diseases such as renal insufficiency, hepatic cirrhosis or the nephrotic syndrome with terminal renal insufficiency. The commonest causes of hypo-osmolar dehydration are renal salt and water loss as a result of diuretic treatment, aldosterone deficiency, or salt-losing nephropathy, as well as extrarenal fluid loss through vomiting or diarrhea. Overflooded osmoregulation is caused by excessive intake of fluid by mouth or by infusion therapy, and is usually disturbed as a result of (inadequate) secretion of antidiuretic hormone (ADH). In this situation, the blood sodium level is low and the extracellular fluid volume normal or increased, but the urine is not maximally diluted, i.e., the urine osmolarity remains higher than the serum osmolarity, as verified by simultaneous estimations *(Schwartz-Bartter syndrome)*.

This condition accompanies various brain diseases or occurs after craniocerebral trauma, myxedema, and some pulmonary diseases including neoplasms and especially small cell carcinoma.

The **signs and symptoms** of hyponatremia occur when the serum sodium concentration falls below 127 mmol/l. They comprise a metabolic encephalopathy, with confusion, drowsiness progressing to coma, muscular fasciculations and myoclonic movements, headaches, sometimes papilledema and less frequently ataxia, pyramidal signs, and occasionally epileptic attacks. Central pontine myelinolysis (p.152) may accompany the form produced by inadequate ADH secretion or cases of hyponatremia corrected too rapidly; the picture may include the locked-in syndrome (p.89) (804). In the CSF, the pressure may be raised and the protein content reduced. The EEG often shows a nonspecific alteration of the background activity and irregular discharges of high-voltage slow waves. In the more chronic forms, clinical signs and symptoms appear when the slowly falling sodium concentration reaches

120–110 mmol/l. These include mental disturbance alternating with lack of drive, adynamia, difficulty in concentration, and eventually hallucinations and delirium, with somnolence progressing to coma. Epileptic attacks occur less frequently than in the acute form. In severe cases, cerebral edema may lead to tentorial herniation. **Histologically,** there is at most a swelling of the astrocytes, with evidence of brain edema and herniation. The **treatment** of hyponatremia consists of combating the underlying cause. If a concomitant dehydration is present, it should be corrected by the infusion of saline solutions – initially hypertonic and later isotonic concentrations, up to a maximum of 4 liters a day. If the hyponatremia is accompanied by a fluid excess (e.g., Schwartz-Bartter syndrome), fluid intake must be restricted and perhaps diuretics prescribed. In this instance also, hyponatremia of acute onset should and must be corrected more promptly than the chronic form.

Disturbances of potassium metabolism, see p.497.

Disturbances of calcium metabolism, see p.291.

Liver and Gastrointestinal Disorders and the Nervous System

Liver Diseases

Portocaval encephalomyelopathy (5, 248) may occur in patients with liver diseases with raised ammonia levels in the blood, as well as in the presence of *portocaval shunts* or surgical anastomoses. **Clinically,** patients show disturbances of consciousness of varying severity with somnolence, confusion, and occasionally hallucinations. Sometimes actual twilight states with complex actions may be present. Epileptic manifestations occur less frequently. Physical examination reveals an irregular tremor which is more severe distally (asterixis), occasionally choreoathetosis, muscular hypertonicity, abnormally brisk tendon jerks, and transient pyramidal signs. In alcoholics, the degree of cerebral atrophy demonstrated by **CT scanning** correlates with the extent of liver damage (5). The **EEG** is usually abnormal and shows characteristic triphasic potentials. Less frequently, spinal symptomatology may be present, including posterior and lateral column signs and the picture of progressive spastic spinal paralysis. Similar changes may be induced experimentally in animals by the injection of ammonia (248). **Treatment** may consist of dietary or antibiotic conversion of the intestinal flora or operative resection of the colon.

Acute Pancreatitis

Patients with acute pancreatitis may show states of agitation, pyramidal signs, rigidity, myoclonic movements, and ataxia, and they may experience epileptic attacks (1101). In this type of *pancreatic encephalopathy* in which the serum amylase level is elevated, histologic foci of demyelination are found in the brain. Antienzyme preparations are recommended in treatment (1101).

Whipple's Disease

This disease is caused by bacterial damage to the cells of the intestinal mucous membrane, mesenteric glands, and reticuloendothelial system. The pathogens, or bacterial rests, consist of PAS-positive mucopolysaccharide material. The general signs and symptoms consist of steatorrhea, weight loss, asthenia, and polyarthritis. Neurologic signs and symptoms occur in about 5% of cases, consisting of increasing apathy, extrapyramidal signs, myoclonic contractions, brainstem signs (disturbances of external ocular movement, nystagmus, trigeminal involvement), and dementia. The histologic cause of these signs is a perivascular nodular encephalitis.

Sprue

See p. 317.

Blood and Blood Vessel Diseases Affecting the Nervous System

Leukemias

These diseases are frequently accompanied by neurologic complications, the most prominent being intracerebral hemorrhage and additional leukemic infiltration of peripheral nerves, nerve roots, brain, and meninges. The latter complication, *leukemic meningitis* (632), occurs in about one-third of cases of leukemia. The signs and symptoms are headache, cranial nerve palsies (especially facial, trigeminal, and optic nerves), meningism, and sometimes mental symptoms and signs of raised intracranial pressure. The CSF shows a high cell count and reduced sugar content; the cytology is diagnostically conclusive. Intrathecal administration of antineoplastic drugs is essential. Paraneoplastic manifestations complicate the leukemias and other reticuloses, as described on p. 156.

Polycythemia Vera (815, 1304)

The subjective complaints include headache, dizziness, tinnitus, and paresthesias, which are common.

Physical examination reveals neurologic signs in about one-fifth of patients with polycythemia, notably cerebrovascular accidents, extrapyramidal signs (parkinsonian signs, chorea), visual disturbances, signs of raised intracranial pressure, epileptic seizures, and mental changes. A polyneuropathy has also been described (1304). The neurologic signs and symptoms usually respond to treatment of the disease itself.

Pernicious Anemia

Subacute combined degeneration of the spinal cord, see p. 227.

Myeloma

See p. 313.

**Hereditary Hemorrhagic
Teleangiectasia
(Rendu-Osler Disease)**

This autosomal dominant disorder is a generalized angiomatosis involving numerous organs of the body. If the brain and spinal cord are involved, neurologic deficits may be present. However, more frequent than direct involvement are the indirect effects on the nervous system of lesions in other sites, e.g., cerebral hypoxia, emboli and abscess complicating pulmonary arteriovenous fistulae, or a portocaval fistula with encephalopathy (1008).

Several Additional Generalized Diseases with Signs of Involvement of the Nervous System

Oral Poliomyelitis Immunization

Neurologic complications only rarely accompany this immunization (Sabin vaccine). Within weeks an acute syndrome appears which may include disturbances of consciousness, swallowing, and breathing, as well as a flaccid paralysis. Polyneuritides may be observed a few days after the immunization. In isolated cases, cranial nerve palsies, paraplegia, and signs of encephalomyelitis may occur, which can be mistaken clinically for multiple sclerosis.

Tetanus Encephalopathy (542)

In the initial weeks of disease, the following signs of an encephalopathy may appear: memory disturbances, irritability, sleep disorders, loss of libido, orthostatic hypotension, and occasionally disturbances of consciousness. Involvement of the anterior horn cells of the spinal cord with permanent quadriparesis may also follow tetanus (394). In the initial weeks of the disease, muscular weakness and atrophy are accompanied by increased blood levels of muscle enzyme and histologically detectable necrosis (90). Nearly all these signs are completely reversible within 2 years.

Special Cerebral Symptoms and Signs

Dementia and Dementing Neurologic Diseases

We define dementia as the secondary loss of intellectual faculties, as opposed to mental retardation (oligophrenia) which is the primary defect. There is a gradual transition from the normal to various (e.g., age-related) states of reduced functional capacity, which end in dementia.

Psychopathologic signs of dementia:
The following signs, which are characteristic features of an *organic mental syndrome* of greater or lesser degree, belong to this group, largely irrespective of the cause:

- rapid exhaustion,
- loss of interest in recent events,
- lack of persistence in carrying out personal tasks,
- disinterest in people and environment, and in extreme cases
- sloppiness in dress, unrestrained and aggressive behavior, loss of insight and a presumptuous and intrusive manner,
- loss of refinement in behavior with improper, crude, and tactless attitudes,
- emotional lability, irritability, and anxiety, and
- hypochondriacal, depressive, or paranoid features.

Subcortical dementia (676): This condition is characterized by prolongation of the thought process ("mental akinesia"), indifference, memory disturbances, and sometimes obsessive behavior. The syndrome accompanies bilateral lesions of the basal ganglia, irrespective of their etiology.

Neurologic signs of dementia: These signs, none of which is necessarily present, may accompany dementia and depend upon the underlying cause of the disease. Focal neurologic findings (often accompanying posttraumatic dementia) need not be present. Neuropsychologic deficits are practically always present (see below). A variety of abnormal reflexes are found in cases of diffuse damage (176, 284, 563), including an accentuated facial reflex (snout reflex), sucking reflex, abnormal nuchocephalic reflex (563), positive grasp reflex, and increased palmomental reflex.

Examination in organic mental syndrome: The following simple procedure and questions will reveal dementia or an organic mental syndrome:

- It should be noted if the patient is oriented in time, place, situation, and person.
- Disturbances in the attention span and memory capacity occasionally become obvious while taking the patient's history. The attention span may be evaluated further by the following: repeating a 6-digit number; recalling a 4-digit number after an interval of 5–10 min; naming 8 diagrams shown to the patient; recalling a 4-word phrase after an interval of 10 min; solving a complex mental arithmetic problem.
- Evaluation of recent memory: menu of the previous evening, names of the doctors, time patient arrived, recent news items.
- Evaluation of concentration ability: months of the year in reverse order; subtracting serial 7s from 100; checking off a particular letter of the alphabet in a long text (Bourdon's test).
- Evaluation of higher intellectual functions including abstract thinking: combining several words into a meaningful phrase; simple questions to verify power of discrimination, e.g., child/dwarf, tree/bush, river/lake, greed/thrift; interpreting a complicated picture; repeating and explaining the meaning of a story.
- Arranging objects according to their size, shape, or mutual affinity.
- In patients with organic mental syn-

Table 1.21   Etiologic causes and differential diagnosis of dementing lesions

Disease	Age	Main Clinical Features	Remarks	See page
Arteriosclerotic dementia	Over 60	Fluctuating	Signs of generalized arteriosclerosis. Often brain CT reveals infarcts. Primitive reflexes	168
Multi-infarct dementia	Over 60	Cerebral infarcts in case history or CT	Similar to arteriosclerotic dementia but infarcts always present	168
Binswanger's disease (subcortical encephalopathy)	Middle age and the elderly	Mood fluctuation, small insults, pseudobulbar signs	Hypertension especially important. Survive up to 10 years. Brain CT shows attenuated density of white matter	85
Thromboangiitis obliterans	60 or younger	Vascular symptoms of other organs	Similar to cerebral arteriosclerosis. Also called Buerger's disease	85
Alzheimer's disease (and senile dementia)	50 or younger	Increasing dementia	Commonest cause of dementia! Over 2–5 years of increasingly severe memory disturbance, periodic confusion, and disorientation	168
Pick's disease	40 or younger	Dementia and focal neurologic deficits	Particularly clear-cut personality change. Apart from diffuse involvement, the brain CT reveals area of focal atrophy	169
Progressive paralysis	30 or younger	Expansive, grandiose ideas	Neurologic deficits, pupillary abnormalities, abnormal CSF	58
Creutzfeld-Jakob disease	Young and middle-aged adults	Pyramidal and extrapyramidal signs, fasciculation, myoclonic features	In about 70% typical EEG. Rapidly progressive coma. Transmissible	169

	Age	Symptoms	Comments	Page
Normal pressure hydrocephalus (nonresorptive hydrocephalus)	Any age	Dementia, apractic gait, disturbances of urination	Seek causes of nonresorptive hydrocephalus. Transient improvement follows LP. Internal hydrocephalus while extraventricular CSF spaces are reduced	19
Brain tumor	Any age	Focal neurologic deficits, epileptic attacks	Especially in slowly growing benign tumors, e.g., meningioma	31
Craniocerebral trauma	Any age	History of injury	Neurologic deficits or abnormal findings in brain CT not essential for the diagnosis. Watch for epileptic attacks!	21
Chronic exogenous poisons	Any age	Contact with toxic substances	e.g., bromice, cannabis, alcohol, barbiturates	
Endocrinopathies	Any age	Other clinical signs	e.g., Cushing's disease, hypercalcemia, hypothyroidsm	
Metabolic disorders	Any age		e.g., Kinnier-Wilson disease	
Malnutrition			e.g., pellagra, vitamin B_{12} deficiency	
As part of another neurologic disease	Preceding illness		e.g., parkinsonian syndrome, Huntington's chorea, myoclonic epilepsy, sphingolipidoses, leukodystrophies, hereditary system degenerations, varicus vascular lesions, chronic meningoencephalitides	

dromes, it is always important to obtain information about their behavior from relatives or friends.

The most important etiologic causes of dementia: The most important etiologic groups for the neurologist are shown in Table 1.**21**, which will serve as a guideline in the assessment of dementia. While most of the clinical syndromes are dealt with in other chapters of this book, only some will be discussed here which belong to the category of *senile or presenile dementia*. Their etiology is not clear. Basically, a genetic defect in the cell structure, a disturbance of the cell metabolism, a slow virus infection, or an autoimmune process have been postulated.

Arteriosclerotic Dementia

In this condition, the onset of the mental symptoms mentioned above is often fluctuating and not infrequently accompanied by physical signs of the underlying disease. The patients are over 60 years of age. The case history and physical examination often reveal evidence of previous vascular accidents. Hydrocephalus is not marked, and it may be absent. Histopathologic study shows the smaller blood vessels to be more severely affected than the larger ones, and small parenchymal lesions are present, usually foci of softening in the cortical gray matter.

Multi-Infarct Dementia

This concept in the modern literature serves either as a substitute for arteriosclerotic dementia or is used in those patients in whom evidence can be demonstrated of previous multiple insults (p. 70). We prefer the latter concept. In a series of 77 patients with multiple infarcts examined by CT scanning, 37 showed dementia (667). Dementia was significantly commoner in lesions of the dominant hemisphere. In ten patients with a clear history of previous insult, the CT revealed evidence only of diffuse atrophy.

Subcortical Encephalopathy (Binswanger)

See p. 85.

Thromboangiitis Obliterans (von Winiwarter-Buerger)

See p. 85.

Alzheimer's Disease

This is a presenile dementia, usually starting after the 50th year of life, but also affecting younger subjects. This pattern of incidence previously served to differentiate it from *senile dementia,* which presents after the age of 65 years. On the basis of transitional patterns and histologic criteria, both forms nowadays are grouped together (629, 1191, 1293) and called senile dementia of the Alzheimer type (SDAT). It is the **commonest cause** of a dementia. The disease is present in about one-fifth of all patients attending psychiatric clinics and is encountered in about 5% of subjects up to the 80th year. Familial cases are not unusual and probably account for 5%–10% of Alzheimer's disease. Women appear to be more commonly affected than men. **Clinically,** the patient initially is often restless and agitated and then within a year exhibits severe progressive memory disturbances, confusion, disorientation, and the other above-mentioned signs and symptoms of a dementia. Neurologic signs are by no means invariably present and may at most be slight: pyramidal signs, extrapyramidal features, anomalies of muscular tone, oral automatisms, etc. The average duration of the disease is 2-5 years. **Autopsy** reveals a diffuse cerebral atrophy involving the frontal and occipital lobes most severely. Histologic study shows the presence of plaques and a great number of neurofibrillary (Alzheimer's) tangles, as well as diffuse cell necrosis, granulovacuolar degeneration, and occasionally a congophilic amyloid angiopathy (436, 629).

Pick's Disease

This disease belongs to the systemic degenerative processes such as Huntington's chorea. It occurs twice as commonly in women as in men, usually in younger individuals than Alzheimer's disease; also, it is far less common. The *personality changes* in Pick's disease are more severe than those in Alzheimer's disease, and the grossly disturbed behavior may occasionally in individual cases give rise to severe ethical problems (differential diagnosis of tertiary neurosyphilis). Apart from these mental changes, **focal neurologic signs** are often present, notably aphasia and parietal lobe involvement (p.178). The disease lasts 2-10 years. Neuroradiologic examination reveals an internal hydrocephalus combined with wide subarachnoid spaces over the surface of the frontal and parietal lobes, with the posterior two-thirds of the first temporal convolution being spared. The caudate nucleus may be atrophic. Apart from loss of ganglion cells and gliosis, the diseased areas of the brain contain Alzheimer's fibrils and senile plaques.

Creutzfeld-Jakob Disease
(620, 637)

This is a rare, rapidly progressive disease which involves men and women with equal frequency. It commences in early adulthood or middle life. The onset is heralded by nonspecific or **uncharacteristic symptoms** such as mood fluctuations, depression, tiredness, sleep disturbances, and increasing forgetfulness. Soon these features are combined with objectively demonstrable **neurologic signs:** anomalies of muscular tone, pyramidal signs, extrapyramidal features, neuropsychologic deficits, muscular fasciculation, and later myoclonic contractions. In parallel, the patient's signs of dementia increase and his mental activity progressively ceases, leading to decorticate status and terminal coma. Diagnostically important is a characteristic **EEG pattern;** however, this may only appear in the later stages. About three-fourths of cases show bilaterally synchronous, diffuse frontal periodic activity comprising sharp polyphasic potentials repeated with a frequency of 1/s (Fig.1.23). In the later stages, these periodic complexes are replaced by diffuse slowing. The disease lasts no longer than 6-30 months.

Pathologic anatomy: Naked-eye examination of the brain reveals spongiform changes of the neuropil with loss of ganglion cells and compensatory astrocytosis. The degree of severity of these changes corresponds to the clinical details and varies from case to case. It has been possible in more than 100 cases to *transmit* the disease to primates and other laboratory animals

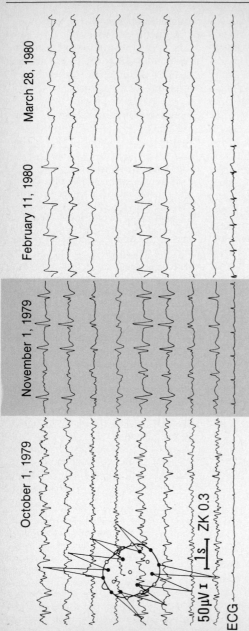

Fig. 1.23 Serial EEG examinations in a 57-year-old with autopsy-proven Creutzfeld-Jakob disease. The examination 6 weeks from the onset of the prodromal stage (October 1, 1979) revealed only periodic activity. One month later (November 1, 1979) this activity was most marked, and in the succeeding months it showed a tendency toward gradual attenuation

(771); human-to-human transfer occurring accidentally during surgical operation has also been observed (119). The etiologic role of virus particles in the disease is nowadays widely accepted (1205, 1207). These particles have been identified as "prions," which are found in laboratory animals infected with scrapie (138). For those in contact with patients, it is recommended that excreta and body fluids should be handled with the same precautions applied to viral hepatitis.

Presenile Spongiform Cerebral Atrophy

This is a rapidly fatal, progressive type of dementia is which choreiform and myoclonic or epileptic features are present. The characteristic pathologic picture, in the presence of intact nerve cells and the absence of signs of Alzheimer's disease, is multiple cystic cavitation of the cerebral cortex. The condition has a complex relationship to Creutzfeldt-Jakob disease (1207).

Prolonged Steroid Medication

Steroid preparations administered over a long period cause diffuse shrinkage of the brain which is visible on CT scanning as surface atrophy and hydrocephalus. This abnormal picture disappears completely upon withdrawal of medication (109).

AIDS dementia has been mentioned on p. 159

Neuropsychologic Syndromes
(935, 960, 961, 962, 1167)

General: Disturbances of complex psychic functions, possessing an organic background, are included in this concept. None of these syndromes presents primarily as disturbances of consciousness, mood, or thought processes – instead they usually manifest as disturbances of recognition and processing of information and secondary effects on the behavior of the individual. These neuropsychologic syndromes are identified by the technique of neuropsychologic testing. The scientific substrate of this field is experiences gained from experimental psychology. It is only partly possible to relate topographically specific syndromes to specific regions of the brain. Experience has confirmed that neuropsychologic testing permits only organic brain damage as such to be demonstrated and evaluated quantitatively (960, 1167), as well as sometimes to be lateralized with a certain degree of accuracy (935). Abnormalities previously accepted as isolated syndromes (finger agnosia, autotopagnosia, right-left confusion, Gerstmann's syndrome) are so closely linked to other basic neuropsychologic disturbances that they cannot be interpreted as independent entities (960, 962). For individual concepts, see below.

One of the complex integrating functions of the brain, of which the abnormalities are particularly striking, is the ability of man to communicate by means of speech and other forms of information transfer with his fellow men and his environment. **Speech disturbances** not caused by cortical lesions must be briefly mentioned in this section, in view of their differential diagnostic importance.

- *Nonorganic speech disturbances* (speech disorders in schizophrenic psychoses, monotonous scant speech in depression, mutism in catatonia, aphonia in hysteria).

- *Developmental speech disorders* are disturbances of speech development, one of which is stammering.

- Lesions of the *speech-forming structures:* the choice of words is correct but there are changes in the tone and clarity of utterance (hoarseness in laryngeal lesions; blocked nasal passages with enlarged adenoids; epipharyngeal tumors or patent nasal passages in cleft palate; spastic dysphonia with irregular phonation accompanied by contractions of the facial and neck muscles – presumably a functional anomaly of phonation).

- Lesions of the *muscles of phonation,* provoking similar symptoms (involvement of muscles of the soft palate in myasthenia gravis with patent nasal passages, progressively increasing exhaustion of the patient, and other myasthenic manifestations).

- Lesions of the *lower cranial nerves,* with paralysis of the muscles of phonation which they supply, causing dysarthria (unilateral hypoglossal palsy affects speech only slightly; paralysis of one vocal cord due to unilateral recurrent laryngeal nerve palsy causes hoarseness but is rapidly compensated; bilateral paralysis of the soft palate, e. g., in diphtheria).

- Lesions of the *nuclei in the medulla oblongata:* "bulbar speech," i. e., nasal, slurred, poorly articulated, and often babbling speech, as if the patient has an egg in his mouth. The consonants "R" and "L" are most likely to be slurred (this type of speech is a typical feature of the bulbar type of amyotrophic lateral sclerosis, see p. 221). A unilateral lesion of the bulbar nuclei, e. g. a vascular accident in the vertebrobasilar territory, produced only transient hoarseness.

- *Upper motor neuron palsy* of muscles of phonation ("pseudobulbar palsy"): articulatory disturbances that cannot be distinguished from those in bulbar palsy (anarthria, dysarthria, p. 85) accompany this type of lesion which usually results from vascular damage to the cortico-bulbar tracts. The onset is usually sudden, unlike that of true bulbar palsy (p. 79). The picture of (childhood) brainstem encephalitis is similar. Paroxysmal dysarthria, see p. 246.

- *Cerebellar lesions:* the coordinating and regulating function exerted by the cerebellum is abolished. Syllables and words are uttered too loudly and too rapidly in an irregular way, i. e., they are articulated explosively. In advanced cases of *multiple sclerosis,* involvement of the cerebellum sometimes leads to scanning speech.

- The parkinsonian syndrome and other *lesions of the basal ganglia* hamper the harmonious and coordinated utterance of speech. The poverty of movement of the parkinsonian patient is expressed as soft and monotonous, slow, and scarcely modulated speech (bradylalia, in extreme cases mutism). Rarely, logoclonia (compulsive repetition of end syllables) and palilalia (repetition of individual words or phrases) may occur. Such repetitive speech may also accompany diffuse cerebrovascular disturbances and senile dementia. The slow slurred speech of general paresis is similar. However, it must be stressed that this early symptom is a nonspecific feature of general paresis.

- Damage in the vicinity of the *periaqueductal gray matter:* failure of the speech impulse with preservation of movement of the organs of speech and no obvious disturbance of consciousness; in extreme cases, akinetic mutism (p. 89); after encephalitis involving the basal ganglia, especially encephalitis lethargica, vertebrobasilar insufficiency, and subarachnoid hemorrhage. A similar clinical picture is produced by lesions of the limbic system. Locked-in syndrome, see p. 89.

- The term *aphemia* is used to describe dysarthria without aphasia. It is observed in left-hemisphere lesions of the pars opercularis, the inferior precentral gyrus, and the white matter immediately below it (1070).

- *Bilateral cortical damage in the anterior operculum* leads to a central diplegia of the mouth and throat muscles, the Foix-Chavany-Marie syndrome (771).

Disturbances of Language, Speech, and Other Allied Forms of Communication
(614, 961, 962, 963)

General: Aphasia, in the context of expressing a disturbance of higher integrative cortical function, should be discussed together with the other complex deficiencies of communication between the individual and his environment which do not directly affect speech (962). Speech is only possible if the information which is hidden in various parts of the brain is integrated. The integrity of various cortical areas and the tracts connecting them is essential for this function. Even if no very precise localizing significance can be attributed to speech disorders, it is justifiable and clinically relevant to attribute certain forms of aphasia and other communication defects to specific areas of the brain (Fig. 1.**24**). In right-handed individuals, the cortical centers responsible for language are nearly always localized in the left hemisphere, and only in 1% on the right side (63). In contrast, only about 25% of left-handed persons have their language center in the right cerebral hemisphere.

Examination of Communication Disturbances

The practical method of testing must be adequate to ensure that any defect encountered can be diagnosed and localized. German physicians use the Aachen aphasia test (962), and the following is a simplified scheme suitable for quick bedside orientation.

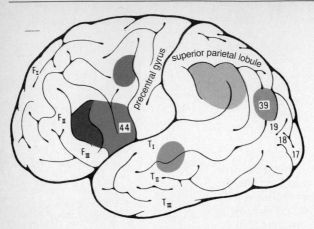

Fig. 1.24   Several areas of the cerebrum significant in speech function

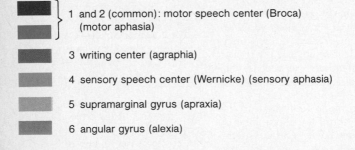

} 1 and 2 (common): motor speech center (Broca)
(motor aphasia)

3 writing center (agraphia)

4 sensory speech center (Wernicke) (sensory aphasia)

5 supramarginal gyrus (apraxia)

6 angular gyrus (alexia)

1. *Preliminary examination:* Verify that
   - the *sensorium* is intact, that no obtundation or stupor is present,
   - no *severe defect of intelligence* is present (retardation, dementia),
   - *hearing* and *vision* are adequate
   - *function of the speech organs* is intact (no severe dysarthria), and
   - no (other) *neurologic defects* are present, e.g., hemianopsia or hemiplegia.

2. *Aphasia testing:* First, *spontaneous speech* should be tested by drawing the patient into conversation.
2.1. Verify that conversation is *fluent,* i.e. consists of a normal speech pro-

duction (more than 90 words a minute), possesses a normal prosody (melody and intonation), and that the sentences have a normal length (more than five words) and no excess of nouns.
2.1.1. If in addition there are no anomalies in the choice or construction of words, then no aphasia is present.
2.1.2. If spontaneous speech is fluent but paraphasias (sense approximately correct but words altered or incorrect) and *neologisms* are present, the picture points to a left-sided postcentral lesion. Greater precision is possible by *testing speech comprehension,* which may be carried out by asking

the patient to point out specific objects, arrange objects in order, answer complex questions, etc.

2.1.2.1. Confirm that *speech reception* is intact, as well as speech repetition (of sounds, words, and sentences).

- If *undisturbed,* an anomic aphasia is present which possesses only slight localizing value (second temporal convolution or angular gyrus?).

- If *speech repetition* is severely *disturbed,* conduction aphasia may be presumed to be present due to damage to the arcuate fasciculus, which connects the posterior part of the temporal lobe to the operculum.

2.1.2.2. If *speech comprehension is disturbed,*

- but *speech repetition* is undisturbed, then a transcortical sensory aphasia is present, localizing the lesion to the angular gyrus,

- and *expression is equally disturbed,* then Wernicke's aphasia is present, and it may be assumed that the lesion lies in the sensory speech center in the first temporal convolution.

2.2. *Spontaneous speech may not be fluent:* speech production may be reduced to less than 50 words a minute, with dysprosody (disturbances of speech melody and intonation of sentences), visible (mimicry) and audible (dysarthria) strained speech, short sentences (fewer than five words), and impaired construction (agrammatism). These features point primarily to a precentral lesion.

2.2.1. If in this situation *speech repetition is intact* (see above), then, in the presence of

- *disturbed expression, Broca's aphasia* is indicated, caused by a cortical lesion in the upper perisylvian region; or in the presence of

- *normal expression, transcortical motor aphasia* is present, caused

by a lesion situated rostrally and more superficially to Broca's area.

2.2.2. If in addition to defective spontaneous speech, *speech comprehension is disturbed,* then either

- a *transcortical sensorimotor aphasia* is present (with marked difficulty in finding names and echolalia), indicating an extensive lesion interrupting the connection of the cortical speech center with the rest of the brain, and particularly cutting off the associated sensory centers (isolation aphasia), or

- a *global (total) aphasia* is present, which is always the result of an extensive lesion in the territory of supply of the middle cerebral artery. The procedure for testing an aphasic speech disturbance is shown in Fig. 1.**25**. The treatment of aphasia continues to undergo intensive development, while its efficacy continues to be challenged, especially in cases of aphasia following vascular accidents (705).

3. *Apraxia examination:* Apraxia is defined as the inability of the patient to execute appropriate movements upon command.

- *Ideomotor apraxia* indicates inability of the face (facial apraxia, in 80% of aphasics) or the extremities to carry out a command or to imitate it by a specific motor response. This inability indicates a lesion of the dominant hemisphere (e.g., Wernicke's region, subcortical beneath the operculum, beneath the motor association center, the commissural tracts to the opposite hemisphere).

- *Ideational apraxia,* far more infrequent, describes the situation in which more complex sequences of movements cannot be successfully executed (e.g., preparing a cup of coffee, opening a letter and filing it, keeping a file in order, etc.).

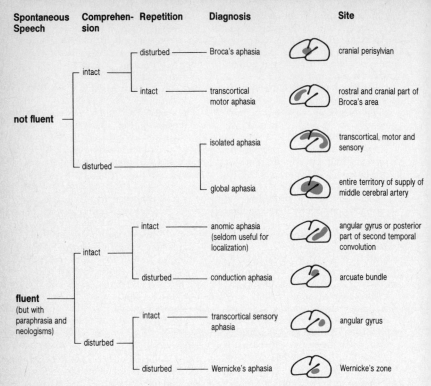

Spontaneous Speech	Comprehension	Repetition	Diagnosis	Site
	intact	disturbed	Broca's aphasia	cranial perisylvian
		intact	transcortical motor aphasia	rostral and cranial part of Broca's area
not fluent			isolated aphasia	transcortical, motor and sensory
	disturbed		global aphasia	entire territory of supply of middle cerebral artery
	intact	intact	anomic aphasia (seldom useful for localization)	angular gyrus or posterior part of second temporal convolution
		disturbed	conduction aphasia	arcuate bundle
fluent (but with paraphrasia and neologisms)	disturbed	intact	transcortical sensory aphasia	angular gyrus
		disturbed	Wernicke's aphasia	Wernicke's zone

Fig. 1.25   Procedure for examining a patient with an aphasic speech disturbance

4. *Agnosia examination:* Agnostic disturbances, i.e., disturbances of recognition, affect the various modalities of sensation. Thus:

- *Visual object agnosias* indicate that although vision is intact, the patient fails to recognize objects which can be identified by touch or hearing (rattling a bunch of keys). The cause is usually a right-sided or bilateral parieto-occipital lesion.
- *Spatial agnosia* implies a disturbance of spatial orientation. It may manifest as follows: the patient loses his way, he is less observant, he is unable to copy simple or more complicated drawings, he is disoriented concerning his own body exhibiting finger agnosia or dressing apraxia. This feature points to a lesion of the posterior part of the right parietal lobe.
- *Prosopagnosia* is the term used to identify an isolated disturbance, namely, failure to recognize familiar faces. It points to a lesion of the occipitotemporal region of the right hemisphere, extending into the cerebral cortex.

- *Anosognosia* is the inability of the patient to recognize an abnormal function of his body, e.g., the patient explains his failure to move a paralyzed left arm as "not wanting to move it." Although mostly seen with lesions of the right hemisphere, in 20% of the cases this symptom also occurs with damage to the left hemisphere. It is not exclusively an expression of a parietal lesion. Rather, it can be the result of diffuse brain damage, combined with a focal lesion (881).
- *Auditory, tactile, and color agnosias* as isolated disturbances are debatable entities.

5. *Disconnection syndrome:* This syndrome is not caused by a lesion of the cortical association centers, but by an interruption of the connections linking these centers. In particular, the connections linking the sensory and motor centers of the right hemisphere with the cortical speech center in the left hemisphere are severed. Some of these disturbances are

- *true alexia*, (alexia without agraphia) i.e., no disturbance of writing, but an inability to read the written word. The lesion may be situated in the splenium of the corpus callosum and left striate cortex.
- Also, *alexia* combined with an *inability to name colors* and *hemianopsia* to the right side may accompany a lesion of the left visual center and the splenium of the corpus callosum (territory of supply of the left posterior cerebral artery).
- *Alexia with agraphia* is not a disconnection syndrome, this combination points to a lesion of the angular gyrus.
- *Pure word blindness* in the presence of intact recognition of nonverbal auditory stimuli and in the presence of an intact cortical Wernicke's area points to a lesion in the left auditory radiation and the commissural fibers of the corpus callosum.

Pain asymbolia is described on p.237.

Syndromes of Individual Areas of the Cerebral Cortex

Lesions of specific areas of the cerebral cortex produce focal neurologic signs as well as a focal and sometimes a generalized mental syndrome (p.164). However, additional specific features point to involvement of specific cortical areas. The description given here of these "lobe syndromes" is summarized from the author's book on this subject (848).

Precentral Region of the Frontal Lobe

Lesions of this region may implicate parts of the pyramidal cell layers and therefore involve motor function of the trunk. Such lesions give rise to focal **paralyses.** The more localized the paralysis, the more superficial is the site of the lesion likely to be, e.g., facial monoplegia or crural monoplegia. The situation may arise, for example, in which a distinction must be made between a central paralysis of the foot and a peroneal palsy. This illustrates the fact that isolated damage to area **4** may be unaccompanied by an increase in muscular tone and present simply as a flaccid weakness. **Disturbances of gaze** accompany lesions of the cortical gaze center at the foot of the second frontal convolution. Gaze is directed initially to the affected side. Sometimes **signs of cere-**

bral irritation may be present in the form of focal motor epilepsy, often referred to as adversive attacks, although the eyes turn away from the discharging focus (aversive movement).

Convexity of the Frontal Lobe

Lesions of the convexity of the frontal lobe give rise to the following disturbances:

Changes in motor behavior: *Grasp automatisms* of the mouth and hand appear at an early stage. The lips and jaws reflexly close when touched or even when an object is brought to the mouth. An object laid in the hand is touched intentionally in a purposeful manner, the fingers following it like a magnet and grasping the object as if obeying a reflex. These features usually affect both hands, but are more marked on the side of the lesion. If the frontopontocerebellar tracts are interrupted, *ataxia* develops, which is most obvious in the lower limbs. Coordination of movements of the opposite side of the body is limited, especially in walking; if the legs are crossed, abduction and adduction are·exaggerated and there may even be abasia. Patients show a type of passive resistance during passive positioning of their limbs, which is called *gegenhalten,* (paratonia), and reaction which may resemble catatonia. Once a limb has been placed in a particular position, that position is maintained for an unusually long time *(postural retention),* and passive repetitive movements are actively continued by the patient (Kral

phenomenon). Also, movements observed may be imitated *(echopraxia),* and words and sentences heard may be repeated *(echolalia).*

Psychopathologic and neuropsychologic features: There is a general *loss of interest and drive, spontaneity, and activity,* leading to an indifferent, unobservant, and detached attitude. Contact with the environment diminishes, and personal initiative and the patient's reaction to external stimuli may disappear. Instead, an impulsive behavioral pattern emerges. Lesions of the basal part of the frontal lobe, the so-called *orbital brain,* bilaterally influence affect and judgmental instincts, especially those concerned with social conventions. This leads to a progressive mental blunting and a picture of impulsive behavior, humorlessness, and moral decay, and ultimately to affective dementia. If the opercular part at the foot of the third frontal convolution (area 44) is also involved, then a lesion of the Broca's speech center leads to *motor aphasia.*

Parietal Lobe

The parietal lobe is not clearly demarcated in the cerebral hemisphere from either the temporal lobe below or the occipital lobe behind. It contains the postcentral gyrus with sensory cortical representation, the circumflex or supramarginal gyrus and the angular gyrus, the latter being important for gnostic function. In lesions involving the postcentral region and upper part of the lobe, the following symptoms and signs may be found.

Neurologic deficits: These include a *sensory* or a *sensorimotor hemisyndrome,* the *avoidance phenomenon* of the contralateral hand (abnormal resting position, clumsy movements, absent grasp reflex on tactile stimulation) (675), homonymous *quadrantic field defect* inferiorly, inattention hemianopsia to the opposite side, and a reduced response of *optokinetic nystagmus* to stimuli, affecting the motion of the eyes toward the contralateral half of the visual field.

Epileptic attacks: These attacks in parietal lobe lesions commence as sensory jacksonian seizures. They may be followed by motor hemiseizures with conjugate deviation of the eyes, head, and trunk to the opposite side. A lesion situated on the medial surface, at the paracentral lobule, causes parasthesias in the anogenital region with urinary and fecal urgency.

Neuropsychologic disturbances: A disturbance of spatial orientation and right-left discrimination may be present, as well as tactile agnosia, a constructional apraxia if the lesion affects the dominant hemisphere, and an amnestic aphasia and dyslexia.

Temporal Lobe

The convexity of the temporal lobe contains cortical areas which are associated with speech comprehension (Wernicke's area in the superior temporal gyrus) and are connected with the sensory auditory pathway and the central pathway of olfaction. The floor of the temporal lobe

forms part of the limbic system, and fibers from the sensory cortex and enteroceptive autonomic afferent pathways terminate here. The visual pathway passes through the basal white matter with fibers arising from the lower half of the retina.

Neurologic deficits: These include homonymous field defects especially of the upper quadrant. No impairment of the senses of smell or hearing accompanies unilateral lesions. Lesions extending into the depth of the globus pallidus present with incoordination of movement and involuntary choreoathetoid movements.

Epileptic attacks: These attacks possess the features of psychomotor epilepsy and may become generalized. Attacks of auditory sensation may occur (Heschl's convolution), also attacks of altered sensations of taste and smell (uncinate fits).

Psychopathologic and neuropsychologic disturbances: Memory disturbances accompany lesions of the mediobasal part of the temporal lobe (hippocampus). Other features are disturbances of mood such as depression and irritability, occasionally disinhibition and aphasic disturbances of the amnestic type. Neglect phenomena are typical. They have in part already been mentioned above. They primarily involve the left side with a right-sided hemisphere lesion, rarely the reverse. This includes not seeing people on the neglected side, not hearing acoustical stimuli, and not feeling sensory stimuli not paying attention to this side of an object during tactile exploration with the eyes closed. One also finds decreased motor activity on the corresponding half of the body and neglect of it, for instance while washing and dressing as well as perhaps an anosognosia (see p.178).

Occipital Lobe

The major part of the occipital lobe lies on the medial surface of the hemisphere and only a small part faces the cerebral convexity. Within it ends the secondary sensory neuron of the visual pathway, the optic radiations terminate in the striate area in the vicinity of the calcarine fissure. In areas 18 and 19, fields are present which are responsible for processing incoming visual stimuli.

Neurologic deficits: Visual defects and optomotor disturbances are described on p. 329. Lesions of areas 18 and 19 lead to a transient conjugate deviation to the side of

the lesion and a gaze palsy to the opposite side. Tracking or pursuit movements of the eyeballs may remain limited for a long period (while the eyes continue to function normally to command). This leads to disturbances of reading (dyslexia).

Signs of irritation take the form of attacks of abnormal visual sensations. In lesions of area 17, they possess a primitive character (flashes, sparks). In lesions of area 18, they consist of hallucinations of objects. In lesions of area 19, they may give rise to complex scenic hallucinations. They may also be combined with conjugate eye and head movements to the opposite side, and they may become generalized.

Neuropsychologic disturbances: Disturbances of visual-spatial orientation, color agnosia or visual agnosia, so-called "psychic blindness," or alexia may occur.

2. Diseases Affecting Mainly the Spinal Cord

Features of a Spinal Cord Lesion

Case History:
- slowly progressive, often subtle disturbance of gait,
- girdle pain, especially a feeling of constriction around the body,
- disordered urination,
- sensory changes confined to the lower extremities
- or truncal sensory changes with a girdle distribution and an upper level in the lower half of the body,
- localized back pains,
- description of electrical sensations passing from the neck into the arms with head movement (Lhermitte's neck flexion sign, p. 246, in cervical lesions or similar sensations from the back into the lower limbs with specific trunk movements.

Physical Findings:
- spastic paraparesis with increased muscular tone, brisk reflexes and pyramidal signs (none of these three signs is essential),
- sensory changes below an upper level on the trunk,
  presence of (spinal) muscular atrophy (sometimes also fasciculation), more frequently in intramedullary lesions than in extramedullary lesions,
- intact cranial nerves, sometimes intact upper extremities.

Ancillary Investigations:
- roentgenograms of the vertebral column,
- positive-contrast myelography,
- CT scanning to demonstrate the spinal cord, if necessary after intrathecal injection of contrast medium,
- MR imaging,
- lumbar puncture (with attention to the Queckenstedt test), sometimes comparison between lumbar and suboccipital CSF,
- somatosensory evoked potentials (SSEP)

Topographic Classification of Spinal Cord Lesions

Transverse Lesion

- Sensory level below which all sensory modalities are abolished to greater or lesser degree (Fig. 2.1),
- spasticity or paraparesis of lower limbs,
- disorder of urination (neurogenic bladder, p. 195; automatic bladder, p. 195,
- sometimes segmental deficit at level of the lesion, thus,
  - segmental deficit of single reflex (Table 2.1)
  - and single muscle or muscle groups (Table 2.1),
  - with radicular or spinal (anterior horn) atrophy,
- sometimes level of lesions indicated by changes in reflexes,
  - knee flexion occurs when patellar reflex elicited, due to damage to the segments below L2 but above L5 (158),
  - reversal of the supinator reflex in C5–6 lesions.
  - "inverted radial reflex".

Unilateral Lesion (Brown-Séquard Syndrome)

This is described in Table 2.2.

Intramedullary Lesion

- spasticity of ipsilateral parts of the body caudal to the lesion,
- segmental (bilateral) dissociated disturbance of sensation of pain and temperature (caused by a lesion of the crossing fibers in the anterior commissure, Fig. 2.2),
- sometimes dissociated sensory disturbance affecting the entire body distal to the lesion (in lesions of the ascending spinothalamic tracts),
- sometimes peripheral paralysis and absent reflexes with atrophy of muscles in lesions of the anterior horn cells at the level of the lesion,
- sensations of movement and deep sensibility more or less intact (due to sparing of the posterior columns),
- disordered urination.

Anterolateral Spinal Lesion (e. g., Anterior Spinal Artery Ischemia)

- paraspasticity or paraparesis,
- dissociated sensory disturbance caudal to the level of the lesion,
- sensations of movement and deep sensibility remain intact,
- disordered micturition.

Column Lesions

- for example, pure spastic paraparesis (spastic spinal paralysis, p. 220),
- disturbed sensation of deep sensibility (e. g., tabes dorsalis, p. 57, or subacute combined degeneration, p. 227),
- combinations.

Further Systematic Spinal Cord Lesions

- for example, spinal muscular atrophy in anterior horn cell involvement,
- combined spinal muscular atrophy and pyramidal tract degeneration in amyotrophic lateral sclerosis (p. 221).

1 Trigeminal nerve
2 Great auricular nerve
3 Anterior cutaneous nerve of neck
4 Supraclavicular nerves
5 Anterior cutaneous branches of intercostal nerves
6 Upper lateral cutaneous nerve of arm (axillary)
7 Medial cutaneous nerve of arm
8 Lateral mammary branches of intercostal nerves
9 Lower lateral cutaneous nerve of arm (radial)
10 Posterior cutaneous branch of radial nerve
11 Medial cutaneous nerve of forearm
12 Lateral cutaneous nerve of forearm
13 Superficial branch of radial nerve
14 Palmar branch of median nerve
15 Median nerve
16 Palmar digital branches of ulnar nerve
17 Palmar branch of ulnar nerve
18 Lateral cutaneous branch of iliohypogastric nerve
19 Anterior scrotal branches of ilioinguinal nerve
20 Anterior cutaneous branch of iliohypogastric nerve
21 Femoral branch of genitofemoral nerve
22 Lateral cutaneous nerve of the thigh
23 Anterior cutaneous branches of femoral nerve
24 Cutaneous branches of obturator nerve
25 Lateral cutaneous nerve of calf
26 Saphenous nerve
27 Musculocutaneous (superfical peroneal) nerve
28 Sural nerve
29 Anterior tibial (deep peroneal) nerve
30 Calcaneal branches of posterior tibial nerve

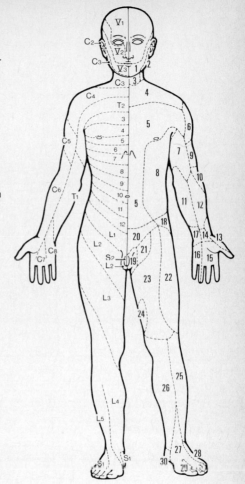

Fig. 2.1 a

Fig. 2.1 a-g The dermatomes. Radicular and peripheral sensory innervation,
a Anterior aspect. Right side: radicular, left side: peripheral innervation

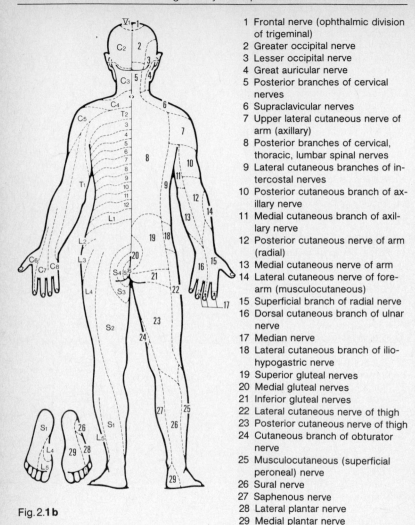

1 Frontal nerve (ophthalmic division of trigeminal)
2 Greater occipital nerve
3 Lesser occipital nerve
4 Great auricular nerve
5 Posterior branches of cervical nerves
6 Supraclavicular nerves
7 Upper lateral cutaneous nerve of arm (axillary)
8 Posterior branches of cervical, thoracic, lumbar spinal nerves
9 Lateral cutaneous branches of intercostal nerves
10 Posterior cutaneous branch of axillary nerve
11 Medial cutaneous branch of axillary nerve
12 Posterior cutaneous nerve of arm (radial)
13 Medial cutaneous nerve of arm
14 Lateral cutaneous nerve of forearm (musculocutaneous)
15 Superficial branch of radial nerve
16 Dorsal cutaneous branch of ulnar nerve
17 Median nerve
18 Lateral cutaneous branch of iliohypogastric nerve
19 Superior gluteal nerves
20 Medial gluteal nerves
21 Inferior gluteal nerves
22 Lateral cutaneous nerve of thigh
23 Posterior cutaneous nerve of thigh
24 Cutaneous branch of obturator nerve
25 Musculocutaneous (superficial peroneal) nerve
26 Sural nerve
27 Saphenous nerve
28 Lateral plantar nerve
29 Medial plantar nerve

Fig. 2.1 b

Fig 2.1 b   Posterior aspect: peripheral, left side: radicular innervation

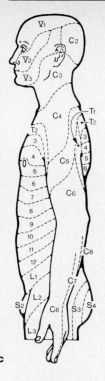

Fig. 2.1c   Lateral aspect: radicular innervation

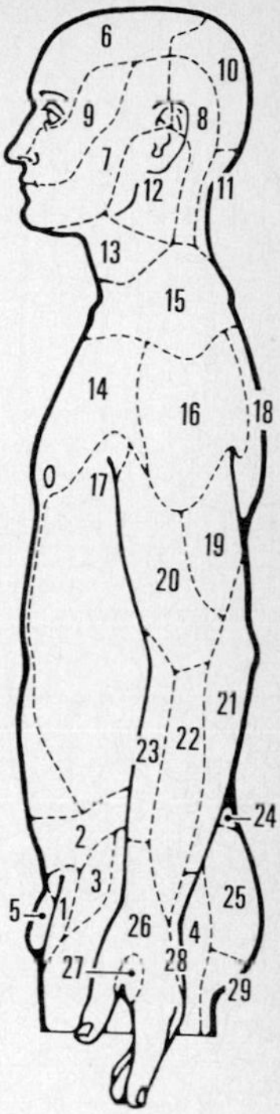

Fig. 2.1d   Lateral aspect: peripheral innervation

c

d

1 Ilioinguinal nerve
2 Iliohypogastric nerve
3 External spermatic branch of genito-femoral nerve
4 Lateral cutaneous nerve of thigh
5 Dorsalis penis branch of pudendal nerve
6 Ophthalmic division of trigeminal nerve
7 Mandibular division of trigeminal nerve
8 Lesser occipital nerve
9 Maxillary division of trigeminal nerve
10 Greater occipital nerve
11 Posterior branches of cervical nerves
12 Great auricular nerve
13 Anterior cutaneous nerve of the neck
14 Anterior cutaneous branches of inter-costal nerves
15 Supraclavicular nerves
16 Upper lateral cutaneous nerve of arm

17 Intercostobrachial branches of inter-costal nerves
18 Posterior branches of thoracic nerves
19 Posterior cutaneous nerve of arm
20 Lateral cutaneous nerve of arm
21 Posterior cutaneous nerve of forearm (radial)
22 Lateral cutaneous nerve of forearm
23 Medial cutaneous nerve of forearm
24 Lateral cutaneous branch of ilio-hypogastric nerve
25 Superior gluteal nerve
26 Posterior cutaneous nerve of forearm (radial)
27 Autonomic innervation in radial nerve
28 Posterior branch of ulnar nerve
29 Inferior gluteal nerve
30 Palmar digital branch of median nerve

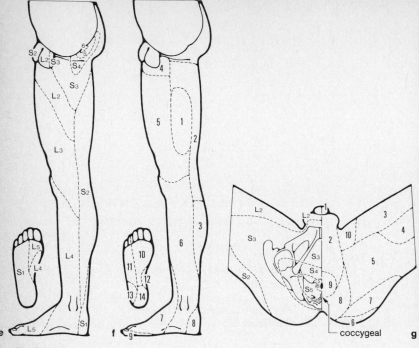

Fig. 2.**1e–g**

1 Cutaneous branch of obturator nerve
2 Posterior cutaneous nerve of thigh
3 Sural nerve
4 Ilioinguinal nerve and external spermatic branch of genitofemoral nerve
5 Medial cutaneous nerve of thigh
6 Cutaneous and medial crural branches of saphenous nerve
7 Musculocutaneous nerve
8 Medial calcaneal branches
9 Medial plantar nerve
10 Medial plantar nerve
11 Lateral plantar nerve
12 Medial cutaneous branches of saphenous nerve
13 Sural nerve
14 Medial calcaneal branches

1 Dorsalis penis (clitoris) branch of pudendal nerve
2 Posterior scrotal (labial) nerves (perineal branches of pudendal nerve)
3 Medial cutaneous nerve of thigh
4 Obturator nerve
5 Posterior cutaneous nerve of thigh
6 Superior gluteal nerve
7 Inferior gluteal nerve
8 Medial gluteal nerve
9 Anococcygeal nerves
10 Ilioinguinal nerve and external spermatic branch of genitofemoral nerve

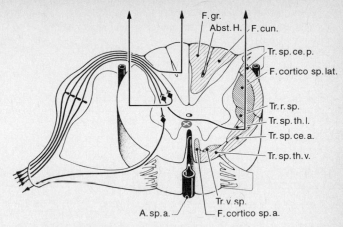

Fig. 2.2   Spinal cord section showing the most important tracts

Abst. H	= descending posterior columns
A. sp. a.	= anterior spinal artery
F. cortico sp. a.	= anterior corticospinal bundle (anterior pyramidal tracts)
F. cortico sp. lat.	= lateral corticospinal bundle (lateral pyramidal tracts)
F. cun.	= cuneate bundle
F. gr.	= gracilis bundle
Tr. r. sp.	= reticulospinal tract
Tr. sp. ce. a.	= anterior spinocerebellar tract
Tr. sp. ce. p.	= posterior spinocerebellar tract
Tr. sp. th. l.	= lateral spinothalamic tract
Tr. sp. th. v.	= anterior spinothalamic tract
Tr. v. sp.	= vestibulospinal tract
✖	= site of lesion in segmental dissociated sensory disturbance

Table 2.**1**   Summary of reflex disturbances, with nerve roots and spinal segments involved. Segmental lesions with motor and sensory deficits

Reflex	Mode and Site of Elicitation	Effect	Muscle Involved
Scapulo-humeral reflex	Blow on inferior part of vertebral margin of scapula	Adduction and external rotation of the hanging arm	Infraspinatus and teres minor muscles
Biceps reflex	Blow on biceps tendon	Flexion of elbow	Biceps brachii muscle
Radial reflex	Blow on distal end of radius	Flexion of elbow	Brachioradialis (plus biceps and brachialis) muscles
Triceps reflex	Blow on triceps tendon proximal to the olecranon with elbow flexed	Extension of elbow	Triceps brachii muscle
Thumb reflex	Blow on tendon of flexor pollicis longus in distal third of forearm	Flexion of terminal thumb joints	Flexor pollicis longus muscle
Finger and hand extensor reflex	Blow on dorsal aspect of wrist joint	Extension of hand and fingers (inconstant)	Hand and fingers extensors
Finger flexion reflex	Blow on examiner's thumb placed in patient's palm; a sudden blow on the pulp of the flexed finger (Trömner's reflex)	Flexion of the fingers	Flexor digitorum superficialis (et profundus) muscles
Epigastric reflex	Rapid downward stroking of the skin of the chest wall in the nipple line	Contraction of the epigastrium	Transversus abdominis muscle
Superficial abdominal reflex	Rapid stroking of the skin of the abdominal wall from lateral to medial	Contraction of the abdominal muscles with umbilical displacement	Abdominal muscles

Peripheral Nerve	Root Segment	Spinal Cord Segment	Motor Involvement in Segmental Lesion	Sensory Level (see Fig 2.1)
Suprascapular nerve (axillary nerve)	C4–C6	C4	Head can be lifted. Quadriplegia. Diaphragmatic paralysis	Shoulders and clavicles
Musculo-cutaneous nerve	C5–C6	C5	Shoulder elevated (intact trapezius, rhomboid and levator scapulae muscles). Weak external rotation of the shoulder remains possible	Shoulder and clavicles, and outer side of upper arm
Radial nerve (musculo-cutaneous nerve)	C5–C6			
Radial nerve	C7	C7	Elevation of arm, adduction of shoulder, flexion of elbow, and extension and flexion of wrist possible. Extension of elbow impossible	Midline of upper limb. Radial side and thumb normal
Median nerve	C6–C8	C8	Shoulder and upper arm muscles, hand extension and flexion possible. Finger flexors and thumb extensors paralyzed as well as interossei	Like C7. Middle fingers usually spared
Radial nerve	C6–C8	T1	Arm spared except small muscles of hands	Hands spared. Ulnar side of forearm and medial side of upper arm involved
Median nerve	C7–C8 (T1)	T4	Arms and hands spared. Sitting up impossible	Nipple line
Intercostal nerve	T5–T6	T8		Costal arch
		T10	Various abdominal muscle groups severely affected	Umbilicus
Intercostal, hypogastric and ilioinguinal nerves	T7–T12	T12		Groin

Table 2.1   (Continued)

Reflex	Mode and Site of Elicitation	Effect	Muscle Involved
Cremasteric reflex	Stroking the skin of the medial side of the thigh (pinching the adductor muscles)	Elevation of testis	Cremaster muscle
Adductor reflex	Blow on the medial femoral condyle	Adduction of the leg	Adductor muscles
Knee jerk (quadriceps reflex)	Blow on the patellar tendon	Extension at the knee joint	Quadriceps femoris muscle
Gluteal reflex	Stroking the skin over the gluteal muscles	Contraction of the buttock (inconstant)	Gluteus medius and maximus muscle
Tibialis posterior reflex	Blow on the tibialis posterior tendon behind the medial malleolus	Supination of the foot (inconstant)	Tibialis posterior muscle
Hamstring (semitendinosus and semimembranosus) reflex	Blow on medial flexors of the knee (patient prone with knees slightly flexed)	Contraction of semitendinosus muscles	Semitendinosus and semimembranosus muscles
Biceps femoris reflex	Blow on lateral flexors of the knee (see above)	Contraction of biceps femoris muscle	Biceps femoris muscle
Ankle jerk (triceps surae or gastrocnemius-soleusreflex)	Blow on the Achilles tendon	Plantar flexion of the foot	Triceps surae (and other flexors of the foot)
Bulbocavernosus reflex	Light pressure on the glans or skin of the dorsum penis	Palpable contraction of bulbocavernosus muscle at root of the penis	Bulbocavernosus muscle
Anal reflex	Stroking or pricking the skin in the perianal region with the patient in lateral position, lying on his side	Visible contraction of the anus	External anal sphincter muscle

Peripheral Nerve	Root Segment	Spinal Cord Segment	Motor Involvement in Segmental Lesion	Sensory Level (see Fig 2.1)
Genital branch of genitofemoral nerve	L1–L2	L2	Abdominal muscles functioning. Hip flexors and thigh adductors paralyzed, as well as other leg muscles	Distal groin
Obturator nerve	L2–L3–L4		Hip flexion spared, thigh adductors only slightly affected, remaining lower limb muscles paralyzed	Anterior and medial aspects of thigh spared
Femoral nerve	L2–L3–L4			
Superior and inferior gluteal nerves	L4–L5–S1	L4	Knee extension only slightly affected, lower leg and foot muscles paralyzed	Anterior surface of thigh spared, posterior and entire lower leg insensitive
Tibial nerve	L5	L5	Quadriceps normal. Dorsiflexion of the foot slightly reduced, but impossible in great toe. Plantar flexion lost	Lateral aspect of lower leg. Sensation lost over foot and posterior aspect of leg
Sciatic nerve	S1	S1	Dorsiflexion of the foot and toes spared. Plantar flexion impossible and gluteus maximus paralyzed	Lateral aspect of foot, posterior aspect of lower leg and thigh and saddle region show sensory loss
Sciatic nerve	S1–S2			
Tibial nerve	S1–S2			
Pudendal nerve	S3–S4	Conus	Disturbances of micturition and defecation	Saddle anesthesia, sometimes dissociated perianal sensory loss
Pudendal nerve	S3			

Table 2.**2**   Brown-Séquard Syndrome

Structure Affected	Ipsilateral Deficits	Contralateral Deficits
Pyramidal tract	Motor weakness	
Vasomotor fibers of lateral columns	Initial overheating and reddening of skin, possibly deficient sweat secretion	
"Overloading" of contralateral spinothalamic tract with touch stimuli?	Transient superficial hyperesthesias	
Posterior columns	Deficient deep sensibility and vibration sense	
Anterior horn and anterior horn cells	Segmental atrophy and flaccid paralysis	
Incoming posterior root	Segmental anesthesia and analgesia	
Lateral spinothalamic tracts		Pain and temperature sense abolished or severely impaired (dissociated sensory disturbance)
Ventral spinothalamic tracts		Touch sensation slightly reduced

Congenital and Perinatal Lesions of the Spinal Cord

Classification

Defective closure of the neural tube may have the following consequences:

- spina bifida occulta (usually defective laminar arch of S1 and L5, often with a tuft of hair on the overlying skin),
- meningocele,
- myelomeningocele or
- meningomyelocystocele.

The last-mentioned two malformations frequently are accompanied by hydrocephalus or an Arnold-Chiari malformation (p. 9) as well as, occasionally, syringomyelia.

Meningocele

Operative treatment within the first few hours of life enables 50%-60% of children to survive 2 years or longer; otherwise, this defect is fatal during infancy. Unfavorable factors in regard to the prognosis and the extent of the remaining defect are a cranial circumference exceeding the 90th percentile by 2 cm or more, very marked kyphosis, or total paralysis of the lower extremities.

Spina Bifida Occulta

This is usually asymptomatic. Occasionally, compression by a spinous process of L5 in the presence of an ununited neural arch of S1 may lead to backache and sciatica (de Anquin syndrome) (280).

Complex Dysrhaphism (34)

A complex pattern of spinal dysrhaphism may be present, with or without intact laminar arches. It may include a dermal sinus, lipoma, or other associated tumors, or a *short filum terminale* (see below). Almost invariably skin pigmentation is present, and abnormal hair overlies the lesion; the child is often incontinent and shows deformities of the feet, abnormal reflexes, and weakness of the lower extremities. The roentgenologic appearances of the vertebral column are rarely normal: spina bifida, sacral malformations, or an abnormally wide spinal canal are present.

Diastematomyelia

In this condition the spinal cord is separated into two halves by the presence of a bony or cartilaginous spur protruding into the spinal canal from its anterior or wall (453). Usually other malformations of the axial skeleton or spinal cord are present. Deformities of the feet, paralysis, and sphincteric incompetence are also seen, which may only be apparent during exercise or become obvious (or worsen) during growth, Operative excision of the spur halts the process, but it fails to reverse those signs and symptoms already present at birth (451).

Short Filum Terminale

This abnormality tethers the spinal cord in the lower reaches of the spinal canal and produces a similar clinical picture.

Birth Trauma

The spinal cord is most likely, but not exclusively, injured during breech birth, the traction on the cervical column usually being responsible for the damage. Actual contusions of the cord may be found, as well as hematomas and areas of traumatic softening.

Traumatic Lesions of the Spinal Cord

Features of (Total) Transverse Syndromes

Acute Total Transverse Lesion

Initially a flaccid paraplegia is present with diminished or absent reflexes and without pyramidal signs (stage of spinal shock, called diaschisis by von Monakow), all sensory modalities are absent, and bladder and intestinal control are lost. This stage is explained by abolition of the tonic action of corticospinal stimuli on the anterior horn cells. The resting potential of the motor neurons of the spinal cord at this stage is 2-6 mV above normal, the membane thus being more stable. This phase lasts 3-6 weeks.

Later Stages, Development of Chronic Transverse Lesion

As a result of neuronal hypersensitivity to denervation, the spinal efferent tracts discharge more easily, and this gives rise to a variety of phenomena which are characteristic of a transverse lesion.

Motor paraplegia with increased muscular tone, abnormally brisk reflexes, and pyramidal signs.

Sensory disturbances in the form of a sensory transverse lesion with a detectable upper level.

Spinal cord automatisms such as a *withdrawal reflex* (elicited by the Marie-Foix maneuver, i.e., forced passive flexion and supination of the foot), a *positive stretch reflex* and magnet reaction (extension of the legs following pressure on the soles, alternating flexion of one limb and extension of the other), and a *mass reflex* including defecation, urination, sweating, and a rise in blood pressure.

Trophic changes, especially of the skin. Together with autonomic dysregulation, ischemia caused by pressure causes *pressure sores* (decubiti) to develop within the first few hours (1239).

Hypotensive changes (when the paraplegic is positioned upright) in lesions above the level of T6 during the phase of initial spinal shock. This is caused by interruption of the sympathetic tracts in the lateral columns, which leave the spinal cord below the level of T4 in the motor roots.

Hypertensive complications. These may occur as a rise in blood pressure after (unnoticed) overdistention of the bladder, starting 8–12 months after the injury, and lead to life-threatening situations. They are ac-

companied by headache, attacks of sweating, and confusion.

Bladder Function

Anatomy: The following features are relevant to normal bladder function:

- the spinal center lies between S2 and S4,
- parasympathetic efferent fibers run in the S2-4 nerve roots, and the pelvic nerve supplies the detrusor and internal sphincteric muscles of the bladder,
- sympathetic efferent fibers run in the upper lumbar and lower thoracic nerve roots and in the sympathetic chain,
- somatic motor (efferent) fibers run in the S2-4 nerve roots via the pudendal nerve to supply the external sphincteric muscle of the bladder, and
- sensory (afferent) fibers accompany the hypogastric, pelvic, and pudendal nerves.

Physiology: Voiding is a spinal reflex but the higher cerebral centers via tracts in the lateral columns of the spinal cord can stimulate or inhibit this reflex. Thus, urination is brought under direct voluntary control.

Disturbances of Bladder Function (745, 1239)

The following disturbances of urination accompany transverse lesions and other neurologic diseases:

Uncontrolled neurogenic bladder: In lesions of the corticospinal tracts, either congenital or following subtotal lesions of the cerebral cortex or pyramidal tracts. Urination is inescapable once started, but it can usually be initiated voluntarily. Incontinence is not always present, there is no resting volume. Uncontrolled neurogenic bladder may accompany diseases such as multiple sclerosis and pernicious anemia.

Reflex neurogenic bladder ("automatic bladder"): The suprasegmental reflex arc is interrupted anatomically and functionally, but the sacral centers as well as the efferent and afferent fibers remain intact. This situation is present in lesions of the spinal cord above the level of the conus, as well as in cases of multiple sclerosis, pernicious anemia, and in normal infants. The bladder empties reflexly when it reaches a specific degree of distention, and no significant residual volume remains. Evacuation usually occurs every 3–6 h and, in spite of the absence of control over initiation and interruption of urinary flow, it can be started by certain manipulations. The instillation of ice water can induce powerful reflex contractions, producing a characteristic curve on cystomanometry – which contrasts with the flat pressure curve of the autonomous bladder (see below).

Deafferented bladder: The sensory fibers accompanying the pelvic nerves are interrupted, e. g., in lesions of the posterior nerve roots, such as tabes dorsalis. Reflex bladder contractions cease altogether, and the bladder becomes overfilled and hypotonic, its wall abnormally thin. Only isolated contractions occur due to the direct response of the smooth musculature of its walls to dilation. The term sensory paralytic bladder may be used to describe this situation, and a so-called overflow bladder results. It may be caused by tabes dorsalis, pernicious anemia, autonomic neuropathy (e. g., in diabetes mellitus), multiple sclerosis, or syringomyelia.

Deefferented bladder: Only the motor component of the bladder reflex arc is interrupted; the term motor paralytic bladder may be used. This picture is seen in poliomyelitis, and also in polyradiculitis. Most patients recover after the acute phase, but retention with overflow may occur.

Denervated bladder ("autonomous bladder"): Both components of the reflex arc are interrupted, either by a peripheral lesion or by damage to the spinal bladder center in the conus terminalis. A flaccid, distended bladder results which empties by overflowing. Small contractions of the muscular wall occur, and occasionally shrinkage and trabecular hypertrophy may distort it. The specific hyperactivity of this type of bladder – pointing to a hypersensitivity of the bladder muscle caused by denervation – allows it to be differentiated from the deafferented bladder. Autonomic bladder may develop after trauma, infection, spinal arachnoiditis, and myelomalacia; it may also accompany spina bifida and cauda equina tumors. The absence of the bulbocavernosus reflex (see Table 2.**1**) is useful for the diagnosis of a lesion of S2-3 segment of the conus, and its afferent and efferent pathways, and serves to differentiate specific neurogenic disturbances of urination from those due to urologic causes.

Clinical Aspects of Traumatic Spinal Cord Lesions (436, 1136)

In spinal trauma, and occasionally also following impact in an axial direction (p. 196), the spinal cord may be injured, with or without detectable damage to the vertebral column, intervertebral disks, or ligaments. The following types of damage may be distinguished:

Spinal Concussion

This term is used to denote an immediate, complete transverse lesion, which cannot be distinguished from the shock phase of complete severance of the spinal cord. However, the typical feature of spinal concussion is complete recovery of the signs and symptoms within hours (or days?).

Spinal Contusion

This term denotes traumatic damage to the tissues of the spinal cord following a direct injury or hemorrhage. It may be caused by fracture dislocation of a vertebra, a loose fragment of bone, a prolapsed intervertebral disk, or a subluxation (with subsequent complete correction) of two adjacent vertebrae so that no roentgenologic abnormality can be detected. The degree of recovery from the initial clinical picture – usually total paraplegia – depends largely on the extent of the mechanical damage. In a series of cases evaluated by experienced colleagues, only 25% of patients with an originally complete transverse lesion and 57% of those with an incomplete lesion showed spontaneous improvement (526). The recovery of sensation appears to be a favorable prognostic sign in respect to the return of motor function (1233). The clinical level of involvement of the cord does not always correspond to the level of the damage to the vertebral column. The levels most frequently involved are C5, T4, T10, and L1, even when the skeletal damage is two or more segments away. The cause is assumed to be an associated vascular mechanism. During recovery, the upper clinical level may migrate downward by several segments.

Myelomalacia

Secondary circulatory phenomena may also explain why the spinal cord may undergo pathologic softening only after a latent interval of hours or days after the trauma. *Syringomyelia* (p. 230) may be a late complication of traumatic paraplegia, occurring months or years later in a cranial segment of the spinal cord and showing a progressive course. This complication merits neurosurgical intervention.

Spinal Cord Compression

This is caused by mechanical factors such as a prolapsed intervertebral disk, a fragment of bone, or an *epidural spinal hematoma*. The last-mentioned condition may also arise spontaneously, complicate anticoagulant treatment, or follow minor trauma or physical exertion. The typical picture is one of very severe localized back pain which after a latent period of hours or days leads to paraplegia. Not infrequently a congenital vertebral malformation is present at the affected level, e.g., Klippel-Feil syndrome.

Hematomyelia

This term is used to denote hemorrhage into the central part of the spinal cord. It usually extends in a longitudinal direction over several segments. The typical clinical deficit is a partial transverse syndrome, sometimes accompanied by dissociated sensory change in the affected segments and distal spasticity or a Brown-Séquard syndrome (p. 182). The commonest cause is trauma, including an axial injury (fall onto the buttocks, diving into shallow water). The signs continue to progress for hours or days, and the clinical level of spinal cord involvement rises through several segments. Local pain is common. The lower cervical cord is the favored site. The CSF is usually, but not always, blood-stained or xanthochromic. Spontaneous hematomyelia is a far less common condition and should always prompt the suspicion of a spinal arteriovenous malformation (p. 212).

Conus Lesion

The conus medullaris lies at the level of the L1 vertebra. The typical features of a pure *conus syndrome* are disturbances of urination (denervated autonomous bladder, p. 195), defecation, and sexual functions in the presence of sphincteric paralysis. Sometimes a dissociated sensory disturbance is present in the lower 3–4 sacral and coccygeal segments, or else there is a disturbance of all sensory modalities in these segments (saddle anesthesia). Motor function may remain intact (however, a gluteal paralysis may be present), and the pyramidal tracts are unaffected. The bulbocavernosus reflex (see Table 2.1) is absent. Apart from trauma, the syndrome is seen in neoplasms and in cases of vascular insufficiency, e.g., aortic aneurysm.

Cauda Equina Syndrome

A pure cauda equina syndrome may accompany fractures, particularly traumatic prolapse of lumbar intervertebral disks below L1-2. Contrary to the picture in conus lesions, this painful condition leads to a flaccid paralysis of the lower extremities with a disturbance of all sensory modalities, usually saddle anesthesia, absent reflexes, and sphincteric paralysis; no pyramidal signs are present. The clinical picture depends on the nerve roots involved, especially the level at which they leave the spinal canal (see Tables 9.1 and 9.2 and Fig. 2.6).

Practical Approach to Acute Traumatic Paraplegia

Diagnostic steps: *Neurologic examination* to determine the segment affected (take care in moving the injured patient!). *Physical examination of the vertebral column* to detect any displacements, gibbus formation, etc.

Roentgenologic examination of the appropriate part of the vertebral column, especially lateral views.
Lumbar puncture with carefully carried out Queckenstedt's test. The amount of blood in the CSF is unrelated to the severity of the lesion or the prognosis.

Myelography is justified only if
- roentgenologically visible evidence is shown of stenosis of the spinal canal (a vertebral body needs to be dislocated by at least one-third of its sagittal width to produce spinal cord compression),

– CT scanning and MR imaging do not give a clear result.

CT scanning – or *MR imaging*, which may replace myelography – in order to detect traumatic stenosis of the spinal canal by hematoma or other soft tissue lesions or by bone fragments not visible in conventional roentgenograms.

Surgical treatment: *Neurosurgical exploration* following laminectomy is an *emergency measure* if neuroradiologic investigation confirms the presence of an obstruction in patients with recent complete or chronic incomplete transverse lesions. However, almost invariably a contusion of the spinal cord is found and the operation is unsuccessful. Only very occasionally does the operation reveal an epidural hematoma or a bone fragment that compromises the blood supply of the cord.

Secondary operation is indicated with delayed onset or a definite worsening of the signs and symptoms or in the presence of the myelographic demonstration of an obstruction. In this situation, also, spinal cord softening or contusion with edema is the usual finding, and the operation is frequently valueless. Numerous useless operations are performed, compared to the few that are potentially useful and have a successful outcome. Stability of the vertebral column, which is so important in the paraplegic, may sometimes be compromised by a surgical maneuver, which consequently delays the start of rehabilitation. For these reasons, experienced colleagues recommend the operative exploration of paraplegic lesions only in exceptional circumstances (526).

Orthopedic operations are always indicated if bone fragments or dislocations of the vertebral column protrude directly into the spinal canal, despite the fact that neurologic deficits (and especially above T12) will not be influenced by it. They are also indicated if the neurologic deficit increases in association with an unstable vertebral lesion, as well as in the presence of instability or pain, in order to accelerate mobilization and rehabilitation.

Rehabilitation of Paraplegics

This commences immediately after the injury (483, 1239). The most important measure is attention to the nursing management of the patient: correct positioning is essential, including a regimen of turning the patient over every 2 h to prevent bedsores. Another obvious aim is to prevent overfilling and infection of the bladder, which leads to infection and chronic inflammation of the bladder wall and stone formation. It is achieved, initially by regular catheterization under stringently aseptic conditions, followed eventually by intermittent self-catheterization. No details of motor rehabilitation can be given here.

Whiplash Injury (1276)

This injury is usually the result of an automobile accident: drivers or passengers struck from behind are at greatest risk, and frontal collision is significantly less often responsible. Lesions of the cervical vertebral column with or without spinal cord signs and symptoms are usually accompanied by prolonged neck and arm pains and headache (p. 457). Often additional distressing autonomic features are present, including dizziness and impotence and long-lasting neurasthenic manifestations. The roentgenologic findings may be completely normal or consist of no more than a limitation of neck extension and a blocking of segmental movements, as well as nontraumatic spondylotic changes. However, occasionally an acute *central cervical cord syndrome* may be observed, which cannot be distinguished initially from hematomye-

lia, although the former condition shows a better tendency to recover. Disturbances of consciousness and a picture of cerebral concussion or even contusion may be present.

Tumors and Other Space-Occupying Lesions of the Spinal Cord

General Principles

Any lesion which mechanically compresses the spinal cord leads to a progressive restriction of its function, and a slowly progressive cord transection syndrome. It is very important that every physician is aware of it when a patient complains of stiffness of the legs, of increasing gauge problems, decreased sensation in legs, a bandlike sensation around the abdomen, or even difficulty voiding. This constellation of cord symptoms due to compression has the following characteristic details:

- *Motor function* is first affected. For example, a slowly growing space-occupying lesion will present for a long time as a purely motor lesion, i.e., muscular weakness and pyramidal signs. However, careful physical examination will usually reveal distal
- *sensory disturbances* (especially epicritic sensibility and vibration sense). A clearly definable sensory level is not always present initially.
- *Disturbances of urination* follow relatively late.

- *Radicular (girdle) sensory changes* occasionally indicate the level of the lesion.
- *Absence of individual superficial abdominal reflexes or tendon jerks* likewise may provide a clue to the level of the lesion.
- *Sciatic-like pains* may be present in the lower limbs, in some cases, even in tumors of the cervical or thoracic cord.
- *The cranial nerves* escape involvement in pure spinal lesions. However, papilledema may be present if the CSF protein content is very high.
- The *vertebral column* may show deformity, gibbus formation, or tenderness to percussion of individual spinous processes.
- *Roentgenograms of the vertebral column* may reveal bone destruction, widening of the spinal canal, destruction of the pedicles or spinous processes, or the presence of a vertebral hemangioma.
- *Lumbar puncture* may yield CSF with very high levels of protein in the presence of total obstruction (Froin's syndrome). No manometric rise in pressure will be obtained with Queckenstedt's test.

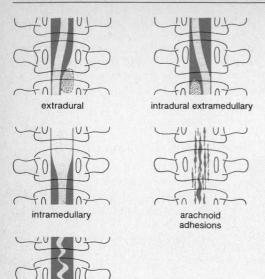

extradural

intradural extramedullary

intramedullary

arachnoid
adhesions

spinal arteriovenous
malformation

Fig. 2.3 Diagrammatic representation of space-occupying and other abnormal intraspinal lesions shown by positive contrast myelography

- *Sensory evoked potentials* may indicate the level of the lesion (581).
- *Myelography or CT or MR scanning* is essential in diagnosis.

Specific fluctuations in the intensity of the signs and symptoms is also encountered in compressive lesions, but there is never true spontaneous recovery. However, treatment with corticosteroids to combat edema will always improve the clinical picture.

Specific Types of Spinal Cord Compression

Tumors of the Spinal Canal

A tumor may be suspected clinically from the *case history* and the clinical *findings* (see above). However, definitive demonstration requires *CT or MR scanning* or *myelography.* Myelography provides, depending on the site and appearance of the space-occupying lesion, a diagnostically definitive picture. As revealed in Fig. 2.3, it defines the relationships between tumor, spinal cord, and dural sac and yields at the very least a topographic diagnosis. The three commonest tumors are neurinoma, meningioma, and metastasis.

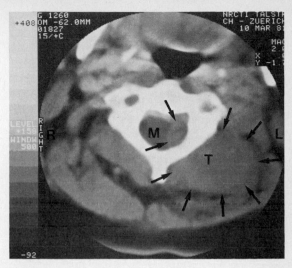

Fig. 2.**4**   CT demonstration of a left-sided neurofibroma (arrows) at the level of C4, partly invading the spinal canal and displacing the cervical spinal cord (M) to the right side. (Image from the Neuroradiological and Computed Tomographic Institute, 65 Talstrasse, Zurich)

Neurofibroma

It accounts for about one-third of all spinal tumors. Although occurring at any level, it is most commonly found in the lower thoracic and lumbar region. Since the tumor often arises from a nerve root, radicular pains or deficits are commonly present. If the tumor develops within an intervertebral foramen and excavates it, oblique roentgenographic projections will show the abnormal canal and enable a diagnosis to be made of intra- and extraspinal growth – the so-called *hourglass (dumbbell) neurofibroma*. These tumors are well demonstrated by CT scanning (Fig. 2.**4**). Spinal neurofibromas may be isolated tumors or one of the manifestations of generalized neurofibromatosis (von Recklinghausen, p. 12).

Meningioma

This benign tumor also accounts for about one-third of intraspinal space-occupying lesions and may lead over the course of years to a terminally severe compression of the spinal cord. The commonest site is the thoracic spine. The spinal meningioma has a very characteristic myelographic appearance, a round mass growing from the dura and displacing the spinal cord (Fig. 2.**5**).

Metastases (1146)

In the majority of cases the deposits are present in the vertebrae and secondarily compromise the spinal cord. The site of *primary growth* in one-third of cases is the lung, in another one-third the breast, in one-fourth there are other sites, and about 10% remain undetected. In at least one-half of cases, the spi-

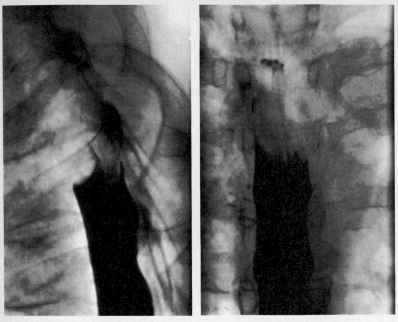

a   b

Fig. 2.5 a, b   Meningioma at the level of T6, shown by contrast myelography. a Lateral, b Anteroposterior view. (Radiographs from the Division of Neuroradiology, Professor P. *Huber,* Department of Diagnostic Radiology, formerly Professor W. *Fuchs,* University of Berne)

nal metastases form the *first clinical manifestation* of the primary tumor. The **clinical picture** is initiated in two-thirds of cases by pain (backache and girdle-like radicular pains). The commonest complaint is weakness of the legs, which may progress rapidly in a few days to paraplegia. Sphincteric disturbances develop later.

Roentgenograms of the vertebral column may initially be normal but in about 80%–90% will be abnormal later, especially in breast cancer.

Treatment: Neurofibromas and meningiomas, which are histologically benign tumors, are treated by radical neurosur-

gical excision. Metastases require a combined surgical and radiotherapeutic approach or are treated by radiotherapy alone. Radiotherapy is the preferred approach in the presence of multiple lesions, if the diagnosis of malignancy is confirmed. The prognosis depends on the nature of the primary tumor. In primary bronchogenic carcinoma, less than 20% respond to treatment; only a few survive 1 year. In carcinoma of the breast, about 50% react favorably to treatment and one-third of patients are alive at the end of 1 year (1146).

Meningeal Carcinomatosis (1131)

In this form of neoplasm, the meninges are diffusely permeated by tumor tissue over many segments. Apart from clinical signs of spinal cord involvement, there is always severe pain and physical signs of polyradiculopathy, which may also involve cranial nerves. The CSF has an increased protein and a reduced glucose content and the cell count is increased; tumor cells may be found in the sediment. In meningeal carcinomatosis as well, adenocarcinoma of the stomach, lung, and breast carcinoma are the commonest primary sources. This variety of neoplasm carries a very poor prognosis, and the average survival time after establishing the diagnosis is 1 month (1131). *Meningeal sarcomatosis* may be a specific form of medulloblastoma.

Nonneoplastic Spinal Cord Compression

Nontumoral Spinal Masses

To this group belongs the *epidural spinal hematoma,* which has already been described on p. 196. An *epidural spinal abscess* (471, 701) usually arises from an adjacent source of infection and may produce compression of the spinal cord of greater or lesser degree (p. 205). *Diseases of the vertebrae* similarly may cause compression of the spinal cord and signs of damage to the cord and nerve roots. *Hemangioma of bone* causes local pain, tenderness to percussion of the spinous process, and radicular pains, and it may compress the spinal cord. The lesion is usually situated in a midthoracic vertebra. *Achondroplasia* (1249), vertebral deformities in *pseudohypoparathyroidism,* osteoporosis with kyphosis and especially *kyphoscoliosis,* all may lead to slowly progressive compression of the spinal cord. Under certain circumstances, most of these lesions are amenable to orthopedic cor-

rection. The kyphosis in *adolescent scoliosis* (Scheuermann) occasionally may cause a transverse lesion (1042).

Myelopathy in cervical spondylosis: the common roentgenologic manifestation of *cervical spondylosis* (469, 1195) may be accompanied by injury to the cervical spinal cord. A similar clinical picture, unassociated with cervical spondylosis or with only slight evidence of it, is found in *congenital stenosis of the cervical spinal canal,* usually in men (616). Patients with rheumatoid arthritis are at particular risk (868). **Pathogenetically,** the signs and symptoms are produced by spondylotic ridges of the posterior surfaces of the vertebral bodies. These ridges impinge directly upon the spinal cord or indirectly impair its function by affecting the blood supply from the anterior spinal or radicular arteries. The **clinical picture** is characterized by muscular weakness in a radicular distribution, sometimes involving several segments because of the oblique downward course of the nerve roots in the lower cervical canal: at the same level, more than one root may be exposed to mechanical damage. Sensory disturbances are present which are often nonspecific and not invariably radicular; they may have a patchy or glove distribution (spinal tract involved). Temperature and pain sensations are most severely affected. Ataxic disturbances occur as a result of damage to the spinocerebellar tracts. Spasticity may be present, particularly of the lower limbs due to pyramidal involvement. Spasticity of the upper limbs when present – occasionally caused in cervical spondylosis of caudal segments by compromise of the anterior spinal artery, and rarely even accompanied by fasciculation – requires differentiation from amyotrophic lateral sclerosis. *Roentgenologic examination* of the cervical spinal canal in the lateral view shows the narrowest segment to have a sagittal diameter of 13 mm or less. *Lumbar puncture* usually reveals no obstruction to the passage of CSF (Queckenstedt's test to be performed with the neck in maximal flexed and extended positions!), and the protein content is normal or only slightly increased. *Lateral cervical myelography or CT scanning* reveals stenosis of the cervical spine canal: the sagittal diameter as measured from the anterior border of the contrast-filled dural sac is 9.5 mm on average, compared with 16–17 mm in normal subjects. *The syndrome of intermittent claudication of the cervical spinal cord* is an unusual manifestation of the condition, which represents fluctuating signs and symptoms of spinal cord compression, resulting from a narrow spinal canal due to congenital and/or degenerative causes. The state of tension of the spinal cord within the canal may also contribute, the compressed cord being more vulnerable to microtrauma through flexion and extension of the neck during increased physical activity. **Treatment** in established cases consists of either wide decompression by multiple-level laminectomy (349 1195) or of anterior spinal fusion (469). Improvement can be expected in about two-thirds of patients in whom the onset of the signs and symptoms is

subacute, and in about one-third of those, the condition is long-standing and slowly progressive (469). In the presence of spasticity of all limbs, the results of surgical treatment are disappointing (1195). The diagnosis of spodylotic myelopathy should be considered in any elderly subject presenting with a chronic progressive spastic-paraparetic syndrome. However, not infrequently it may be due to an unassociated disease such as multiple sclerosis. MR scanning may be helpful in such cases.

Nonmedullary clinical signs of cervical spondylosis, see p. 378.

Myelopathy due to a narrow thoracic canal: This form of cord compression is rare but rather typical (1299). It occurs also with the specific diseases of the spine listed on p. 203. Spastic gait disturbance, sensory disturbance, and sometimes difficulty voiding develop with gradual progression over months or years.

A claudication intermittens forces the patient to stop or change his position. The myelogram or computer tomography are diagnostic. A generous dorsal decompression.

Differential Diagnosis of Spinal Cord Compression

The following diseases are the conditions that must most frequently be differentiated from a mechanical cause, in patients with suspected compression of the spinal cord:

- Multiple sclerosis, spastic progressive spinal form (usually bouts of illness and nonmedullary features in the history, no clear-cut sensory level).
- Familial spastic paraplegia (pure motor lesion).

- Syringomyelia (look for dissociated sensory disturbances).
- Specific metabolic disorders, e.g., subacute combined degeneration.
- Vascular spinal syndromes and myelitides (these usually run an acute course, although occasionally a sub-acute or chronic variety may be seen.)
- Rarely, reversible spastic paraplegia may appear in hyperthyroidism (401).
- Spastic myelopathy in association with an anterior horn cell lesion has been described in lathyrism (246).

Inflammatory, Allergic, and Toxic Diseases of the Spinal Cord and its Coverings

Infective Lesions of the Spinal Cord

Septic Diseases

Intramedullary abscess is very rare.

Spinal subdural abscess presents with backache, radicular involvement, a transverse lesion, or paraplegia of sudden onset. A previous history of infection is common, and osteomyelitis of a vertebral body may be present. The ESR is usually elevated. The prognosis depends on early diagnosis, antibiotics, and operation.

Spinal epidural abscess (471, 701) was found once in 250–350 neurological in-patients and is encountered at an early age. In about one-half of cases the causative primary infection is known — boil, lung infection, septic abortion, osteomyelitis, endocarditis, otitis media, etc. The microorganism is usually a *Staphylococcus aureus.* Neurologic signs and symptoms appear 15–20 days after the primary infection and comprise initially severe back pains with fever failing to respond to treatment and a high ESR. Later on, root signs develop and almost invariably a picture of spinal cord (or cauda equina) compression. The CSF is always abnormal, the cell count being raised. Roentgenograms of the vertebral column may reveal a diskitis. Antibiotic treatment is best com-bined with laminectomy, but it may be successful without this operation (701).

Acute Anterior Poliomyelitis

Epidemiology: Acute anterior poliomyelitis (infantile paralysis) has become rare in those countries in which active preventive immunization of the population has been practiced. Previous experience with this endemic and epidemic virus infection, which is transmitted in early life in conditions of filth and poor hygiene, but also at a later age, when sanitary practices are better, has shown it to cause neurologic signs and symptoms in only 1%–2% of the individuals affected.

Pathologic anatomy: The pathologic lesion affects the gray matter, particularly the anterior horn cells of the spinal cord, which are replaced by glial tissue.

Clinical picture: After an incubation period of 3–20 days, the patient usually experiences a nonspecific *febrile illness* which, after a latent period of several days, leads to the *main* *phase* of the disease. This phase, also febrile, begins with by general malaise, headache, and meningism, followed 1–4 days later by paralysis. The *pattern of the paralysis* is one of progressive spread over the course of several hours or days. Neither paresthesias nor specific sensory disturbances form part of the picture of anterior poliomyelitis, although sometimes the affected muscles are painful and tender. Apart from the commoner spinal variety of the disease, other forms occur. There may even be exclusive involvement of the bulbar and pontine muscles, with paralysis of deglutition and respiration. Facial palsy, and disturbances of external ocular movement have been reported, but are atypical. The encephalitic variety is very rare.

CSF findings: At the start of the second phase, the CSF contains several hundred cells, mostly polymorphonuclear leukocytes, but soon the pattern changes. In the course of 1–2 weeks, the cell count diminishes and round cells predominate, and the protein content increases, sometimes leading to definite albuminocytologic dissociation.

Differential diagnosis: The differential diagnosis from Guillain-Barré polyradiculitis is discussed on p. 297. Apart from the poliovirus, other virus diseases produce anterior horn cell damage, specifically echo and coxsackie virus infections. Isolation of the virus is required to identify the cause.

Prognosis: The prognosis in patients with bulbar involvement and respiratory paralysis is poor, the mortality being as high as 50%. The recovery stage may commence at the peak of the paralysis so that a considerable improvement or complete recovery of the paralyzed muscles is possible within a few weeks. The retention of some residual functions, however slight, is a prognostically favorable sign. After the initial few months, the changes of significant further recovery are slender. In most patients only a partial recovery occurs, leaving a residue of motor weakness, muscular atrophy, and absent reflexes as well as in those cases affecting young children, retarded growth of the affected extremity.

Immunization: Active oral immunization with a live vaccine (Sabin) has resulted in the virtual disappearance of paralytic forms of the disease in many countries. The complications of immunization, which are rare (p. 164), are outweighed by the practical benefits of eliminating the disease.

Late complications: Occasionally the residual paralysis may be observed to increase in patients many years after the acute infection. This *increased residual paralysis* ("post-polio syndrome") is presumed to result from a further degeneration of the initially infected anterior horn cells or from a secondary associated myopathy of partially denervated muscle elements. Children vaccinated against poliomyelitis, all of them under 10 years of age, have been observed to develop muscular weakness a few days after an acute attack of *bronchial asthma*. This weakness develops suddenly and affects one or other extremity to a varying degree. Secondary atrophy occurs but there is no sensory deficit. Occasionally muscular pains and meningism are encountered. The CSF shows an increased cell and protein content. The muscular weakness usually fails to improve, or does so only unsatisfactorily (1264).

Myelitis

General: The term "myelitis" is used to describe any involvement of the spinal cord, either isolated or within the context of an infectious disease, as a result of an allergic reaction or an "allergic" demyelinating process. Most myelitides affect the various columns of the spinal cord, in addition to presenting sometimes as an encephalitis, and this process may give rise to a variegated pathologic picture.

Lesions of the spinal cord may be multifocal and involvement of the entire cross section produces a transverse myelitis (see below). Myelitides occasionally follow leptospiral, spirochetal, *Legionella,* or rickettsial infections, as well as measles, mumps, herpes simplex, and other viral infections. They also occur after active smallpox and antirabies immunization, and as a paraneoplastic process (500). Myelitis may occur in the context of multiple sclerosis (p. 243). The cause of many cases remains unexplained.

Transverse Myelitis (Acute Transverse Myelitis) (117, 1012)

Epidemiology: The annual incidence amounts to about 1.3 per 1 million inhabitants (117). It may appear at any age but two definite peaks occur in patients 10–20 or over 40 years of age. Men and women are equally affected. No seasonal incidence is known.

Precipitating factors: Only one-third of patients give a history of preceding illness, usually an upper respiratory tract infection 5–21 days before the onset of the neurologic signs and symptoms. Immunization does not appear to be a precursor.

Clinical features: The initial symptoms – often fever, muscular pains, backache, and girdle pain – worsen within 24 h in about one-half of cases to a transverse lesion which is more or less complete; the time scale varies from 5 min to many weeks in duration. A slow improvement commences after an interval varying from a few weeks to 3 months; thereafter, no further improvement can be expected. Patients who have experienced one attack of transverse myelitis seldom experience a fresh attack; in particular, its reoccurrence in multiple sclerosis is very rare, even in patients with a long history (117, 1012). If an optic neuritis appears, the condition is referred to as neuromyelitis optica (Devic's disease) (p. 253). It is impossible to differentiate an *acute necrotizing myelopathy,* a disease which has a very poor prognosis, from the attacks of transverse myelitis accompanying demyelinating diseases.

Toxic Myelopathies

Myelopathy in Heroin Addicts

Various neurologic complications are described in heroin addiction, including brachial plexus neuropathy, polyradiculitis, polyneuropathy, injection damage to a peripheral nerve, rhabdomyolysis, brain abscesses, mycotic aneurysms, stroke, tetanus, and epileptic seizures. The myelopathy, which is of special interest in this section, usually appears immediately after a self-injection and may follow an unconscious state. Physical examination shows a transverse lesion at the thoracic level, often total but occasionally only partial in extent. The prognosis is poor. Suggested causal mechanisms include hypertension, an extended position of head in coma, toxic or allergic factors, and embolic or other vascular lesions.

Myeloneuropathy After Nitrous Oxide Inhalation

Signs and symptoms may appear in addicts after months or years and rarely after repeated involuntary inhalations (dentists!) (682): The polyneuropathy produces sensory changes distally in the extremities, ataxia, impotence, brisk reflexes and pyramidal signs, sphincteric disturbances, and mental changes. The prognosis is poor.

Other Toxic Myelopathies

The myelopathies accompanying *chronic alcoholism* (1050) (p.151) and *lathyrism* (p.221) are described elsewhere.

Circulatory Disturbances of the Spinal Cord

Blood Supply of the Spinal Cord

The blood supply of the spinal cord is shown diagrammatically in Figs.2.6 and 2.7. The fetal pattern of a separate pair of radicular arteries in each segment is reduced in adults to six to eight anterior and posterior segmental arteries of supply of the spinal cord. The largest of these is the great radicular artery (artery of Adamkiewicz), which enters the spinal canal between T10 and L2, usually on the left side. The segmental arteries reach the spinal canal through the intervertebral foramina and penetrate the intradural space in the root sleeves. They feed an anastomotic chain, the anterior spinal artery and the paired posterior spinal arteries. These three arteries are connected with each other by a network linked at the various segmental levels in the transverse plane, the vasocorona. Local conditions within these arteries and general pressure relationships may combine to reverse the flow so that the blood in the various longitudinal arteries may be flowing in different directions. The boundary zones appear to be particularly vulnerable to ischemic changes.

Spinal Cord Ischemia (140, 560, 952, 1168)

Pathophysiologic mechanisms: *Ischemic softening of the spinal cord,* so-called *myelomalacia,* may be caused by a pathogenetic mechanism similar to that responsible for ischemic softening of the brain. These changes may result from local lesions of the walls of feeding or radicular arteries, or as a result of hemodynamic factors. The causes of an inadequate blood supply are:

- a *steal phenomenon,* e. g., in Paget's disease of bone (505),
- a lesion of the *abdominal aorta* (dissecting aneurysm, fusiform aneurysm, severe atheromatosis, syphilitic arteritis, thrombosis),
- iatrogenic occlusion of a *large lumbar artery* during aortography, either plugged by the catheter or during injection of the contrast medium,
- mechanical damage to a *radicular artery,* e. g., during sympathectomy, external compression by spondylotic constriction of an intervertebral foramen (especially thoracolumbar),
- a *local atheromatous lesion,* or thrombosis of a radicular artery,

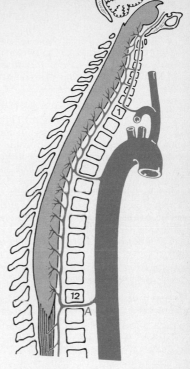

Fig. 2.6 Blood supply of the spinal ▷ cord from the radicular arteries. A = Great radicular artery of Adamkiewicz (after *Lazorthes*)

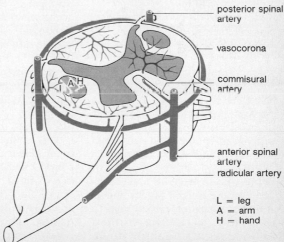

posterior spinal artery

vasocorona

commisural artery

anterior spinal artery

radicular artery

L = leg
A = arm
H = hand

Fig. 2.7 Blood supply of the spinal cord (cross section)

- *generalized arterial hypotension,* e.g., circulatory collapse or perioperative complication,
- *anoxemia,* e.g., cardiac insufficieny (140), cor pulmonale, or CO intoxication, sometimes combined with local narrowing of a radicular or spinal artery.

The arteriosclerotic process involves only the large feeding arteries, and it is not seen in the intrinsic vessels of the spinal cord. These vessels may exhibit fibrosis of the adventitial layer, but this lesion does not lead to occlusion. Pathologically, symmetrical areas of softening are found in the gray matter with lumbosacral predominance, after anoxic cardiocirculatory complications (70). Spinal cord infarction is a rare complication of venous thrombosis (619).

Clinical Syndromes

Depending on the extent and duration of the ischemia, very different clinical syndromes may result. Intermittent circulatory insufficiency, apart from producing fully reversible spinal deficits, may lead to complete softening of a segment of the spinal cord, with clinical features appropriate to the timing and the site of the lesion.

Intermittent Spinal Circulatory Insufficiency

This term is used to describe repeated, transient ischemic signs such as paraparesis, pyramidal signs, paresthesias of the legs, and sensory disturbances. For example, the severity of these signs may correspond to the degree of decompensation in a case of cardiac insufficiency (140, 581). Somatosensory evoked potentials, elicited in the brain upon stimulation of the lower half of the trunk, may sometimes reveal a level which is not demonstrable upon clinical examination (581).

Intermittent Claudication of the Spinal Cord

Symptoms and signs caused by a lesion in the blood vessel walls may appear during exercise. The vast majority of such patients are elderly males. A transverse lesion which may appear to be virtually complete and remain present for several days (or weeks) can regress completely. However, permanent deficit may occur in patients with circulatory insufficiency whose signs and symptoms were initially intermittent and potentially transient.

Anterior Spinal Artery Syndrome
(952)

This is caused by an ischemic lesion of the spinal cord, the damage being confined to the territory of supply of the anterior spinal artery. Certain prodromal signs and symptoms (pains and girdle paresthesias at the level of the subsequent lesion) may precede the paralysis by hours or days. The onset is rapid, although not necessarily apoplectiform, and an initially flaccid paraplegia develops within the space of 1 h and usually within a few minutes. A pure dissociated sensory disturbance is present, in that the modalities of passive movement, position sense, and vibration remain intact and only those of pain and temperature are affected. It is important to note that, if physical examination does not include pain and temperature testing, an erroneous diagnosis of psychogenic paralysis may be made since pyramidal signs may initially be absent. Sphincteric disturbances may be present. The neurologic picture can be explained by a lesion in the territory of supply of the anterior spinal artery and the sulcocommissural arteries. The cause may be any of the arterial or circulatory lesions mentioned above. Direct compression of the anterior spinal artery by a space-occupying lesion such as a prolapsed intervertebral disk is another cause to be considered. Some patients show partial regression of the clinical deficit; few recover completely.

Infarct in Territory of Posterior Spinal Artery

In contrast to the anterior spinal artery syndrome, this is a very rare lesion. Total deficit of all posterior column sensory modalities is present, as well as a paraplegia.

Sulcocommissural Artery Syndrome (1168)

This syndrome results if one-half of the area of the spinal cord is involved at a specific level – in effect, a vascularly mediated incomplete Brown-Séquard syndrome.

Global Myelomalacia

Focal myelomalacia, i.e., ischemic softening of the entire cross-sectional area of the spinal cord at a specific level, may have a painful and sudden, although not always stroke-like onset. A march of signs over several days may be observed. The paralysis remains virtually complete, although exceptions occur. The likely causes of this lesion have been mentioned above. Some cases of so-called necrotizing myelitis or acute paraplegic myelitis belong to this group. The lesion may also occur at the level of the conus medullaris.

Centromedullary Softening

Occasionally focal softening of the cross-sectional area of the spinal cord at a specific level (with corresponding clinical syndrome, including sometimes a dissociated sensory level) may be combined with a further area of softening involving the centromedullary part of the spinal cord lying caudal to it. As a result of involvement of motor neurons, a syndrome of permanent flaccid paraplegia results (849).

Chronic Progressive Myelopathy

This syndrome may follow a chronic circulatory insufficiency of the spinal cord in the context of arteriosclerosis. Although it may cause spastic paraparesis, the signs and symptoms may be indistinguishable from amyotrophic lateral sclerosis. In chronic hypoxia associated, for example, with chronic respiratory insufficiency, electrophysiologic signs of an anterior horn cell lesion may be present (1222). For pathologic changes following anoxia, see above.

Venous Infarction of the Spinal Cord

A rare cause of a circulatory disturbance of the cord is a venous thrombosis which may or may not be hemorrhagic (618). A transection syndrome develops in a stepwise or continuous progression. Inflammatory involvement of the spinal venous channels, spinal phlebitis, is another vascular cause of paraplegia.

Arteriovenous Malformations of the Spinal Cord

Definition: "Subacute necrotizing myelopathy of Foix and Alajouanine" and "spinal cord varicosities" are terms used to describe a circulatory disturbance of the spinal cord caused by an extra- or intramedullary arteriovenous malformation, e.g., angioma racemosum venosum (716, 1199).

Clinical features: The signs and symptoms usually appear between the 2nd and 4th decades of life. The most frequent level of involvement is the thoracolumbar junction. The onset is usually sudden or subacute, rarely slowly progressive. Local or radicular pains may be present initially, followed rapidly by signs of a transverse lesion. Men are significantly more often affected than women. A disorder of urination often occurs early in the course of the disease, and this feature may be diagnostically useful in differentiating it from spinal cord tumors and other compressive lesions. The clinical picture may amount to a complete transverse syndrome or assume a more incomplete form, corresponding to a Brown-Séquard syndrome. Not infrequently the course may be episodic, punctuated by partial or complete remissions. Each new attack affects the same segment, which facilitates the differential diagnosis from an acute attack of multiple sclerosis. A spinal arteriovenous malformation (and exceptionally also a spinal tumor) is a rare cause of *acute subarachnoid hemorrhage* (p. 90). The presence of backache and signs and symptoms pertaining to the spinal cord are useful in diagnosis, helping to differentiate bleeding caused by an intracranial aneurysm. Other factors claimed to trigger the clinical signs and symptoms are trauma, physical exertion, and menstruation.

Ancillary investigations: The CSF in 75% of cases shows an increased cell and protein content, less frequently xanthochromia. Myelography reveals the presence of varicose, tortuous blood vessels on the surface of the spinal cord (subdural injection of the contrast medium may mimic this appearance!). Spinal arteriography always demonstrates the pathologic vessels.

Differential diagnosis: If the signs and symptoms have a rapid onset, a myelitis should be considered, and if prolonged a compressive lesion. If after recovery the patient experiences a fresh attack, multiple sclerosis is a diagnostic possibility. However, this condition is made less likely by involvement of the same level and the presence of pain, which usually accompanies the attack. *Hematomyelia* has been discussed on p. 196.

Prognosis: The prognosis in most cases is poor. However, if patients exhibit intermittent signs and symptoms, which are likely to regress, surgical measures may be considered.

Treatment: Operative extirpation of the superficial veins by means of microsurgical techniques with the operating microscope is possible in many cases (1300, 1301), embolization in others.

Degenerative and Heredodegenerative Diseases Principally Involving the Spinal Cord

Damage to Anterior Horn Cells

General Characteristics

So-called *spinal muscular atrophy* is characterized by:

- flaccid, purely motor weakness,
- muscular atrophy,
- fasciculation,
- tendon jerks reduced or absent, no pyramidal signs,
- intact sensorium,
- muscle serum enzymes usually normal, but
- enzyme levels increased in the presence of so-called accompanying myopathy,
- EMG: giant potentials and reduced interference patterns progressing to single oscillations in maximal voluntary innervation,
- CSF usually normal, but occasionally slight increase in protein content,
- muscle biopsy: groups of fibers possessing the same degree of atrophy without overall structural changes (in exceptional cases, accompanying myopathy).

Pathophysiology and Particular Features

The Motor Unit

The *peripheral motor neuron* comprises the motor (anterior horn) cell and its axon with its ramifications. The *motor unit* expresses the totality of all those muscle fibers depending on the same anterior horn cell (Fig. 2.8). This population of muscle fibers contracts synchronously. The number of fibers dependent on one such anterior horn cell varies from muscle to muscle, e.g., 10–12 in the eye muscles, up to 1600 in the gastrocnemius muscle. Anatomically, these fibers are evenly distributed across a part of the cross section of the muscle: in the human biceps brachii they occupy an area with a cross-sectional diameter of 5 mm. Within this zone in healthy muscle, all the individual fibers belonging to the same motor unit are randomly distributed.

Denervation and Reinnervation

Damage to a motor ganglion cell, e.g., in spinal muscular atrophy, leads to degeneration of its axon and *denervation* of the muscle fibers belonging to the axons. The adjoin-

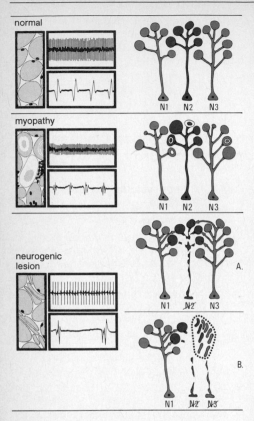

Fig. 2.8   Motor unit. *Top:* The fibers of normal muscle have the same caliber, as drawn in the three motor units shown. The electromyogram shows a complete interference pattern and normally formed motor unit potentials. *Middle:* In myopathies, individual muscle fibers of the various motor units are affected. Electromyogram: Complete interference pattern is still present but lower amplitudes and smaller, deformed motor unit potentials are also present. *Below:* Neurogenic lesions. Death of motor ganglion cells (or an axon lesion). The component muscle fibers degenerate and are partly taken over by the adjacent units. When one neuron of one of these newly enlarged motor units dies, a histologic picture of groups of muscle fibers which show the same degree of atrophy can be found. Electromyographically, a reduced interference pattern is present in voluntary innervation, with wider and deformed potentials. (See also Fig. 10.2)

ing axons, which remain linked to intact ganglion cells, then show sprouting. The denervated muscle fibers of the diseased unit become partly *reinnervated* from the adjoining axons. This leads on the one hand to an *increased number of muscle fibers in the adjoining healthy motor unit* and produces on the other hand a new grouping of the old, together with the newly innervated fibers, so-called *subunits.* These altered motor units themselves may later be denervated through degeneration of the ganglion cells to which they are linked. This process explains the changes shown by EMG and muscle biopsy, in which the processes of denervation and reinnervation may parallel each other (see Fig. 2.8).

Electromyography

In electromyography normal biphasic and triphasic action potentials and interference patterns are obtained with maximal voluntary innervation. In chronic neurogenic muscular atrophy, the EMG reflects the enlarged motor unit (see above) by revealing large, partially polyphasic potentials and an incomplete interference pattern. In *myopathies* the muscle fibers of more than one motor unit are affected. The resulting diminution of muscle units - the motor units are not numerically reduced - is reflected by the EMG as small, partially split individual potentials. They may combine upon maximal voluntary effort to produce a complete interference picture of low amplitude potentials (see Fig. 2.**8**).

Muscle Biopsy

The results of muscle biopsy enable a distinction to be drawn between neurogenic muscular atrophy and primary myopathy. In a *neurogenically damaged* motor unit, a certain number of the atrophied fibers are grouped together, corresponding to the subunit involved. They are usually elongated or distorted polygonally but their structure is intact; the nuclei are marginal and appear normal, and the interstitial tissues are not increased. In *primary myopathies,* the affected fibers are irregularly distributed, showing varying degrees of atrophy and most appear round and show - often in the absence of atrophy - structural changes (waxy degeneration, loss of longitudinal and cross-striations, floccular changes with disintegration of muscle fibers, macrophages, etc.). The nuclei, which are often increased in number, are centrally situated and form chains. The connective and fatty tissues may be increased. An inflammatory cellular infiltration is present in polymyositis as well as in certain other conditions. Some diseases have specific histologic appearances which enable their nature to be diagnosed from the biopsy material (Fig. 2.**9a** and **b**). Frequently, but by no means always, in slowly progressive spinal (and neural) muscular

atrophies, muscle biopsy reveals "myopathic" changes in the fiber structure, connective tissue proliferation, and cellular infiltration. This finding is described as an accompanying myopathy (841). In such cases the serum creatine kinase level is often raised (4).

Fasciculation

The fasciculations occurring in chronic anterior horn cell degeneration are involuntary synchronous contractions of single muscle fiber groups which are visible with the naked eye. They may be provoked or increased by tapping of the muscle or the intravenous injection of 10 mg of Tensilon. However, it is not certain that this test is a specific sign of anterior horn cell degeneration. This type of fasciculation can be distinguished only with difficulty from the *benign fasciculations* following an infection or some other undetermined cause. This is usually accomplished by studying the associated signs and symptoms or by observing the patient further. A syndrome of muscular pain and fasciculation has been described (534), see p. 486.

Contraction Fasciculations

The newly reshaped and enlarged motor unit contains an increased number of muscle fibers. Therefore, the recruitment of such units provokes the activation of a larger number of muscle fibers and thus a more powerful contraction. This causes more marked and thus visible excursions of the limb, e.g., small movements of the straightened fingers (*signe de l'index,* "polyminimyoclonus").

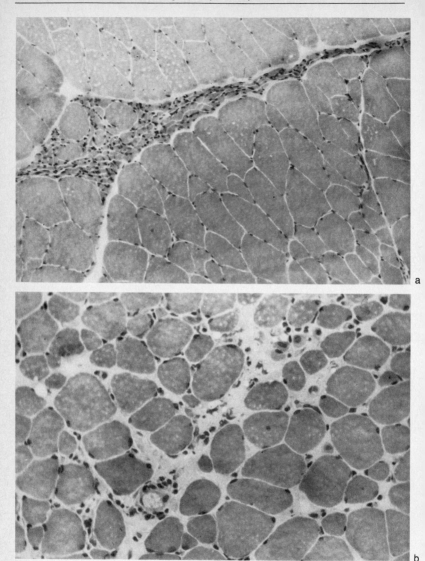

Fig. 2.**9a, b**   Muscle biopsy **a** In spinal muscular atrophy, histology reveals a field of uniformly atrophied fibers **b** In progressive muscular dystrophy, the muscle fibers vary greatly in size, some being hypertrophied and partly atrophic. Proliferation of central nuclei and regenerated fibers. Slight increase in connective tissue

Clinical Disease Pictures

The "degenerative" disease pictures (some of them familial) discussed here are often indistinguishable on clinical grounds from the rarer symptomatic forms of spinal muscular atrophy in malignant diseases, dysproteinemias, certain types of poisoning, and disturbances of glucose metabolism. Also, spinal muscular atrophy is a feature of a wide variety of diseases which are discussed elsewhere: amyotrophic lateral sclerosis, the parkinsonism-dementia complex, Creutzfeldt-Jakob disease, Friedreich's ataxia, spinal space-occupying lesions, orthostatic hypotension, etc. In hexosaminidase deficiency a complex syndrome is encountered comprising encephalopathies, ataxias, and neurologic deficits including a pure spinal muscular atrophy (577). The true primary spinal muscular atrophies are classified in Table 2.3 and will be considered further below.

Infantile Spinal Muscular Atrophy (Werdnig-Hoffmann)

This disease is **genetically** linked and appears to be inherited as an autosomal recessive. Occasionally several siblings may be affected, but there is never a history of the disease in the patient's ancestors. **Clinically,** the disease may already manifest itself in utero by a reduction in fetal movements. Occasionally it may be the cause of congenital arthrogryposis multiplex. The majority of cases are seen after birth, usually in the first 6–12 months of life. The child shows flaccid paralysis and adopts an unusual posture:

he lies with his arms flexed laterally (handle position), and his legs apart, and exhibits only small distal movements; he cries feebly. Paradoxical respiration is present and later he may have difficulty in swallowing if the bulbar nuclei become involved. Fasciculation is most marked in the tongue and less visible in the extremity muscles, where the infantile fat pads make the atrophy less obvious. More frequently fasciculation of the eyelids is visible (1116). Under certain circumstances, the fasciculations may be audible with a stethoscope. The muscular atrophy is clearly demonstrable by soft-tissue roentgenography or CT scanning.

The **prognosis** is hopeless and most patients succumb before their 5th birthday; many die earlier. However, individual cases may show a much slower progression of the disease and survive longer – up to the age of 20 years. Such cases may represent a transition – if not already manifested in the earlier years of life – toward the localized cervical and scapulohumeral form (Vulpian-Bernardt) of the disease or toward pseudomyopathic spinal muscular atrophy (Kugelberg-Welander), which will be discussed below. No **treatment** is known.

Differential diagnosis: The following must be considered: congenital muscular dystrophies, cases of the astatic-atonic syndrome (Foerster), cerebral palsy, and rare myopathies which may be benign. The syndrome of marked hypotonia and poverty of movement present at birth or in the first months of life is

Table 2.3 Principal diseases with chronic involvement of anterior horn cells

Name	Affected Structures	Symptoms	Details	Etiology
Infantile spinal muscular atrophy (Werdnig-Hoff-mann)	Anterior horn cells of spinal cord	Atrophy and paralysis of muscles. Hypotonia. Fasciculation of tongue	Infants or small children. Rapidly fatal	Inherited. Autosomal recessive (?)
Pseudomyopathic spinal muscular atrophy (Kugelberg-Welander)	Anterior horn cells of spinal cord	Atrophy and fasciculation of muscles. Progressive disturbance of gait. No bulbar symptoms	Children and adolescents. Starts proximally, usually in the lower limbs. Slow progression	Irregular dominant
Spinal muscular atrophy of the adult (Aran-Duchenne)	Anterior horn cells of spinal cord	Atrophy and paralysis of muscles. Fasciculation	Young adults. Starts distally (hands!)	Usually isolated, etiologically unexplained. Occasionally syphilis
Proximal spinal muscular atrophy of the shoulder girdle (Vulpian-Bernhardt)	Anterior horn cells of spinal cord	Atrophy and paralysis of muscles as well as fasciculation of the shoulder girdle	Adults. Slowly progressive	Unknown. Occasionally syphilis
Amyotrophic lateral sclerosis (sometimes combined with a true bulbar palsy)	Anterior horn cells of spinal cord, sometimes involvement of the bulbar motor nuclei. Pyramidal and corticobulbar tracts	Atrophy and paralysis of muscles, fasciculation, bulbar palsy with difficulties of swallowing and speech. Spasticity and pyramidal signs	Adults. Rapidly progressive and fatal. Rarely, juvenile (familial) and relatively benign cases	Usually isolated forms. Seldom genetically determined

Various rare affections with involvement of the anterior horn cells as an additional feature: Creutzfeldt-Jakob disease, orthostatic hypotension, diabetic amyotrophy (?), carcinomatous myelopathy, organic mercury poisoning, etc.

known as amyotonia congenita (Oppenheim's disease). It consists of an etiologically heterogeneous group of conditions which is unsatisfactory and should probably be abandoned. Clinical follow-up examination of such cases and the use of ancillary diagnostic methods such as EMG and muscle biopsy permits a precise etiologic classification to be reached in most cases.

Pseudomyopathic Spinal Muscular Atrophy (Kugelberg-Welander) (652)

This type of spinal muscular atrophy (type III), which is not rare, is a **hereditary** disease. It is inherited as an autosomal recessive, and more rarely as a dominant, trait. In the past, cases of the disease have been misdiagnosed as progressive muscular atrophy. **Clinically,** the disease usually commences in children aged between 2 and 10 years or in adolescents. The patients – in contrast with the cases of Werdnig-Hoffmann disease – have therefore learned to walk normally. The first signs are weakness and atrophy of the proximal muscles, usually of the lower extremities. The knee jerk disappears early. Pseudohypertrophy of the calves may occur. Fasciculation is common. As a rule, there are no signs of bulbar or pyramidal involvement. Exceptionally, an ophthalmoplegia may develop. Cardiac involvement, with conduction disturbances and signs of failure, is described (1186). The clinical course is only slowly progressive. **Ancillary investigations** such as EMG and muscle biopsy reveal the presence of neurogenic muscular atrophy and

are essential for the diagnosis. Occasionally "myopathic" changes, in the sense of an accompanying myopathy, are visible in the biopsy sections (4, 841), and occasionally the serum creatine kinase content is increased.

Adult Spinal Muscular Atrophy (Aran-Duchenne)

This variety is usually an isolated disease and familial cases are rare. **Clinically,** the disease commences in the 3rd decade of life or even later. A feature is the distal distribution of the atrophy, particularly of hand muscles, which is accompanied by fasciculation. The **clinical course** is only slowly progressive and may extend over several decades. The signs spread slowly in a proximal direction to involve the arms, and also the trunk and legs. Such a chronic course prompts description of the disease as *chronic poliomyelitis*. In this context it should be pointed out that patients who in childhood developed a true acute anterior poliomyelitis (p. 205) from which they largely or completely recover may sometimes in later life develop into a progressive motor weakness (268). This is associated with progressive muscle atrophy and electromyographic signs and biopsy findings of a spinal muscular atrophy. The progression, however, is limited and the condition is not life-threatening. There have been reports that an amyotrophic lateral sclerosis (1011) may develop. It should be distinguished from the symptomatic forms (p. 223), as well as from amyotrophic lateral sclerosis.

Adult Proximal Spinal Muscular Atrophy (Vulpian-Bernardt)

This form of the disease, which appears to be transmitted as an autosomal recessive (926), is viewed as a separate entity. **Clinically,** the signs and symptoms usually start in the 4th decade of life. The picture of atrophy and paralysis has a symmetric pattern and is largely confined to the trunk muscles. The disease is only very slowly **progressive** and does not reduce life expectancy, although the patient's gait becomes impaired over the course of years.

Monomelic Amyotrophy (433)

This rare form of spinal muscular atrophy affects only one extremity. It starts in young adult life or middle age, and is only slowly progressive; after many years, other muscle groups remain unaffected.

Spastic Spinal Paraplegia and its Differential Diagnosis
(477, 517, 1308)

Concept: After symptomatic causes of spastic paraplegia in other spinal cord diseases have been excluded (see below), the entities remaining are mostly the genetically determined forms, in which the presenting clinical picture is one of spastic paraplegia with brisk reflexes and no sensory loss.

Transmission: In two-thirds of cases the disease is transmitted as an autosomal dominant (477, 517), less frequently as an autosomal recessive (479). Males and females are therefore equally affected.

Incidence: Of 672 patients to whom a diagnosis of spastic-paretic syndrome was attached in a university hospital, only 16 were eventually classified as cases of familial spastic paraplegia, and 44 were labeled as "spastic paraplegia of undetermined origin" (1218).

Clinical aspects: The disease may commence at any time between childhood and old age, usually as a very slowly progressive spastic weakness of the lower extremities. The initial feature is a very specific, later on frankly spastic gait abnormality. Work capacity is only slightly diminished, despite the severe spasticity. About 20% of cases exhibit associated findings (223, 479) such as amyotrophy, fasciculation, ataxia, extrapyramidal signs, optic atrophy, or dementia. Even distal sensory neuropathies with trophic changes have been described (223).

Histopathology (436): Most cases show no more than a degeneration of the lateral columns of the pyramidal tracts below the level of the decussation (Strümpell's "primary lateral column sclerosis"). Less commonly, the anterior pyramidal tracts and the posterior columns are affected.

Differential diagnosis: One of the rare symptomatic forms of spastic paraplegia is seen in *ectodermal dysplasia* (Bloch-Sulzberger type or incontinentia pigmenti) (1220). This is a familial disease which affects mainly women. In early childhood, linear pigmentation of the skin is visible, and later atrophic zones appear which are horizontal on the trunk and vertical on the backs of the thighs. Frequently dental anomalies, corneal and lens opacities, alopecia, and nail changes develop. Intelligence is frequently reduced. A metabolic anomaly, *hyperglycinemia,* may present in a familial form as a paraspastic syndrome, combined with atrophy of individual leg muscles, high arched foot, and absent ankle jerk – somewhat resembling Friedreich's ataxia or Charcot-Marie-Tooth disease. Paraparesis progressing rapidly to paraplegia may also be combined with an *abnormal aminoaciduria* (78). In *lathyrism,* a disorder seen in times of hunger following the use of the chick pea, spasms of the leg muscles parasthesias, tremors of the extremities, and urinary frequency, are followed by memory disturbances, fasciculations, and a rapidly progressive paraparesis; sensation remains intact. An acute myelopathy may accompany *heroin addiction* (334). A myelopathy and occasionally a pure progressive quadriparesis or spastic paraparesis may be caused by spinal arteriovenous malformations, less commonly by an intracranial dural arteriovenous fistula with drainage into the spinal veins (1296). In the *Sjögren-Larsson* syndrome (751), which is transmitted by an autosomal recessive gene, congenital ichthyosis is combined with spastic quadriparesis, dementia, and sometimes a disturbed function of peripheral nerves with dysalbuminemia. *Rud's syndrome* is a congenital ichthyosiform erythrodermia combined with mental deficiency and epileptic attacks, but without spasticity. Myelopathy with spasticity in *alcoholism,* see p. 151. Leukodystrophies with spastic paraparesis, see p. 143. *Adrenal insufficiency* with spastic paraparesis, see p. 144. Spastic-paretic forms of *multiple sclerosis,* see p. 245. Spastic paraparesis with hyperthyroidism, see p. 154.

Motor Neuron Disease (ALS)
(151, 837, 838, 1031)

Definition: One of the various titles of this disease – amyotrophic lateral sclerosis – indicates that it combines features of

– spinal muscular atrophy (following anterior horn cell degeneration) and
– spasticity with pyramidal signs (reflecting involvement of the cor-

ticobulbar and pyramidal tracts in the lateral part of the cord).

Epidemiology: The disease usually appears between the ages of 40 and 65 years, and men more often affected than women. Adolescents and children are only rarely involved.

Etiology and pathogenesis: A small group of cases is **genetically** determined, being described in families, as a disease with a dominant transmission. Several such families of *juvenile familial and relatively benign amyotrophic lateral sclerosis* are known, in which the disease began in childhood and ran a slowly progressive course over several decades. A form that has been considered possibly hereditary is found on the island of Guam among the Chamorro tribe, in whom the disease was, until recently, 100 times commoner than among Western Europeans. The association with parkinsonism and dementia has already been described (p. 106). In this connection, the question of a toxic cause has been repeatedly raised.

Most cases occur **sporadically**. A *large number of pathogenic theories* have been advanced (1303). The role of an increased exogenous manganese intake has also been discussed (1032). The serum of patients with amyotrophic lateral sclerosis contains a substance which is toxic to mouse anterior horn cells in tissue culture, and this substance has not been found in patients with other neurologic diseases (1292). A substance has been identified in the blood of patients which influences the sprouting of collateral fibers and the reinnervation of muscle cells in botulin-treated mice (451). Careful examination has failed to confirm the presence of any disturbance of pancreatic function, as previously suggested (1219). However, abnormal glucose tolerance is present, as well as a reduced insulin response following glucose loading and tolbutamide administration (1143). In the plasma of ALS patients a significantly elevated level of glutamate was found, which increased even more after a glutamate challenge (953). Abnormal liver function tests are present, and pathologic changes in hepatic cells are commonly found electron-microscopically (773). A loss of androgen receptors of the motor ganglion cells is thought to be responsible for the disease (1255). The normal presence of thyrotropic releasing hormone at the synapses connected to motor neurons forms the rationale of a form of treatment (see below). Isoenzyme deficiency of the DNA repair enzyme in the motor neurons may be responsible for the presence of abnormal DNA, resulting in the failure of normal transcription in the motor neurons of ALS patients (160). It is claimed that disturbances of circulatory perfusion of the spinal cord and brainstem may play an etiologic role, or at least be a constant contributory factor (1164).

Clinical features: *Subjectively,* the patient usually first notices a *muscular weakness* which, contrary to popular belief, affects not only the distal muscles but commonly begins in the proximal groups as well. The process can retain a unilateral distribution for many months. Later, other muscle groups become affected. Sometimes the patients by chance notice *muscular atrophy,* especially of the small muscles of the hand. On questioning, many patients will admit to painful *muscular spasms,* usually experienced at night and in the calf muscles, present initially or coincidentally with the muscular weakness and/or they may report that they had observed *fasciculations* in individual muscles.

Physical examination reveals *paralysis of muscles,* the distribution as a rule being asymmetric, distal, or proximal. Systematic testing soon reveals additional weakness of other muscle groups in addition to those noticed by the patient. Occasionally the muscles exhibit myasthenic features which are improved by cholinesterase inhibitors. *Fasciculations* must be sought systematically and patiently. They may be elicited by tapping, or provoked or made more definite by injection of a cholinesterase inhibitor (edrophonium chloride, 10 mg i.v., p.490). Paralysis may precede visible signs of *muscular atrophy* by a long period. The additional presence of *spasticity, brisk reflexes, and other pyramidal signs* is essential to the diagnosis of ALS, which cannot be accepted simply on the basis of muscular atrophy. Not infrequently, signs of spasticity manifest only late in the course of the disease and they may remain discrete. In some cases they may be extinguished to a certain extent by the subsequent spinal atrophy and paralysis ("pseudoneuritic form of amyotrophic lateral sclerosis"). Despite gross pyramidal signs, the spasticity is often remarkably mild; indeed, none may be present. Conversely, in other cases the spasticity may precede signs of involvement of the anterior horn cells so that the disease presents as a spastic paraplegia or quadriplegia. Sphincteric function is retained. There is no sensory loss. The respiratory muscles in the course of the disease show progressively more severe involvement and respiratory insufficiency develops. *Bulbar signs* usually appear at a late stage of the disease. However, in one-fourth of cases they are prominent from the outset: *increasingly severe slurred speech, swallowing disturbances,* and reduced mobility of the facial muscles. *Fasciculations of the tongue* are present, associated with restricted movements of the lips. Ocular movements remain intact. Damage of the corticobulbar tracts produces *abnormally brisk facial reflexes* (snout reflex, nasopalpebral reflex, mental reflex). For the same reason, *uncontrollable laughing* and *crying* may occur, and the latter should not be misdiagnosed as incontinence of affect.

Ancillary investigations: The *CSF* is normal. *Electromyography* makes an important contribution to diagnosis in revealing the fasciculation and fibrillation potentials, as well as a reduction in the number of motor units with increased potentials and a virtually normal conduction velocity in the peripheral nerves. *Muscle biopsy* may reveal, apart from the typical picture of neurogenic muscular atrophy, an association myopathy, and there is a raised creatine kinase level (4, 841),

Prognosis: The prognosis is poor. The disease runs a steadily progressive course, and 80% of patients die within 3 years. Of the patients with bulbar palsy, 60% die within 1 year. Sometimes the course is slower: about 20% remain alive after 5 years, 6% after 10 years. Remissions have been observed (838).

Treatment: No treatment has been found to be effective. Successful management with thyrotropic releasing hormone (TRH) has yet to be confirmed (341); intravenously, it appears not to be effective (1161). A pilot study suggested a favorable influence of oral ingestion of an amino acid mixture on the course of the disease (956).

Differential diagnosis: *Pure motor weakness with atrophy of muscles* accompanies myopathies. Fasciculations are observed in radicular lesions, but they may also be harmless benign fasciculations (p. 215). *Spasticity* accompanies a wide variety of neurologic diseases, e. g., paraplegia (p. 220). Real problems of differential diagnosis arise only with the *combined presence of muscular atrophy and spasticity or fasciculations.* Similar pictures are encountered as paraneoplastic manifestations of a neoplasm (500) and usually run a more prolonged course. This combination of signs may also be observed in diabetes mellitus and hyperparathyroidism (920), poisoning with organic mercury compounds, exposure to lead (153), and after trauma, electrocution, and gastric resection. *Chronic progressive vascular myelopathy* is discussed on p. 211. Muscular atrophy and spasticity may also occur in isolated cases of Creutzfeld-Jakob disease. A picture similar to ALS may be observed after burnt-out poliomyelitis (1011) (p. 219), as well as in macroglobulinemia with a paraproteinemic lesion of the nerve roots (1034). Like the latter, the acquired multifocal demyelinating polyneuropathy represents a neuroimmunological process. In this neuropathy, which at least initially was purely motor, fasciculations and cramps are additional symptoms, and may well imitate the picture of amyotrophic lateral sclerosis (918). Electromyography reveals multifocal conduction blocks. More details on p.321. Muscular atrophy with paralysis, fasciculation, and brisk reflexes may complicate hyperthyroidism and simulate ALS (833). A tumor of the craniocervical junction may produce bulbar features with bulbar atrophy, uncontrollable laughing, and pyramidal signs.

Spinocerebellar Ataxias

Definition: The majority of the entities in this group are hereditary diseases, the so-called spinocerebellar heredoataxias (436, 478, 479, 1016). This term refers to hereditary diseases first manifesting clinically in childhood or adolescence and showing a gradually progressive course. Diagnosis is based on the involvement of specific tracts in the spinal cord and specific parts of the cerebellum, occasionally also of the optic nerves and other CNS structures. Various combinations of signs and symptoms are possible, of which ataxia, disturbances of gait and movement coordination, speech disorders, and abnormal tendon jerks are prominent.

Classification: Harding's classification according to symptomatology, mode of inheritance, and age of clinical onset (479) is reproduced in Table 2.**4**.

Most Important Forms

Some predominantly cerebellar forms have already been mentioned (p. 134), and several other forms will be described here.

Friedreich's Ataxia (335, 377, 436, 478, 479, 1016)

This form is a *familial*, progressive degenerative disease of the spinocerebellar and corticospinal tracts and the posterior columns. Although assumed to be inherited as an autosomal recessive, the disease, which can be observed in generation after generation in the same family, does not appear to follow a simple Mendelian rule. Men are more commonly affected than women. The disease appears at the same age in each generation, but the age of onset varies considerably from generation to generation. Usually the *signs and symptoms* begin in childhood, occasionally there is a history of difficulty with learning to walk or the patient later experiences progressive difficulty in walking. In all cases, the appearances are typical: the first sign of the disease is an uncertain, broad-based, and jerky gait. In the course of years, unsteadiness of the hands occurs, accompanied by increasing difficulty in articulating words. The advanced cases show movement ataxia, a broad-based unsteady gait, explosive speech with an irregular rhythm, altered or absent position, movement, and vibration sense (with retained normal superficial sensation), a typical "Friedreich's foot" (clubfoot with hammer toes) (Fig. 2.**10**), scoliosis, sometimes nystagmus, muscular hypotonia, ab-

Table 2.4 Classification of hereditary forms of ataxia and spastic paraparesis (after Harding [434])

Entity	Inheritance	Decade of Life
1. Diseases with established causes		
1.1 Metabolic disorders		
1.1.1 Progressive unremitting ataxias		
Abetalipoproteinemia (Bassen-Kornzweig disease)	Autosomal recessive	1st and 2nd
Hypobetalipoproteinemia	Autosomal recessive	2nd and 4th
Hexosaminidase deficieny	Autosomal recessive	1st
Glutamate dehydrogenase deficiency	Autosomal recessive	2nd to 4th
Cholestanolosis	Autosomal recessive	Ataxia, 3rd–6th
1.1.2 Intermittent ataxias		
Pyruvate dehydrogenase deficiency	Autosomal recessive	1st
Hartnup disease	Autosomal recessive	1st
Intermittent branched chain keto-aciduria		
Deficiencies of urea cycle enzymes (ornithine transcarbamylase deficiency, citrullinemia, argininomia, argininosuccinylaciduria)	Autosomal recessive X-chromosome-linked dominant	
1.2 Disorders characterized by defective DNA repair		
Ataxia teleangiectasia (Louis-Bar syndrome)	Autosomal recessive	1st
Xeroderma pigmentosum (de Sanctis Cacchione syndrome)	Autosomal recessive	2nd
Cockayne's syndrome	Autosomal recessive	1st
2. Disorders of unkown etiology		
2.1 Cerebellar ataxias of early onset (before 20 years)		
Friedreich's ataxia	Autosomal recessive	1st and 2nd
Cerebellar ataxia of early onset with retained tendon reflexes with hypogonadism and sometimes deafness and/or dementia	Autosomal recessive	1st–3rd
With congenital deafness	Autosomal recessive	Ataxia, 2nd and 3rd
With childhood deafness and mental retardation	Autosomal recessive	1st
With pigmentary retinal degeneration and sometimes retardation/dementia/deafness	Autosomal recessive	1st

Table 2.4   (Continued)

Entity		Inheritance	Decade of Life
	With optic atrophy and retardation and sometimes deafness and spasticity (Behr's syndrome)	Autosomal recessive	1st
	Marinesco-Sjögren syndrome (with cataract and mental retardation)	Autosomal recessive	1st
	With myoclonus (Ramsay Hunt syndrome)	Autosomal recessive/ autosomal dominant	1st and 2nd
	X-linked recessive spinocerebellar ataxia	X-chromosome linked	1st and 2nd
	Cerebellar ataxia with essential tremor	Autosomal dominant	1st–3rd
2.2	*Cerebellar ataxias of late onset (after 20 years)*		
	Cerebellar ataxia with optic atrophy/ ophthalmoplegia/dementia/amyo- trophy/extrapyramidal signs (prob- ably including Azorean ataxia)	Autosomal dominant	3rd–5th
	Cerebellar ataxia with pigmentary reti- nal degeneration and sometimes ophthalmoplegia and/or extra- pyramidal signs	Autosomal dominant	2nd–4th
	Pure cerebellar ataxia with later onset	Autosomal dominant	6th and 7th
	Cerebellar ataxia with myoclonus and deafness	Autosomal dominant	Ataxia, 2nd–5th

(For further reading, see reference 434)

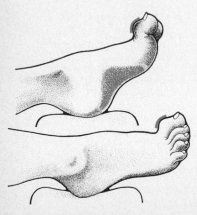

Fig. 2.**10**   Friedreich's foot

sent tendon jerks and later extensor plantar responses, atrophy of muscles, dysphagia, and bulbar signs. Optic atrophy is also described, and careful examination often reveals disturbances of ocular motility and the otovestibular apparatus, the latter giving rise to abnormal brainstem auditory evoked potentials (335). Occasionally a dementia may also be present. The ECG reveals evidence of myocardial damage, often marked interstitial fibrosis with focal degeneration of myocardial fibers. The disease follows an uninterruptedly **progressive course** and usually incapacitates the patient after a number of years, but some patients show only slow progression. Even in this respect, the disease follows an identical pattern in siblings. Apart from the identical ataxic features, each sibling exhibits accessory signs and symptoms of the disease which vary significantly in degree, and also from case to case. It is understandable, therefore, that some authors prefer to speak of *"Friedreich's syndrome"* (1016) and include in this description a group of etiologically variable diseases.

Treatment is limited to physostigmine, which appears to produce symptomatic benefit in cases of Friedreich's syndrome as well as in patients with other spinocerebellar degenerative disorders (598).

Roussy-Levy Syndrome

These authors described a progressive disease of dominant inheritance, so-called *dytasie aréflexique héréditaire*. It is characterized by clubfeet, gait ataxia, and absent tendon jerks, but the sensory modalities, muscular function, speech, and cerebellar functions remain intact (878). Occasionally posterior column signs, tremor and, exceptionally, also transient pyramidal signs, sphincteric disturbances, and skeletal anomalies may appear.

Familial Clubfoot with Absent Tendon Jerks

Sir Charles Symonds applied this descriptive title to a hereditary anomaly in which no other abnormal features are present. The disease causes scarcely any disability.

Rarer Forms

A pure *hereditary posterior column ataxia* has been described. The *alipoproteinemias,* heralded by ataxia, absent reflexes, and occasionally pyramidal signs, are described on p. 140. Transitional forms link Friedreich's ataxia and other diseases with a similar clinical picture, such as Charcot-Marie-Tooth muscular atrophy. *Sensory radicular neuropathy with analgesia of the distal extremities,* see p. 236. Other forms, see Table 2.4.

Metabolic Disturbances Involving the Spinal Cord

Subacute Combined Degeneration of the Spinal Cord

Pathophysiology: Animal products, especially liver and meat and only to a slight degree eggs and dairy products, serve as a *source of vitamin B_{12}* in the human body. Vitamin B_{12} participates in numerous metabolic exchanges in the body, notably the synthesis of nucleic acids. Vitamin B_{12} (extrinsic factor) combines with a secretory product of the mucus glands of the fundus of the stomach (intrinsic factor) to form a hematopoietic factor. Only in this combination can vitamin B_{12} be absorbed through the mucous membrane of the intestine and reach its destination in the metabolic exchanges of the body. If a disturbance of absorption leads to a deficiency of vitamin B_{12} in the body, various abnormalities arise such as a megaloblastic hyperchromic anemia, as well as neurologic signs.

Causes of vitamin B deficiency: These are usually connected with *abnormal absorption,* e.g., deficient intrinsic factor (atrophy of the gastric mucous membrane, carcinoma, total gastrectomy) or disease of the small intestine (sprue, steatorrhea, Crohn's disease, extensive small bowel resection). *Abnormal utilization* of vitamin B_{12} in the small intestine occurs in carriers of the tapeworm Diphyllobothrium latum or abnormal bacterial populations. *Inadequate intake* is exceptional, e.g., strict vegetarian diet. In such cases, the body's supply of vitamin B_{12} lasts for about 2½ years.

Clinical signs and symptoms: *General and hematologic signs and symptoms* consist of: gastric complaints, general lassitude, a burning tongue, glossitis, sometimes enlargement of the liver and spleen; hyperchromic megaloblastic anemia with macrocytosis, leukopenia, a relative lymphocytosis and platelet deficiency, yellow serum, and a pale complexion; all cases of true pernicious anemia with neurologic signs exhibit a histamine-refractory achlorhydria (achylia), with the exception of certain childhood cases.

Neurologic signs and symptoms do not parallel the hematologic signs in any respect: severe neurologic deficits may be present without any evidence of anemia. In some cases, the neurologic changes appear suddenly, while in others they develop in a slow progressive way: they comprise severe disturbances of deep sensibility and sometimes also of other sensory modalities. The situation may arise within a few weeks so that the patient can no longer walk. In other cases, the course of the disease is far slower, and the initial *sensory changes in the lower extremities* may precede the muscular weakness by several months. In many the presenting feature is a symmetric, painful paresthesia of the lower extremities. Soon an *ataxic gait disturbance* occurs. Neurologic examination shows that position sense is grossly abnormal, as well as vibration sense. Areas of tactile hypesthesia and hypalgesia may also be found, which progress rapidly to complete analgesia. The *tendon jerks* are reduced, and *pyramidal signs* are present. However, the latter features may be absent so that "tabetic" and "polyneuritic" forms of the disease are described. Careful examination reveals a *polyneuropathy* in two-thirds of cases, in which vitamin B_{12} deficiency appears to play a part (256). A positive *neck flexion sign* (p. 246) may sometimes be present (590, 1180). *Visual defects* and central scotomata occasionally occur, particularly in men. Vitamin B_{12} deficiency plays an important part in so-called tobacco-alcohol amblyopia (p. 330). In about 4% of cases, *mental changes* are present, and they are always combined with objective neurologic signs. They include neurasthenic symptoms, depression, confusional states, paranoid psychoses, amnesia, and dementia. The *CSF* is usually normal. The *EEG* reveals nonspecific abnormalities, which do not parallel the severity of the clinical picture, in about 50% of cases.

Diagnosis: *Hematologic examination* and the search for an *achylia* (see above) play an important part, but the diagnostic key is confirmation of a vitamin B_{12} deficiency. Estimation of the *vitamin B_{12} concentration in the serum* (normal values between 100 and 900 ng/l) becomes invalid once treatment has been started. For this reason, the *vitamin B_{12} absorption test* (Schilling test) is necessary. After oral administration of 0.1–0,5 μCi of ^{57}Co-labeled vitamin B_{12}, an intramuscular injection of 1,000 μg of vitamin B_{12} is given (to saturate the binding capacity of the plasma), not earlier than 1 h and not later than 2 h after the oral dose. In normal subjects, the vitamin B_{12} is absorbed from the intestine and 10%–30% is excreted within 24 h in the urine; its radioactivity can be monitored. In the presence of a disturbance of absorption, the orally administered dose of labeled vitamin B_{12} is excreted in the intestinal tract and less than 10% appears in the urine; in true pernicious anemia less than 5% is found. If the intrinsic factor is deficient (and there is no local disturbance of intestinal absorption), the absorption and urinary excretion of vitamin B_{12} return to normal if intrinsic factor is added by mouth to the labeled vitamin B_{12} dose. The Schilling test may also be performed after vitamin B_{12} treatment It remains persistently positive in cases of true pernicious anemia.

Pathologic anatomy: Initially the histopathologic lesion consists of a reversible degeneration of the myelin sheath, later an irreversible disintegration of the axons with secondary neuroglial proliferation. The changes in the spinal cord are first seen in the posterior columns, usually at the midthoracic level, then in the pyramidal tract and other columns. Small foci of perivascular demyelination may be found in the brain (436, 1217).

Prognosis: Insofar as the subjective sensory changes, mild ataxia, and motor signs are concerned, the outlook is good if treatment is started early. In the later stages, irreversible changes are present.

Treatment: Whenever the suspicion of subacute combined degeneration exists, treatment should be started immediately. For the first 2 weeks 1,000 ng of vitamin B_{12} should be injected daily in order to fill up the depot. Thereafter, once monthly injections should be given.

Differential diagnosis: *Subacute ataxic signs* are encountered in a variety of diseases, e.g., specific types of poisoning such as phenytoin or in an acute polyneuropathy such as porphyria. *Combined involvement of various tracts* of the spinal cord may be part of the picture of paraneoplastic disease of the spinal cord (500), see p.156. Disturbances of deep sensation, spasticity, and pyramidal signs have been described as a rare complication of hypocalcemia, e.g., of renal origin, and also very exceptionally in portocaval shunts (p.162).

Syringomyelia and Syringobulbia (332, 402, 435, 503, 1080)

Definition and pathologic anatomy: The characteristic feature of *syringomyelia* is the conversion of the spinal cord into a hollow organ over several segments by the presence of a tubular or slitlike cavity within it (435). In *syringobulbia* a similar process deforms the medulla oblongata and sometimes the pons, although only a small proportion of cases involve this site. The abnormal cavities are filled with yellowish fluid. In cross section they usually extend from one posterior horn of the spinal cord to the other and forward to the anterior commissure. In the thoracic cord, not infrequently they are unilateral, involving only one posterior horn. The medullary lesion commonly consists of a fissure extending forward and outward from the floor of the fourth ventricle. The walls of the cavities often have irregular outlines, and in their vicinity degenerative changes may be present in the nerve cells and neuroglia; the myelin shows poor staining characteristics. Later, gliosis occurs. If the walls of the cavities communicate with the central canal of the spinal cord, they may be lined with ependyma. This condition should be differentiated from *hydromyelia,* i.e., simple enlargement of the central canal, in which the tubular cavity is always lined by ependyma. In syringomyelia, pressure effects of the syrinx on the axons cause secondary degeneration of the ascending and descending spinal tracts. In some cases, a glial plug is present instead of a syrinx.

Clinical aspects: The *first signs of disease* usually occur in the 2nd and 3rd decades of life. The exception is *infantile syringobulbia,* in which stridor or difficulties with drinking and swallowing may be present shortly after birth. This lesion is often associated with other anomalies, e.g., spina bifida or a malformation of the craniovertebral angle. Torticollis may be present from an early age (see below).

Most common and typical signs and symptoms: These will depend on the level and site of the cavities within the spinal cord. In individual cases the following grouping of signs and symptoms may be possible:

- Pressure of a cavity on adjacent descending and ascending tracts may damage the motor fibers, leading to *spastic weakness* with pyramidal signs and *sensory disturbances including a clinical level* at the site of the lesion. These sensory changes may be confined to a single modality, depending on the particular tract which has been damaged, i.e., a dissociated sensory loss.
- Pressure of the cavity on adjacent anterior horn cells produces a lower motor neuron lesion, leading to flaccid paralysis, *muscular atrophy,* and later to fasciculation. The posterolateral cell groups of the anterior horn in the lower cervical cord are preferentially involved, therefore atrophy of the hand muscles is most commonly seen.

- Damage to the decussating pain and temperature fibers in the anterior commissure leads to *segmental dissociated sensory disturbances* (see Fig. 2.2).
- Cavitation in the vicinity of the posterior horn may damage all afferent sensory fibers in the posterior root, producing a disturbance of *all sensory modalities* in the corresponding segments.
- *Pain* may be a prominent symptom for a long time, sometimes the initial symptom of syringomyelia. It is usually confined to the cervicobrachial region. Careful examination of such patients invariably reveals objective sensory disturbances, although other neurologic deficits may not appear for months or years.
- Damage to the intermediolateral tract in the upper thoracic cord produces marked disturbances of autonomic function, e.g., abnormal sweat secretion, puffy swelling of the hands etc. The latter, combined with the additional risk of (painless) injury and infection, leads to the condition of succulent hand with *mutilation of the fingers* (Morvan type).
- In the same way, the disturbances of autonomic and trophic function are responsible for the mutilating *arthropathies* present in 20% of patients. These lesions may lead to painless destruction of the intracapsular part of joints and the adjacent bone, e.g., total destruction of the humeral head. Spontaneous fractures may occur. A particularly severe degree of cervical spondylosis may be present. Patients in whom the clinical

picture has appeared early in life invariably exhibit roentgenologic evidence of an abnormally wide sagittal diameter of the cervical spinal canal, due to adaptation of the bony vertebral canal to its contents.
- Secondary *kyphoscoliosis* is usually present.
- Common *associated findings* are spina bifida, basilar impression, dolichocephaly (p. 20), high arched palate, etc. A fixed torticollis in children may be an early sign of the disease (621)

Pathogenesis: The following factors play a part in the development of syringomyelia:

- *Disturbances of embryogenesis*, as reflected by the constancy of the topographic distribution of the cavities along the suture line between the alar and basal laminae, associated with other congenital malformations, especially an Arnold-Chiari malformation (see below).
- A remarkably frequent finding in syringomyelic patients is a history of a *complicated birth* (332).
- A *disturbance of the normal CSF drainage* from the fourth ventricle leads through various mechanisms to bulbocervical cavitation (402), occasionally combined with an anomaly of the craniovertebral angle and often with an Arnold-Chiari syndrome. Successfully treated tuberculous meningitis should be included among the causes of scarring (arachnoiditis) of the basal meninges producing obstruction of CSF drainage (933).
- Reference has already been made above (p. 196) to syringomyelic lesions occurring as a late complication of *spinal cord trauma*, at a level above that of the injury.

Course: The clinical course of the disease is either slowly progressive or stationary for a long period. Transient improvement of the signs and symptoms of long-tract deficit is sometimes described and can be explained by a temporary pressure reduction within the abnormal cavities. Conversely, clinical progression may be attributed in part to an increased pressure and greater fluid content of the cavities.

Treatment: Neurosurgical treatment is essential in cases of clear-cut progression (1224). On the basis of the theory that the CSF pressure waves which are synchronous with the pulse propel the CSF from the fourth ventricle through an existing patent channel into the cavity in the cervical cord, lateral ventricular shunting is advised. If the passage of CSF from the fourth ventricle is obstructed, operative decompression of the craniocervical angle (and of an existing Arnold-Chiari malfor-

mation) is carried out to restore patency to the occluded exit foramina of Luschka and Magendie (746). Individual cases may be submitted to the Poussepp operation, i.e., posterior laminectomy and release of CSF contents from a high cavity. Permanent drainage may be established by means of a catheter into the subarachnoid space (1187). Since the central canal in syringomyelia often extends caudally into the filum terminale, exposure of the canal by "terminal ventriculostomy" has produced clinical improvement (300). It is claimed that X-irradiation relieves the pain.

Differential diagnosis: This must include other intramedullary lesions, particularly tumors, hematomyelia, and postirradiation myelopathy. Other causes of dissociated sensory loss are lesions of the thalamus or dorsolateral medulla oblongata (e.g., Wallenberg's syndrome), the Brown-Séquard syndrome, and the various causes of disturbed pain sensation described on p.236.

3. Diseases Affecting Mainly the Autonomic Nervous System (53, 80)

General symptomatology: The following *functional disorders* accompany lesions exerting their main effect on the autonomic nervous system:

- blood pressure regulation,
- regulation of heart rate,
- pupil and lens function,
- sweat secretion,
- secretion of saliva and tears,
- urination and function of the gastrointestinal tract, and
  male sexual function.

The various *tests* used to verify disturbances of the autonomic regulatory mechanisms are given in Table 3.1.

Pathologic signs: The abnormal phenomena accompanying autonomic dysregulation include, with greater or lesser prominence and in various combinations:

- orthostatic hypotension including syncope (845), without simultaneous rapid pulse,
- medium-sized pupils not reacting to light or other stimuli,
- absence of sweating and
- reduced salivary and lacrimal secretion,
- disturbances of urination, constipation, or diarrhea, and
- impotence in males.

Acute Pandysautonomia (53, 55, 80, 898, 1202, 1307)

Pathogenetically, acute pandysautonomia is an acquired disturbance probably caused by an isolated lesion of the pre- or postganglionic nonmyelinated fibers (30, 871). Many of the cases described have been attributed to infection with the Epstein-Barr virus (392, 1297).

Clinical features: The disease picture is characterized by orthostatic hypotension, constant heart rate, defective secretion of sweat and tears, dry mucous membranes, pupils that are nonreactive and fixed in midposition, impotence,

constipation, and hypotonic bladder. No muscular weakness or reflex changes are present. Dysesthesias and pains may be present (871), as well as hypoventilation and a sleep apnea syndrome (381). The CSF may contain an increased amount of protein. Sural nerve biopsy reveals unusually thin unmyelinated fibers which are increased in number (55, 1307).

Course: The disease has a subacute onset extending over several weeks, and runs a course over many months. Recovery is usually complete.

Table 3.1 Methods of Testing the Regulatory Mechanisms of the Autonomic Nervous System (After *Weidmann* [1150]; *Fujii* et al. [351])

Function	Test	Method	Result
Blood pressure regulation (complete reflex arc)	On tilting table or patient getting up	BP and pulse with patient lying down for 8, 9, and 10 min. Thereafter every 2 min to 10 min after getting up	Systolic BP levels equal or lower, diastolic levels higher. Pulse rate increased 10–20/min
Blood pressure regulation (efferent sympathetic)	Cold pressure test	A hand and forearm submerged in iced water (4 °C) for 1 min, and BP levels recorded before and afterward until maximal response. ECG if available	BP level rises, heart rate slows
	Hand grip test	Pumping a hand manometer for 3 min or longer with about 30% of maximum contraction power. BP levels recorded before and during the test	BP level rises (diastolic more than 10 mm Hg)
Pupillary reaction (noradrenalin in terminal sympathetic nerve endings)	Size of pupil	0.2 ml of a 2.5% tyramine solution instilled into the conjunctival sac	Pupil enlarges
Pupillary muscles	Size of pupil	2.5% methacholine drops instilled into the conjunctival sac	No constriction
Pulse rate (efferent vagus)	Atropine test	0.04 mg atropine/kg i. v., and pulse rate monitored	Pulse rate increases
Pulse rate (afferent vagus)	Carotid sinus test	Unilateral carotid massage under ECG control	Pulse rate slows
Sweating	Heat test Pilocarpine iontophoresis	Heat With 20 mg pilocarpine	Diffuse sweating Local sweating
Lacrimal secretion	Schirmer's test	After conjunctival anesthesia insert strips of filter paper (5 × 0.5 cm) into the conjunctival sac	After 5 min, at least 3 cm should be damp. Abnormal result if less than 1.5 cm damp or more than 30% difference with opposite side
Salivary secretion	Secretion test	Probe in the parotid duct	0.4–0.8 ml/min

Treatment: In view of the tendency to spontaneous regression, none is required. Postural precautions will prevent syncopal disturbances. Carbamazepine is advised for painful dysesthesias (871).

Differential diagnosis: The syndrome should be differentiated from botulism (see below), as well as those polyneuropathies particularly involving the autonomic fibers, e.g., the diabetic form (p. 311).

Familial Dysautonomia (Riley-Day Syndrome) (927, 999)

Pathogenetically, this is a rare hereditary disease of autosomal recessive pattern, which appears to be caused by defective synthesis of noradrenalin. It is virtually confined to patients of Eastern European Jewish ancestry.

Clinical features: The disease presents in infancy as a feeding difficulty caused by a disturbance of swallowing. Signs of autonomic dysfunction are prominent, and other signs may be present: absence of tears while crying is a constant feature, orthostatic hypotension, excessive sweating, disturbances of swallowing, ataxia, dysarthria, absent or reduced sensitivity to pain, and abnormal mental lability occur. Commonly there is also abnormal temperature regulation, absence of tendon jerks, vomiting, frequent attacks of bronchopneumonia, and impaired growth.

Prognosis: This is poor, more than one-half of the patients fail to reach adulthood.

Pathologic anatomy: The CNS shows no changes. Histologic changes are present in the peripheral autonomic ganglia and plexuses, and the peripheral sensory nerves show a reduction in the number and thickness of myelinated fibers (18).

Orthostatic Hypotension (Shy-Drager Syndrome)
(80, 1108)

Pathogenesis: This is a primary neurologic disease, being a form of system degeneration.

Pathologic anatomy: Microscopic study reveals cell degeneration in the cerebral cortex, cerebellar cortex, substantia nigra, and other basal ganglia, as well as in the dorsal root ganglia. The number of ganglion cells in the lateral horns of the spinal cord is reduced by 60%–80% (723).

Clinically, the disease begins in middle-aged or elderly subjects, twice as frequently in men as in women. Initially, only the signs of orthostatic hypotension are present: dizziness, weakness, and disturbances of vision or consciousness upon standing up. In contrast to idiopathic orthostatic circulatory collapse, no increase in pulse rate, yawning, or sweating accompanies the hypotension in this condition. Neurologic signs appear many months or years later, although they may precede the hypotension. Thus, the following signs may be found: absence of sweating, impotence, incontinence, pyramidal signs, rigidity, akinesia, tremor, muscular atrophy, fasciculations, external ocular palsies, and atrophy of the iris. The clinical picture does not include dementia. Death follows after 1 or more years. Progression of the neu-rologic signs does not cease if the hypotensive situation is corrected.

Treatment: Fludrocortisone and indomethacin favorably counteract the hypotension but fail to influence the course of the disease.

Botulism

Pathogenesis: The disease is caused by the action of toxins of the anaerobic microorganism, *Clostridium botulinum*, which may survive in canned food. Apart from food poisoning, botulism may also complicate wounds of the soft tissues and give rise to signs of poisoning (232).

Clinically (231), the picture includes ocular palsies and disturbances of accom-modation, a dry mouth, bulbar signs, and evidence of a polyneuropathy. The toxin of the type B of the microorganism is especially likely to give rise to a mild form of poisoning which disturbs only cholinergic autonomic innervation – disturbances of ocular accommodation, dry mouth, and reduced lacrimal secretion, signs which recede in the course of months (566).

Loss of Pain Sensation

In several diseases, inability to appreciate the sensation of pain may be the principal clinical deficit.

Congenital Absence of Pain Sensibility

Various names are applied to this condition, e.g., pain asymbolia, and several clinical variants exist.

Congenital Sensory Neuropathy with Anhidrosis

In this condition, which may often be familial, the failure of sweat secretion accompanies the absent sensation of pain. Small infants present a picture of self-mutilation and fever. Pathoanatomically, there is marked cellular depletion of the dorsal root ganglia (228), which contrasts with the presence of only trivial changes in the central nervous system. Electrophysiologic examination including evoked potentials point to a lesion of the first sensory neuron. A familial form is characterized by a reduction of the myelinated fibers coupled with a mosaic arrangement of the Schwann's cells (54). These changes can be shown by sural nerve biopsy.

Sensory Radicular Neuropathy (Acropathie ulcéro-mutilante of Thévenard, Acrodystrophic Neuropathy)

This disease is caused by changes in the neurons of the dorsal root ganglia which also affect the posterior roots, peripheral nerves, and posterior columns. It is an autosomal dominant, hereditary syndrome which may manifest in childhood but usually appears between the 2nd and 4th decades of life. The main features are a dissociated sensory loss combined with indolent ulcers of the feet. In addition, the other sensory modalities may be disturbed, the patient complains of lancinating pains and numbness, tendon jerks are absent, and there is muscular atrophy and involvement of the upper extremities. A raised IgA is often present, which may result from increased production in the jejunal mucosa (1266).

Pain Asymbolia

This acquired condition is characterized by a loss of protective reflexes in response to painful stimuli in the entire body and the absence of an appropriate emotional reaction to pain. It is caused by a lesion which interrupts the connections between the sensory cortex and the limbic system (122).

Sympathetic Syndromes (53, 77, 1079)

Anatomy and Pathophysiology

The *central sympathetic* tract probably arises in the hypothalamus. At this level, the emotional impulses from the opposite cortex converge with the thermoregulatory impulses. The sympathetic impulses then run in the ipsilateral column of the spinal cord and synapse, between T3 and L2-3, with a second neuron in the lateral horn of the gray matter. The axons of these cells leave the spinal cord with the anterior root of the corresponding thoracic and upper lumbar nerves: Sweat fibers supplying the head and neck leave in the T2-4 roots, those for the thorax in T5-7, and those for the rest of the trunk and the lower extremities in T8-L2/3. The sympathetic fibers pass along white rami communicantes to the sympathetic chain. Here the change to the third distal neuron takes place. The latter again makes communication with the spinal nerve root through the gray rami communicantes and passes in the sensory part of the peripheral nerve to the skin and also the sweat glands. Sweat secretion, piloerection, and vasomotor activity are controlled by nerve fibers running within the sympathetic chain and passing peripherally with the sensory nerve branches, as shown in Fig. 3.1a and b.

Typical Signs and Symptoms
Disturbances of Sweat Secretion

Lesions of a sensory or mixed peripheral nerve may show, in addition to sensory loss, a loss of sweat secretion in the territory of distribution of the nerve. The disturbance may be confirmed with the aid of a sweat secretion test (p. 390). Excessive focal sweating can occur in paroxysms. As causes, a compensatory excessive sweating of individual body parts after partial resection or destruction of the sympathetic trunk during surgery, or due to a disease process, hypothalamic has to be considered. It occurs in cord dis-

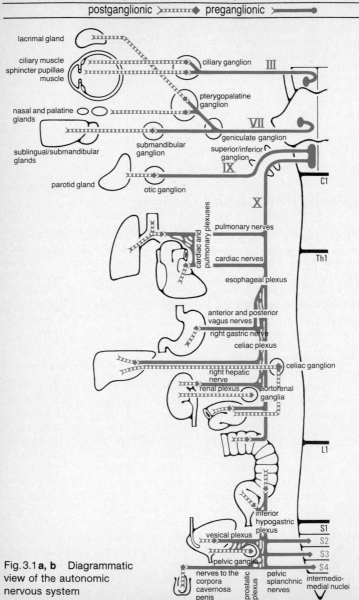

Fig. 3.1 **a, b** Diagrammatic view of the autonomic nervous system

Sympathetic nervous system

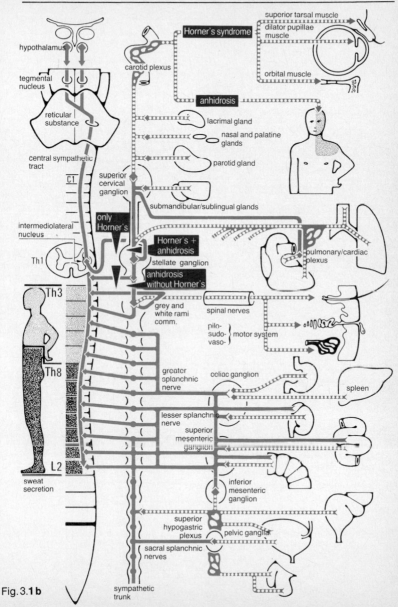

hypothalamus

tegmental nucleus

reticular substance

central sympathetic tract

C1

intermediolateral nucleus

Th1

Th3

Th8

L2

sweat secretion

carotid plexus

Horner's syndrome

superior tarsal muscle
dilator pupillae muscle

orbital muscle

anhidrosis

lacrimal gland

nasal and palatine glands

parotid gland

superior cervical ganglion

submandibular/sublingual glands

only Horner's

Horner's + anhidrosis

stellate ganglion

anhidrosis without Horner's

grey and white rami comm.

spinal nerves

pilo-
sudo-
vaso-
} motor system

greater splanchnic nerve

celiac ganglion

lesser splanchnic nerve

superior mesenteric ganglion

pulmonary/cardiac plexus

spleen

inferior mesenteric ganglion

superior hypogastric plexus

pelvic ganglia

sacral splanchnic nerves

sympathetic trunk

Fig. 3.1 b

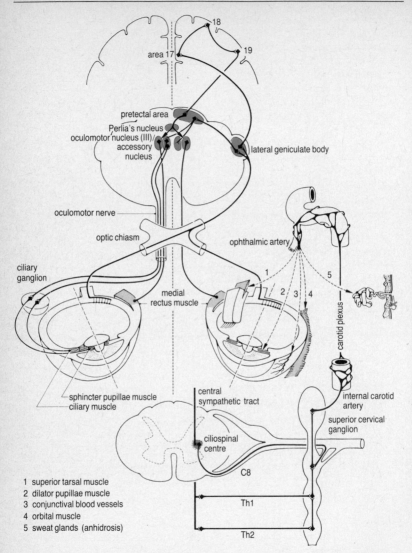

Fig. 3.**2**   Anatomic basis of ptosis and Horner's syndrome, as well as the nerve supply of the pupil (from *Mumenthaler* [772])

eases such as syringomyelia, in tabes dorsalis, cord tumors, cord trauma, and also with hypothalamic lesions. Localized excessive sweating has also been described with peripheral nerve lesions, such as cervical rib, osteomas of the vertebral bodies, with bronchiogenic carcinoma and pleural endothelioma, testicular teratomas, and the socalled sudoriparous nevus. In rare cases, an idiopathic form without any recognizable etiology may be encountered. It appears to respond to clonidine (655).

Horner's Syndrome

The characteristic features of this syndrome are a constricted pupil, ptosis, and enophthalmos. If these signs are present without disturbance of sweat secretion, then the lesion affects the (anterior) roots of C8-T2 proximal to the sympathetic chain, because the sweat fibers leave the spinal cord only below T2 in the spinal roots. However, if in addition to the classic signs of the syndrome mentioned above, there is an absence of sweating over the face, neck, and arm on the corresponding side, the stellate ganglion has been damaged. Disturbed sweat secretion of the upper part of the body may be found without signs of Horner's syndrome, and this picture indicates a lesion of the sympathetic chain immediately caudal to the stellate ganglion. Pharmacologic tests are used to verify the site of the lesion (788). With a central Horner's syndrome (i.e., lesions of the first sympathetic neuron) and in normal subjects, the local application of hydroxyamphetamine (Paredrine)

causes pupillary dilatation. In chronic lesions of the postganglionic portion of the sympathetic chain, noradrenalin secretion is exhausted, therefore hydroxyamphetamine can release no noradrenalin and consequently no pupillary dilatation occurs. This test allows the condition to be clearly differentiated from other causes of miosis, e.g., common anisocoria which is present in 15%-30% of the normal population, in the elderly (1198). Fig. 3.2 reviews the nerve supply of the pupil.

Paratrigeminal Paralysis (Raeder Syndrome) (759, 1245)

This syndrome is produced by a lesion of the sympathetic oculomotor fibers together with a trigeminal palsy, and sometimes associated with double vision. It is caused by a lesion situated between the pituitary fossa and the gasserian ganglion. Characteristic features are unilateral miosis, ptosis, and facial pain, as well as weakness of masticatory muscles and sometimes disturbances of ocular motility.

Lesions of the Sympathetic Chain

These lesions are usually caused by tumors invading the paravertebral gutter. They produce a clinical picture of absent sweat secretion over the trunk and lower extremities without sensory loss. On the other hand, in cases of sensory loss in the lower lumbar or sacral segments, the absence of sweat secretion rules out a proximal root lesion, e.g., lumbar disk herniation. In such cases, the lesion must lie more distally and particularly in the lumbar plexus since the sweat fibers for the lower extremities leave the spinal cord at a higher level, above L2-3 (see Fig. 3.1a and b). Lesions of the sympathetic chain and Horner's syndrome, see above.

4. Demyelinating Diseases

The diseases classified under this heading possess a common feature in showing pathologic changes and degeneration of the myelin sheaths in the CNS. They are caused partly by a congenital defect in the enzyme system which controls the normal manufacture and metabolism of myelin. To these diseases belong the leukodystrophies, which have already been discussed. Others may result from a secondarily acquired abnormality, the cause of which remains imperfectly understood.

Review of the Origin, Significance, and Metabolism of Myelin (1065)

The myelin sheath is built up in the peripheral nerve by Schwann's cells arranged around its axon and in the CNS by oligoglial cells. To a certain extent, the axon becomes embedded in a Schwann's cell so that the cell membranes serve as a covering for the axon. This double membrane, a so-called unit membrane, is called the mesaxon, in which the axon is finally enveloped and which is eventually covered by a multi-layered myelin sheath. Schwann's cells appear to fulfill the active role. A simple unit membrane measuring 0.0075 μm consists of four monomolecular layers, two lipid (e. g., cholesterol) and two nonlipid (protein) comprising phosphatides and cerebrosides. Each change in the structure of the membrane, such as alterations in the monomolecular protein layer, may lead to changes in the membrane formation or to its degeneration. Allergic reactions, autoimmune processes, or lipotropic substances may play a part. Since the myelin sheaths are concerned in the transmission of stimuli along the axon, any such degenerative process will alter the conduction properties of the axon. These changes may be reflected clinically as paralysis or sensory deficit, and they remain reversible as long as the axon itself is intact and remyelination can take place.

Multiple Sclerosis (466, 735, 740)

Typical Clinical Features

- *Numerous attacks occurring at irregular intervals,* with complete or partial recovery from the signs and symptoms between each attack in about 60% of cases.
- *Scattered sites of involvement* throughout the CNS, accounting for the very varied clinical picture.
- *At the same time,* signs may be present indicating demyelinating foci in various sites, e.g., optic atrophy accompanied by paraplegia.
- *Successive attacks* of the disease may cause involvement of various systems, e.g., ocular palsy followed 1 year later by a disturbance of voiding.

Epidemiology (466): In the latitude of Northern Europe, multiple sclerosis is the commonest neurologic disease. Its prevalence, i.e., the number of cases simultaneously present in a population, is highest in Northern and Middle Europe, including Switzerland, in Soviet Russia, Canada, and the northern United States, New Zealand, and the southwestern part of Australia. In these countries, multiple sclerosis is present in 30–80 per 100,000 of the population. In other parts of the world, the prevalence drops to below 5. Among multiracial populations, whites are at greatest risk. When moving to a low-prevalence country, only immigrants over the age of 15 years carry the higher risk of their country of origin. In the reverse situation, only immigrants to a high-prevalence country under the age of 15 years are at risk. In Switzerland and the Federal Republic of Germany, multiple sclerosis accounts for one per thousand of all autopsies, and the frequency has probably risen in the past decade. In the Faroe Islands, no case of multiple sclerosis was registered before 1939. British troops occupied the islands during the Second World War, and between 1943 and 1960 24 cases were registered (603). A variable *familial incidence* (between 3% and 12%) is claimed. The risk of multiple sclerosis is 15 times greater if the disease is present in a close relative.

Clinical Symptomatology

General features: The first signs and symptoms appear in young adults in two-thirds of cases. In about 60% individual *bouts of illness* are found which occur irregularly over the course of many years. Each lasts a few weeks. They affect different locations of the CNS and thus give rise to *variable clinical features*. In the beginning these regress more or less completely. Later on, increasingly obvious *residual signs and symptoms* remain after attacks. The later phases are characterized by disability, especially progressive spasticity, without obvious new bouts of illness occurring. This is the commonest pattern of the disease, but variants are found: *frequent attacks,* occurring one after the other and leading in the course of months or a few years to a severe degree of invalidism; *benign forms,* which produce mild disability over the course of a decade or more; and a form with a *progressive course from the outset* without individual attacks, usually starting over the age of 50 years (887). Multiple sclerosis tends to involve several specific sites in the CNS, giving rise to *typical signs and symptoms,* which will be discussed in greater detail below. These are retrobulbar neuritis, internuclear ophthalmoplegia, nystagmus, cerebellar ataxia, intention tremor, spastic paraparesis and a spastic-ataxic gait disturbance. The degree of *disability can be quantified* by rating neurologic impairment according to the expanded disability status scale (EDSS) of Kurtzke (658).

Individual Clinical Features

Ocular signs (1245): *Retrobulbar neuritis* (250, 917, 1245) is recognized by severe visual impairment which is initially usually unilateral and progressive over the course of a few days. The patient may not be able to count the fingers of his outstretched hand. Eye movements may cause eyeball pain and sensations of light. Both the fundus and the optic nerve initially show a normal appearance ("neither the patient nor his doctor sees anything"). If the inflammatory process affects the distal part of the optic nerve, a picture of papillitis develops, followed 3-4 weeks later by optic atrophy, particularly temporal pallor. However, the latter sign is far too frequently diagnosed by the inexpe-

rienced. Visual acuity begins to improve within 1-2 weeks and may return completely to normal. About one-third of patients with retrobulbar neuritis develop other signs of multiple sclerosis in subsequent years (250), and almost 80% show signs of this disease 15 years later (540). This group, i.e., those who go on to develop signs of multiple sclerosis, are significantly more often HLA-RT-1a positive (250). Retrobulbar neuritis may be an isolated finding, and in about 15% of patients it is the presenting symptom of multiple sclerosis. The statistics mentioned above do not apply to cases of retrobulbar neuritis simultaneously involving both optic nerves. A follow-up study of bilateral cases pursued for more than 30 years revealed no children and very few adults who subsequently developed signs of multiple sclerosis (917). Visual evoked potentials, see below. The Marcus Gunn pupillary phenomenon and "swinging flashlight" test after retrobulbar neuritis, see pp. 348 and 349. *Uveitis* is less common, see p. 252. *Disturbances of external ocular movement* are very common signs (466, 858, 991, 1245). Transient *double vision* usually appears in an early phase of the disease and it is not infrequently caused by a sixth cranial nerve palsy. Later, clinical and oculographic examination reveal disturbances of the ocular movements in 80% of cases of multiple sclerosis (991, 1127), in whom an internuclear ophthalmoplegia (p. 342) is present in about one-third of cases (858). A "one-and-a-half" syndrome (p. 342) is less common. These disturbances of ocular motility are frequently accompanied by *nystagmus* which, once present, is unlikely to disappear. Diagnostically, a dissociated nystagmus is particularly suggestive of multiple sclerosis. In contrast to nystagmus due to other causes, the nystagmus of multiple sclerosis may be provoked – and confirmed by means of electronystagmography – by increasing the body temperature (571).

Brainstem and cerebellar signs: *Trigeminal neuralgia* is seen in 1.5% of patients with multiple sclerosis; therefore, it is 300 times more frequent than in the general population (537). It is twice as often *bilateral* as in patients with other causes of trigeminal neuralgia. Continuous pain is seen with particular frequency between individual neuralgic attacks. Moreover, pain outside the trigeminal distribution sometimes occurs, and in addition facial palsy or other signs of a focal lesion of the pons. Sudden *deafness* or acute *attacks of vertigo*, similar to an acute vestibular crisis, are less frequent presenting signs of the disease. *Cerebellar signs and symptoms* are present in three-fourths of cases (661). A movement *ataxia* is often a prominent sign involving particularly the patient's gait, which is not only spastic but also ataxic. Particularly impressive and highly characteristic in multiple sclerosis is the *intention tremor* which accompanies voluntary movements, e.g., finger-nose test (see Fig. 1.20). The tremor indicates a lesion of the dentate nucleus involving its efferent fibers. A dysdiadochokinesia and dysmetria on

movement are present, usually accompanied by signs of spasticity and increased tendon jerks. The *speech disturbance* is described as scanning in type, and explosive (p. 171).

Pyramidal tract signs: Over 80% of patients with multiple sclerosis show a spastic paraplegia, i.e., bilateral pyramidal signs and increased reflexes (661). Those cases starting at an advanced age are especially likely to present monosymptomatically as a progressive paraparesis with a tendency to rapid progression (887). Other causes of this picture may be ruled out by the presence in multiple sclerosis of oligoclonal IgG in the CSF (709) and sometimes the demonstration of involvement of other locations in the central nervous system – mainly by utilizing refined investigative methods to demonstrate abnormality, such as visual evoked potentials, electro-oculography, (1127) or MR scanning. *Absent superficial abdominal reflexes* may be an expression of spasticity: however, since these reflexes are absent in 20% of normal adults, this clinical sign is valueless as a solitary finding. Their absence becomes significant if the reflexes of the abdominal muscles are also simultaneously increased. The *spastic gait* in the later stages of multiple sclerosis is typical, not infrequently showing an ataxic component, as stated above.

Sensory disturbances: Such changes are present in about 50% of patients early in the disease (661). Occasionally the presenting symptom may be spontaneous abnormal sensations (paresthesias) or as an abnormal feeling upon stroking the skin of the extremities (dysesthesia). The hands sometimes may exhibit a severe astereognosis. Less frequently dissociated sensory disturbances are present. *Painful sensations* are not uncommon.

Seizure-like phenomena (778, 906, 1211): The occurrence of *epileptic attacks* in multiple sclerosis has been repeatedly claimed (342) and disputed (1001). The author in his own group of multiple sclerosis patients has found epilepsy to occur 4 times more often than in the general population. *Paroxysmal brainstem attacks* should raise the suspicion of multiple sclerosis, especially in younger subjects (342, 778); they are discussed on p.276. They may occur as presenting signs of the disease, in the same way as attack-like *loss of muscular tone* which causes the patient to fall down or as a *paroxysmal dystonia* (113). Less frequently repeated attacks lasting 15–45 s may occur, accompanied by a *paroxysmal dysarthria* and ataxia (778, 906, 1288).

Bladder and rectal disturbances: By the time of first hospitalization, 20% of patients show these signs (661). The most common is an *uncontrollable urge to void,* which may lead to bed-wetting or wetting of the clothing. Other forms of incontinence are less common.

Mental disturbances: The multiple sclerosis patient not infrequently exhibits an inappropriate euphoria and lack of insight in regard to his disease. The longer its course, the more likely are psycho-organic changes to appear which, particularly in cases with a protracted course, can be expected to produce a state of dementia in one-fourth of patients (924). Mental changes may be the presenting feature in multiple sclerosis, usually in association with signs of brainstem involvement (1305); indeed, a psychotic picture may be early evidence of the disease. In the early stages, mental signs are likely to be observed in about 3% of cases (661).

Specific signs and forms: A clinical sign (actually, a symptom) which is typical but not pathognomonic of multiple sclerosis is *Lhermitte's sign.* This neck flexion sign is observed in about one-third of multiple sclerosis patients, and in about one-half of these during the first attack of the disease (590). It is characterized by the feeling of an electric charge passing down the vertebral column, and perhaps into the arms and legs, upon forced flexion of the neck. A similar response may be elicited in the presence of other cervical cord lesions, e.g., space-occupying lesions, arachnoiditis, subluxation of the atlantoaxial joint, after X-irradiation, and in subacute combined degeneration. Lhermitte's sign after cranial trauma, see p.28. Less frequently, cases are described of *peripheral neuropathy* with muscular atrophy, absent reflexes, and fasciculation involving particularly the hand muscles (371). Rarely, forceful flexion of the neck produces a transient exacerbation of the spastic leg weakness and the gait disturbance. The term "McArdle sign" has been suggested for this phenomenon (902). In the *hemiplegic type,* which is usually encountered in younger subjects, a complete hemiplegia may develop within hours without accompanying coma or pain, and may disappear completely within days or weeks. In rare cases an *abnormal fatigability of muscles,* similar to myasthenia, may be observed. This symptom can be reversed clinically and electrophysiologically by the administration of cholinesterase inhibitors (921). Symptoms of the disease may be increased by *raising the body temperature* (167) – a feature which is explained by a reversible conduction block affecting partially demyelinated fibers. For example, the patient may not be able to help himself out of a hot bath or mistake the acute signs of a febrile illness for a new "attack." This feature may also be utilized to diagnostic advantage, e.g., testing the patient's ability to identify two closely spaced visual stimuli while raising the body temperature (396). (Caution! Permanency of symptoms thus induced has been reported.)

Ancillary Investigations in Multiple Sclerosis

CSF Examination

A lumbar puncture should always be performed if greater diagnostic certainty is considered necessary. No deleterious effects on the course of the disease have been observed from it. About one-third of patients show an increased *total protein,* but only rarely is the level above 75 m%. About two-thirds show a relative increase in the gamma globulin content. Previously this was demonstrated by a shift to the left of the colloidal gold curve, but nowadays immunoelectrophoresis is relied upon. These studies reveal a significant increase in the IgG, IgA, and IgM levels which are less abnormal with steroid medication or during a remission (668).

Proof of intrathecal antibody production in multiple sclerosis is yielded by the demonstration with immunoelectrophoresis of increased IgG levels in 70% of cases, and with isoelectric focussing of *oligoclonal bands* in 90% of cases (573). The total *cell count* is slightly raised in less than one-half of cases, rarely over 40 cells, and plasma cells which are not present in normal CSF are found in at least two-thirds of cases. No direct correlation exists between the individual abnormal findings in the CSF.

Evoked Potentials (235, 1163)

This technique enables lesions to be demonstrated in the corresponding sensory tracts, without providing information about their nature. *Visual evoked potentials* (VEP) in most patients reveal a prolonged latent interval of the cortical evoked potentials following visual stimulation. This finding is almost invariably present in all patients who give a history of an episode of retrobulbar neuritis, but it is also present in about 70% of those without such history (64, 225, 354, 465). The supplementary technique, *auditory evoked potentials* (AEP), yields abnormal results in a defined group of multiple sclerosis patients and confirms the presence of a plaque of demyelination of the brainstem.

CT and MRI

Computed tomography (CT) may reveal demyelinating plaques which show abnormal enhancement after the injection of an iodine solution (987).

Magnetic resonance imaging (MRI) is a more sensitive technique, showing more plaques than CT, as well as lesions as small as 4×3 mm (310, 1306) (Fig. 4.1). With an MRI study with gadolinium enhancement, fresh plaques can be identified which will disappear after the exacerbation has subsided (811). This expensive examination is justified only in the small group of cases in which the clinical and ancillary investigations mentioned above fail to establish the diagnosis.

Additional Investigations

Other ancillary investigations can usually be dispensed with. *Electroencephalography* in at least one-third of cases reveals nonspecific abnormalities which bear no correlation with the patient's mental picture. The *blood serum* shows an increased gamma globulin level and immunoelectrophoretic changes only during an acute attack. Serologic tests have little use at the time of the clinical diagnosis, despite the fact that circulating brain antibodies can be demonstrated in one-fourth to one-third of patients. Unfortunately these antibodies are nonspecific, be-

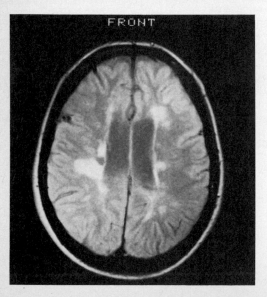

Fig. 4.1 A 29-year-old woman known to have been suffering from multiple sclerosis for several years. In the T$_2$-weighted double-echo sequence on a transverse projection, extensive patchy disturbances of the signal can be seen in the white matter in both hemispheres. The ventricular system is noticeably enlarged on both sides; a periventricular pattern predominates. (MR image courtesy of the Brunnhof Röntgen Institute, Berne – Dr. Fritschy, Dr. Cerny, and Dr. Porcellini)

ing encountered in other diseases in which cerebral tissue is destroyed. A significantly greater proportion of multiple sclerosis patients show high antibody titers against the measles virus than is encountered in the general population. Lymphocytes from these patients more often show a rosette grouping than epithelial cells injected with measles virus (769).

Prognosis: Ten years after their first attack, 80% of patients are alive compared with 100% of a similarly structured normal population. An unfavorable prognostic sign in respect to improvement is paraparesis with bilateral extensor plantor responses. Other unfavorable prognostic factors are a higher age at onset, rapid initial progression, and male sex (291). A frequency of 0.5 new disease episodes per patient year is assumed during the first 5 years. The clinical picture 5 years after the onset correlates well with the picture after 10 and 15 years, especially in respect to cerebellar and pyramidal signs (466). Of male patients with established multiple sclerosis, 8% succumb to the disease or its effects within 10 years, and 20% within 20 years (660). Isolated individual cases may run a very acute course, with death occurring within weeks, particularly cases of neuromyelitis optica (see below) and those with rapidly progressive brainstem signs. Despite these statistics, about one-third of patients remain free of significant disability 10 years after the first attack and a smaller percentage 25 years later. So-called *benign forms* of multiple sclerosis

are described, the patients experiencing remarkable recovery from the signs and symptoms of individual attacks (irrespective of their frequency) and showing no progression between the attacks (152). Evaluation for the purpose of life insurance is extremely difficult. In some patients, notably those with marked disability, the prognosis for life depends directly on the quality of nursing care.

Pathologic anatomy (436, 466, 1217): The pathoanatomic lesion of multiple sclerosis is typical, viz. plaques or foci of demyelination without accompanying axonal destruction, except in very acute foci. These changes may occur throughout the CNS, but they are found most often around the aqueduct, in the floor of the fourth ventricle, and in the subpial part of the spinal cord. The plaques often appear as sharply defined, pale areas. The neurons in the gray matter are often intact and the astrocytes slightly increased in number. In the white matter, old plaques show marked neuroglial proliferation, fibrillary gliosis, and a network of reticulum fibers so that they appear as gray and hardened areas. These "multiple" and "sclerotic" foci give the disease its name.

Etiology and pathogenetic mechanisms (251, 466, 693, 740, 1240): The **cause** of multiple sclerosis remains unknown, despite intense research activity in this field. Countless hypotheses have been advanced. The majority of multiple sclerosis patients in Europe are types HLA-A3, B7, DW2, and DR2. During the acute attack, the number of suppressor cells in the peripheral blood is reduced. Experimental studies favor the theories of a *slow virus infection* (640) or an *autoimmune reaction* (93). The inoculation into sheep (in Iceland) of brain tissue removed from multiple sclerosis patients has provoked an attack of scrapie, a transmissible disease of the CNS in sheep in the animals after a latent interval of about 18 months. Two other chronic progressive CNS diseases of humans are known to be transmissible to chimpanzees – Kuru (p. 137) and Creuzfeldt-Jakob disease (p. 169). Although a raised measles titer is often present in multiple sclerosis patients, the measles virus cannot be viewed as the responsible agent. This pathogenesis of multiple sclerosis partly complements and partly contradicts the theory of autoimmune mechanisms. These are supported by the model of experimental allergic encephalomyelitis (EAE) in animals. In recent years, a recurrent course of the disease has been reproduced in animal models (1284). A delayed sensitization to "encephalitogenic protein" of the CNS has been shown to occur through a cellular immune reaction. Sensitized lymphocytes are the most important carriers of this process. Some support exists to suggest that a herpes simplex 1 virus infection occurs in childhood, which leads either to persistence of the virus in a clinically silent form or to an abnormal immunologic situation which is initially latent. An additional subsequent herpes simplex 2 infection might be responsible for the flare-up of the viral infection or

for the development of an autoimmune reaction (769).

Current scientific concepts allow the following *assumptions* to be profitably discussed (740):

– Following an infection of the neuroglia during childhood, the causal agent remains present as a genome and is periodically activated. The effect on the oligodendroglia is responsible for the bouts of demyelination, the CNS signs of demyelination and antibody production being secondary consequences. The effects outside the CNS can explain the lymphocyte changes.
– Infection provokes a cellular autoimmune response against normal CNS tissue or CNS components damaged by the virus.
– Multiple sclerosis is a single reaction to more than one causal factor, with which the various identifiable manifestations and courses are compatible.

Factors provoking the disease: The above-mentioned ignorance of the actual causes of multiple sclerosis inevitably reopens discussion on whether external toxins and other influences provoke the *onset of the diseases* or acute attacks. A combination of circumstances associated with military service is usually dismissed. Exceptionally, an acute traumatic incident may coincide in time and site with an acute attack of multiple sclerosis and merits serious consideration. Direct brain trauma may determine the site of a plaque of the disease. Pregnancy and childbirth appear to hasten the onset of the first attack of the disease, but they do not increase the frequency of the attacks themselves. Therefore, only very exceptionally is the disease an indication for terminating pregnancy.

Treatment: Of the countless suggested forms of treatment (175, 206, 466, 735, 1015, 1166), management with corticosteroids and especially ACTH and immunosuppression with azathioprine in selected cases appear to be the only measures to influence individual attacks or alter the course of the disease.

In individual cases – after excluding other contraindications – the *acute attack* may be treated by: intravenous infusion of 0.5 mg of synthetic ACTH in 500 ml of physiologic saline or 80 units of corticotropin daily for 10 days. For the next 2-3 weeks intramuscular injections of ACTH gel are given, the dose and frequency of injection being progressively reduced. The intramuscular route may be used from the start. Oral treatment with dexamethasone or other corticosteroid preparations in equivalent doses may be used according to the following regimen: for the first 3 days 2.5 mg 3 × daily of dexamethasone, 4th day 25 units of ACTH, 5th through 8th day 0.5 mg of dexamethasone 3 × daily. This may be followed by ACTH gel in reducing doses, as above. Potassium replacement and prophylactic antibiotics may also be given, if required. Intrathecal hydrocortisone 25-75 mg 2-3 times a week, introduced by lumbar puncture into the subarachnoid space, appears at best to exert only a transient effect on signs of spasticity. Although ACTH treatment hastens regression of the symptoms during the acute attack, it exerts no effect on the general course of the disease.

In specific patients, especially those who fail to recover after attacks and who show *stepwise deterioration* (1014) and exceptionally *frequent attacks* (702, 802), intensive immunosuppressive therapy appears to be justified for a year or more, in order to attempt to stabilize the course of the disease (426, 1000, 1044). The efficacy of immunosuppression in progressive cases has not been proved (1044): 10% of these patients develop malignant tumors after 5 years or more (702).

Spasticity may be treated with diazepam or the GABA derivative baclofen (Lioresal R) 10-50 mg at night (199). Treatment with vincristine in order to provoke a neuropathy (and thus lessen the spasticity) has also been suggested (343). Trials with intrathecal baclofen are in progress.

Other measures include the low-fat Evers diet (1176). Additionally, physiotherapy plays a significant part. This includes active measures, careful nursing, and the treatment of secondary complications (bedsores, urinary infections). A sign which is particularly difficult to treat is intention tremor, often disabling to the patient. Isoniazid has been recommended (1045), and beneficial results have been reported with stereotactic operations. Appropriate psychologic support for the patient is very important. Openness and sincerity are essential; at the same time, the physician must adopt a careful and hopeful attitude toward his patient.

Differential diagnosis: This includes a wide variety of diseases and depends upon the presenting signs and symptoms.

Forms with cranial nerve deficits must be differentiated from a brain tumor, e.g., dermoid of the base of the skull base, cerebellar tumor with ataxia and nystagmus, optic glioma or sphenoid wing meningioma, brainstem glioma, or brainstem encephalitis (1213).

Hemiplegic forms require differentiation from tumors of a cerebral hemisphere or an ischemic brain lesion.

Spastic-paretic forms always raise the possibility of a spinal cord tumor or myelopathy due to cervical spondylosis.

Recurrent parapareses are a feature of spinal cord arteriovenous malformations.

The simultaneous presence of pyramidal signs, cerebellar and brainstem features raises the possibility of a space-occupying lesion or malformation of the brainstem or the craniovertebral angle. These lesions are particularly frequently liable to be misdiagnosed as cases of multiple sclerosis. The same is true of brainstem vascular malformation which occasionally presents a fluctuating course and then manifests clinically for the first time in middle-aged or elderly subjects (162).

Multisystem involvement may also mislead the physician, including systemic affections, vasculopathies, and infectious and toxic encephalomyelitides, as well as hypothyroidism and subacute combined degeneration of the spinal cord.

Involvement of the eyes combined with neurologic signs raises the possibility of an infectious or vascular lesion. For example, a uveitis combined with neurologic deficits is found in *uveoencephalomyelitis* (Vogt-Koyanagi-Harada syndrome). This viral disease presents, in addition to a uveitis, as a disturbance of hearing, leukodermia, premature graying of the hair, and encephalitic or sometimes meningeal signs. *Behçet's disease* may show signs of CNS involvement, particularly brainstem encephalitis in addition to the aphthous and ocular features, (489, 1028, 1169). Arguments have been advanced that the CNS deficits are produced by multiple areas of softening occurring as the result of a vasculitis (643). Occasionally a myopathy may accompany the disease. Another ocular lesion, *Eales' disease,* consists of recurrent retinal and corneal hemorrhages with periphlebitis, and occasionally a severe subacute myelopathy followed by an encephalopathy (1113).

Other Demyelinating Diseases

Concentric Sclerosis (Balo's Disease)

This disease, also known as concentric periaxial encephalitis (220, 436, 735), involves both sexes and all age groups. **Pathoanatomically,** the demyelination is grouped in concentric zones around a central point, separated by layers in which the myelin is preserved. In addition, small plaques of demyelination may be found similar to those in multiple sclerosis. **Clinically,** the disease runs a slowly progressive course, sometimes commencing with focal deficits followed by increasing paralysis and dementia accompanied occasionally by signs of raised intracranial pressure.

Diffuse Sclerosis (Schilder's Disease)

The condition described in children by Schilder was characterized by symmetric demyelination involving particularly the centrum semiovale, producing rapidly progressive mental deterioration and neurologic signs. It may be a leukodystrophy (1058), but the likelihood exists that the cases Schilder described belonged to several etiologic groups.

Acute Disseminated Encephalomyelitis

This is a descriptive term applied to rapidly progressive cases of multiple sclerosis. Histologic examination of the demyelinating lesions in the brain and spinal cord reveals evidence of degeneration of the axis cylinders and a perivascular round cell infiltration. The onset is acute, sometimes with fever, leukocytosis, and a raised CSF cell count (up to $400/mm^3$). The disease runs a rapidly fatal course, death occurring within a few weeks.

Neuromyelitis Optica (Devic's Disease)

In this condition lesions of the spinal cord and optic nerves appear in rapid succession. It may be viewed as an incident of acute multiple sclerosis involving a specific site. Children or adolescents are usually involved, the onset being rapid and the spinal cord and optic nerve involved simultaneously or in rapid succession. Often both optic nerves are affected by retrobulbar neuritis or papillitis. The level of the myelitis progresses upward to the cervical cord and may involve the bulbar centers. The prognosis is poor, but some patients survive.

Subacute Myelo-Optic Neuropathy (SMON)

Japanese authors have described a disease entity which is rather common in Japan, subacute myelo-optic neuropathy (SMON) (866, 1122). **Clinically,** ascending paresthesias, muscular weakness of the lower extremities, and optic neuritis (in about one-third of cases) appear days or weeks after gastrointestinal symptoms or after an abdominal operation. The patients seldom recover and most remain significantly incapacitated; recurrences are described. **Pathologically,** changes in the anterior and posterior spinal nerve roots and spinal ganglia have been consistently shown, as well as symmetric plaques of demyelination and axonal degeneration of the corticobulbar tracts and posterior columns, particularly in the cervical region. Occasionally the optic nerves also show demyelinating plaques (1122). **Pathogenetically,** an association with oxyquinoline is suspected, although only 75% of sufferers have taken this drug. A viral etiology has also been discussed (867). Cases of SMON after oxyquinoline have been reported outside Japan but they are rare (586), so that a particular genetic-enzymatic predisposition of the Japanese or other concomitant factors must be considered. A similar disease picture is said to be produced by *thallium poisoning* (98). SMON should be viewed as an example of a group of diseases with demyelination as their presenting feature, which have been designated *central distal axonopathy syndrome* (1197). Amnestic episodes after oxyquinoline intake, see p. 80.

Congenital Demyelinating Diseases

See p. 143.

5. Damage to the Nervous System by Specific Physical Agents

Electrical Damage to the Nervous System

Physical factors: The effects of industrial electricity and natural lightning upon the nervous system (172, 846) depend on
- strength of the current
  - a function of the voltage and
  - resistance, the latter depending on
  - size, shape, and skin resistance of the point of entry,
- duration of contact, and
- points of entry and exit of the current in the body.

Mechanism: The effects on the nervous system are produced by
- direct and immediate effect of the local burn,
- delayed changes resulting from secondary scarring caused by the local burn,
- damage to the part of the nervous system through which the current flowed, e.g.,
  - disturbances of consciousness and seizures during the acute episode,
  - paralysis, and
  - delayed epileptiform seizures.

Clinical features: Heat damage, i.e., *electrical burns,* may be caused at the *point of entry of the current,* and the nervous tissue lying directly be-

neath it may be affected. Such injuries usually accompany lightning or contact with a high-tension current of more than 5,000 V. The lower the resistance of the skin (wet skin!) and the longer the flow of the current, the lower will be the voltage necessary to produce an electrical burn; under certain circumstances, ordinary alternating household current may do so. The nervous system is a relatively good conductor of electricity, and it may be damaged other than by direct burning or coagulation necrosis, along the path of flow of the current through the body. If the *brain* lies within the circuit, unconsciousness and tonic or clonic seizures may occur. If there is also a high heat flow, permanent damage may be produced in the form of a focal cerebral lesion, e.g., hemiplegia, quadriparesis, cerebellar signs, a parkinsonian syndrome or, subsequently, symptomatic epilepsy. Passage of the current through the *spinal cord* (e.g., the cervical cord, if the current flows from arm to arm) may lead to a severe and complete transverse lesion. Muscular atrophy and various spastic clinical syndromes are described, as well as a classic picture of amyotrophic lateral sclerosis following electrotrauma. Damage to the *peripheral nerves* produced by electricity is rare (172, 846). Paresthesias, sensory disturbances, or peripheral motor weakness have been observed in only 3,6% of 10,000 cases (172). These cases can be explained on the basis of a local burn or as a reversible paralysis of peripheral nerve trunks (343). The neurologic signs following electrotrauma may often regress, but permanent damage is known to occur.

Acceptance of causal relationship: It is justifiable to accept a causal relationship only under the following circumstances:

- if the abnormal signs are topographically related to the site of entry of an electric current;

- if the clinical signs are present immediately after the electrotrauma, especially if the affected parts of the nervous system lie within the line of passage of the electric current through the body;

- conversely, the greatest possible reserve must be exercised if no immediate connection in time exists between the injury and the onset of signs, the latter possibly being caused by a coincidental and unassociated disease of the nervous system developing at the same time, and if the signs grow worse later;

- nonspecific signs and symptoms such as headache, autonomic lability, neurasthenic complaints are sometimes an "indirect" effect, the result of a fright reaction.

Damage During Decompression

Caisson Disease

This term describes the signs and symptoms in divers who ascend from the deep too quickly. The **pathogenetic mechanism** is gas embolism, because blood gases are released early as a result of oversaturation during rapid decompression. **Clinically,** the most serious effects are various transverse lesions of the spinal cord (197, 462). However, not to be ignored are the widespread lesions of the brain, which may later manifest as a neuropsychologic deficit, often with neurasthenic or psychosomatic features (939). **Treatment** by immediate recompression is justified, even hours after the rapid ascent. Additional late treatment with hyperbaric oxygen even when given with a delay of 48 hours up to 8 days, may have a beneficial influence on the resolution of the cord symptoms (197).

Damage by X-Irradiation

Introduction: Damage to the brain, spinal cord, and peripheral nerves may be produced during X-irradiation. This damage depends on several factors, including the size of the single and total dose applied and the timing of individual treatment sessions. It is expressed by the formula

$$NSD_{RET} = TD \times N^{-0.24} \times T^{0.11}$$

in which the normal standard dose (NSD) expressed in rad equivalent therapy (RET) is related to the total dose (TD) multiplied by the number of individual doses (N) and the duration of treatment (T). Depending on the NSD, the radiation damage appears, after a latent period which varies between months and years.

Irradiation Damage to the Brain

This requires a dose of at least 2,800 rad (= 28 Gy), and under certain circumstances radionecrosis of the brain may occur. The signs and symptoms develop after a latent period of many months or years; both the length of the latent period and the tissue effects depend upon the size of the dose. The **pathologic lesion** is a fibrinoid necrosis of the blood vessels with perivascular exudation of plasma and erythrocytes, lymphocytic infiltration, and massive necrosis of the white matter. Since irradiation is usually applied to patients with neoplasms, the onset of signs and symptoms nearly always necessitates a differential diagnosis from tumor recurrence. Radiation-induced clinical deficits may also arise indirectly, as a result of occlusion of the larger blood vessels such as the middle cerebral and internal carotid arteries.

Irradiation Damage to the Spinal Cord

Analogous to the brain damage that may follow X-irradiation is a myelopathy which may complicate conventional roentgen therapy and irradiation with fast electrons. This complication is usually seen after the application of more than 3,500 rad within 28 days. Instances have been described following irradiation of pharyngeal and laryngeal tumors, lymphomas, malignant mediastinal masses, and bronchial tumors. The latent period between irradiation and the onset of clinical signs varies from 2 months to 5 years, usually about 1 year. The **clinical picture** may vary greatly. Most patients develop cervical myelopathy. The first sign is usually paresthesias of the lower extremities, sometimes accompanied by Lhermitte's sign, and the clinical picture may not progress. However, in other patients a progressive paraparesis or quadriparesis may develop. In at least one-half of the patients, a pure Brown-Séquard syndrome develops. The modalities of deep and superficial sensation are usually abnormal. The role of X-irradiation in the development of a myelitis with myoclonic involvement of the lower extremities remains a controversial subject. The lesion may be arrested at an early stage, but most cases advance over the course of weeks or months as a progressive transverse syndrome. About 50% of the patients die within months or years of the effects of the myelopathy, while in the remainder the lesion may remain stationary for years or may even exhibit only transient clinical features. The **pathologic lesion** (561) involves the white matter more than the gray matter. Spongy demyelination and reactive astroglia are present initially; later focal or diffuse demyelination and necrosis are characteristic features. Vascular changes are always present, varying from fibrinoid necrosis with fluid passage through the walls of the blood vessels to telangiectatic malformations. The nerve cells are usually spared. **Therapeutically,** the administration of a protein-free blood extract is recommended in chronic progressive cases (533).

Damage by Generalized or Local Hypothermia
(366, 846)

General remarks: Hypothermia of the entire body is a very rare complication of simple exposure to cold – at least in the latitudes of Continental Europe. In most cases, other accidental factors have contributed to the patient failing to find shelter from exposure to cold (366).

Clinical Features

Central Nervous System

The level of consciousness is altered roughly according to the degree of hypothermia, which is accompanied by a fall in blood pressure, pulse rate, and respiratory rate. The pupillary reactions and tendon jerks become weaker, muscular tone may be increased, and pyramidal signs may appear. Meningism may be encountered, even if the CSF findings are normal. Patients who survive hypothermia do not usually exhibit specific long-term neurologic deficits (366).

Peripheral Nervous System

Laboratory experiments have shown that cooling prolongs conduction time in peripheral nerves and alters their ultrastructure (889). Clinical evidence was produced during the World Wars that local cooling of peripheral nerve injuries in trench or shipwreck victims led to paralysis and sensory disturbances. The heavily myelinated fibers are particularly sensitive to cold. During open heart operations involving cooling of the myocardium, phrenic nerve damage has been observed in 7% of cases as a result of the hypothermia; it is not always reversible (173).

6. Epilepsies and Other Diseases Presenting as Attacks or Disturbances of Consciousness

Epilepsies (505, 544a, 555, 596, 712, 777, 882, 1175)

Definition: The epileptic diseases are characterized by disturbances which

- occur in attacks,
- are usually, but not always accompanied by disturbances of consciousness,
- and/or other attack-like motor, sensory, or autonomic phenomena,
- are produced by an abnormal focus of excitation in the brain,
- can usually be observed during an attack as an abnormal electrical discharge by means of EEG recordings made with surface or deep leads, and is
- caused by a (metabolic) abnormality of the brain which is usually structural but may sometimes be functional.

Pathophysiology and Etiology

Pathogenetically, a disturbance of function of the cerebral neurons plays a part. Electrophysiologic study reveals an abnormal synchronous discharge from groups of neurons which may sometimes, but not invariably, be reflected by the EEG. Local perfusion measurements show an increased regional blood flow in focal epilepsy during an attack, as well as upon local stimulation without attacks or in the absence of EEG changes (527). The idiopathic and particularly the familial forms of epilepsy show a tendency to low IgA values in the blood serum, even an IgA deficiency during phenytoin treatment (364). The significance of these findings is uncertain.

Etiology: In principle, any brain will respond to appropriate stimulation or provocation through epileptic seizures. In some cases of epilepsy, a morphologic abnormality may be detectable, such as a congenital malformation of the brain, perinatal or subsequently acquired traumatic damage, a disturbance of perfusion, or a neoplasm. In other patients, metabolic disturbances such as hypoglycemia may be present. However, often no cause is found.

Epidemiology

Epilepsy is one of the commonest diseases of the nervous system and affects about 0.5% of the population. If a family history is present, the risk of attacks is greater than in

Table 6.**1**   Classification of epileptic seizure forms recommended by the International League Against Epilepsy (from Epilepsia 22: 1981, 493–495)

1.   Partial (Focal, Local) Seizures

1.1   *Simple partial seizures* (consciousness not impaired)

1.1.1 With motor signs
- Focal motor without march
- Focal motor with march (jacksonian)
- Versive
- Postural
- Phonatory (vocalization or arrest of speech)

1.1.2 With somatosensory or special-sensory symptoms (simple hallucinations, e.g., tingling, light flashes, buzzing)
- Somatosensory
- Visual
- Auditory
- Olfactory
- Gustatory
- Vertiginous

1.1.3 With autonomic symptoms or signs (including epigastric sensation, pallor, sweating, flushing, piloerection and pupillary dilatation)

1.1.4 With psychic symptoms (disturbance of higher cerebral function). These symptoms rarely occur without impairment of consciousness and are much more commonly experienced as complex partial seizures
- Dysphasic
- Dysmnesic (e.g., déjà vu)
- Cognitive (e.g., dreamy states, distortions of time sense)
- Affective (fear, anger, etc.)
- Illusions (e.g., macropsia)
- Structured hallucinations (e.g., music, scenes)

1.2   *Complex partial seizures* (with impairment of consciousness; may sometimes begin with simple symptomatology)

1.2.1 Simple partial onset followed by impairment of consciousness
- With simple partial features followed by impaired consciousness
- With automatisms

1.2.2 With impairment of consciousness at onset
- With impairment of consciousness only
- With automatisms

1.3   *Partial seizures evolving to secondarily generalized seizures* (this may be generalized tonic-clonic, tonic, or clonic)

1.3.1 Simple partial seizures evolving to generalized seizures

1.3.2 Complex partial seizures evolving to generalized seizures

1.3.3 Simple partial seizures evolving to complex partial seizures evolving to generalized seizures

Table 6.1   (Continued)

2.	**Generalized Seizures (Convulsive or Nonconvulsive)**
2.1	*Absence seizures*
	• Impairment of consciousness only
	• With mild clonic components
	• With atonic components
	• With tonic components
	• With automatisms
	• With autonomic components
2.2	*Atypical absences*
	May have:
	• Changes in tone that are more pronounced
	• Onset and/or cessation that is not abrupt
2.3	*Myoclonic seizures* Myoclonic jerks (single or multiple)
2.4	*Clonic seizures*
2.5	*Tonic seizures*
2.6	*Tonic-clonic seizures*
2.7	*Atonic seizures*
3.	**Unclassified Epileptic Seizures**

the average population. If one parent is epileptic, the risk of the disease in his descendents is 1 in 25 if he suffers from the idiopathic form and 1 in 67 in the symptomatic form. If both parents are epileptic, the risk is greater than 1 in 25 (565, 777).

Classification of Epilepsy

Epileptic seizures may be classified according to
- etiology,
  • genuine, genetic,
  • symptomatic, on the basis of an existing brain lesion,
- clinical picture (Table 6.1),
- EEG correlation,
- onset of first attack (e.g., delayed epilepsy after the age of 30 years).

No constant relationship exists between the clinical characteristics and these criteria of classification. For example, generalized epileptic seizures that are clinically identical may be provoked by genuine idiopathic epilepsy or, on the other hand, by a localized lesion such as a brain tumor, while in another patient the same tumor may provoke focal or jacksonian attacks. The classification of epilepsy will be discussed and described in the next section which deals with the clinical aspects. The revised recommendations of the commission on classification and terminology of the International League Against Epilepsy (48, 557, 1134, 1286) are given in Table 6.1. The approach recommended by this body, namely of relying upon the symptomatology of the seizures, can lead to descriptive confusion and circumlocution. Consequently this nomenclature does not always enjoy clinical currency and its value continues to be challenged (594). The EEG characteristics are related to the clinical manifestations. General approach to epilepsy, see p. 277.

Generalized Seizures

Grand Mal Epilepsy

Clinical aspects. This is the classic form, familiar to the layman, typified by severe, and generalized convulsions and unconsciousness. The attack may be preceded by a premonitory subjective sensation, the so-called aura. Suddenly, a generalized tonic convulsion occurs with respiratory arrest, the patient falls to the ground and may utter a cry; after 10 s, clonic convulsions follow. The patient may foam at the mouth, bite his tongue, and be incontinent of feces and urine. The clonic convulsions may last for several minutes, and they are followed by a period of unconsciousness which passes into a state of postictal confusion. Finally, normal consciousness returns. Amnesia lasting 10 min or longer is present for the attack and the postictal phase. Frequent attacks may lead to personality changes which are typically a slow, fussy, overprecise "cloying" attitude, but they may take the form of episodic agitation and irritability. These changes are exceptional if the therapeutic regimen is adequate.

EEG and other ancillary investigations: The *EEG* is normal in at least one-fourth of patients with generalized epilepsy between attacks and shows the characteristic features of epilepsy in only 50%. The typical picture is that of episodic discharges of very slow waves in all leads, with individual spikes and sharp waves (Fig. 6.1). However, cases with documented focal lesions of the brain are encountered which give rise to generalized seizures and/or bilaterally synchronous spikes and waves. During an attack, the EEG remains permanently abnormal – the changes are nonspecific and a clinical attack of grand mal epilepsy may, for example, be reflected in the EEG as a focal epileptic change (see below). The *CSF* sometimes reveals a pleocytosis of up to 100 cells after repeated generalized attacks (1081).

Etiologic or provoking factors: The cause may be defined as either a change in the function of an individual part of the brain without visible morphologic change ("genuine epilepsy," primary generalized epilepsy), in which inherited factors play a part, or it may be symptomatic, in which specific factors (see below) are responsible for focal changes, the resulting attack of epilepsy being generalized. The focal nature of the discharges is usually revealed by the EEG made during the attack, but in some cases careful clinical observation shows the seizures to have a focal distribution initially (see below) and to become generalized subsequently. An *inherited predisposition* and exogenous factors may contribute to a varying

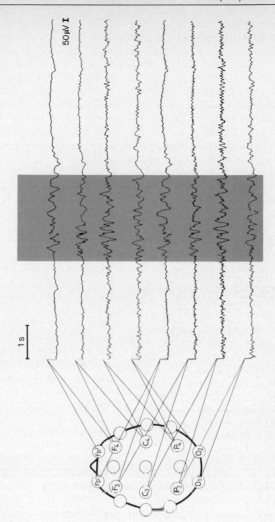

Fig. 6.1   Interictal EEG in a patient with grand mal attacks. All leads show simultaneous generalized paroxysmal bursts, partly atypical spikes and waves

extent in individual cases. Sleep deprivation or repetitive light stimulation (disco, traveling through an artificially illuminated tunnel, television, etc.) may trigger attacks. A first-time onset of epileptic seizures in *pregnancy* (565, 624) is commoner than eclamptic attacks. The first seizure usually occurs between the 26th and 36th week. The ratio of seizures of symptomatic epilepsy to simple pregnancy attacks and to an attack of a spontaneous idiopathic form of epilepsy is 1:2:5. Nevertheless, a careful search for any organic cause is always advisable (624). In the puerperium, epileptic seizures may be a clinical sign of cerebral venous thrombosis (p.97).

In a woman with established epilepsy, the frequency of attacks usually increases during her pregnancy; thus, her demand for appropriate medication increases. This heightens the risk of intoxication after delivery. Since antiepileptics (particularly phenytoin) as well as the pregnancy itself may provoke a folic acid deficiency and osteopenia, prophylactic folic acid and vitamin B supplements are essential. Antiepileptics and fetal malformations, see p.282.

Alcohol intake may trigger attacks in an established epileptic or be the actual etiologic cause of epileptic attacks. Thus, 30% of patients with delirium tremens suffer from epileptic attacks. The seizures usually predate the delirium tremens, occur 12 h or longer after the last intake of alcohol (946) ("rum fits"), and recur only after further alcohol abuse or a new episode of delirium. On the other hand, elderly chronic alcoholics may develop a genuine epilepsy with repeated seizures. **Additional causes** of generalized epileptic seizures will be discussed when the individual etiologic disease pictures are considered. Tumors, see p.31; posttraumatic forms, see pp.28 and 275; brain atrophy, see p.171; cerebral circulatory disturbances, see p.67.

Status epilepticus and sudden death: *Status epilepticus* is a condition which may accompany primary generalized or primary focal attacks. The term denotes a succession of attacks, none of which need be generalized in a classic sense since some may consist of solitary contractions of individual muscle groups. The important fact is that the patient does not fully regain consciousness between attacks. Status epilepticus is a life-threatening condition which may cause sudden death by central hyperpyrexia, aspiration, electrolyte disturbances, or hypoxic cerebral necrosis. Treatment is discussed on p.278. *Sudden death* may occur in epileptics, even when there has been no status epilepticus. Only in about one-third of such cases does autopsy examination provide a satisfactory explanation of the cause of death. In a series of 37 sudden deaths in epileptics, nearly all of whom had experienced more than one attack a month, only 3 showed a blood concentration of antiepileptic agent in the therapeutic range, and in about 50% none was present (1190).

Absences

Definition: This heading includes a variety of epileptic manifestations in the group of patients suffering from generalized attacks. They are characterized by a very brief period of disturbed consciousness without loss of postural support, and usually accompanied by transient focal motor phenomena. The seizures appear for the most part in children, and a specific type of attack can be related to a specific age group. They exhibit highly characteristic EEG changes and respond to specific medical treatment.

Simple Absences

This is the *petit mal epilepsy of childhood,* the attacks starting between the 2nd and 14th years. **Clinically,** they begin with by disturbances of consciousness lasting no more than a few seconds, which suddenly interrupt the individual in his action or speech. He stares vacantly ahead for a moment and then resumes the activity that was interrupted. Occasionally these attacks are viewed in schoolchildren as "absentmindedness." Girls are more affected than boys, and the attacks may be provoked by hyperventilation. If the absences are the only abnormality, the term *pyknolepsy* is used. Actual loss of consciousness, falling about, or other coarse motor phenomena do not form part of the typical picture of absences. When mouth and tongue movements, pill-rolling, and other more delicate motor signs occur, the term *petit mal automatisms* is used, and it must be differentiated from temporal lobe epilepsy. Ab-

sences occur with considerably greater frequency than attacks of temporal lobe epilepsy – often dozens an hour. Also, they are usually far briefer. Physical examination shows no abnormality. The **EEG** reveals the typical 3–4/s spike and wave pattern, which appears suddenly in all leads, superimposed on a normal pattern (Fig. 6.2). If these abnormal bursts last less than 3 s, the aberration will not manifest itself clinically. For this reason, the EEG is an essential part of the diagnosis of absences, and when performed during hyperventilation is abnormal in 90% of cases. Similar EEG changes are described – albeit rarely – in focal brain lesions in children, which suggests that absences are age-dependent. The **incidence** is low and accounts for less than 10% of cases of childhood epilepsy. At least one-third of patients have a family history of epilepsy. The most likely explanation appears to be that absences are a genetically or metabolically determined form of epilepsy. Regarding the **course** of absences, about one-fourth are symptom-free by the time of puberty or soon after. However, other patients continue to show absences, and at least one-half begin to experience grand mal attacks. The term *mixed epilepsy* is then used, although this condition may be primarily present, the EEG showing evidence of both types. Treatment, see p. 277.

Absence Status

This condition (petit mal status, status pyknolepticus) is a difficult clinical diagnosis which may be impossible to make without EEG. The

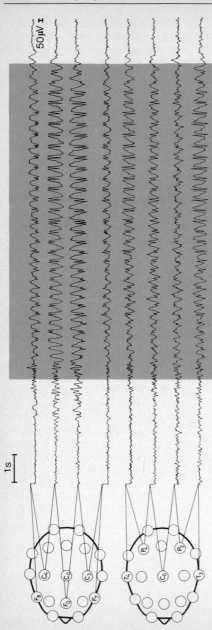

Fig. 6.**2**   EEG in absence epilepsy. Hyperventilation produces generalized 3–4/s spikes and waves

patient appears to be confused or in a dream state. His reactions and answers are slow but often his behavior is not abnormal. Only adults are affected.

Salaam Spasms

This type belongs to the atypical absences recorded in Table 6.1 and is also known as propulsive petit mal, infantile spasms, or the West syndrome (555, 608, 776, 998). They usually appear in the 1st year of life and are seen to be an age-specific reaction of the brain to a variety of causes (malformations, perinatal lesions, congenital brain lesions, leukodystrophies, etc.). **Clinically,** the disease picture consists of rapid, jerky forward movements: the patient nods his head and then sweeps both arms forward and sideways spontaneously, or else immediately experiences a convulsion of the whole body with flexion and elevation of the arms and flexion of the legs. The attacks occur frequently – up to 100/h. The *EEG* consists typically of mixed high slow waves with peaks and spikes in various sites (hypsarrhythmia, mixed epilepsy potentials) (316, 555). **Treatment** consists of ACTH combined with antiepileptics for several weeks (see Table 6.2). The **prognosis** is poor (776, 998): the mortality amounts to about 20%, and of the survivors less than one-fifth are normal, 50% are severely retarded, and in more than one-half various attacks persist. Favorable factors are the absence of any specific cause for the attacks, a previously normal mental development, and the absence of other attacks before the onset of the salaam spasms. Transitional forms with myoclonic and astatic petit mal (see below) are described. Treatment, see p. 277.

Myoclonic and Astatic Petit Mal

This variety is also known as akinetic seizures, drop attacks, or the Lennox-Gastaut syndrome (555, 1087), and are another variety of atypical absences. It affects children, particularly boys aged between 1 and 9 years (commonest 2–4 years). Symptomatic cases are slightly less often seen than in salaam spasms (1087). **Clinically,** the attack may consist merely of a brief nod of the head; the child may, however, fall to the ground (depending on his center of gravity at the time of the attack) by simply collapsing or by striking the floor violently, a myoclonic component being present. Consciousness is not lost during brief attacks, but short absences or longer periods of confusion may occur even if the patient does not fall down. During the drop attacks, three-fourths of patients experience tonic-clonic or simply clonic convulsions. A *myoclonic astatic status* develops in one-fourth of patients and predisposes to the development of dementia (306). The **EEG** shows generalized, somewhat irregular 2/s bursts of spike waves ("petit mal variant") (597). The typical EEG changes may not be present at the start of the illness (597).

Myoclonic Attacks

This variety is also known as impulsive petit mal or bilateral epileptic myoclonia (555). Although the attacks may begin in childhood, they usually begin in adolescence; thereafter, they tend to decrease in frequency. Myoclonic epilepsy is rarely seen in adults. **Clinically,** the attacks may be described as consisting of severe, brief, jerky, irregular convulsive movements. They may be solitary or repeated, isolated or symmetric, and involve particularly the neck, shoulders, and upper extremities. They are more frequent after sleep deprivation or upon waking. Precipitating factors include shock, emotional upset, or flashing lights. The patient does not lose consciousness. More than one-half of patients subsequently develop additional grand mal attacks, which are particularly likely to occur on waking in the morning ("waking epilepsy"). Physical examination reveals no abnormality. Psychopathic traits are remarkably common. The **EEG** shows, especially with photic stimulation, high amplitude slow waves interpolated with numerous spike potentials during an attack. Nitrazepam is particularly useful.

Myoclonus Epilepsy (Unverricht's Syndrome)

This familial disease should not be confused with the variety mentioned above. **Clinically,** it consists of severe epileptic attacks, progressive dementia, and myoclonic spasms. The latter are symmetric, usually affecting muscle segments or groups without provoking much movement, nonrhythmic, and triggered by intentional movements and sensory stimuli. The disease pursues an unrelenting course to death. The cause is believed to be a genetically determined disturbance of carbohydrate metabolism manifested by intracytoplasmic Lafora bodies: inclusion bodies

typical of the disease. This inclusion material may also be observed in muscle and liver cells. The sensory evoked potentials are abnormally long-lasting (464), while those in myoclonic attacks are normal.

Partial Attacks

General Remarks

Clinical features: This type of attack does not give rise to generalized involvement of the whole body. As a rule it involves either

- motor or sensory phenomena, being the *elementary symptomatology* of involvement of one part of the body only (e.g., focal clonic jerking of a particular extremity), or it is
- a *complex event* (e.g., confusional state).

Secondary generalization is always a possibility.

Etiology: Partial seizures are always caused by local abnormalities of the brain; thus, they are a form of *symptomatic epilepsy.* Their presence always prompts a diligent search for an underlying pathologic lesion. The fact should be stressed yet again that generalized seizures also may be the clinical manifestation of a focal change in a specific part of the brain.

Topographic localization of focal lesions: The nature of the onset of the attack, i.e., the presence of any particular focal features, is vitally important for topographic diagnosis, and it should be carefully studied. Accurate topographic attribution to a specific region of the brain is possible (Fig. 6.3). The initial

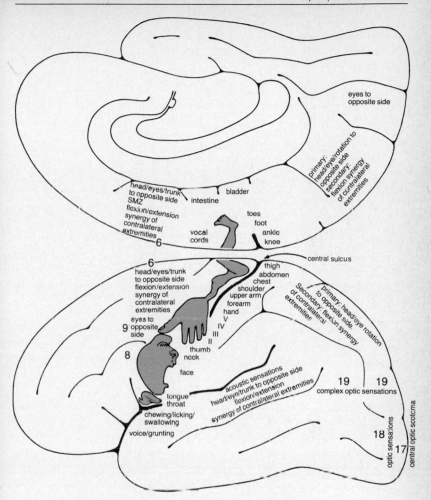

Fig.6.**3** Focal epileptic attacks. The type of attack depends on the site of the focal lesion. SMZ = supplementary motor zone (after *Foerster*)

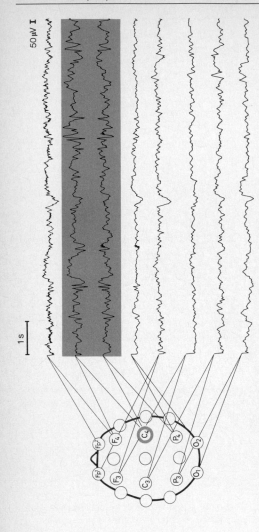

Fig. 6.4   EEG made during a focal epileptic attack. Epileptogenic focus in right central region, with spikes as well as sharp and slow waves. Phase reversal in C4

phase of the attack, which is the important part for reaching a topographic diagnosis, may be very brief or poorly observed, and therefore remain hidden. Occasionally an EEG will reveal the focal nature of the disturbance (Fig. 6.4).

Partial Seizures with Simple Symptomatology

Focal Motor, Focal Sensory, and Focal Somatosensory Epilepsy

These are characterized **clinically** by clonic seizures and/or sensory phenomena confined to one part of the body. Usually the attack *starts* in a hand, corresponding to the relatively large cortical representation of the hand in the anterior part of the central convolution; sometimes the attack starts in the face, rarely in the foot. The latter accompanies lesions of the cortical edge (e. g., parasagittal meningioma). The attack may begin with motor or clonic jerks or by paresthesias, less frequently by other symptoms such as flashes of light or optic hallucinations, which point to a focal lesion in an occipital lobe (see below). The attacks may last from several seconds to several minutes. The patient may not lose consciousness at all, or only later when the attack becomes generalized. It may lead to a transient *postictal hemiparesis* (473). This condition, a hemiplegia usually following an attack of ipsilateral focal epilepsy and disappearing in the course of a few days (Todd's paralysis), must be distinguished from a *hemiparesis arising from a constant epileptogenic focus* in the contralateral hemisphere, in which only mild

clonic seizures occur (473). The reverse situation is the occurrence of epileptic attacks as part of a severe hemisyndrome caused by perinatal brain damage, the so-called HHE syndrome (hemiplegia-hemiatrophy epilepsy). A *neurologic deficit* may be present, which depends on the focal nature of the disturbance and the circumstances of the attack. The interictal **EEG** reveals either an epileptogenic focus or a delta wave focus, but in some cases it is not abnormal. During the attacks, however, an epileptogenic focus is constantly present (Fig. 6.4). Lesions in appropriate sites may provoke *attacks starting with sensory signs and symptoms,* e. g., visual hallucinations, auditory sensations, and abnormal gustatory and olfactory sensations (see below; follow also Fig. 6.3). These initial symptoms may be followed by other focal symptomatology, e. g., jacksonian seizures, or go on to a grand mal attack. *Focal status epilepticus,* i. e., a series of focal attacks occurring in rapid succession, may also develop.

Jacksonian Epilepsy

This type of epilepsy starts, in a similar way to the forms described above, as a focal attack which spreads slowly to involve adjacent parts of the body ("march of convulsion") and finally encompasses half of the body or becomes a generalized grand mal attack. In the *differential diagnosis* of jacksonian epilepsy, *migraine accompagnée* (p. 278) should be considered (959). In the latter condition, the first attack always occurs before the age of 50 years. The foot is seldom involved initially and progression from the starting point to the rest of the body is slow, lasting minutes or hours (in jacksonian seizures, within seconds or minutes), the affected side may change from one attack to the next, and clonic seizures neve occur. Headache is common in *migraine accompagnée* and not the exception, as in jacksonian epilepsy.

Epilepsia Partialis Continua (Kozhevnikov's Syndrome)

This is a variety of clonic or myoclonic seizures, often remaining strongly localized, which continue for hours or days and are not abolished by sleep (791, 1196). In autopsy cases of this condition, a lesion has always been found in the motor cortex or immediately adjacent to it (1196). The EEG shows correspondingly strong focal epileptic discharges. The focal attacks may occur only many years after the causative lesion manifests. However, in another group of patients, mostly children with a progressive lesion, the myoclonic attacks occurred in an early phase of the disease, and they were more diffusely spread and accompanied by neurologic deficits (76).

Benign Focal Epilepsy of Adolescents (590, 1230)

Here the attacks involve children or adolescents, particularly during sleep. Consciousness is unaffected in the waking attacks. Generalized seizures develop in only about one-third of cases; 20% of children experience only one attack. In one-third the attacks are frequent. **Neurologic examination** is negative and the children- show normal intellectual and emotional development. The **EEG** invariably exhibits abnormal unilateral centrotemporal activity which consists of slow biphasic spikes of high amplitude *(rolandic*

spikes). The **prognosis** is good, and after puberty the attacks regress spontaneously, as do the abnormal EEG findings. It is questionable if this condition can be differentiated from a solitary focal seizure with a normal EEG (717). However, a small group of patients must be differentiated from this variety, namely those in whom the attacks start in the first 6 years of life, in whom absences are present as well as atonic seizures and the sleep EEG shows a continuous generalized spike and wave activity. In this group of patients, the attacks also appear to regress spontaneously (20).

Adversive Attacks

"Adversive" (more accurately, aversive) seizures occur in the presence of a *focal lesion* in the precentral part of the frontal lobe or the supplementary motor area on the medial surface of the cerebral hemisphere (see Fig. 6.3). **Clinically,** the patient's eyes, head, and sometimes a shoulder are rotated suddenly to the opposite side. Consciousness is initially preserved, but it may be lost if the attack becomes generalized. If the focal lesion involves the temporal, occipital, or parietal region, a sensory aura may herald the attack and the patient may lose consciousness before the turning movements take place.

Partial Seizures with Complex Symptomatology

Nomenclature: This form of epilepsy is also designated psychomotor epilepsy or temporal lobe epilepsy.

Causes: The attacks accompany lesions in the vicinity of the limbic system, especially in the temporal lobe. The usual cause is perinatal brain damage, although the attacks may only manifest clinically many years later, in adulthood.

Clinical features: The clinical features of these epileptic manifestations are an abrupt onset, which is brief or lasts minutes or hours, and complex phenomena which the patient may find difficult to describe. Often premonitory autonomic reactions occur, such as tachycardia, dyspnea, epigastric pressure, and nausea. These may be followed by feelings of anxiety, depersonalization, a déjà-vu sensation, or difficulty with thought processes. Sometimes, but not always, the patient exhibits oral automatisms with licking, swallowing, and lip-smacking movements or more complex motor phenomena with stereotyped movements. Finally, brief or longer-lasting twilight states may occur which may be more complicated and organized - *fugue épileptique*.

The symptoms and signs described above may be grouped as follows:

Sensory disturbances, isolated or occurring as an aura before an attack. These include giddiness, dysmorphopsias (macropsia, micropsia), abnormal taste sensations, or unpleasant odors (uncinate fits, p. 179).

Autonomic phenomena, e.g., palpitations, nausea, increased salivation, dry sensation in the mouth, a feeling of hunger, or a desire to urinate. Paroxysmal abdominal pains are described as an attack equivalent, particularly in children. An attack of this type, *abdominal epilepsy* (71), is usually brief, lasting only a few minutes. Consciousness may be altered but it is never lost. The EEG is nearly always abnormal.

Motor phenomena, comprising tonic and clonic jerks as well as complex motor movements such as stereotypical repetition of a gesture, undressing, rubbing or wiping movements, abnormal activity related to the autonomic nervous system such as disturbed respiration, chewing, licking, lip-smacking, choking or swallowing movements, urination, etc. Any attack of temporal lobe epilepsy may finally progress into a generalized epileptic attack.

Mental and psychomotor manifestations, including changes in the level of consciousness. Sometimes the patient lives in an unrealistic dream world and he may experience compulsive ideas or an abnormal clarity of thought. He may appear to have experienced the present previously (déjà-vu experience). He may exhibit groundless anxiety or outbursts of anger or experience actual hallucinations. If the paroxysmal nature of these disturbances is overlooked, an incorrect diagnosis of schizophrenic psychosis may be made.

Twilight states are a typical feature of psychomotor epilepsy, in which the patient carries out complex movements while apparently awake and fully conscious. These states may be brief and may be difficult to recognize *(twilight attacks)*. On the other hand, a twilight state may last for hours or days, during which the patient may carry out a series of complicated actions, such as a journey, a true *fugue épileptique,* and for which he will have amnesia.

Temporal syncope is the name applied to the brief episodes of loss of consciousness, with collapse but no motor activity, seen in temporal lobe epilepsy.

Psychomotor status epilepticus may also accompany temporal lobe epilepsy.

Findings on Examination: *Physical examination* is usually normal, although focal signs such as a homonymous field defect may sometimes be present. In about 70%, slight weakness of the perioral muscles is said to be present on the side opposite to the EEG focus (989). *Neuroradiologic investigation* may reveal an enlarged temporal horn. The *waking EEG* is abnormal in only 30% of patients, while sleep tracings reveal abnormalities in 70%. The typical finding is a focus in the anterior part of a temporal lobe, often with high theta and delta waves, and less frequently, spikes as well.

Differential diagnosis: Differentiation may not be easy from a severe case of *autonomic disturbances,* from *hyperventilation tetany,* and from *psychogenic attacks.* Similarly, the possibility of *beta-adrenergic hyperactivity* (327) (panic disorder) may not be easy to dismiss. This disturbance, which may begin spontaneously or be provoked by an infusion of isoproterenol hydrochloride, presents a picture either of circulatory disturbances with tachycardia and a feeling of chest pressure or the combination of anxiety, nervousness,

dyspnea, and shivering. The attacks appear out of the blue and recur up to several times a week, lasting for minutes or hours. They are abolished by propranolol 160 mg a day. Occasionally a case of *hypovigilance in narcolepsy* has to be distinguished from twilight attacks of temporal lobe epilepsy, and, because of the daytime drowsiness, sleep apnea has to be considered in the differential diagnosis (p. 285).

Specific Forms and Causes of Attacks

Pyridoxine-Dependent Seizures (555, 721)

Clinically, these generalized seizures start a few hours after birth. They fail to respond **therapeutically** to antiepileptics without a vitamin B_6 supplement in the form of pyridoxine hydrochloride. When the pyridoxine supplement is subsequently withdrawn, further attacks may occur. A delay in starting treatment may lead to psychomotor retardation.

Febrile Seizures

This term is applied **clinically** to generalized attacks occurring in children under the age of 6 years as a complication of a febrile illness, usually an upper respiratory tract infection (876). A febrile convulsion is an epileptic seizure which may be followed by further seizures, even when the patient is afebrile. The long-term prognosis is better if the initial febrile convulsion occurs between the first 6 and 18 months of life, and definitely before the 7th year; if the attack is generalized and not focal; if it lasts less than 5 min;

if the EEG is normal after 10 days; if no abnormal physical signs are found on neurologic examination; if there is a family history of febrile convulsions (nearly 50% of cases!); and if there is no sign of birth defect or other brain damage. If all these criteria can be fulfilled, there is a 90% probability that the febrile convulsion will not be followed by subsequent seizures. **Long-term treatment** is justified after the third attack, usually with phenobarbital dipropylacetate, but it should be started after the second or even after the first attack if aggravating features are present. These include a prolonged attack, neurologic deficit, signs of cerebral damage, family history of epilepsy, or epilepsy-specific EEG changes.

Startle Epilepsy (1047)

This rare form belongs to the reflex epilepsies. It is encountered in brain-damaged subjects especially in association with perinatal lesions. The attacks, which are provoked by fright, may be generalized or focal, in the latter instance involving the side of the body appropriate to the brain damage. These patients may benefit from treatment with carbamazepine.

Posttraumatic Epilepsy

Epileptic attacks after craniocerebral injuries (37, 224, 439, 564, 913) possess no uniform clinical features, and may appear as partial attacks or (secondarily generalized) grand mal attacks. They occur particularly commonly after open brain injuries and are seen in about one-third of such patients, and in 5% of patients with closed head injuries, especially

if coma has been prolonged. The interval between the traumatic episode and the first epileptic attack varies between minutes and many years. However, at least one-half occur within 6 months and 80% within 2 years: 5% of all cases at risk experience the first attack within the 1st week, 10% in the first 3 months, 16% in the first 6 months, 22% within the 1st year, and 29% within the first 3 years. Even beyond this time and up to 20 years, further seizures occur. Only about 65%–75% of cases remain free from epileptic attacks if observed for long enough (224). Of the 5% with early-onset epilepsy, 25%–30% will have attacks later on (564). Children in the early years of life may develop epilepsy as a complication of a very mild head injury. The more frequent the attacks, the more likely will they occur later. About 50% of patients with posttraumatic epilepsy will be symptom-free within 5 years, with or without treatment, while about 8% will continue to have attacks which are resistant to treatment. Comparison of the results of large series of patients with head injuries – victims of war (224) and civilian life (37) – show a clinical course with a uniform pattern. Improved patient care and the prophylactic use of antiepileptics in the Vietnam War appear to have had no effect on this pattern (224). With correct treatment, the prognosis is not unfavorable. Predisposing (inherited) factors contribute to the onset of posttraumatic epilepsy (224): 15% of patients with depressed fractures have early seizures, but more of them later develop epilepsy (439).

After mild craniocerebral trauma with concussion, brief loss of consciousness, and no signs of contusion, the incidence of epileptic attacks is 0.1% in the 1st year and 0.6% in the first 5 years – figures not exceeding those in the general population (37). The attacks, depending on the primary local cause, are purely focal in about 10% of cases and become generalized in the remainder; in about 25% they are generalized from the outset. The existence of posttraumatic absences has not been conclusively proved and they remain a source of discussion – as does the possibility of posttraumatic myoclonic-astatic petit mal (see below).

Further Types of Epilepsy with Specific Etiologic Factors

To this group belong the *toxic and drug-induced epilepsies*. A very large number of therapeutic agents may provoke epileptic attacks (818, 967). A series has been reported in which 0.8‰ of nonepileptic patients developed drug-induced seizures (966), the substances heading the list being penicillin, i.v. insulin, lidocaine, tricyclic antidepressants, and neuroleptics.

Brainstem Seizures

Despite the occasional description of these attacks as "brainstem epilepsy," the inclusion of this entity in the group of epileptic diseases is not undisputed. **Clinically,** these attacks occur suddenly, sometimes provoked by movement or a change in posture and sometimes by hyperventilation. Each attack consists of tonic and almost invariably painful contractions of all muscles of one side of the body; it lasts less than 1 min. The patient does not lose consciousness. Less frequently the attacks occur without tonic muscular contraction, and consist of sudden *unilateral pains* or focal *atonic states,* e.g., sudden inability to open the eyes. Dozens of attacks may occur in the space of a day. **Etiologically,** these attacks may accompany multiple sclerosis (906), vascular brainstem lesions, or tumors of the basal ganglia, and sometimes they occur in patients in whom no primary lesion can be found. **Physical examination** is usually normal or reveals evidence only of the underlying disease. The EEG shows no epileptic changes. The **differential diagnosis** of these seizures includes hyperventilation, tetany due to a metabolic disturbance, and reflex epilepsy caused by a lesion of the cerebral cortex. **Treatment** with antiepileptic medication, especially carbamazepine, is usually successful.

Paroxysmal Choreoathetosis

The appropriateness of classifying this attack-like motor disturbance as an epileptic disease is also questioned. A *familial* form exists which starts in childhood. Choreoathetotic movements occur in attacks which begin distally in the extremities and spread finally to involve the whole body. These attacks, which may last only a fraction of a minute and which are followed by a refractory stage lasting several minutes, are not accompanied by a loss of consciousness. They may be provoked by sudden movements, especially after long periods of sitting or lying still. Various transitional forms and associations exist between this condition and brainstem epilepsy. Apart from the familial form, *symptomatic forms* are described in association with phenytoin intoxication, neuromyelitis optica, multiple sclerosis (p.243), perinatal asphyxia, hypoparathyroidism and hyperthyroidism (365), and with hypoglycemia (880). **Treatment** of both familial and symptomatic forms with antiepileptics, especially carbamazepine is successful.

Practical Approach to a Case of Epilepsy

Case History

Questions should be asked about

- family history of epilepsy,
- events which are relevant to fetal brain damage:
  - difficult birth,
  - meningitides and encephalitides,
  - craniocerebral trauma,
- seizures early in life, particularly in infancy, e.g.:
  - febrile convulsions,
  - bed-wetting as a sign of infantile nocturnal epileptic attacks,
- nature of the attacks (description of a third person is essential):
  - timing of the first attack,
  - timing of the last attack,
  - average frequency of attacks,
  - trigger factors such as loss of sleep, alcohol intake, visual stimuli such as television, frightening experiences, reflex epilepsy caused by specific movements, etc.
  - Specific features of the attack such as aura, loss of consciousness, motor phenomena, identical onset in the same part of the body, tongue-biting and other injuries, incontinence, and concurrent postictal disturbances (confusional states, pareses, marked tiredness or amnesia).
- Drug treatment:
  - which drug,
  - dose,
  - how long,
  - regularity, and
  - efficacy.

Physical Examination

- Neurologic examination should include a check for
  - focal lesions of the brain,
  - signs of raised intracranial pressure,
  - systemic disturbance,
  - heart disease, and
  - evidence of seizures such as tongue-biting.
- EEG:
  - Baseline examination with each first evaluation of epilepsy. However, the diagnosis of epilepsy as such does not usually depend on a concurrent EEG finding.
  - Repeat examination only if the EEG is required for further therapeutic evaluation, e.g., reduction or cessation of medication.
  - EEG examination required for medicolegal purposes (permission to drive).
- Neuroradiologic examination
  - in all cases of focal epilepsy, and all cases of generalized epilepsy with a focal EEG discharge,
  - in all patients with neurologic deficits, provided that these have not remained unaltered for a long period or that a satisfactory explanation is not available,
  - in cases of late-onset epilepsy (first attack after the age of 30 years),
  - sometimes in patients who are resistant to treatment.

Treatment of epilepsy (206, 555, 712, 777, 819, 1083, 1166, 1175): *Elimination of specific causes:* The first step in all symptomatic cases is to identify a treatable specific cause of the attacks, e.g., neoplasm or chronic alcoholism. Precipitating events should be eliminated, e.g., lack of sleep, alcohol abuse, and in rare cases visual stimuli produced by flickering lights, such as television.

Choice of optimal treatment: Before medical treatment can be started, the nature of the attacks must be clearly defined since specific seizure forms respond to specific medications. Second, a meticulously accurate record must be compiled by the patient of all existing or previous drug therapy (preparation, dose, duration of administration). A variety of preparations prescribed for the various types of seizure are listed in Table 6.2.

Principles of antiepileptic prescription: First, the importance must be impressed upon the patient of regular intake of the prescribed dose and of keeping a written record of drug intake and the occurrence of further

Table 6.2 Types of epileptic seizures and their treatment

Type of Seizure	Medication
Grand mal (tonic-clonic seizure), primary or secondary generalized	Phenytoin, phenobarbital, primidone, carbamazepine (especially in secondary generalized seizures), dipropylacetate
Absences (simple absences)	Valproic acid (dipropylacetate), ethosuccimide, methsuccimide (with additional phenobarbital, especially in mixed epilepsy)
Salaam spasms (propulsive petit mal) Myoclonic-astatic petit mal (akinetic seizures, Lennox syndrome)	Clonazepam, nitrazepam, corticotropin
Bilateral epileptic myoclonia (impulsive petit mal)	Valproic acid, clonazepam, primidone
Partial seizures with simple symptoms (focal attacks; jacksonian seizures; adversive seizures, etc.) Partial seizures with complex symptoms (psychomotor epilepsy, temporal lobe epilepsy)	Carbamazepine, phenytoin, phenobarbital, primidone
Brainstem seizures	Carbamazepine, phenytoin
Status epilepticus Petit mal status Grand mal status	Clonazepam i.v. Diazepam, clonazepam i.v. Phenytoin i.v.

seizures. Second, a preparation which is expected to be efficacious in a particular type of epilepsy is first prescribed in small doses. After 3 days, and on each 3rd day following, the dose is increased until a therapeutic effect is obtained or noteworthy side effects occur which rule out a further increase in dose. (Exception: patients with frequent seizures or status epilepticus, in whom prompt saturation is justified.) The time taken to achieve a steady state in the serum, i.e., a constant concentration, may be as long as 10 days with constant daily doses. This factor must be kept in mind when evaluating the "usefulness" of a specific dose. If the effect is genuinely inadequate, the dose should be increased stepwise until the drug is effective, or until toxic side reactions occur. Only when the latter are observed should another drug be substituted and the dose again increased stepwise. The aim should always be to try to achieve the therapeutic objective with one drug and to consider combinations only if no single drug is found to be effective. (However, mixed epilepsy and absences, sometimes from the start, require a combination of drugs; see below.) Chemically pure preparations (Table 6.3) are preferable to combined preparations. If a particular type of antiepileptic treatment is prescribed and embarked upon after a careful analysis of the situation, it should be carried through to its logical conclusion. An attempt to reduce the dose in the absence of attacks should be instituted only after 2 years.

Antiepileptic levels in the serum: Although monitoring of the drug concentration in the serum is possible with most antiepileptics (356, 662, 719) and useful in some cases, it seldom is essential to the drug management of the seizures. Usual therapeutic range, see Table 6.**3**. No fixed relationship exists between the dose taken and the serum concentration of the drug. It is possible to achieve long-term freedom from seizures with a serum concentration below the therapeutic range (356). Estimations are made only if

- suspicion exists in the presence of an inadequate clinical effect that the drug dose is too low (only about one-fourth of the cases studied in a large series showed any useful serum concentration of antiepileptic [719]), there is lack of compliance or that
- toxic side effects are suspected,
- if combinations of the various antiepileptic drugs are used or antiepileptics combined with other medications, which influence the serum concentration and exert this effect through enzyme induction (662). For example, carbamazepine, primidone, and dipropylacetate reduce the serum concentration of phenytoin in this way (1281).
- Under certain circumstances when high doses are already being used without adequate clinical effect, and a further increase in dose is considered.
- Required in some countries by driver's license regulations in patients receiving antiepileptic drugs.

Table 6.3 Antiepileptics, dosage, therapeutic serum concentration, side effects, and indications

Generic Name	Average Daily Dose in mg/kg	Adult Daily Dose in mg	Serum Half-Value Time in Hours	Therapeutic Serum Concentration in μg/ml	Side Effects and Details	Indications
Phenobarbital and derivates	1–5	150–300	100–300	10–30	Sedation, allergies, ataxia, dizziness, nystagmus	Basic medication, especially for grand mal and combined forms (morning and waking epilepsy)
		200–400	Like phenobarbital of which this is a by-product		Less hypnotic than phenobarbital	Like phenobarbital
Primidone	10–25	750–1500	12	2–15 (cf. 10–30 phenobarbital)	Less hypnotic than phenobarbital	Like phenobarbital
Diphenylhydantoin	3–7	200–300	22 (10–40)	7–15	Sedation, allergies, gingival hypertrophy, nystagmus, dizziness, ataxia, skeletal changes, macrocytic anemia	Basic medication for grand mal (especially sleep epilepsy) and combination forms, also focal and psychomotor epilepsy, phenytoin i. v. for status epilepticus, 500 mg i. v. slowly, 250 mg i. m.
Carbamazepine	10–20	600–1200	40	2–8	Allergies, leukopenia, liver damage, dizziness	Basic medication for psychomotor epilepsy (temporal lobe epilepsy), other focal epilepsies, and grand mal epilepsy

Ethosuximide	20–30	500–700 a day for babies, 700–1500 a day for adults	30–40	40–100	Allergies, nausea vomiting, anorexia	True absences
Methsuximide	10–20	600–1200		2	Sedation, leukopenia	
Dipropylacetate (valproic acid)	20–40	200–400 for babies, 600–1200 for adults	8–15	40–100	Allergies, elevated phenobarbital concentration in the serum	Absences, grand mal epilepsy, mixed epilepsy, myoclonic epilepsy
Diazepam	0.15–2	10–150	1–2		Sedation, respiratory depression, short-acting	Status epilepticus 10–20 mg i.v. in adults
Clonazepam	0.1–0.3 mg/100 ml for babies and children				Sleepiness, mucous congestion	Salaam spasms, myoclonic-astatic petit mal, petit mal status
Nitrazepam	0.1–1 mg/kg for babies; 3 × 2.5–5 mg a day for children				Like clonazepam	Like clonazepam
Corticotropin (ACTH)	40–60 U				Allergies, psychoses	Salaam spasms, impulsive petit mal

Routine determination of the drug concentration in the serum is foolish and expensive, and fastidious attention to the "therapeutic value" is often a bar to useful therapy.

General life-style: An epileptic should live as normal a life as possible, and needlessly severe restrictions on his activity should be avoided. The discussion with the patient, and his family, as well as other participants to the patient's care, is important. As a rule in most countries, epileptics may drive an automobile after an attack-free interval of at least 2 years, in the absence of epilepsy-specific EEG, and if drug treatment is reliably and regularly maintained. Rules in various States differ from the above: it is important to consult the Department of Motor Vehicles for regulations that apply locally.

The *commonest antiepileptics* are listed in Table 6.3, together with their usual dosage, proprietary names, and indications. Individual types of epilepsy and the commonest antiepileptic drugs used in their control are given in Table 6.2.

Patients with focal epilepsy who do not respond satisfactorily to medical treatment may be suitable candidates for *neurosurgical excision,* if a focus can be identified by electrocorticography. Similarly, early investigation with deep electrodes and possible neurosurgical treatment should be considered in every case of adolescent temporal lobe epilepsy, which produces frequent and therapy-resistant attacks (707).

Grand mal status is a life-threatening event and should be aborted with diazepam (Valium) 10–20 mg i.v. Instead or in addition, a water-soluble phenytoin preparation (Dilantin) may be useful; 250 mg is administered once or twice, slowly i.v., or as an infusion of 750 mg and an injection of 250 mg i.m. at the same time. *Petit mal status* responds immediately – clinically and electrophysiologically – to clonazepam, 2–4 mg administered slowly i.v. in adults, 0.5–1 mg in infants, and 1–2 mg in schoolchildren.

The *side effects of antiepileptics* may take the form of *acute allergic reactions* and exanthemata or *granulocytopenia,* which may require withdrawal of the drug. Therefore, regular monitoring of the blood smear is necessary, particularly at the time of prescribing a new antiepileptic. Other side effects may take the form of a *chronic intoxication,* which is reversible: the signs and symptoms can be made to disappear by reducing the dose. Ataxia and other signs following phenytoin medication are described on p.149. An upsetting tiredness may accompany treatment with phenobarbital, diazepam, and clonazepam, but it usually diminishes after a few weeks and then disappears. Vertigo is particularly likely to affect elderly subjects after carbamazepine. The effect of anticoagulants is reduced by phenobarbital, phenytoin, and carbamazepine, and the efficacy of oral contraceptives by phenytoin.

A greater incidence of *fetal malformations* is said to accompany antiepileptic medication of the pregnant mother – about 6% as compared with a risk of malformation of 2.5%

in normal adults. However, a direct relationship appears to exist between epilepsy per se and malformation (1100) because children of epileptic parents, even without antiepileptic medication, carry a risk of malformation of 4.2% (555). The somewhat higher incidence of malformation in mothers treated with antiepileptics compared with untreated mothers may perhaps be related to the fact that only the most severely affected cases receive treatment. In each case, the risk to the fetus of an epileptic attack in the mother, as well as the risk to the fetus of medication, must be carefully weighed.

Among the many interactions when anticonvulsants are being given in combination (50), only a few shall be mentioned: diphenylhydantoin, combined with carbamazepine decreased the carbamazepine effect: in combination with valproate, phenytoin toxicity is increased. The effect of valproate is diminished in combination with carbamazepine and increased with diazepam.

Nonepileptic Disturbances of Consciousness, Syncopes, and Motor Attacks

Diseases which may be mistaken for epilepsy are those which present with

- a disturbance of the level of consciousness,
- attacks of motor or sensory disturbances,
- collapse,
- or a combination of these phenomena.

Table 6.4 provides a review of the epileptic and nonepileptic paroxysmal disturbances of consciousness of a syncopal nature. For a more detailed discussion, the reader is referred to the author's definitive work on the subject (845). In the following section, only the commonest and diagnostically most severe clinical syndromes are described.

The Narcolepsy-Cataplexy Syndrome and Its Differential Diagnosis (447, 506, 589, 845, 879, 1041)

Etiology and pathogenesis: These are known only in the rarer symptomatic forms (trauma, encephalitides, vascular lesions, multiple sclerosis). Much commoner are the idiopathic forms of narcolepsy, which in many cases involve a genetic factor. In about one-third of cases, the narcolepsy (and a hypersomnia) are inherited as an autosomal dominant (879). Familial forms of cataplexy have been described. 95% of narcoleptics have the HLA-DR2 type. In the remainder, a disturbance of midbrain function is assumed, which involves the waking centers.

Epidemiology: The disease may affect both sexes, but men are far

Table 6.**4**   Etiologic classification of seizure-like disturbances of consciousness of a syncopal nature and/or drop attacks

1. Primary Cerebral Causes

1.1. *Epilepsies*

    1.1.1. Grand mal seizure

    1.1.2. Absences of childhood
        Pure absences
        Complex absences

    1.1.3. Salaam spasms (West syndrome)

    1.1.4. Myoclonic astatic seizures (Lennox-Gastaut syndrome)
        Primary generalized myoclonic astatic seizures

    1.1.5. Bilateral epileptic myoclonias (myoclonic petit mal)

    1.1.6. Partial seizures with complex symptomatology (especially "temporal syncope")

1.2. *Other primary cerebral causes*

    1.2.1. Narcolepsy-cataplexy syndrome

    1.2.2. Cryptogenic drop attacks of the female *(maladie des genoux bleus)*

    1.2.3. Parkinsonian drop attacks

    1.2.4. Vestibular cerebral syncope

    1.2.5. Other
        – Atonic brainstem attacks
        – With tumors
        – With syringomyelia
        – With basilar impression
        – With normal pressure hydrocephalus
        – Toxic or metabolic disorders

2. Cardiovascular Causes

2.1. Heart diseases

2.2. Extracardiac organic lesions and anomalies of blood vessels

2.3. Vascular and vascular-neurologic dysfunction

2.4. Reflex circulatory syncope

2.5. Pressor-postpressor syncope

3. Psychogenic Involvement and Upset Accompanying Acute Disturbances of Consciousness

3.1. Attacks in childhood with respiratory anomalies

    3.1.1. Crying spells (breath-holding syncope)

    3.1.2. Sobbing syncopes
        – Cyanotic
        – Noncyanotic

3.2. Hysteroepilepsy

3.3. Psychogenic syncope

3.4. Simulation

more often affected than women. Because of the missed diagnoses, the incidence of the disease is difficult to estimate. Of the author's series of neurologic patients, they accounted for 0.6% of cases (506). In a population study in the United States, their prevalence was estimated to be 0.06%–0.1% (286). The disease is usually present in youth, but first becomes noticeable in young adulthood when daily pressures become more pronounced.

Signs and symptoms: Only about 10% of patients exhibit at the same time the four cardinal features

- disturbances of alertness,
- cataplectic attacks (loss of affective tone),
- sleep disturbances ("waking attacks," sleep paralysis),
- hypnagogic hallucinations and other rarer symptoms.

In the majority of patients, one or other of these clinical features is either absent or present in a milder form.

Disturbances of Alertness

Typical sleep attacks occur even in rested patients in sleep-provoking situations (pleasant warmth, comfortable position, satiety, boredom). They cannot be volitionally avoided and may last 10–15 min, rarely as long as 1 h. The patient can be aroused normally. About one-half of narcoleptics exhibit *partial hypovigilant states,* e.g., a disturbing sleep-drunkenness, a type of twilight state with automatic movements which are either appropriate or purposeless, and associated with

an amnesia. In this situation, twilight states caused by temporal lobe epilepsy are an important differential diagnosis.

Cataplexy

This type of attack is characterized by a sudden loss of muscular tone. It does not occur in all patients with sleep attacks; however, it does not occur in their absence either. An individual muscle group or, indeed, the entire musculature may suddenly lose its normal tone so that the parts affected fall limply to the side of the body or the patient himself collapses to the ground. For a brief period, usually less than 1 min, the patient is unable to move the affected parts. These attacks may dominate the clinical picture, and only detailed interrogation uncovers a history of mild episodic disturbances of alertness. If the attacks are triggered by emotion (hearty laughter, sudden fright), the term *affective loss of tone* is used. However, the attacks of muscular atonia with collapse eventually occur without emotional stimulation and may accompany simple acts such as assuming a particular bodily posture, i.e., triggered by motor innervation. The patient remains conscious throughout the attack.

Sleep Disturbances

Disturbances of nocturnal sleep are common. So-called *sleep paralysis* ("waking attacks") is the term used to describe a specific phenomenon which affects the patient when he is either about to fall asleep or wake up. These attacks are true cataplectic states, which are associated with an oppressive feeling of helplessness.

The abnormal state usually lasts for a few seconds or minutes. It ceases at once if the patient is touched or spoken to. Another, often severe disturbance of which these patients complain is *nocturnal dreaming* or *nightmares.*

Rarer signs and symptoms: Under this heading belong *hypnagogic hallucinations,* i.e., hallucinations occurring during the transitional phase from waking to sleeping; actual psychotic states, sleepwalking (somnambulism), double vision during an attack of sleep paralysis, and nocturnal sleeplessness.

Examination methods and diagnosis: *Neurologic examination* is normal, apart from rare symptomatic cases. *General physical examination* sometimes shows a patient who is stocky in build and obese, frequently with a low basal metabolic rate, a labile blood pressure, lymphocytosis, and hypogonadism. The *EEG* findings possess great significance. The waking EEG may be completely normal. However, recordings made during attacks exhibit the typical sleep characteristics. More informative is *polysomnography,* with simultaneous recording of the eye movements and muscular activity in the evening or during the night. It shows that the patient falls asleep very quickly and documents the onset within the 1st h of so-called rapid eye movement (REM) sleep, which repeatedly alternates with typical deep sleep.

Treatment: This is not always necessary. The sleepiness is best countered by methylphenidate 10–80 mg/day, phenmetrazine 25–75 mg, amphetamine 5–40 mg, or mazindol 2–8 mg/day. Cataplexy, sleep disturbances, and nightmares and hallucinations respond to clomipramine 25–75 mg, imipramine 25–100 mg, or protriptyline 10–20 mg/day. Sleep attacks and the cataplexy may be abolished by beta-blocking with large doses of propranolol in specific cases (589), although the effect is transient. But L-Tyrosine in a dose of 100 mg/kg of body weight per day reportedly alleviates the narcoleptic attacks and cataplexy with few side effects (834).

Differential diagnosis of sleep disturbances: Nearly all patients with the *sleep apnea syndrome* (447, 775) are male. Strikingly frequent features are loud snoring, sleep restlessness, difficulty to arouse and spells of respiratory cessation lasting up to 1 min with resumption of respiratory activity after being startled. Repeated impairment of the free air passage in the upper airway, the so-called obstructive sleep apnea syndrome, is responsible. The rarer central nervous form, with arrest of the activity of the respiratory muscles, is central sleep apnea syndrome. In nocturnal sleep, recurrent apneic periods of more than ten seconds' duration, which can be demonstrated by polygraphy, occur in REM and NREM sleep with concomitant lowering of the O_2 saturation in the blood. The patients are tired during the day, repeatedly fall asleep, engage in automatic activities, experience hypnagogic hallucinations, and may show intellectual decline or even a (reversible) dementia. Children may also be affected, in whom likewise an acquired disturbance of the autonomic nervous system should be suspected (381). Treatment spans the spectrum from avoidance of hypnotic substances, to the correction of an anomaly of the laryngopharynx, from a retainer to correct an overbite to the very successful nocturnal continuous positive airway pressure (CPAP) with individually adjusted pressure.

The *pickwickian syndrome* (406) is a state of episodic somnolence (hypersomnia) and drowsiness with irregular respiration in very obese subjects. Occasionally headaches and papilledema may be present.

The *Kleine-Levin-Critchley syndrome* (459) is characterized by recurrent episodic sleep disturbances lasting several days, autonomic disturbances, and especially abnormally increased appetite (polyphagia, bulimia) and disturbances of sexual function. There are mental abnormalities including confusion and agitation. Men are mostly affected, usually in their 20s, but occasionally also women. If the disease is prolonged, the attacks become less frequent and shorter. As a rule, they cease spontaneously when the patient is in his 30s. Neurologic examination is usually normal. The EEG during the attack shows a slow background rhythm. The syndrome may be caused by a midbrain disturbance.

Drop Attacks

Sudden collapse may be a consequence of a loss of consciousness (epileptic and nonepileptic disturbances of consciousness, see above). However, drop attacks may occur without loss of consciousness or after a disturbance of consciousness so brief that it goes unobserved (see also Table 6.4).

Drop Attacks in the Parkinsonian Syndrome

Drop attacks may occur in the akinetic forms of parkinsonism when prompt reflex corrective movements fail to materialize and the patient loses his balance. Such drop attacks may be an early manifestation, occurring as one of the first signs of an as yet unrecognized parkinsonian syndrome (623).

Cryptogenic Drop Attacks in Women (1160)

Previously called menopausal drop attacks, these sudden drop attacks affect women between the ages of 40 and 60 years. Many of these women will have experienced similar attacks when younger. They occur sporadically, and the women do not always lose consciousness. During an attack, the patient without warning or accompanying symptoms falls suddenly forward, and she may hurt herself and bruise her knees (French: *maladie des genoux bleus*). The drop attacks may occur only a few times a year and may later gradually disappear. The pathogenesis is unclear.

Vestibulocerebral Syncopes (653)

The patient falls to the ground, often on the same side, as if struck by a flash of lightning. A split second previously he will have been overcome by a severe and brief sensation of giddiness – the surroundings appear to slip away. Sometimes the attacks may be provoked by sudden movements of the head. Some patients after the drop attack exhibit other vestibular signs. *Benign parox-*

ysmal vertigo of childhood (201), also lasting for only a few seconds, may also cause sudden drop attacks and recur several times a week.

Further causes of drop attacks (845): The *atonic forms of brainstem attacks* have already been referred to (pp.245 and 276). Occasionally *brain tumors* (especially frontal and midline) may present in this way. In *syringobulbia, colloid cyst* of the third ventricle, *Arnold-Chiari malformation,* and *basilar impression,* syncopal attacks are described. Cardiovascular diseases producing drop attacks, see below.

Cardiovascular Causes of Syncopes and Drop Attacks

Only some of these causes will be discussed below. In a series of patients admitted to a hospital because of syncope, a cardiovascular cause was demonstrated in more than one-half of the patients (593).

Cardiogenic Syncopes

Syncope with loss of consciousness and drop attacks may be caused by a sudden and transient reduction of cerebral blood flow. The causes are listed in Table 6.5, the commonest being a disturbance of rhythm. This may lead to an Adams-Stokes attack 5–12 s after the cardiac arrest (see also p.62 and Fig.1.6). Complete recovery under such circumstances will occur only if the cerebral circulation can be restored to normal within 5 min. In any unexplained syncope, careful search for a cardiac cause is essential.

In a heart which is structurally intact, a disturbance of the reflex regulation of cardiac activity and blood pressure may lead to syncope.

Reflex Circulatory Syncopes

Excessive vagal stimulation caused by various afferent impulses may lead to bradycardia and/or vasomotor collapse, and both may cause syncope.

Vasovagal Syncopes

In subjects with a corresponding disposition, emotional stress (sight of blood, repulsive scene), pain, heat, or cold may cause syncopal attacks. Knowledge of this tendency usually heightens the anxiety and correspondingly increases the tendency to suffer a syncopal attack.

Swallow Syncope (27, 697)

The act of swallowing can provoke syncope in the presence of glossopharyngeal neuralgia, after irradiation, or in the presence of a tumor. The pathophysiologic mechanism is probably related to ephapses which, by generating increased afferent impulses, provoke exaggerated vagal efferent discharges.

Carotid Sinus Syndrome

Pathophysiology: The normal carotid sinus reflex can be described as follows: stimulation of the pressor receptors in the carotid sinus gives rise to afferent impulses which pass along carotid sinus nerves and the glossopharyngeal nerve. They produce reflex efferent impulses in the vagal and sympathetic fibers and thus reduce the heart rate and alter the vascular peripheral resistance. An increased sensitivity of the carotid sinus, e.g., in arteriosclerosis, hypertension, or diabetes mellitus, leads to an excessive reaction as

Table 6.5   Syncopes of cardiac origin [845]

1. *Heart diseases without disturbance of cardiac rhythm*

   1.1. Incomplete emptying of the left ventricle
   - Valvular aortic stenosis
   - After aortic valve replacement
   - Hypertrophic obstructive cardiomyopathy
   - Disturbances of myocardial function

   1.2. Incomplete filling of the left ventricle
   - Myxoma or thrombus of left auricle
   - After mitral valve replacement
   - Mitral stenosis
   - Prolapse of mitral valve
   - Cardiac tamponade

   1.3. Lesions of the pulmonary circulation and the right side of the heart
   - Congenital malformations
   - Acute massive pulmonary embolism
   - Chronic pulmonary hypertension

2. *Disturbances of Cardiac Rhythm*

   2.1. Bradyarrhythmias
   - AV block, grade 3
   - After pacemaker implantation
   - AV block, grade 2
   - Chronic bi- and trifascicular blockage
   - Sick sinus syndrome
   - Other bradyrhythmias

   2.2. Tachyarrhythmias
   - Supraventricular paroxysmal tachycardia
   - Paroxysmal chamber tachycardia
   - Tachycardia accompanying Wolff-Parkinson-White syndrome
   - Prolonged QT syndrome and *les torsades de pointes*
   - Auricular fibrillation and flutter

a result of local pressure or forced movements such as violent rotation or extension of the neck. A reduction of sinus rhythm by more than 50% or a fall in the systolic blood pressure of more than 40 mm Hg is considered to be abnormal. The carotid sinus syndrome may be subdivided into a cardioinhibitory type, a vasodepressor type, and a central or cerebral type. **Clinically** (593, 803), the syndrome affects mainly elderly men, often those suffering from one of the above-mentioned diseases. A brief feeling of dizziness or nausea may precede the loss of consciousness. The latter lasts only for a few seconds, exceptionally as long as 1 min. **Diagnostically,** it is important to search for and identify the above-mentioned trigger mechanisms and risk factors. The important investigation is the carotid sinus pressure test, which requires ECG monitoring and should be carried out on one side only. A syringe filled with atropine should be available, as well as a pacemaker device.

Treatment: Implantation of a permanent pacemaker. In the vasodepressor form of the syndrome, surgical denervation of one or both carotid sinuses may be performed.

Post-Pressor-Reflex Syndrome

Pathophysiologically, these attacks are due to a mechanism by which the venous return to the heart is reduced. Other factors almost invariably are also responsible for reducing the blood supply to the brain. *Cough stroke* and *laughing stroke* (ictus laryngis and geloplexy) (997) are events most likely to overtake males who are emphysematous, of a pyknic build, and who are smokers. Because of a severe bout of coughing or prolonged laughing, there occurs simultaneously a fall of blood pressure and a reduction of the heart rate (Valsalva maneuver). In addition, the venous return is reduced by compression of the inferior vena cava at the level of the diaphram. Unconsciousness with a feeling of dizziness and weakness supervenes within 30 s.

Micturition syncope occurs when the patient, awakened from sleep, empties a distended urinary bladder while standing erect; often he may be half asleep and hung over from alcohol. A reduction in sympathetic vasoconstrictor tone leads to a fall in blood pressure, and the patient collapses. A contributory factor is the Valsalva mechanism at the start of urination, and the loss of the support afforded by the full bladder to maintaining the blood pressure.

Stretch syncope: This well-known pathophysiologic mechanism is used by wayward schoolboys to provoke an attack: first they induce intense hyperventilation, through which the cerebral vessels are constricted by the hypocapnia, then they suddenly stand up from a crouching position, provoking a corresponding orthostatic fall in blood pressure. Powerful compression against the constricted vocal cords, as well as passive pressure exerted on the thoracic cage by bystanders, provokes the syncope ("fainting lark"). *Supine hypotensive syndrome,* which affects pregnant women when lying in the supine position, is thought to be caused by disturbed venous return resulting from compression of the inferior vena cava by the gravid uterus.

Syncopes Resulting from Disturbed Orthostatic Circulatory Regulation

Pathophysiologically, failure of one or more of the mechanisms regulating blood pressure and the circulation produces a pool of blood in the periphery (845), and the cardiac minute volume becomes inadequate. Additional factors such as orthostasis, may also contribute.

Idiopathic Vasomotor Collapse of Adolescents (845)

Most patients are rapidly growing youths, and the predisposing factors appear to be overtiredness, emotional situations, poor physical health, or excessive heat. The patient first becomes dizzy, experiences darkness before his eyes, perspires profusely, and then loses consciousness and falls down. However, he does not fall heavily to the ground like a patient during an epileptic seizure; rather, he collapses passively. Sometimes he remains aware of his surroundings but fails to react. He may exhibit discrete nonsystematic movements, or he may shiver. Exceptionally, he may be incontinent of urine. The typical picture is a patient with a pale complexion, cold sweat, and widely dilated pupils reacting to light. The period of unconsciousness lasts for a few seconds only and no more than a minute, and the patient recovers immediately in the horizontal position. Observers may mistakenly ask him to sit or stand up. This may cause – as in other types of syncope – a so-called *convulsive syncope* associated with epileptiform convulsions and urinary incontinence. After the attack, the patient either recovers immediately or remains exhausted for a while. However, the period of transient confusion observed after a genuine epileptic attack does not occur. These vasomotor forms of collapse occur most often in schoolchildren, the incidence showing two peaks, at 6 years and 11–12 years of age; thereafter, their incidence decreases.

Orthostatic Hypotension

This form of hypotension – and, as a consequence, syncope – may accompany various pathologic conditions, all of which influence the normal regulatory mechanism of the blood pressure. These conditions include hypovolemia, sodium depletion, Addison's disease, hypothyroidism, autonomic denervation in diabetes mellitus, Parkinson's disease, the Shy-Drager syndrome, and other autonomic disturbances. Some pharmaceuticals may also induce orthostatic hypotension with syncope, notably diuretics, antihypertensives, and tricyclic antidepressants.

Syncope Produced by Disease of Blood Vessels

This type includes the transient cerebral circulatory disturbances, particularly basilar artery ischemia, caused by the aortic arch syndrome and other structural abnormalities of the cervicocranial arteries. These circulatory disturbances have already been discussed elsewhere: drop attacks in basilar circulatory insufficiency (p. 78) and unconsciousness in the subclavian steal syndrome (p. 78).

Metabolic Causes of Loss of Consciousness

These diseases are also dealt with in other sections. Hypoglycemia (p. 142), electrolytic disturbances, and particularly hyponatremia (p. 161), hypothyroidism (p. 154), and hypoparathyroidism.

Tetanic Syndromes

These may be the reflection of *hypocalcemia* in a metabolic disturbance of calcium metabolism, in hypoparathyroidism (p. 155), or in sprue. There is a metabolic alkalosis, and the serum phosphorus level is elevated. *Normocal-*

cemic tetany always presents with a normal serum phosphorus picture. It may be accompanied by a metabolic alkalosis (e.g., when bicarbonate is given) or by a respiratory alkalosis. *Hyperventilation tetany,* a condition to be considered in the differential diagnosis of epilepsy, is heralded **clinically** by a *tetanic attack* and accompanied by vague anxiety and muscular pains. Tingling of the fingers and the mouth next follow, as well as tonic contractions of muscles. The fingers are pressed together, the thumbs are rongly adducted (obstetrician's hand), the wrist and elbow joints are flexed (Trousseau's phenomenon). The lower limbs are extended, the feet are plantar-flexed and internally rotated, the toes flexed (carpopedal spasm). The lips are pursed. Occasionally laryngeal spasm and stridor occur, as well as spasm of the gastric cardia, bronchi, and blood vessels. The attacks, which may persist from a fraction of a minute to hours, may be very disturbing. Sometimes the patient experiences clouding of consciousness which may resemble true unconsciousness, although in general he remains aware of events. *Between the attacks,* signs of latent tetany are present: mechanical overreactivity of the peripheral nerves, e.g., contraction of the facial muscles on tapping the trunk of the facial nerve (Chvostek's sign), extension and abduction of the foot on tapping the peroneal nerve against the head of the fibula (Lust's phenomenon), or contraction of fingers into the obstetric position on compression of the nerve trunks of the upper arm by means of a tourniquet (Trousseau's phenomenon). *Needle electromyography* reveals, in the course of one of the provocation methods described above, repetitive discharges of motor units, particularly so-called doublets and triplets. The tetanic syndrome must be distinguished from brainstem attacks (p. 276).

Psychogenic Association and Aspects of Attack-Like Disturbances

Under appropriate circumstances, emotional factors may lead to a true epidemic situation and facilitate the appearance of vasovagal attacks with syncope (96). In other patients, the picture is dominated by the psychologic aspects of the case.

Childhood Attacks Induced by Emotion

Respiratory Affect Seizures (Reflex Anoxic Seizures)

Breath-holding spells, also known as crying fits, are usually encountered in rebellious and hyperactive infants aged 6–18 months or in young children; they have usually disappeared by the age of 6 years. In so-called *cyanotic affective seizures,* fright, anger, pain, or other situations provoke a bout of increased crying and weeping. During the expiratory phase, breathing suddenly stops, the child becomes cyanotic and collapses or becomes stiff, then starts breathing deeply 5–30 s later. He may be confused but only rarely does he lose consciousness or exhibit brief clonic convulsions. The underlying mechanism is assumed to be a hypocapnia induced by hyperventilation resulting in cerebral ischemia. In so-called reflex anoxic seizures *("white-breath-holding")* (1157), the child utters a sudden cry, or may jerk. A fright or a fall may trigger the attack. The crying phase may be absent. Within a few seconds the child becomes flaccid and unconscious; he may become stiff and exhibit myoclonic contractions. The pulse rate may be arrested by vagal stimulation, leading to cerebral hypoxia. The *EEG* in both forms is always normal between attacks. During attacks, initial theta activity is present which gives way to high-voltage delta activity during the period of unconsciousness. The **prognosis** is favorable. No connection with epilepsy. Some patients later develop vasovagal syncopes.

Sobbing Syncope

Pain or emotion is the trigger factor. The infant sobs for several minutes, then breathes shallowly and uses deadspace air. He becomes cyanotic and his level of consciousness is disturbed. Occasionally the child may become unconscious and exhibit muscular spasms. The condition is harmless.

Startle Disease

This name is used to describe an abnormal reaction which is always precipitated by fright (61). The entity differs from hyperexplexia (p. 127) in tic disease, which is an organically determined excessive reaction to external stimulation. Most cases of startle disease occur in brain-damaged children. For a few seconds after the fright, the child has an alarmed expression and remains immobile as if frozen, then falls to the floor with arms stiff and outstretched, and lies there. Within seconds he recovers, and weeps or laughs in an embarrassed way. These attacks may recur throughout the day. This condition must be distinguished from true epilepsy provoked by external stimuli, from true affective convulsions, and from hysteria.

Psychogenic Attacks and Hysteroepilepsy

Psychogenic Epileptiform Attacks

These attacks possess a demonstrative and appellative character and occur in specific situations, such as the presence of spectators (289, 650). Purposeless and dramatic movements are a feature. Differentiating signs from true epilepsy are (289): the movements deviate from the pattern of known seizure types, the interval EEG is always normal and exhibits no slowing postictally, and the incidence of attacks fails to diminish in the presence of a rise in the blood concentration of an antiepileptic.

Psychogenic Fainting

Here the patient appears to be asleep with normal respiratory and circulatory parameters. Regular swallowing movements are visible. Attempts to open the eyelids passively usually encounter resistance, and the eyes stare at the examiner. If the examiner attempts to elicit the vestibulo-ocular reflex by lifting the lids and rapidly rotating the head, no physiologic response occurs – instead, the eyeballs remain fixed at a point in the distance or rotate excessively in the direction of the head. Neurologic examination and EEG are normal (of course, the latter is also normal in so-called alpha coma accompanying brainstem lesions [p. 276]).

7. Polyradiculitis and Polyneuropathies

The feature common to these diseases is simultaneous involvement to a greater or lesser degree of numerous peripheral nerve roots or trunks. Consequently the signs and symptoms are dominated by extensive sensory and motor deficits, as well as absent tendon jerks and later muscular atrophy. The two main groups show perceptible differences in clinical course and accent.

Acute Polyradiculitis (Landry-Guillain-Barré Syndrome)
(308, 309, 446, 492, 715, 1021)

The polyradiculitis described by Guillain, Barré, and Strohl in 1916 does not appear to be distinguishable from the paralysis described by Landry in 1859.

Epidemiology: Any age group may be affected, even small children (1021). Males are slightly more commonly affected than females. The annual incidence varies between 0.5 and 2 per 100000 of the population.

Case history: In about three-fourths of cases the neurologic picture is preceded by nonspecific generalized symptoms, particularly those referable to the upper respiratory or gastrointestinal tract. After 2–4 days, rarely a week or more, about one-half of the patients develop paresthesias in the feet, legs, and hands; occasionally there is also pain (1013). At the same time or immediately afterward, weakness of the lower limbs appears which may progress within a day or so to complete paralysis or even quadriplegia ("Landry's ascending paralysis"). The upper level of paralysis may continue to ascend and, due to involvement of the upper cervical nerve roots, the diaphragm may be immobilized (C4) and respiratory paralysis may follow. Not infrequently intense pains occur during the phase of progressive paralysis. Bladder and bowel incontinence is exceptional, even if the paralysis is severe.

Physical examination: A flaccid paralysis is present with absent reflexes, and in the advanced stages, muscular atrophy. Sensations may remain intact, and about 10% of patients neither possess demonstrable sensory changes nor complain of paresthesias. More than 50% show involvement of the lower cranial nerves, including paralysis of swallowing and bilateral facial palsy, so-called facial diplegia. Myokymias of the facial muscles are also described (1228). Occasionally choreiform and athetotic movements appear, as well as other forms of central nervous involvement, reflecting the presence of an associated encephalitis. The markedly raised CSF protein level (see below) may occasionally produce papilledema. General complications requiring attention are the secondary effects of respiratory paralysis and prolonged immobility. Surprisingly often there are disturbances of autonomic regulation with hypertension, orthostatic hypotension, and abnormal sweat secretion (1210).

Ancillary investigations: The *CSF* shows a so-called albuminocytologic dissociation, i.e., an elevated protein level which may exceed 300 mg%, in the presence of a normal cell count. This finding, which may appear as late as 2–3 weeks after the onset of the paralysis (492), can be repeatedly confirmed over many subsequent weeks and gradually recedes as the clinical picture improves. Very exceptionally, the cell count may be slightly increased, but this finding should always prompt a careful search for an alternative diagnosis. *Electrophysiologic examinations* (742) confirm typical changes of demyelination in periph-

eral nerves. A decreased conduction rate and increased terminal latency are found in 50% of cases if several nerves are examined. These findings also may appear late in the course of the disease. Fibrillation potentials are rare and, if present in the first 4 weeks, point to a poor recovery (978).

Course and prognosis: Most patients experience a gradual recovery, the symptoms disappearing in reverse order of their appearance. Complete recovery may be expected within weeks or months, the interval depending on the severity of the weakness. In exceptional cases, 2 or more years elapse before maximal recovery is achieved. The overall mortality of the disease depends largely on the quality of the nursing care and the respiratory assistance which is required. In a large personal series (715), the mortality amounted to no more than 3% and there were no fatalities among the children, who comprised 30% of the cases. Follow-up examinations reveal physical deficits in nearly 50% of patients, especially absent reflexes and distal lower limb weakness. Only 5%–15% of patients remain handicapped to some degree in their daily lives (715, 1021). The longer the interval between maximal paralysis and the onset of recovery, the more likely is the persistence of residual signs (715).

Pathologic anatomy (436, 452, 972): Changes are found in the junctional area of the anterior and posterior nerve roots but occasionally also in the anterior roots. This finding may explain those cases which present with purely motor signs. Other parts of the peripheral nervous system also may be involved and show myelin degeneration in sites in which lymphocytes and macrophages are in contact with the myelin sheath. Occasionally, axonal loss is also found. Sural nerve biopsy is likely to reveal demyelination (743, 891).

Etiology and pathogenesis: The **etiology** of the syndrome is not clear. It appears to be a toxic or neuroallergic manifestation, provoked by a wide variety of noxious agents. In most cases no specific etiology can be detected. However, in other cases the disease picture described above may appear in infectious mononucleosis, *Mycoplasma pneumoniae* (424), herpes zoster, or mumps. In one-third of cases a mixed titer of complement-fixing antibodies against cytomegalovirus has been observed (309), in others against a herpes virus (308). In the United States, a link with influenza vaccination has been discussed (1088). Other cases have followed a *Borrelia* infection transmitted by a tick bite, or febrile diarrhea caused by *Campylobacter jejuni.*

Pathogenetically, immunologic factors play an important part. Antimyelin antibodies are more commonly present in the blood and CSF of patients with polyradiculitis than in controlled cases, and a cell-mediated immunity also plays a part. No explanation of the precise mechanism has yet been given (252, 544).

Treatment: The good prognosis for spontaneous recovery in the majority of cases allows treatment to be confined to careful nursing and the prevention of secondary complications. Corticosteroids as a rule are not indicated (535, 715), except in cases of chronic recurrent (inflammatory) polyradiculopathy (see below). Plasma exchange is desirable in cases showing a rapidly progressive course and respiratory insufficiency; it may help to shorten the patient's stay in the intensive care unit.

Differential diagnosis: Clinically, acute peripheral polyneuropathies must be considered, such as the forms associated with typhoid fever, porphyria, or acute poisoning (e.g., triorthocresylphosphate). After an infection treated with penicillin, an *acute sensory neuropathy* may be observed 4–12 days later (1158). This condition is heralded by a feeling of numbness, painful paresthesias over the whole body surface, ataxia, absent reflexes, and profound sensory disturbances. Electrophysiologic tests confirm that the sensory conduction time is correspondingly slowed; however, no motor weakness occurs. The CSF shows an increased albumin level but the cell content is always normal. A severe sensory deficit can be expected to remain present for several years. Infectious lesions involving the anterior horn cells may mimic polyradiculitis clinically, particularly if pain is present at the onset and if, after several days, the initial pleocytosis returns to normal and the protein level rises. Polyradiculitis after tick bite is described on p. 321. In *acute anterior horn cell infectious diseases,* e.g., poliomyelitis, the deficit is purely motor, and the CSF always shows an increased cell count. The typical CSF syndrome of *albumino-cytologic dissociation* may give rise to differential diagnostic problems. Readers should again be reminded that these CSF findings combined with chronic polyneuropathy are encountered in a variety of conditions, such as specific paraproteinemias, diabetes mellitus (p.308), paraneoplastic syndromes (p.320), and in Refsum's disease (p.139). Also, specimens of CSF from cases of thecal obstruction or hypoliquorrhea may show marked elevation of protein without increase in cells.

Atypical Polyradiculitides

Associated with, but not identical to the Guillain-Barré syndrome, are the following lesions.

Chronic Inflammatory Relapsing Polyradiculoneuropathy
(265, 266, 267, 319, 320, 896)

Clinical aspects: The **course** differs from the Guillain-Barré syndrome in various respects. It may be chronic or slowly progressive in a stepwise fashion, i.e., characterized by specific acute attacks with interval remissions. Pains are more often present. Of the physical findings, asymmetric involvement and recurrent cranial nerve palsies are noteworthy. A coarse and irregular tremor may also be present and appears to point to recurrence (267). Tendon jerks are absent. The CSF findings are similar to the Guillain-Barré syndrome, often with an unusually high protein content. Electrophysiologic testing frequently reveals axonal involvement. The **prognosis** is poor (319): 10% die, 25% remain bedridden or chairbound, and only about 60% walk again and return to work. Recurrences occur in 5%–10% of cases.

Pathogenesis: Abnormal immunoglobulins in the CSF and immunoglobulin deposits in the sural nerve biopsy point to a dysimmunopathy. Cases of monoclonal gammopathy have been observed (265), which correspond clinically to a more chronic form of polyneuropathy. Similar mechanisms may underlie motor polyneuropathy with multiple conduction block sites, as described on p.307 (918).

Treatment: A prolonged course of corticosteroids is indicated in these cases, as well as immunosuppressives and plasmapheresis (265, 320, 896).

Cranial Polyradiculitis and Fisher's Syndrome

Cranial Polyradiculitis

As a rule, this condition is part of a Guillain-Barré syndrome, but sometimes it may herald the disease. It begins with headache and has a good spontaneous prognosis, although relapses may occur.

Fisher's Syndrome
(24, 132, 369, 790, 793, 1215)

This is a disease picture common in adolescents. It is characterized by ophthalmoplegia with ataxia, absent reflexes including pupillary involvement and facial palsy, in which high CSF protein levels are present. The neuro-ophthalmologic findings – the presence of Bell's phenomenon despite the absence of voluntary upward gaze and the presence of Adie's pupil – point to a central lesion in the sense of an accompanying brainstem encephalitis (24, 605, 790, 793). The prognosis is usually good (84), but cases complicated by respiratory paralysis have been described (132).

Cauda Equina Polyradiculitis (Elsberg's Syndrome)

In 1913 Elsberg described a lesion of the sacral roots which was progressive over the course of months or years (336). Physical examination revealed backache, distal weakness or paralysis, and absent reflexes of the lower extremities as well as sphincteric disturbances. Operative exploration revealed a red appearance of the affected roots with no sign of a tumor, and syphilis could be excluded. The patients recovered slowly in the course of years. The author has seen similar cases with raised protein content and increased cell count in the CSF, usually pursuing a more rapid course. The possibility of a borreliosis (753, 851) was considered. Careful exclusion of a spinal space-occupying lesion is essential, as well as a stenotic lumbar spinal canal (p. 473) or infection with *Borrelia burgdorferi* caused by tick bite.

Polyneuropathies (Peripheral Neuropathies)
(322, 413, 583, 730, 877, 1067)

Definition and general characteristics: This term refers to a group of diseases involving a number of peripheral nerves. They are caused by a wide variety of (non-mechanical) pathogenic factors (see Table 7.2). This widespread disturbance usually involves a number of peripheral nerves in a more or less symmetric way. The polyneuropathies are usually slowly progressive and develop in the course of weeks, months, or years, and this is a clear point of differentiation from the Guillain-Barré type of polyradiculitis (p. 297).

Typical clinical features: *Paresthesias and sensory disturbances* are the presenting features of most polyneuropathies. They begin
- usually symmetrically,
- distally and
- start in the lower extremities,
- as stocking distribution in the lower extremities,
- and glove distribution with distal accentuation in the upper extremities,
- an especially reliable sign is loss of vibration sense distally, or
- disturbed epicritic sensibility of the fingertips.

Motor deficits are less frequent, much less disturbing, and appear late. They are

- usually symmetric,
- begin in the lower extremities, and especially in the dorsiflexor muscles of the feet and toes,
- involve the hand later, and
- may produce atrophy of the anterior tibial and interosseous muscles.

Absent tendon reflexes are an essential part of the clinical diagnosis of polyneuropathy

- initially both ankle jerks are absent, and
- later the knee jerks or the reflexes of the upper extremities are absent.

Trophic changes are always present and may be the marked feature of certain types of polyneuropathy:

- muscular atrophy, see above,
- reduced sweat secretion, and
- dry, smooth skin,
- trophic ulcers (see especially diabetic polyneuropathy),
- or dystrophic deformity of the toe phalanges.

Peripheral nerves painful to pressure is a common finding, e.g., painful calf muscle pressure. Ataxia usually accompanies severe disturbances so that a picture is produced of so-called pseudotabes polyneuropathica.

Ancillary investigations: These studies contribute to the diagnosis as well as to the etiologic classification. Table 7.1 lists the investigations which are recommended.

Electromyography (needle myography) enables the presence of denervation to be detected very early (724, 730):

- fibrillation potentials,
- signs of reinnervation,
- an irregular interference pattern on maximal voluntary contraction.

Nerve conduction velocity (NCV) studies. Measurement of the sensory and motor conduction velocity of peripheral nerves may be useful (729):

- Sensory nerve conduction disappears very early.
- Motor nerve conduction may under certain circumstances be severely impaired, despite the fact that only minor changes are found in the myelin sheaths at this stage.
- The group of polyneuropathies with electromyographically detectable changes can be further enlarged by determining the extent of scatter of the conduction velocity in the motor fibers. It is also possible with this method to differentiate between a polyneuropathy and a polyradiculitis.

Muscle biopsy may reveal
- a picture of neurogenic muscular atrophy, and
- under certain circumstances a vasculitis.

Nerve biopsy, usually sural nerve biopsy, may

- distinguish between axonal involvement and demyelination,
- demonstrate the deposition of foreign material (e.g., amyloid),
- reveal a vasculitis,

Table 7.**1**   Useful laboratory tests for the etiologic diagnosis of polyneuropathies

Electrophysiology: Nerve conduction velocity (to establish the diagnosis of polyneuropathy), somatosensory evoked potentials (to determine involvement of the posterior columns), electromyography (to differentiate between neurogenic and myopathic paralysis of muscles)

Blood sedimentation rate: Collagen diseases, infections, paraproteinemias, neoplasms

Blood smear: Inflammations, lead poisoning (basophilic stippling), leukemias, polycythemia

Blood sugar, glucose tolerance: Diabetes mellitus

Creatinine, urea: Uremia

Liver function, liver enzymes: Hepatic lesions, disturbances of coagulation or anticoagulant hemorrhage (Quick test), alcoholism

Thyroid function: Hypothyroidism

Serum Levels of vitamin B$_{12}$, folic acid, thiamine, vitamin E: Malabsorption

Schilling test: Treated vitamin B$_{12}$ deficiency

Uro- and coproporphyrins: Porphyria

Rheumatic serology, antinuclear antibodies, circulating immune complexes: Rheumatoid arthritis, collagen diseases

Phytanic acid level: Refsum's disease in the differential diagnosis of hereditary motor and sensory neuropathies

Serum electrophoresis: Collagen diseases and paraproteinemias (M gradient?)

Gas chromatography: To demonstrate specific toxins and heavy metals in cases of suspected toxic neuropathy

Microorganisms, serology: Infectious and parainfectious agents

Bone marrow: Leukemia, myeloma, Waldenström's disease

Lumbar puncture: Albuminocytologic dissociation in Guillain-Barré syndrome. Total protein elevated in many polyneuropathies and cauda equina neurofibromas. Pleocytosis: meningoradiculoneuritis (Garin-Bujadoux-Bannwarth syndrome in Lyme disease). Neoplastic cells: carcinomatous meningitis, leukemia

Roentgenology: Paraneoplastic (chest, barium enema and swallow examinations, intravenous urography), osteolytic and osteosclerotic myeloma (skull, vertebral column), lead (long bones, lead line)

Nerve biopsy: Vasculitis?, special questions concerning formal and causal pathogenesis

Muscle biopsy: Distinction between neurogenic and myopathic weakness of muscles

- show specific characteristic histologic details (e.g., onion bulb structure of Schwann cells in hereditary motor and sensory neuropathy).

Lumbar puncture: This is least productive. It may be

- normal,
- rarely abnormal, revealing a nonspecific increased protein content (e.g., diabetic neuropathy or Refsum's disease).

General physical and serologic findings may be essential for an etiologic diagnosis, e.g.,

- diabetes mellitus,
- chronic alcoholism,
- porphyria,
- a paraproteinemia.

Histopathology of the polyneuropathies: Brief mention should be made of the pathologic changes in the polyneuropathies (730). As a rule a sural nerve biopsy is undertaken, by means of teased preparations, paraffin sections for light microscopy, and thin sections for electron microscopy. The severity of the clinical picture in no way corresponds to the severity of the morphologic changes. A number of endogenous and exogenous diseases of the peripheral nerves exhibit initial morphologic changes in the distal segments; only subsequently are the proximal segments involved, and finally the perikaryon. In lead neuropathy and also in experimental diphtheritic polyneuropathy, patchy destruction of the nerve fibers leads to demyelination. The changes often affect only one segment between two nodes of Ranvier and often possess a focal distribution so that some nerve fibers remain intact while others can be shown to be diseased. A further group is characterized by primary changes in the interstitial tissue, e.g., acute por-

phyria, in which changes are present in the central as well as in the peripheral nervous system. Acute and chronic cell changes may be observed in the spinal ganglia, and the CNS shows diffuse and focal, acute and chronic nerve cell damage as well as focal patches of gliosis. The most severe disintegration of the nerve fibers occurs in thallium intoxication, in which the fiber may be affected in its entire length from the spinal cord to the periphery. True inflammatory changes in the nerves are rare: this group includes leprosy and the polyneuritis of infectious mononucleosis and leprosy. Changes in the vessel walls may be present in periarteritis nodosa, diabetic polyneuropathy, and the polyneuropathy of syphilis.

Table 7.2 is an etiologic classification of the commonest polyneuropathies. This list is not complete, but represents one of the possible classifications.

Genetically Determined Polyneuropathies

The following diseases, resulting from genetically determined metabolic abnormalities, may give rise to signs and symptoms of a polyneuropathy. Some of these diseases remain unexplained. A careful family investigation, including history-taking from, and examination of, siblings, electrophysiologic studies, nerve biopsy, and biochemical metabolic investigations is particularly important for etiologic classification.

Hereditary Motor and Sensory Neuropathies (HMSN)
(322, 796, 909)

This group comprises a variety of diseases leading to hereditary disorders – although in individual cases

Table 7.**2**   Review of the common polyneuropathies

P. genetically determined
- Hereditary motor-sensory neuropathies, see Table 7.**3**
- Neuropathy with a tendency to compression paralysis
- With porphyria
- With primary amyloidosis

P. accompanying metabolic disturbances
- With diabetes mellitus
  - Symmetric, mainly distal form
  - Asymmetric, mainly proximal form
  - "Mononeuropathy"
  - Amyotrophy or myelopathy
- With uremia
- With hepatic cirrhosis
- With gout
- With hypothyroidism

P. accompanying undernourishment and malnutrition

P. accompanying vitamin B_{12} absorption deficiency

P. in dysproteinemias and paraproteinemias

P. accompanying infectious diseases
- Leprosy
- Parotitis
- Infectious mononucleosis
- Typhus and paratyphus
- Typhoid fever
- Diphtheria
- Botulism
- After tick bite

P. accompanying arterial diseases
- Polyarteritis nodosa
- Other collagen diseases
- Arteriosclerosis

P. accompanying sprue and other disturbances of intestinal absorption

P. accompanying exogenous toxic disturbances
- Ethyl alcohol
- Lead
- Arsenic
- Thallium
- Triaryl phospahte
- Solvents (e. g., carbon disulfide)
- Drug intoxications (isoniazid, thalidomide, furadantoin)

Other P.
- Serum sickness
- Neoplasms
- Sarcoidosis
- HIV infection

not always definable defects – in which a symmetrical progressive polyneuropathy is the dominant feature. The classification proposed by Dyck (322) is not entirely satisfactory, and individual cases may be difficult to incorporate (Table 7.3). Only a few of these entities will be discussed below.

Hereditary Motor and Sensory Neuropathy Type I (Charcot-Marie-Tooth Disease)
(322, 481, 797)

This disease, labeled either peroneal or neural muscular atrophy, has a *prevalence* of about 2 per 100000. It is inherited as an autosomal domi-

Table 7.3 Hereditary motor-sensory neuropathies (after *Dyck* 1975, see *Meier* and *Tackmann* [797])

Type I (hypertrophic form of Charcot-Marie-Tooth disease)
- Autosomal dominant inheritance
- Starts in 2nd–4th decades of life
- Develops distally as muscular atrophy and deformity of the feet
- Slight distal sensory deficit
- Slowed nerve conduction velocity
- Peripheral nerves thickened and of increased consistency
- Sural nerve biopsy reveals signs of axonal degeneration, de- and remyelinization, onion bulb formations

Type II (neuronal type of peroneal muscular atrophy)
- Autosomal dominant inheritance
- Starts in 2nd–4th decades of life
- Distal atrophy of the feet and calf muscles with pes cavus, hands less affected
- Slight sensory deficit
- Slightly slowed or normal nerve conduction velocity
- Peripheral nerves not thickened and of normal consistency
- Sural nerve biopsy reveals signs of axonal degeneration with mild (secondary) segmental demyelinization, no sign of onion bulb formation

Type III (hypertrophic neuropathy, Dejerine-Sottas)
- Autosomal recessive inheritance
- Starts in 1st decade of life
- Delayed motor development, rapidly progressive, obvious weakness of the hand muscles
  Sensory disturbances well marked, distal distribution
- Markedly slowed nerve conduction velocity (slower than type I)
- Peripheral nerves thickened and of softer consistency
- Sural nerve biopsy: hypomyelination, de- and remyelination, onion bulb formations and only small caliber myelinated (up to 4 μ in diameter), endoneural interstitial tissue markedly increased
- Biochemistry: increased content of ceramide monohexoside sulfate in the liver (observed in some cases)

Type IV (hypertrophic neuropathy accompanying Refsum's disease)
- Autosomal recessive inheritance
- Begins in first 3 decades of life

Table 7.3   (Continued)

- Retinitis pigmentosa, sensorimotor neuropathy, disturbances of hearing, cardiac and skin manifestations, skeletal deformities
- Markedly slowed nerve conduction velocity
- Sural nerve biopsy; axonal degeneration, segmental de- and remyelination, onion bulb formations, accumulation of lysosomes in the Schwann's cells
- Biochemistry: phytanic acid accumulation in various tissues

Type V (with spastic paraparesis)
- Autosomal dominant inheritance
- Begins in 2nd decade of life or later
- Slowly progressive course with spastic paraparesis and a virtually normal life expectancy
- No sensory disturbances, subjectively or on clinical examination
- Nerve conduction time normal or slightly reduced
- Sural nerve biopsy: individual patients exhibit marked reduction in myelinated fibers

Type VI (with optic atrophy)
- Autosomal dominant or recessive inheritance
- Onset very variable
- Loss of vision, progressive blindness, atrophy of peripheral muscles
- Neurophysiologic findings not known
- Individual patients exhibit hypertrophic nerve changes

Type VII (with retinitis pigmentosa)
- Probably autosomal recessive inheritance
- Variable onset
- Weakness and atrophy of peripheral muscles
- Slight peripheral sensory disturbances
- Nerve conduction time reduced
- Biopsy findings not known

nant, rarely also as an autosomal recessive (480), with a gene penetration claimed to be 70%–80%. The gene appears to be linked to the Duffy locus of the chromosome (448). The *first signs of the disease* occur in childhood or adolescence. **Clinically**, a deformity of the feet is found, which has usually been present since childhood, and which in 70% of cases is a true clubfoot (436). Thereafter, a progressive atrophy of the lower limb muscles occurs, in particular those innervated by the peroneal nerves. The resulting dorsiflexor weakness produces difficulty in walking since the strength of the plantar flexor muscles is preserved. A steppage gait is nearly always found. The ankle jerks disappear early, and later other tendon reflexes also are absent. The atrophy and paralysis of the calf muscles may increase but the thigh muscles are seldom involved so that the powerful thigh muscles contrast with the profoundly atrophic calf muscles ("stork leg," "inverted champagne bottle") (Fig. 7.1b). The distal muscles of the upper extremities, especially the small muscles of the hands, may in time become involved (Fig. 7.1c). Only one-fourth to one-half of cases show sensory changes involving the modalities for touch and especially vibration sense, which is diminished. Occasionally slightly thickened nerve trunks can be palpated, especially the subcutaneous trunks of the neck (322) or dorsum of the foot. Rarely, other neurologic deficits are present, such as proximal muscular atrophy, nystagmus, posterior column signs, optic atrophy, or pupillary abnormalities either singly or in combination with essential tremor (1054). If pyramidal tract signs are present, the case belongs to HMSN type V (482). *NCV testing* provides diagnostic information. The nerve conduction time is severely reduced in all patients, as well as in affected family members, even before the onset of clinical signs. *Nerve biopsy* shows a typical finding, thickening of the endoneural interstitial tissue, signs of chronic segmental demyelination, and regeneration with an increase in Schwann cells which are arranged in onion skin formation, as well as axonal degeneration. *Muscle biopsy* reveals, in addition to signs of neurogenic muscular atrophy, an accompanying myopathy which may be severe (841). The *course* of the disease is, as a rule, only very slowly progressive, and the patient becomes gradually disabled, although usually after a long period, and he remains able to work until middle or advanced age.

Hereditary Motor and Sensory Neuropathy Type II

The *neuronal type of peroneal muscular atrophy* (322) is inherited as a dominant disease. It is very similar in clinical respects to neural hypertrophic neuropathy (see below), although the signs and symptoms appear later in life and affect the hands less convincingly. The peripheral nerve trunks do not appear to be thickened, and the nerve conduction time is not markedly prolonged. Electromyographic studies show evidence of anterior horn cell damage. Histologic examination of the peripheral nerves reveals changes similar to, but less well-marked, than those observed in type I. Comparative electrophysiologic and biopsy examinations in patients with types I and II indicate that they are two independent and unrelated inherited diseases (192). Variants are described with an earlier onset in childhood, more rapid progression, and autosomal recessive mode of inheritance (909).

Hereditary Motor and Sensory Neuropathy Type III (Déjerine-Sottas Disease)
(322, 797, 1067)

This form is inherited as an autosomal recessive disease. The clinical picture is comparable with HMSN type I, but usually commences earlier in life so that the motor development of the child is affected. Motor involvement is more marked, especially in the proximal muscles, and the disease progresses more rapidly. The reflexes are absent. The peripheral nerves and large nerve trunks

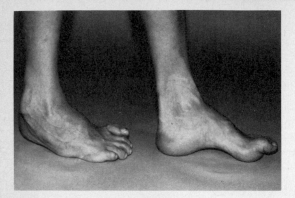

Fig. 7.1a–c Typical appearances of the hereditary motor and sensory neuropathies, type I (**a** and **b**) and type II (**c**). **a** Equino-varus deformity. The clawed toes are produced by the predominating action of the long flexor tendons over the dorsal extensor tendons

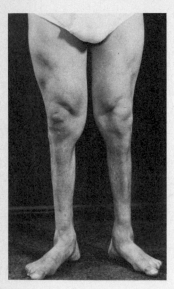

b Typical stork legs. The severe atrophy of the calf muscles contrasts with the well-preserved state of the quadriceps muscles

are usually thickened; thick nerve roots may lead to spinal cord compression. The CSF protein is often increased.

The motor conduction time is more markedly slowed than in type I. Nerve biopsy shows onion bulb formations to be prominent. Biopsies of sural nerve and liver have revealed abnormal amounts of cerebrosides and sulfatides (318). A systemic defect of ceramine hexoside and ceramide hexoside sulfate is presumed to be present.

Hereditary Neuropathy with Liability to Pressure Palsies ("Tomaculous Neuropathy") (796)

This disease is *inherited* as an autosomal dominant and produces recurrent *pressure palsies* of individual peripheral nerves or the brachial plexus. These lesions follow light pressure and may regress completely. Well-marked *prolongation of the conduction time* of unaffected peripheral nerves is a characteristic feature. *Histologically,* a sausage-shaped (= "tomaculous") internodal thickening of the nerve sheath is present, combined with segmental myelin atrophy.

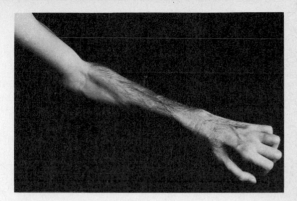

c Atrophy of the distal forearm muscles and small muscles of the hand (from *Meier* and *Tackmann* [797])

Polyneuropathy in Porphyria
(322, 730)

Porphyria is *inherited* as a dominant disease. **Clinically**, it may cause acute *abdominal symptoms* (colic, constipation, vomiting) as well as arterial hypertension; not infrequently these attacks are precipitated by barbiturate intake. *Neurologic examination* reveals signs principally of a polyneuropathy – either mononeuritis multiplex (p. 315) or a severe, rapidly ascending mainly motor polyneuritis and polyradiculitis, which gives rise to a rapidly ascending flaccid quadriplegia. Often the patient complains of pains and paresthesias of the extremities, but the pareses are hardly ever accompanied by sensory loss. Cranial nerve palsies may be present, as well as transient blindness (retinal artery spasm) and various CNS symptoms. As expressions of involvement of the autonomic nervous system, tachycardia, arterial hypertension, constipation and bladder dysfunction occur. Agitation, hallucinations, clouding of consciousness, and mental changes such as hysteria may be encountered, and the patient may experience epileptic attacks. The *CSF* is usually normal, exceptionally an albuminocytologic dissociation is found. The **prognosis** is poor, and about one-third of patients die sooner or later in the disease during an attack, usually with bulbar signs and respiratory paralysis (912a). **Treatment** consists in the careful avoidance of barbiturates. Adenosine-5-monophosphate is perhaps useful.

Pathophysiologically, porphyria represents a genetically determined disturbance of pyrrole metabolism, a partial failure of uroporphyrinogen synthetase, causing an increased production of delta-aminolevulinic acid and porphobilinogen, as well as uro- and coproporphyrins which are excreted in the urine. The diagnosis can be made by detecting dark urine, which may appear normal when fresh, but changes to a dark red-brown color upon standing for some hours (uro- and coproporphyrins) through the action of light. Porphobilinogen may also be suspected from the red color produced by the addition of Ehrlich's aldehyde reagent: in contrast to that produced by urobilinogen, this color is not extracted by chloroform. *Histopathologic examination* shows patchy myelin degeneration with intact axons of the peripheral nerves and secondary (retrograde) ganglion cell degeneration as well as focal vascular damage.

Polyneuropathy in Primary Amyloidosis

Primary amyloidosis is rare. Most cases are familial in type, inherited as an autosomal dominant trait, and only rarely are isolated cases found (661).

Signs and symptoms, most commonly a chronic polyneuropathy, are present in about 15% of patients. This lesion may commence at any time between the 2nd and 6th decade of life, usually in men. It consists initially of distal paresthesias and a sensory disturbance in the lower limbs which is often dissociated and accompanied by loss of normal sweating. Later a progressive motor neuropathy develops which is more marked distally and associated with muscular atrophy which is initially asymmetric. Signs of automatic involvement are not uncommon, particularly orthostatic hypotension, abnormalities of sweat secretion, impotence, and trophic ulcers.

Gastrointestinal signs and symptoms are invariably present, either diarrhea or constipation, sometimes also hoarseness, cardiac and renal signs, and vitreous opacities. The course of the disease may extend over many years.

Diagnosis is confirmed by biopsy – gingival, rectal mucous membrane, muscle, or peripheral nerve.

Giant Axonal Neuropathy (931)

This autosomal recessive disease develops in childhood as a severe polyneuropathy, progresses slowly, and eventually exhibits features of central nervous involvement. The axons show segmental dilatation caused by the heaping up of neurofilaments. The children have wiry, curly hair.

Polyneuropathies in Metabolic Disorders

Diabetic Polyneuropathies (40, 181, 1218)

Incidence: Statistics concerning the incidence of neurologic complications in diabetes mellitus vary greatly and depend upon the thoroughness with which they are sought. In an unselected series of diabetics, between 20% and 40% showed abnormal tendon jerks or sensory disturbances. The most frequent age of onset of diabetic neuropathy is the 6th decade of life, and the diabetes then lasts 5–10 years. In at least 10% of patients the diagnosis of diabetes is made only after the onset of the neurologic deficit. Men and women appear to be equally affected.

Pathogenesis: The pathogenesis involves metabolic disturbances as well as angiopathic factors. Abnormalities of the blood supply of the vasa nervorum have been demonstrated. These may explain the sudden onset of individual episodes. A particularly strong indication of the significance of the vascular lesions is the observation that hyalinization and the deposition of abnormal material in the walls of the vasa nervorum are significantly more common in diabetic patients with a neuropathy than in those without a neuropathy or in nondiabetic subjects (379). Favoring the pathogenetic importance of the metabolic disturbances is the fact that the sensory nerve fibers are affected frequently and early (paresthesias, pains, absent reflexes), while these thin and poorly myelinated fibers are, on the oth-

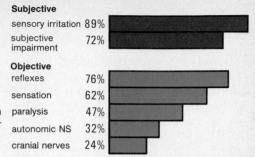

Subjective

| sensory irritation | 89% |
| subjective impairment | 72% |

Objective

reflexes	76%
sensation	62%
paralysis	47%
autonomic NS	32%
cranial nerves	24%

Fig. 7.2 Neurologic deficits in 200 diabetics (from A. Bischoff: *Die diabetische Neuropathie.* Thieme, Stuttgart 1963)

er hand, particularly resistant to ischemic damage. Moreover, many of the disturbances, such as the external ocular palsies, are completely reversible – which would be unlikely following ischemic infarction of the peripheral nerves. Despite the pathogenetic importance of abnormal peripheral nerve metabolism in the development of the neuropathy, no simple quantitative relationship exists between the severity of the metabolic disturbance and that of the neurologic picture. Indeed, neuropathy may be present in a mild or well-compensated diabetic. The important fact is that any diabetic condition, even the latent variety in which the disease is proved only by the presence of an abnormal glucose tolerance test, may be accompanied by signs of neuropathy. Measurements of peripheral nerve conduction velocity in diabetics have shown that the conduction is slower if the blood sugar is out of control. The signs and symptoms regress, or at least do not get worse, if optimal therapeutic control is maintained over the diabetes (40, 516).

General remarks: The *prevalence* of individual symptoms and signs in 200 diabetic patients with neurologic complications is shown in Fig. 7.2. It can be seen that subjective and objective sensory disturbance predominate. The pain is more often proximal than distal, and more commonly unilateral than bilateral.

Electrodiagnostically, a prolonged peripheral conduction time may be shown in motor nerve fibers, even in the absence of a clinically recognizable motor deficit. The *CSF* also is often abnormal. Diabetics without signs of peripheral neuropathy may show a raised albumin level. About two-thirds of diabetics with a neuropathy have an increased total protein content, and values as high as 400 mg have been recorded. The cell count is invariably normal so that an albuminocytologic dissociation is present. In 75% an abnormally high glucose level is found.

The *combination and pattern of individual clinical signs and symptoms* may in individual cases vary greatly. The signs and symptoms are often grouped in characteristic syndromes, and it seems justifiable to define the following clinical pictures.

Sensorimotor Diabetic Neuropathy

The (symmetric) presence of a predominantly distal diabetic polyneuropathy, often referred to as diabetic polyneuritis, is by far the commonest neurologic complication of diabetes mellitus. The *most discrete form* is usually found in late-onset diabetes. Symmetric paresthesias and burning sensations are present, usually affecting the lower limbs and much less often the upper limbs. Neurologic examination reveals that the ankle jerks are almost invariably absent, sometimes other tendon jerks as well. Vibration sense is usually diminished distally, and occasionally also position sense. Motor involvement as a rule is absent. A *severe form* of polyneuropathy is found which affects particularly young diabetics and poorly controlled diabetics. This form starts slowly in the lower extremities and may sometimes be unilateral. In the hyperalgesic form, the burning sensations and dysesthesias are often unusually intense, particularly at night. The bedclothes can scarcely be tolerated and the patient seeks relief by moving about or, less often, by remaining still. Exposure to cold may also provoke the pain. Unpleasant cramps, particularly affecting the calf muscles, may appear. Distal sensory disturbances are always very definite and sometimes the presence of ataxia produces the picture of *diabetic pseudotabes*. The tendon jerks are invariably diminished or absent, and sometimes muscular weakness may be observed. These features lead to a steppage gait and difficulty in climbing stairs.

Proximal Asymmetric Diabetic Polyneuropathy (57)

This form occurs far less frequently than the distal form described above. The entity is subdivided into several forms. The first of these is an asymmetric form caused by unilateral involvement of several nerve roots or a nerve plexus. The clinical picture is characterized by a sudden onset and dominated by pains which are often intense and worse at night; they are usually proximal and affect the lower limbs more than the upper limbs. An initial diagnosis of sciatica is often made. Simultaneously muscular weakness appears which is followed by atrophy, causing the patient difficulty in climbing stairs or in rising from a chair. The symptoms and signs usually occur in the distribution of the femoral nerve and stretch pain accompanying hyperextension of the hip joint ("reversed" Lasègue's sign) is a striking feature (547). The knee jerk is usually absent. Signs of a distal polyneuropathy may also be present, but they are inconstant; in particular, sensation remains intact. The cause appears to be ischemia of parts of the nerve plexus. Asymmetric proximal neuropathies are especially common in poorly controlled diabetics, but they may also occur in patients without glycosuria or other clinical features of diabetes. Patients with this form of the disease tend to recover spontaneously.

Symmetric Proximal Muscular Weakness

From the rapid-onset, unilateral form described above, various transitional forms exist to slowly progressive, symmetric muscular weakness affecting the lower limbs and pelvic girdle. These forms progress without sensory disturbance, and they are therefore called *diabetic amyotrophy* (57, 239). This disease picture is caused by a metabolic disturbance and not ischemic infarction of the nerves. Both types of proximal diabetic neuropathy show a tendency to good recovery. An exception is any patient with chronic anoxic damage of anterior horn cells. Such patients exhibit fasciculation and are similar to ischemic forms of spinal muscular atrophy or amyotrophic lateral sclerosis (p. 221).

Mononeuropathies in Diabetes

These lesions are caused either by mechanical factors compressing the nerves already damaged by ischemic infarction of the nerve trunks or an underlying metabolic disturbance. Support for the concept of local (mechanical) nerve damage is provided by the observation that electrophysiologic abnormalities in such cases can be demonstrated only in affected nerves. A careful search should always be made for a local cause which may be amenable to treatment, e.g., carpal tunnel syndrome.

Cranial Nerve Palsies in Diabetes Mellitus

Paralyses of the extraocular muscles (1192, 1245) are observed in about 0.5% of diabetics. The third and sixth cranial nerves are affected with equal frequency, but the fourth nerve only rarely. The onset is acute, often accompanied by intense local pain. In contrast to the oculomotor palsies seen in other diseases, the form accompanying diabetes mellitus spares the internal ocular muscles. The paralyses usually affect only one eye and are transient, but they may be bilateral. Sometimes these ocular palsies are the presenting clinical feature of the diabetes. They point to ischemic lesions of the peripheral nerve trunks (58) and usually regress spontaneously within 2–3 months. *Pupillary anomalies* are present in 10%–20% of diabetics. Anisocoria and an abnormally slow light reaction are the most common ones. A paralysis of the pupil to light with normal contraction on accommodation – like the true Argyll Robertson pupil – if present, is usually unilateral, unlike the syphilitic form. *Other cranial nerve palsies* in diabetic subjects occur less frequently, and they do not always appear to be related to the metabolic disturbance. Disturbances of olfaction, optic atrophy, facial palsy, and deafness have been described.

Disturbances of the Autonomic Nervous System in Diabetics

Autonomic disturbances in diabetic patients are usually associated with other deficits, but they may be present in the absence of involvement of the voluntary nervous system. These changes take the form of *bladder disturbances,* either sphincteric insufficiency or bladder atonicity, resulting in a painless large residual volume of urine. Attacks of *diarrhea,* especially at night, are well known. One-fourth of young male diabetics are *impotent,* experiencing retrograde ejaculation. Other signs of autonomic involvement are tachycardia, orthostatic hypotension, edema of the feet and ankles, and an absence of sweating especially in areas of normal sensation. A reddish-yellow atrophy of the skin *(necrobiosis lipoidica diabeticorum),* commonly affecting women, appears to be specific to diabetics: it has a focal distribution and a painless course. *Joint and bone disturbances* involve almost exclusively the lower extremities. Roentgenologic examination reveals foci of osteolysis and destruction, particularly in the region of the tibiotarsal and tarsometatarsal joints and less often distally. These skeletal lesions, as well as the intractable *perforating ulcers* of the soles, are usually painless. The skin of the sole of the foot is strikingly thin, smooth, and dry.

Disturbances of the Central Nervous System in Diabetics

These will be briefly explained here. The existence of a diabetic myelopathy as indicated above, is not universally accepted. The pathologic changes in the anterior horn cells, which may be observed histologically, may represent retrograde changes secondary to the peripheral neuropathy. Cases of amyotrophic lateral sclerosis have repeatedly been observed in diabetic patients, but no proof has yet been advanced of a statistically significant frequency of this association. In contrast, there is no doubt about the greater incidence of *cerebrovascular accidents* in diabetic patients as a result of diabetic angiopathies. Deep hypoglycemic coma may be heralded by *convulsions,* which were reported in about 7% of a group of juvenile, insulin-dependent diabetics. In one-third of this group, true epileptic seizures followed prolonged hypoglycemic crises (539).

Treatment: The basis of therapy is treatment of the underlying disease, i.e., optimal control of the diabetic condition (516). If treatment is successful, some of the above-mentioned clinical syndromes such as the proximal asymmetric neuropathies and external ocular palsies tend to regress spontaneously. Other syndromes appear to be refractory, including cases of severe symmetric polyneuropathy, of which the paresthesias and burning sensations may cause the patient much misery. Antiepileptic agents such as carbamazepine and thioctanic acid apply in this situation. The most useful combination appears to be clomipramine with small doses of neuroleptics (674). Other therapeutic measures to be recommended are vitamin B complex, vasodilators, and sedatives, as well as avoiding tobacco smoking.

Uremic Polyneuropathy

Polyneuropathies occur in chronic renal insufficiency. About 25% of the patients in a dialysis unit will show the pertinent signs and symptoms. An arteriovenous fistula associated with the dialysis may lead to a focal ischemic neuropathy of the median nerve.

Polyneuropathy in Hepatic Cirrhosis

Polyneuropathy, on rare occasions, is associated with *primary biliary cirrhosis* and may be present prior to signs of the hepatic lesion – for example, as a pure sensory neuropathy (227).

Polyneuropathy in Gout

While other evidence of nervous system involvement is not unusual (carpal tunnel syndrome, ulnar neuropathy, or compression of the spinal root or cord), polyneuropathy is a great rarity (285).

Polyneuropathies in Undernourishment and Malnutrition (272, 415)

These forms are rare in Westernized countries. A rigid vegetarian diet may cause vitamin B_{12} deficiency that leads to subacute combined degeneration of the spinal cord with polyneuritic components. In thiamine deficiency (vitamin B_1), polyneuropathy may develop as part of the picture of beriberi. Similarly, polyneuropathy and other neurologic signs may follow niacin deficiency in pellagra (dermatoses, diarrhea, agitated states, organic psychosyndromes). In disturbances of vitamin E absorption, polyneuropathy may occur in addition to ophthalmoplegia, ptosis, muscular weakness, nystagmus, and pyramidal signs (1253). The pathogenesis of all these cases is complex and involves a deficiency of protein and other factors apart from the vitamin deficiency. Nutritional factors also play an important part in causing the neurologic signs and symptoms associated with alcohol abuse (p.151).

Occasionally the neuropathies following malnutrition may persist for years or even decades. For example, peripheral neuropathies such as burning feet, optic atrophy, and disturbances of hearing have been identified in 5.5% of Far Eastern prisoners of war several decades after the cessation of hostilities (415).

Polyneuropathies in Disturbances of Vitamin B_{12} Absorption

This disease has already been discussed in connection with subacute combined degeneration of the spinal cord (p.227). It rarely occurs in isolated form, although careful examination including electrodiagnostic tests shows involvement of the peripheral nervous system to be present in two-thirds of untreated cases of pernicious anemia. Thiamine deficiency is usually also present (256). *Folic acid deficiency* may lead to polyneuropathy, sometimes combined with signs of subacute combined degeneration of the spinal cord.

Polyneuropathies in Dysproteinemias and Paraproteinemias

In *multiple myeloma* as well as *solitary myeloma deposits* (612), isolated infiltration of individual peripheral nerves or the CNS organs may occur ("myelomatous paraplegia"). In addition, a painful, progressive neuropathy may be found which particularly affects the lower extremities and may be confined to motor involvement (612) or be sensorimotor (1246). These lesions usually precede the discovery of the myeloma and respond fairly well to radiotherapy (276) but not to chemotherapy. Pathogenetically, amyloid deposits have been observed in the interstitium of peripheral nerves, but this finding may not be relevant. The cause is far more likely to be the presence of immunoglobulins, of the type observed in other *polyneuropathies with monoclonal gammopathies,* which react with components of peripheral nerves – for example, with myelin-associated glycoprotein (MAG) (794, 799, 1148). Electron microscopy reveals demyelination and degeneration of the myelin lamellae, and an abnormal Schwann cell reaction. Attempts to transmit anti-MAG antibodies to laboratory animals have failed (1149). Changes have also been observed in the endothelium of blood vessels, sometimes producing obliteration of the vasa nervorum (969). These changes may be partly responsible for the changes in the peripheral nerves. A syndrome which is described to occur in solitary myeloma, under the term POEMS, constitutes a special form (990). Aside from the neuropathy, this syndrome includes an organomegaly, (e.g. hepatomegaly or spleenomegaly), endocrine disturbances, and skin changes such as hyperpigmentation or cyanosis. Radiotherapy of the myeloma causes regression of the symptoms. *Waldenström's macroglobulinemia* may also be accompanied by polyneuropathy. The cause is attributed to occlusions of the smaller vasa nervorum by the sludging of erythrocytes, and also to a competitive ef-

fect of the neoplastic process upon the nervous system with respect to cocarboxylase requirements.

Polyneuropathies in Infectious Diseases

These polyneuropathies have an acute onset, but they may appear only after the acute phase of the infectious disease has subsided.

Diphtheria

The infection has usually abated – it may not even have been recognized as such – when the neuropathy appears. Polyneuropathies occur far more commonly after severe diphtheria, and myocardial involvement is not unusual. Palatal paralysis heralds the onset, usually between the 5th and 12th day of the illness. Other cranial nerve palsies follow, typically with paralysis of accomodation. These early signs regress within 1–2 weeks, but a second stage of the illness may appear in patients who have recovered from diphtheria. This phase takes the form of a sensorimotor polyneuropathy of the extremities, in a patient who has no fever and is no longer unwell. It has a good prognosis, recovery commencing within 1–3 weeks and leading to complete cure.

Mumps (Epidemic Parotitis)

Mumps may be accompanied by involvement of peripheral nerves as well as signs of myelitis or encephalitis (p. 48). Cranial nerve palsies and nerve root involvement may occur, as well as an ascending polyradiculoneuritis with increased CSF protein (p. 294).

Other Forms

Infectious mononucleosis is a well-known cause of polyradiculoneuritis (p. 294). *Abdominal typhoid, paratyphoid fever, typhus, syphilis,* and *leprosy* may be complicated by polyneuropathy. Leprosy is the only polyneuropathy – in the true sense of the word, a polyneuritis – in which an inflammatory lesion of the peripheral nerves can be demonstrated. Botulism, see p. 236.

Polyneuropathies Accompanying Arteriopathies

Various collagen-vascular diseases, as well as *rheumatoid* arthritis, may lead as a result of the accompanying arteritis to signs and symptoms of polyneuropathy, in addition to CNS involvement.

The polyneuropathy develops as a *mononeuritis multiplex.*

- Initially the ischemic damage is confined to a single nerve trunk,
- later other nerves are involved so that
- the classic picture of a diffuse polyneuritis results, following step-wise onset over a varying length of time.

Polyarteritis Nodosa

Pathogenesis: Ischemic lesions of the nervous system and internal organs are produced by arterial thrombosis. Histologic examination shows the vascular occlusion to be produced by a combination of fibrinous exudation, damage to the medial layer of arteries and arterioles, and inflammatory infiltration of the vessel wall.

Clinical features: Examination reveals both **generalized features** of the disease and neurologic signs. The general signs include febrile attacks, lassitude, joint pains, cardiac irregularities, renal insufficiency, skin rashes, anemia, and frequently a raised ESR. In about one-half of cases, the **neurologic signs** are the presenting clinical features of the disease (221). The CNS manifestations of polyarteritis nodosa are described on p. 157, but the commonest neurologic sign of the disease is polyneuropathy. The characteristic feature of involvement of the peripheral nervous system is mononeuritis multiplex. Usually, the nerve trunks of the lower extremities are first to be involved, accompanied initially by paresthesias or pains and then by weakness which progresses rapidly to paralysis. The individual peripheral palsies eventually summate; however, a symmetric and progressive polyneuropathy may be present from the start (221). Occasionally, peripheral involvement of a cranial nerve is a prominent clinical feature (68), usually described as Cogan's syndrome (p. 363). Polyarteritis nodosa may also present as an isolated sciatica (798). The diagnosis is confirmed by the other clinical features and the results of muscle biopsy.

Treatment and prognosis: Despite the short-term efficacy of steroid medication, the long-term prognosis remains very poor.

Other (Necrotizing) Arteritides and Arteriopathies

Clinical pictures similar to that seen in polyarteritis nodosa may be exhibited by other necrotizing angiitides.

Rheumatoid Arthritis

Two types of vascular polyneuropathy are described in this disease (1017). The more common is mononeuritis multiplex with necrotizing arteritis which is indistinguishable clinically and histologically from that of polyarteritis nodosa. It involves other organs as well and has a somewhat better prognosis than periarteritis nodosa. Previous cortisone medication appears to be a significant factor, and it is wise to replace it with another form of treatment. The second type is a slowly developing symmetric polyneuropathy more severe in the periphery and associated with a non-necrotizing arteritis.

Lupus Erythematosus

In this disease, in which CNS complications are most common (p. 157), a slowly progressive demyelinating polyneuropathy may develop (982).

Sjögren's Syndrome

The main features of this disease are a keratoconjunctivitis, rhinitis sicca, parotid swelling, and rheumatic joint pains. Polyneuropathies, including cranial nerve palsies, as well as primary myopathies (p. 502) may be found, apart from CNS deficits (25).

Scleroderma

Polyneuropathies may be present in this disease, of which paresthesias may be one of the presenting clinical features. Myopathies with the histologic picture of polymyositis are rare (429).

Wegener's Granulomatosis

See p. 502.

Thrombotic Microangiopathy

Polyneuropathies are not infrequent in this disease, which is described on p. 158.

Polycythemia Vera

Polyneuropathies are described as a rare complication of this disease (1304). Other neurologic complications, see p. 163.

Arteriosclerosis

Arteriosclerotic arteriopathy may produce a polyneuropathy (325). Following experimental arterial occlusion, histologic examination shows the development of focal changes in myelin sheaths, followed by secondary changes in axons. Within 10 days, sign of incipient regeneration are visible. Sudden or rapidly progressive deficit in function of a single peripheral nerve or part of a plexus is a feature of arteriosclerotic polyneuropathy. Isolated lesions of a brachial or lower limb plexus as well as cases of sciatic paralysis. These deficits remain isolated to a nerve trunk or plexus and do not broaden into a true polyneuropathy. The syndrome described by Wartenberg, so-called *migrant sensory neuritis* (779), also appears to have a vascular basis. It is characterized by transient attacks of pains and sensory deficits in the distribution of various peripheral sensory nerves. Ischemic necrosis of muscle is another mechanism responsible for acute ischemic damage to peripheral nerve trunks, e.g. in the so-called compartment syndromes. In Volkmann's contracture (193, 579), ischemic necrosis of the wrist and long finger flexors is accompanied in about two-thirds of cases by a reversible lesion of the median nerve and less often by a lesion of the ulnar nerve. In the *tibia-*

lis anterior syndrome (p. 436), the anterior tibial (deep peroneal) nerve may be temporarily affected.

Polyneuropathies in Sprue and Other Disturbances of Intestinal Absorption (77)

Nontropical Sprue

Polyneuropathies are the commonest neurologic complication in this disease, as well as in idiopathic steatorrhea or celiac disease of adults – syndromes characterized by fatty stools, emaciation, and anemia, as well as diverticulosis. An associated subacute combined spinal cord degeneration and cerebellar signs may be present, as well as myopathies due to vitamin D deficiency and osteomalacia and tetany in hypocalcemia. The neurologic signs may precede the intestinal manifestations. Not all patients respond to vitamin B_{12} treatment, and sometimes a gluten-free diet or antibiotics are necessary (intestinal flora!) (see also pp. 227 and 313).

Extensive Small Bowel Resections

This postoperative state may lead to deficient vitamin E absorption, a condition which may be associated with a complex neurologic syndrome which includes sensory disturbances and brisk reflexes, as well as symptoms referable to the muscle, ataxia, eye movement disturbances, atrophy and fasciculations of the tongue, or areflexia (1061, 1253). Abetalipoproteinemia, more commonly than resection of the small intestines or a chronic cholestasis (671) can cause a vitamin E deficit. The symptoms can be alleviated by administration of vitamin E, 200 mg/kg of body weight per day. The symptoms can be expected to improve or at least plateau (171).

Artificially Restricted Gastric Emptying

A nutritional sensory neuropathy (782) may follow the surgical treatment of obesity by stenosis of the outlet of the stomach. Other gastroenterologic causes may lead to similar signs and symptoms.

Polyneuropathies in Exogenous Toxic Disorders (132, 730)

Exogenous causes are responsible for about one-fourth of all polyneuropathies; they are the largest etiologic group. They include stimulants, medicaments, industrial poisons, and other substances. Several of the more important of these substances will be discussed in detail, including their additional effects on the nervous system.

Chronic Alcoholism (132, 461, 1236)

Pathophysiology: The total amount of alcohol consumed is responsible for the ill effects on the body. Thus, the risk of hepatic cirrhosis increases from 3-fold with a daily alcohol intake of 20–40 g to 600-fold with a daily intake of 140 g. Moreover, individual and genetically and racially determined factors – responsible for determining alcohol dehydrogenase and aldehyde dehydrogenase activity – influence the susceptibility of the body to damage by alcohol. A slightly raised acetaldehyde concentration may point to a (genetic) defect of both dehydrogenases and thus to an increased risk of a toxic effect of chronic alcohol intake. Disulfiram (Antabuse) inhibits aldehyde dehydrogenase activity. In addition to the toxic effects of ethanol and acetaldehyde, malnutrition is nearly always a major clinical factor in the chronic alcoholic.

Clinical aspects of neurologic complications other than polyneuropathies: The effects of alcohol on the nervous system are summarized in Table 1.**19**. *Psychopathologic phenomena* will not be considered further. Epileptiform manifestations, see p.152. Wernicke's *encephalopathia haemorrhagica superior,* see p.152. *Cerebellar ataxias,* see p.134. *Myopathy,* see p.504. *Amblyopia,* see p.329.

Polyneuropathy (100, 132): The clinical picture is dominated by the *subjective* features including intense neuralgic pains, mainly in the lower extremities, and occasionally accompanied by nocturnal cramps; less often the patient first complains of weakness. *Neurologic examination* shows absent or diminished tendon jerks; in about one-half of patients both ankle jerks are absent. Abnormal deep sensation and stocking hypesthesia are present, as well as muscular weakness, especially of the flexor muscles of the ankle. Electric studies show a slow, 3 cycles/s tremor of the legs, and the auditory evoked potentials may be delayed (1018). Peripheral nerve conduction also is delayed, particularly in the peroneal nerve. Involvement of the *autonomic nervous system* leads to disturbances of sweat secretion, in particular increased sweat secretion of the soles of the feet, and to disturbances of blood pressure as well as hypothermia, impotence, and trophic skin changes (658). Comparative electrophysiologic and *histologic examinations* of the sural nerve show decay (mainly axonal) of myelinated and unmyelinated fibers (100).

Lead Neuropathy

See p.148.

Arsenic Poisoning (859)

The commonest *cause of poisoning* is the accidental intake of a specific insecticide, but poisoning may result from the excessive absorption of arsenic-containing drugs. **Clinically**, after 1–2 weeks a neuropathy appears, which is accompanied by severe dysesthesias and muscles that are painful to pressure; distal muscles may be paralysed. Some patients experience diarrhea, trophic changes and altered pigmentation of the skin, loss of hair, and cross-striations of the nails (Mees' lines). This sign, although it is typical, is not pathognomonic of arsenic poisoning. The cranial nerves are not involved and encephalopathies and myelopathies are rare. The signs of polyneuropathy reach their clinical maximum after about 4 weeks, electrophysiologic evidence of delayed conduction lasts about 3 months. The **prognosis** for complete recovery is poor. The patient may continue to complain of burning soles of the feet for many years. Accordingly, **treatment** with chelating substances should be undertaken even before signs of polyneuropathy appear.

Thallium Poisoning (277)

Thallium is an ingredient of certain rat poisons. This tasteless, odorless, heavy-metal salt produces signs similar to arsenic poisoning. Histologic examination reveals axonal degeneration.

Triarylphosphate Poisoning

Triarylphosphate is a chemical substance present in certain lubricants. It was also used in the production of the parsley extract apiol, an abortifacient. When triarylphosphate is accidentally used in the preparation of food, an epidemic of food poisoning may result. Individuals who eat food containing this toxic substance experience diarrhea and nausea initially, followed by a clinically silent latent period which may last 1–5 weeks. This is followed by a prodromal phase with a slight fever, catarrhal and intestinal symptoms. The paralysis, which follows 10–38 days after the actual poisoning, is usually flaccid and symmetric, involving first the toes and spreading after a few hours to the feet. Within days the fingers and hands also are affected so that the full picture of involvement of the proximal muscle groups is reached within 8–10 days of the onset of paralysis. The initial picture of flaccid paralysis, absent reflexes, muscular atrophy, and a stocking distribution of sensory deficit may later regress, but the *subsequent course* varies. Some patients develop spasticity and pyramidal signs with increasing frequency; after 1 year at least one-third of adult patients have brisk knee jerks. Experimental studies during the early phase have shown pathologic changes in the axoplasm, as well as changes in the nervous system and individual muscles.

Medications

Thalidomide

This hypnotic (unavailable because of its teratogenic effects) after only a few regular doses, produces clinical signs and symptoms within a few weeks. *Subjectively,* paresthesias and neuralgic pains appear, as well as muscular weakness. The paresthesias are constant and a prominent feature, affecting the toes and aggravated at night by the warmth of the bedclothes; they may have a causalgic character. *Objectively,* a glove and stocking distribution of the sensory disturbances is present, and the ankle jerks are invariably absent. Clinically, thalidomide neuropathy appears to be a sensory polyneuropathy. The **prognosis** is poor, in that polyneuropathic signs and symptoms may persist for a long time, even for many years, despite withdrawal of the drug.

Isoniazid (INH)

The polyneuropathy of isoniazid usually occurs only if a *dose* of more than 15 mg/kg body weight/day is administered. Over 50% of patients receiving such a dose develop polyneuropathy. Usually the **subjective symptoms** develop 6–8 weeks after the start of treatment, with numbness and paresthesias of the toes and feet which gradually worsen and spread to involve the hands. They are followed by painful sensations. **Objective** signs show the final picture to be one of severe distal polyneuropathy which is predominantly sensory and accompanied by vasomotor disturbances. Psychotic and other CNS signs may also follow isoniazid intake. *Pathophysiologically,* the toxic effect of isoniazid on the nervous system is mediated by a disturbance of pyridoxine metabolism. INH intake leads to an increased excretion of pyridoxin in the urine. *Prophylactically* the development of polyneuropathy may be forestalled by the daily administration of 50–100 mg of pyridoxine. **Treatment** of the polyneuropathy consists in withdrawing or reducing the dose of INH, combined with the daily injection of pyridoxine 200–400 mg.

Nitrofurantoin

Even with conventional doses this substance, which is used in the treatment of urinary tract infections, may lead to a polyneuropathy in the presence of a renal insufficiency. The severity of the neurologic signs and the prognosis itself depend directly upon the severity of the renal insufficiency. If the insufficiency is severe, nitrofurantoin may within 1–2 weeks produce **clinical features** of a marked motor and sensory polyneuropathy which shows no tendency to recover.

Other Medications

Rarely *meprobamate, hydralazine,* or *disulfiram* (Antabuse) (404) causes a polyneuropathy. Disulfiram in high doses when associated with alcohol intake may provoke a fulminating polyneuropathy (1026). *Vincristine* medication (273) provokes a polyneuropathy which is sometimes accompanied by alopecia and constipation. A rare observation in the course of a polyneuropathy of unknown etiology is the development

of a pronounced *corticosteroid dependency:* the polyneuropathy largely regresses provided the corticosteroid is continued, and a relapse occurs if it is withdrawn. A severe polyneuropathy has been described following *lithium poisoning* (911), as well as with the thyrostatic *carbimazole* (691).

Other Exotoxic Polyneuropathies

A severe polyneuropathy occurring in epidemic proportions has been described following the use of *Spanish olive oil* containing a toxic agent, the nature of which has not been identified (262). Between 4 and 8 weeks after ingestion of the oil, the polyneuropathy affected three-fourths of the oil users, but eventually 92% exhibited neurologic signs and symptoms. The illness is an axonal neuropathy presenting as muscular pains, cramps, pareses, and atrophy, with absent reflexes and disturbances of sensation. Many patients remained disabled by the neurologic deficits 12 months later.

A variety of solvents may produce neuropathies which are mainly sensory in nature, e.g., *trichlorethylene* (Tri) and *carbon disulfide.* Polyneuropathies are also described in *carbon monoxide poisoning* and in "glue sniffers" after they have inhaled *n-hexane* solvent.

Polyneuropathies Due to Other Causes

Serogenetic Polyneuropathy

This form is especially associated with antitetanus injections and always occurs within the framework of a generalized serum sickness, i.e., 4–12 days after the injection. It may present in a localized form near the site of injection, simulating a neuralgic amyotrophy of the shoulder (p. 409) or a peroneal palsy of the lower extremity, or as a generalized acute polyradiculoneuropathy with quadriparesis and cranial nerve palsies.

Proximal Motor Neuropathy with Multifocal Conduction Block

This condition is characterized clinically by chronic progressive asymmetrical, initially purely motor weakness, by fasciculations, by pain or cramps, and at times by myokymias (159, 700, 918, 1025). The weaknesses gradually accumulate over months and years, and lead to progressive impairment. Differentiation from a spinal muscular atrophy or amyotrophic lateral sclerosis is necessary and not always easy (918). The demonstration of multiple mainly proximal, segmental conduction deficits of peripheral nerve trunks by electromyography is the definitive diagnostic test (1025).

Meningopolyneuritis After Tick Bite (Lyme Disease)

Epidemiology: This is an illness transmitted by the bite of ticks, usually *Ixodes ricinus* and sometimes other insects. The picture is easily recognizable. The neurologic signs and symptoms may be those of viral spring meningoencephalitis when a virus is transmitted (p. 50) or of a spirochetal disease such as *Borrelia* infestation (Lyme disease). It occurs most commonly in summer and autumn, particularly in geographical areas infested with ticks.

Nomenclature: Accompanying skin involvement prompts the use of the following: *erythema chronicum migrans, Lyme disease, meningopolyneuritis,* or the *Garin-Bujadoux-Bannwarth syndrome* (6, 839).

Clinical features: Immediately after the insect bite – but not in all cases – a circular patch develops at the site and, in the course of days or weeks, gradually grows larger: *chronic migrating erythema*. A few weeks after the tick bite, *intense pain* is felt at the location of the bite. This is followed by a polyneuropathy or polyradiculopathy, often asymmetric, and not infrequently accompanied by bilateral *facial palsy*. The distribution of the paralysis may vary greatly, from a painful *Guillain-Barré polyradiculitis* to a cranial polyradiculitis. This neurologic picture is nearly always accompanied by CSF changes: elevated protein and pleocytosis (up to 400 cells or more). The condition is therefore a true *meningoradiculitis* (1006, 1084) or lymphocytic meningoradiculitis (945). Associated non-neurologic manifestations include *monoarthritic pains* which are typical of Lyme disease (839), as well as cardiac signs. The CNS symptoms of neuroborreliosis were referred to on p. 52.

Prognosis and treatment: Although the course of the disease may be prolonged, eventually recovery is complete. The value of penicillin and the tetracyclines has been established in Lyme disease (1152), and they have also been successfully used to treat tick bite meningoradiculitis.

Tick Paralysis

A disease entity that is probably different is a partial paralysis with absent reflexes which occurs

4-14 days after a tick bite. The distribution of the clinical lesions varies: they may be confined to the affected extremity, or they may be rapidly progressive and involve all skeletal muscles (463, 925). They are caused by a disturbance of conduction in peripheral nerves at the neuromuscular end plate, similar to the lesion in botulism (654).

Polyneuropathies in Malignancy (500)

Malignant tumors may manifest paraneoplastic features without local spread. The cerebellar and CNS signs (p. 156), as well as the myopathies (p. 503), are discussed in other sections.

Clinical features: In the peripheral nervous system, a *sensory polyneuropathy* is most often observed. The initial picture is that of radiating pains, paresthesias, and sensory disturbances in the distal extremities, particularly the calves, feet, and hands. Deep sensation is disturbed to the extent that ataxia is evident on movement. Physical examination reveals hypotonic muscles and absent reflexes without marked weakness of muscles. The same clinical picture may occur in patients without a carcinoma (602). A rarer form, mononeuritis multiplex, develops on the basis of a vasculitis confined to the nervous system (574).

Pathologic anatomy and pathophysiology: Study reveals degenerative changes in the spinal ganglia, the posterior roots, the posterior columns, and the peripheral nerves. The pathophysiologic mechanisms are not always clear. While bronchogenic carcinoma is the malignant neoplasm that causes neurologic complications most often, other malignant lesions should not be forgotten, notably Hodgkin's lymphoma.

Prognosis: The disease is progressive. Regression of the neurologic deficits after operative removal of the carcinoma is exceptional.

Hypothyroidism

A polyneuropathy may be observed (795), in addition to CNS (p. 154) and muscular (p. 502) disturbances. The polyneuropathy is present in 15%-60% of patients with hypothyroidism, the true incidence depending on the enthusiasm of the search. The polyneuropathy has a symmetric, distal pattern. The patient experiences unpleasant paresthetic sensations in the distal extremities, muscular pains especially in the calves, lancinating pains in the feet, and sensory disturbances are clinically demonstrable in the distal extremities. Muscular weakness, although often mentioned, is usually a myopathic feature.

Pathoanatomically, an axonal degeneration is present (795).

Treatment: The polyneuropathy responds well to treatment of the hypothyroidism.

8. Diseases of the Cranial Nerves

Of the 12 pairs of cranial nerves, the first two are parts of the brain evaginated during embryogenesis, and not peripheral nerves. Table 8.1 provides a review of the cranial nerves, their function, and their method of examination. Fig. 8.1 illustrates the nuclei of cranial nerves III through XII in the brainstem. The symptomatology produced by lesions of the brainstem requires careful analysis for topographic localization accord-

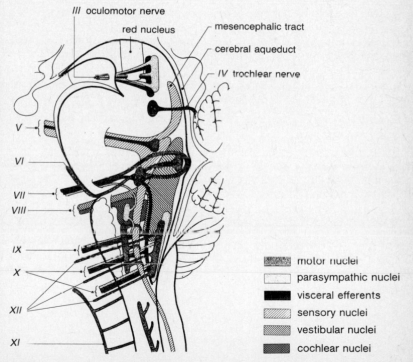

III oculomotor nerve
red nucleus
mesencephalic tract
cerebral aqueduct
IV trochlear nerve

V
VI
VII
VIII
IX
X
XII
XI

motor nuclei
parasympathetic nuclei
visceral efferents
sensory nuclei
vestibular nuclei
cochlear nuclei

Fig. 8.1   The cranial nerves. Positions of their nuclei in the brainstem (after *Braus* and *Elze*)

Table 8.1 Cranial nerves. Function and method of examination

Cranial Nerve	Function	Function Tested	Remarks
I Olfactory	Sense of smell	Ability to smell substance (coffee, cloves, oil of menthol)	Trigeminal stimulants (ammonia) as test for simulation and for local mucosal changes
II Optic	Pathway for visual stimuli from the retina	Visual acuity: evaluating the appearances of the optic fundi with the ophthalmoscope; plotting the visual fields digitally or instrumentally	Visual field defect also accompanies lesions of the optic tract or optic radiation
III Oculomotor	Innervation of the levator palpebrae, 3 rectus muscles (medial, superior, and inferior) and inferior or oblique muscles, also the sphincter pupillae and the ciliary muscle	Controlling visual axis, following an object with the eyes, pupillary reflexes (light and convergence)	Nuclear and supranuclear disturbances of external ocular and pupillary disturbances in ocular lesions are significant in differential diagnosis
IV Trochlear	Innervation of the superior oblique muscle. Eyeball directed downward and medially	Following an object with the eyes	Paralysis is accompanied by head tilt to the opposite side
V Trigeminal	Innervation of the masticatory muscles, sensation of the face, and mucosal surfaces of the eyes, tongue, and parts of the nasopharynx	Opening the mouth (deviation to the paralyzed side), clenching the teeth (palpation of the masseter and temporal muscles). Sensation tested by touch. Corneal reflex	Corneal reflex also diminished in cases of facial palsy and upper motor neuron and sensory disturbances
VI Abducent	Innervation of lateral rectus muscle. Eyeball directed to temporal side	Following an object outward	Differentiation from nuclear and supranuclear paralysis

VII Facial	Innervation of the muscles of expression and the lacrimal and salivary glands. Carries taste fibers from the anterior 2/3 of the tongue	Furrowing the brow, screwing up the eyes, sniffing, whistling, Schirmer's lacrimation test (p. 356), taste test (p. 355)	Differential diagnosis with upper motor neuron facial palsy (p. 355)
VIII Auditory and vestibular	Sense of hearing. Sense of balance	Counting whispered numbers. Tuning fork tests (Weber's and Rinne, p. 361). Observe nystagmus during eye movements. Balance tests (Romberg, p. 364, standing on one leg: Unterberger test, Babinski-Weil walking test, p. 365)	Differential diagnosis of central disturbances of balance
IX-X Glossopharyngeal and vagus	Innervation of the muscles of the soft palate, pharynx, larynx (through the vagal recurrent nerve), sensation of soft palate, fauces, tonsilar fossae, inner ear; supplies fibers to the parotid gland. taste fibers from the posterior 1/3 of the tongue	Deglutition, the gag reflex (palata symmetry, "curtain" phenomenon displacing the posterior pharyngeal wall from the paralyzed side), hoarseness, pharyngeal sensation (comparison of the two sides)	
XI Accessory	Innervation of the sternomastoid muscle and upper part of the trapezius muscle	Turning the head against resistance: strength reduced toward the side opposite to the sternomastoid paralysis (p. 370). Trapezius paralysis causes shoulder drop and a tilted scapula. Raising the shoulder against resistance	
XII Hypoglossal	Motor innervation of the tongue	Appearance of the tongue (wrinkled surface, irregular puckered margin). Deviation of the protruded tongue to the paralyzed side	Acute upper motor neuron paralysis with deviation of the tongue to the paralyzed side is soon compensated

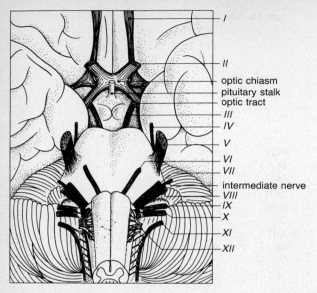

I
II
optic chiasm
pituitary stalk
optic tract
III
IV
V
VI
VII
intermediate nerve
VIII
IX
X
XI
XII

Fig. 8.**2**   The cranial nerves shown in relation to the base of the brain

ing to the particular nerve roots that are damaged. Fig. 8.**2** illustrates the relationship of the cranial nerves to the base of the brain, and Fig. 8.**3** shows their relationship to the skull base. In many lesions, these topographic relationships determine the clinical signs and symptoms.

Disturbances of Olfaction (1071)

Anatomy: Axons from the olfactory nerves pass from the 10–20 million receptor cells of the olfactory mucous membrane through the lamina cribrosa to the olfactory bulbs. The first neuron ends at this level in the dendrites of the mitral cells, from which the second neuron passes through the olfactory striae to the amygdala and other regions of the temporal lobe. Examination of olfactory perception is successful only if the test substance is brought in contact with the receptor cells.

Technique of testing: The sense of smell should be tested separately in each nostril with the subject's eyes shut. Coffee will be recognized by about 70% of patients; remarkably often it is called "tobacco" or "smoke." If the patient states that he can smell "nothing," an empty container should be held up for comparison. If he then chooses the test substance but fails to indicate the nature, the result can be regarded as normal. However, if he fails to differentiate between the empty container and a test

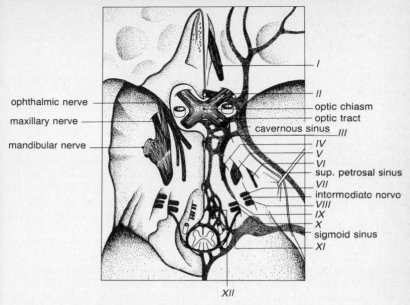

Fig. 8.3 The cranial nerves shown in relation to the base of the skull, covered by dura (left), with the venous sinuses exposed (right). The cranial nerves exit through the following foramina:

I	cribriform plate	VII	} internal auditory canal
II	optic canal	VIII	
III	} superior orbital fissure	IX	} jugular foramen
IV		X	
VI		XI	
V/i	superior orbital fissure	XII	hypoglossal canal
V/ii	foramen rotundum		
V/iii	foramen ovale		

substance with an intense smell (e.g., asafoetida), anosmia is present. By contrast, if household ammonia (which is not a test substance for olfaction but a trigeminal nerve stimulant) can be recognized, a lesion of the olfactory nerve is present. If the patient fails to recognize ammonia, or does so only after deep inspiration (bronchial stimulation), a lesion of the nasal mucous membrane or – in the absence of any reaction – a psychogenic disturbance is present.

Terminology: A reduction of the sense of smell is called *hyposmia,* and this finding is irrelevant to neurologic diagnosis. *Parosmia* is the failure to recognize proffered smells, *cacosmia* is the abnormal sensation of disagreeable, often stinking smells; sometimes no cause can be demonstrated. Only the complete absence of the sense of smell, *anosmia,* will be analyzed here.

Anosmia

Complete loss of the sense of smell may accompany *nasal disorders,* e.g., rhinitis sicca, and it may be unilateral if only one side is occluded. Anosmia which is not rhinogenic may be an isolated manifestation of an *olfactory groove meningioma.* The commonest cause of anosmia is *craniocerebral trauma,* in which the olfactory nerves are severed or the olfactory bulbs are contused. Usually posttraumatic disturbances of the sense of smell are observed after a latent period of weeks or months, possibly as a result of secondary fibrotic changes in the meninges. The incidence of posttraumatic anosmia correlates directly with the duration of posttraumatic amnesia. In about one-third of cases the anosmia disappears within 1 year at the latest. After *viral influenza,* three-fourths of patients experience some impairment of the sense of smell, and one-third a complete anosmia. Only two-thirds of those severely affected improve within 6–12 months; an even smaller proportion recover completely. Often parosmias and kakosmias may be permanent (501). Similar effects may follow common colds. *Rarer causes* are a diminished sense of smell in Paget's disease, occasionally in diabetes mellitus, and after laryngectomy. Intermittent impairment of the olfactory and gustatory functions were described above in the section on sarcoidosis (p. 53).

Anosmia caused by aplasia of the olfactory bulb is part of the congenital anomaly known as Kallmann's syndrome (hypogonadotrophic hypogonadism with eunuchoidal dwarfism, delayed puberty, and occasional color blindness).

A **restricted sense of taste** (ageusia) often accompanies anosmia. It is usually an *indirect* effect and indicates the importance of the sense of smell in taste perception. True ageusia (1071) may be caused by the local action of a toxic substance on the mucous membrane of the tongue, e.g., wetting the tip of a pen. A transient ageusia may accompany the oral administration of certain drugs, e.g., penicillamine, L-dopa, phenindione, the thyrostatic substance thiamazole (630), the H_2 receptor antagonist ranitidine (Zantac) (associated with headache and cough), and the coronary vasodilator Ildamen (975). A deficiency of zinc ions, which may occur during the treatment of scleroderma with histidine, may cause ageusia and anosmia (497), in addition to mental changes and cerebellar disturbances. Loss of the sense of smell has been described following tonsillectomy (372). Hypogeusia has been reported in diabetes mellitus, Sheehan's syndrome, and hypothyroidism. Gustatory disturbances are not uncommon in elderly subjects; they may be the result of an arteritis and may be an early sign, together with a burning tongue, of rheumatoid polymyalgia in giant-cell arteritis. Intermittently, disturbances of olfactory and gustatory function occur in sarcoidosis. A classic finding is unilateral ageusia of the anterior two-thirds of the tongue in cases of peripheral facial palsy (p. 352).

True Combination of Anosmia and Ageusia

This rare simultaneous finding after craniocerebral trauma (exceptionally also an isolated ageusia) may be attributed to a contusion of the diencephalon in the vicinity of the wall of the third ventricle.

Cacosmias

These spontaneous attacks of an abnormal odor indicate damage of the olfactory bulb, amygdaloid nucleus, or uncus. They may occur as the aura of an epileptic attack (uncinate fit) and then indicate a lesion in the anterior and basal part of the temporal lobe (p. 179).

Disturbances of Vision as a Neurologic Problem

Only a few topics from the large field of neuro-ophthalmology (486, 530, 1245) will be discussed in this section, as common problems facing the neurologist.

Loss of Vision

Unilateral Visual Loss of Sudden Onset

This may be a *traumatic event* following a fracture through the optic canal (Rhese radiographic projection!). Amaurosis fugax is observed in *carotid artery occlusion*. Changes in the optic nerve caused by arteriosclerosis lead to pseudopapilledema, on the basis of *ischemia* (*ischemic optic neuropathy* or malacia of the optic nerve). A sudden fall in arterial blood pressure or hemorrhage may trigger visual loss, as may *temporal arteritis* (p. 456). In *papilledema* a gradual loss of vision is observed over weeks or months, although amblyopic attacks with transient blindness may occur; the latter may

end in permanent blindness. *Intracranial mass lesions* without papilledema may lead to sudden visual disturbances through compression of the posterior cerebral artery at the tentorial edge and secondary occipital ischemia (513).

Bilateral Visual Loss of Sudden Onset

This event may sometimes indicate a bilateral *retinal ischemia,* e.g., on the basis of an aortic arch syndrome. However, it is usually caused by *ischemia of the occipital cortex* in vertebrobasilar arterial insufficiency. The prodromal signs are typical: loss of color vision, hemianopic episodes, and relative preservation of central vision; sometimes a patient denies any visual disturbance despite obviously severe disability. Sudden release of fluid under pressure in hydrocephalus, particularly in a seated patient, may provoke immediate irreversible blindness caused by ischemia of the optic nerve.

Rapid or Gradual Visual Loss in One or Both Eyes

This event has a wide variety of causes. In *retrobulbar neuritis* and *papillitis,* the visual loss appears in the course of one or several days and disappears after a few weeks, although exceptions are possible. Both eyes may be simultaneously affected. The vascular lesions of the optic nerve discussed above may also produce visual disturbances of gradual onset. In *hemorrhagic anemias,* usually associated with blood loss from the gastrointestinal tract in men and the genital tract in women, vision may be reduced within hours or days, usually in both eyes; about 10% of patients are blinded in one eye. The visual defect usually takes the form of symmetric loss of the lower half of the field. The prognosis is poor (220). *Toxic causes* include methyl alcohol poisoning and tobacco-alcohol amblyopia. The latter condition causes bilateral visual loss characterized by an early inability to distinguish between red and green. Vitamin B_{12} deficiency is a significant etiologic factor. *Compression of the optic nerve* by a mass lesion (tumor, carotid aneurysm) leads to a visual field defect and optic atrophy combined with slowly progressive visual loss. An *optic glioma* – common in children, particularly girls – causes gradual visual loss in the presence of an enlarged optic canal (Rhese radiographic projections, CT scan) and leads to unilateral proptosis.

Disturbances of the Visual Fields (486)

Examination technique: As a rule, the visual fields are tested in both eyes at the same time (homonymous defects) and occasionally in each eye separately. The patient is seated at a distance of about 1 m in front of the examiner and fixes his gaze on the examiner's nose. The visual fields are then mapped out, first with one finger alone and then with one finger of each hand simultaneously (visual neglect or inattention hemianopsia) (Fig. 8.4). The examiner can verify, by reference to the borders of his own visual field, when the patient should see his moving finger. Occasionally early visual field lesions affecting the red isopters can first be demonstrated by the use of a red-topped needle which is brought from the periphery of each field, as in the finger test.

Topographic Classification of Visual Field Defects

Various field defects are shown diagrammatically in Fig. 8.5, including their topographic significance. From this information, etiologic conclusions are possible when considered in conjunction with the case history and other clinical signs. The patient may be unaware of his *homonymous field defect,* including a complete homonymous hemianopsia. With *visual neglect* or inattention hemianopsia, the stimulus applied upon simultaneous testing of right and left visual fields is not noticed on one side; however, testing of each half of the visual field alone reveals no hemianopsia. This finding accompanies lesions of the parietal lobe of the appropriate hemisphere, usually the nondominant one. The *Riddoch phenomenon* refers to the observa-

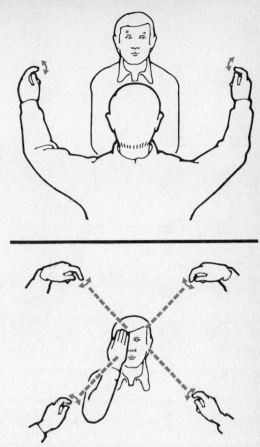

Fig. 8.4 Manual testing of the visual fields. Above: simultaneous testing of both eyes in a patient with visual neglect. Below, testing one eye

tion of movement within the boundaries of a visual field in which stationary objects are not seen. A positive Riddoch phenomenon in a case of hemianopsia is a favorable prognostic sign, heralding recovery. *Palinopsia* or visual perseveration may be encountered in patients with right-sided temporo-occipital le-

sions (810). This phenomenon describes the situation in which, after the visual stimulus is removed, objects seen during the visual stimulus are "observed" again after an interval. The imaginary picture is incorporated into the real visual milieu. A monocular remnant in the temporal part of the visual field, the so-

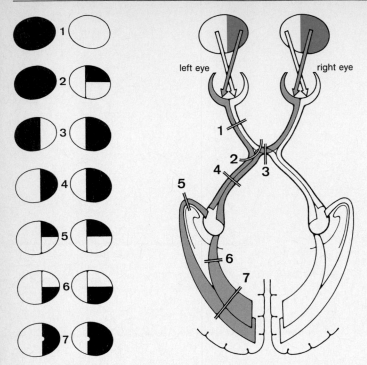

left eye   right eye

Fig. 8.5   Visual field disturbances, according to the site of the lesion in the pathways

called *temporal crescent,* remains when hemianopsia is caused by a lesion (usually cerebral softening) in the contralateral occipital lobe, if the central part of the calcarine fissure is spared (789). The *chiasmal syndrome* is described on p. 38.

Abnormal Findings in the Disks

Papilledema

The *differential diagnosis* of papilledema includes an engorged optic disk, inflammatory papillitis, and vascular papillitis related to hypertension. Clinical details are given in Table 8.2. In doubtful cases, fluorescein angiography may be useful.

Optic Atrophy

The degree of optic atrophy, if it is present, need in no way parallel the degree of visual loss. The following causes must be considered: *optic glioma* or *optic nerve compression* by an adjacent space-occupying lesion, *traumatic damage* to the optic nerve, a previous *retrobulbar neuritis* (temporal pallor), a previous *choked*

Table 8.2 Papilledema and its differential diagnosis

Pathologic Condition	Appearance of Fundus	Vision	Visual Field	Other Signs and Symptoms	Etiology	Side
Papilledema	Blurred margins. Disk enlarged and prominent. Hyperemic, engorged veins, leading to splinter hemorrhages. Retina normal in other respects	Usually vision remains normal for long time	Blind spot enlarged	Amblyopic attacks of short duration	Brain tumors in 75%. Thrombosis of cerebral veins. Other causes of raised intracranial pressure	Almost invariably bilateral
Hypertensive retinopathy	Disk appearance similar to above. However, the vascular changes involve the entire retina and include A-V crossing phenomena, variations in caliber, silver-wiring and yellowish-white exudates. Peripheral hemorrhages common	Sometimes reduced	Normal	Signs of hypertension (in part, similar to symptoms of a brain tumor), raised blood pressure, renal signs	Hypertension, nephropathy	Almost invariably bilateral
Central vein thrombosis	Disk blurred, edematous, and prominent. Veins enormously engorged, corkscrew appearance. Hemorrhages extending into the periphery, some superficial	Very rapid, but visual loss not abrupt	Variable	Bulbar pain	Hypercoagulation states	Usually unilateral

Table 8.2 (Continued)

Pathologic Condition	Appearance of Fundus	Vision	Visual Field	Other Signs and Symptoms	Etiology	Side
Papillitis	Ophthalmoscopically often indistinguishable from papilledema. Disks slightly more prominent and veins more dilated	Severe visual failure within a few days. Recovery after a week or so	Early central and paracentral scotoma. Sometimes segmental peripheral scotoma	Pain in region of eye, accentuated by movements of eyeball. Also flashes of light	Focal infection? Multiple sclerosis	Almost always initially unilateral, may become bilateral within weeks
Retrobulbar neuritis	Similar to papillitis, but disk findings normal					
Drusen	Disk enlarged and prominent with blurred margins, but with a yellowish color. Veins normal, no hemorrhages. If *drusen* are superficial, disk has a glistening granular appearance	Normal	Occasionally slight defects	None	Congenital deposition of hyaline substance (often hereditary)	Usually unilateral
Persistent medullated fibers	Extension of snowy white medullated fibers of the disk beyond its margins. Disk normal in other respects	Normal	Normal	Sometimes in the retina as well, independently of the disk	Congenital disturbance	Bilateral in 20%
Pseudopapilledema (= pseudoneuritis)	Optic nerve fibers heaped up. Disk prominent and widened. Grayish-white color without hyperemia. Veins may become tortuous but not engorged	Normal	Normal	Often hypermetropic	Congenital excessive overgrowth of glial tissue. Occasionally familial	Bilateral or unilateral

disk, syphilis, or Leber's *familial optic atrophy* (in males). In the latter condition, a concomitant encephalitis has been described and the theory advanced of a slow virus transmission from mother to son which depends on a genetically controlled resistance in the child (1242). Optic atrophy, sometimes bilateral, accompanies *turricephaly*. Bilateral optic atrophy has been observed following *X-irradiation* of the chiasmal region. *Opticochiasmatic arachnoiditis* – a mechanical lesion of the optic pathway caused by arachnoid adhesions – is probably too frequently diagnosed. The *Foster-Kennedy syndrome* consists of ipsilateral optic atrophy (due to compression of the optic nerve) and engorgement of the contralateral optic disk in a tumor of the middle cranial fossa.

Disturbances of Ocular Movement (59, 242, 468, 929)

Function of External Ocular Muscles and Examination Technique

Function of Individual Ocular Muscles

These are illustrated in Fig. 8.6 and in Table 8.3. It may be noted, for example, that the right superior rectus muscle in the starting position adducts the globe and turns the vertical meridian inward. Its elevatory function is minimal and only becomes important after abduction of the globe by other muscles (external rectus, inferior oblique, and superior oblique).

Analysis of Paralyzed Muscles

Evaluation may take the following form:

– Double vision (diplopia) is accentuated if the patient looks in the direction of function of the paralyzed muscle. For example, if the distance of the double vision is greatest on looking to the left,

then the paralysis involves either the left external rectus or the right internal rectus muscle. The image of the normal eye is designated as the true image, that of the paralyzed eye as the false image. The latter is more peripherally situated, compared with the true one.

– If the patient looks in the direction of maximal double vision and one eye is then covered, the corresponding image is obscured and the patient can indicate whether the latter is peripheral (false, i.e., the paralyzed eye) or central (true, i.e., the healthy eye).

– Differentiation can be further facilitated by placing a colored glass over one eye and using a rod-shaped light source.

– Diplopia is described as crossed when the image in the right eye lies to the left of the image in the left eye (and the reverse). For example, in left abducent palsy, the two images diverge further when the patient looks to the left side. The image falling on the macula

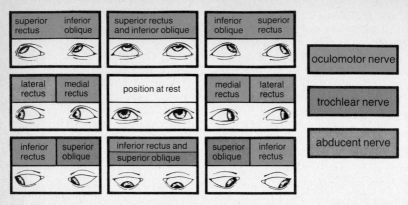

Fig. 8.6   Hering's diagram, indicating the direction of gaze in which individual eye muscle functions are most prominent. Other ocular muscles are first activated to reach this position of maximum function

Table 8.3   Principal and subsidiary functions of the external ocular muscles (after *Stern* et al.)

Muscle	Principal Function	Subsidiary Function
Superior rectus	Elevation. Action is enhanced if the eye is abducted. Conversely, muscle is inactive if eye is adducted	Adducts the eye and rotates the vertical meridian inward. This action is enhanced if the eye is adducted. Raises upper lid
Inferior oblique	Elevation. Action is enhanced if the eye is adducted. Conversely, the muscle is inactive if the eye is abducted	Abducts the eye and rotates the vertical meridian outward. This action is enhanced if the eye is abducted
Inferior rectus	Moves eye downward. Action is enhanced if the eye is abducted. Conversely, the muscle is inactive if the eye is adducted	Adducts the eye and rotates the vertical meridian outward. This action is enhanced if the eye is adducted. Depresses the lower lid
Superior oblique	Moves eye downward. Action is enhanced if the eye is adducted. Conversely, the muscle is inactive if the eye is abducted	Abducts the eye and rotates the vertical meridian inward. This action is enhanced if the eye is abducted
Medial rectus	Adducts the eye	None
Lateral rectus	Abducts the eye	None

of the normally mobile right eye is projected onto the nasal half of the immobile left eye. The image seen by the left eye is thus seen on the left side of the visual field, therefore it is uncrossed.

- In cases of vertically divergent diptopia, the distance may be greatest if the affected eye is directed outward. This indicates involvement of a rectus muscle (see Fig. 8.6). If the distance between the double images is greatest in the upward-inward direction, paralysis of an oblique muscle is present.

Practical Examination of Ocular Motility

Ocular movements may be tested by requesting the patient, whose head has been fixed by the examiner, to follow the examiner's finger through a range of motion. If a visible defect of motility is present, or if the patient volunteers that he has double vision, further testing should be undertaken to elucidate its nature. The use of a light source as a fixation point and of a colored glass enables the examiner to establish which picture is seen by which eye. The examiner also observes the reflexes of the reflected images of a light source on the cornea of the patient's eyes: they will appear on the same spot in each cornea if the eyeballs are parallel, but on different spots if the motility of one eye is disturbed.

Symptomatology of Abnormal Ocular Movements

Disturbances of ocular motility are found with or without dislocation of the bulbs from their normal parallel position. Double vision is (nearly) always present with dislocation, but absent if the bulbs remain parallel. The main categories are listed in Table 8.4.

Paralytic Strabismus (Paralytic Squint)

This disturbance of ocular motility is **caused** by

- failure of one or more ocular muscles (e. g., myasthenia, myopathy),
- a lesion of one or more nerves of the external ocular muscles,
- a lesion in the vicinity of the nuclei of the nerves of the external ocular muscles.

In paralytic strabismus, the following features are found:

- an abnormal position of the paralyzed globe,
- a restriction of globe movement, and
- sometimes a compensatory abnormal posture of the head (see Fig. 8.8).

The restricted movements resulting from the muscular palsies can be studied in Figs. 8.6 and 8.8; they are most clearly seen when the patient looks in the direction which places the greatest demand on the particular paralyzed muscles. If the paralysis is not severe, the patient may reduce the degree of diplopia by adopting a compensatory posture of

Table 8.4   Disorders of ocular mobility. Classification

Axis of Globe	Diagnosis	Site of Lesion	Remarks
Divergent	Paralytic strabismus	External ocular muscles or their nerves or nuclei	Accompanied by double vision
Divergent	Concomitant strabismus (may be alternating)	?	Unilateral amblyopia present from childhood, no double vision
Intermittently divergent	Internuclear ophthalmoplegia	Medial longitudinal fasciculus	Absent (or more commonly, delayed) adduction. Nystagmus especially of the abducted eye. Convergence is maintained despite defective adduction. Double vision usually absent in incomplete cases
Parallel	Supranuclear disturbances of motility (conjugate paralysis)	e. g., paramedian pontine reticular formation, frontal visual center (area 8); occipital visual center (area 18)	No double vision

the head which enables him, albeit to a reduced extent, to look in various directions without double vision.

Concomitant Strabismus (Concomitant Squint)

This form is caused by weakness of vision of one eye that is congenital or acquired in early life. Weakness of vision of one eye. Simultaneous movement of both eyes produces a strabismus, although individual testing reveals that each eye possesses a normal range of movement. This may be confirmed by the so-called cover test; one eye is covered (but left open) and the gaze of the other eye is fixed on an object. If the cover is now removed and placed over the opposite eye, a significant degree of movement will be demonstrated in the uncovered eye which is now the eye fixed on the object. No double vision occurs because of the weakness of vision of one eye.

Principles of External Ocular Movements

Conjugate Gaze Movements

Command Movement

The term command movement is applied to the voluntary act of directing gaze in a specific direction. The *cortical visual center* is situated in areas 6 and 8 of the second frontal convolution and in the paravisual association fibers (59). The visual tract passes via the anterior limb of the internal capsule to the cerebral peduncle. It then crosses the midline along a circuitous cerebellar pathway to end in the paramedian pontine reticular formation of the brainstem, a sort of pontine gaze center. This center also receives afferent fibers from the vestibular nuclei. From this site, the ipsilateral external rectus muscle is innervated via the abducens nucleus, the contralateral internal rectus muscle via the medial longitudinal fasciculus and the oculomotor nucleus. Lesions of this system are recognized clinically by the presence of permanent parallel deviation of the eyeballs to one side and the patient's inability to direct his gaze across the midline to the opposite side.

Vertical Gaze Movements

The center for vertical movements is situated in the vicinity of the corpora quadrigemina, that for upward gaze in the rostral part, and that for downward gaze in the caudal part. The center is linked to the oculomotor nerve via the tecto-ocular tracts.

Focusing or Scrutiny Movements

Gaze movements may be triggered visually or acoustically. Retinal stimuli pass along the optic tracts and the calcarine sulcus to the occipital visual center in the visuomotor area (area 19). Impulses pass from it via the medial part of the optic radiations to the vicinity of the quadrigeminal bodies (vertical eye movements) or via the corticotegmental tracts to the opposite pontine reticular formation. Auditory stimuli may also lead to reflex eye movements as a result of noise. Fibers pass from the auditory visual center in the posterior and temporal transverse radiation of the insula via the retrolenticular field of the internal capsule to the system controlling conjugate eye movements.

Following (Pursuit or Tracking) Reactions

The term "visual tracking" is given to the normal capacity of the subject to fix a slowly moving object in his gaze. An essential requirement is an intact visual cortex. *Compensatory vestibular eye movements* ensure a reflex, opposite movement of the eyes to any movement of the head, guaranteeing an unaltered visual perception. Fibers pass from the vestibular nuclei to both the ipsilateral and contralateral medial longitudinal fasciculi (MLF), as well as to the vestibulospinal tract. In this way, vestibular stimulation leads not only to reflex eye movements but also to corresponding head and trunk movements. This reflex may be elicited in unconscious patients as well (87). If rapid rotation of the head shows that the eyeballs remain fixed in the original direction in space, it can be assumed that the vestibular apparatus as well as its connections to the oculomotor system are intact; for example, paralysis of an external ocular muscle can be ruled out. (However, compare the doll's eyes phenomenon, Table 1.1). Slow passive sideways and forward movement of the head produce reflex conjugate movements of the eyeballs, the *oculocephalic reflex,* which is impaired by brainstem damage (1003).

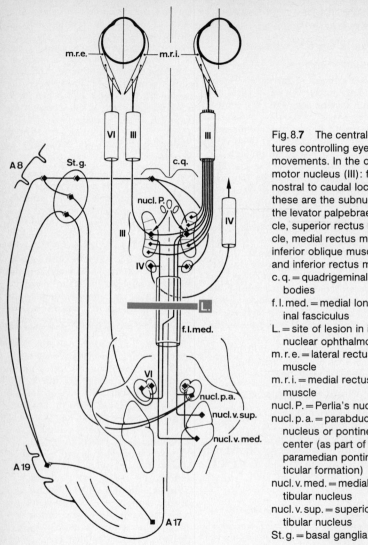

Fig. 8.**7**   The central structures controlling eye movements. In the oculomotor nucleus (III): from nostral to caudal location, these are the subnuclei of the levator palpebrae muscle, superior rectus muscle, medial rectus muscle, inferior oblique muscle, and inferior rectus muscle

c. q. = quadrigeminal bodies

f. l. med. = medial longitudinal fasciculus

L. = site of lesion in internuclear ophthalmoplegia

m. r. e. = lateral rectus muscle

m. r. i. = medial rectus muscle

nucl. P. = Perlia's nucleus

nucl. p. a. = parabducent nucleus or pontine gaze center (as part of the paramedian pontine reticular formation)

nucl. v. med. = medial vestibular nucleus

nucl. v. sup. = superior vestibular nucleus

St. g. = basal ganglia

The Most Important Supranuclear Disturbances of Eye Movement

Anatomic basis: This group of syndromes is caused by lesions situated central to the nuclei for the nerves of the external ocular muscles, i.e., *supranuclear structures* responsible for ocular motility (59). These are illustrated in Fig. 8.7.

Lesions of the Frontal Gaze Center

In trauma as well as cerebral hemispheric insults involving the precentral region, damage to the gaze center in areas 6 and 8 lead to dominance of the contralateral center. In an acute lesion, this produces tonic deviation of gaze and the head to the side of the lesion *(déviation conjuguée);* the patient "shows you his injury." After hours or days, a gaze movement as far as the midline again becomes possible, but not beyond it. Completely free gaze movements return much later, an irregular nystagmus remaining visible at the extreme end of gaze toward the opposite side, as the last remaining sign of the lesion. The nystagmus beats away from the side of the focus.

Lesion of the Visuomotor Region in the Parieto-Occipital Part of Hemisphere (Area 19)

Damage to this region and its efferents results in a failure to bring objects moving in the field of vision reflexly into focus. *Optokinetic nystagmus* also disappears, i.e., rapid back-and-forth movements of the eyes following a moving object or a measuring tape that is passed in front of patients' eyes. Nystagmus is *lost* (or impaired) when the fixation stimulus moves *from* the side of the visual field that is opposite to the lesion in the hemisphere, i.e. moves *toward the lesion.*

Lesion of the Paramedian Pontine Reticular Formation

Previously described as a disturbance of the "pontine gaze center" or "parabducent nucleus." A lesion leads to deviation of the eyes to the opposite side and inability to direct gaze across the midline to the side of the lesion. An additional distinguishing feature from frontal gaze paralysis is the absence of *déviation conjuguée* of the head. As a rule, clinical evidence is present of damage to other pontine structures, e.g., abducent palsy, nystagmus, or pyramidal signs.

Paralysis of Vertical Gaze

A *lesion of the pretectum* leads to a paralysis of upward gaze, while damage to the rostrally situated *interstitial nucleus of the medial longitudinal fasciculus* leads to a paralysis of downward gaze. A supranuclear gaze palsy combined with progressive dementia may be the presenting sign of Whipple's disease (p. 163) (362). In *Parinaud's syndrome,* a conjugate paralysis of upward gaze is present, combined with a weakness of convergence and sometimes an absent pupillary response to light. Bell's phenomenon is always retained. The causes are tumors, particularly of the pineal gland, as well as vascular lesions and encephalitides. A bilateral lesion situated medially and dorsally to the red nuclei may produce an *isolated paralysis of downward gaze* without affecting upward gaze (548).

Internuclear Ophthalmoplegia

In this particular form of supranuclear disturbance of ocular movement, movement of the eyes in specific directions produces strabismus. A *lesion of the medial longitudinal fasciculus* (MLF) is responsible (see Fig. 8.7) (1072, 1245). Diplopia may be present in complete lesions, but is absent in the more common incomplete form. If a *bilateral lesion* is present, the patient when requested to look to one side is unable to rotate the contralateral eye beyond the midline, while convergence (and therefore contraction of both internal rectus muscles) upon close accommodation remains intact, unless a lesion is present which is localized far rostrally. If the lesion is situated caudad in the MLF, nystagmus is present, in all cases, and there is also a paresis of the lateral rectus muscle; convergence remains intact. Because of the internal rectus palsy, horizontal nystagmus is more marked in the abducted eye. Damage to the rostral part of the MLF may also impair convergence, but the external rectus muscle is not paralyzed and there is no nystagmus. In a *unilateral lesion,* the signs are confined to inadequate or slowed adduction of the homolateral eyeball, with dissociated nystagmus of the abducted eyeball.

The *best examination technique* for demonstrating internuclear ophthal-moplegia is the following: The patient is encouraged to make a sweeping gaze movement, in which his gaze passes from the one side to the other. *Etiologically,* internuclear ophthalmoplegia is especially common in multiple sclerosis. It is also observed after cerebrovascular insults of the brainstem, in tumors, and in Wernicke's encephalitis.

The *one-and-a-half syndrome* (1241) is a specific variety: with lesions of the caudal part of the MLF and the paramedian pontine reticular formation, a conjugate horizontal gaze palsy exists to the homolateral side and an internuclear ophthalmoplegia on contralateral gaze. The syndrome is usually caused by multiple sclerosis.

Other More Complex Supranuclear Disturbances of Ocular Motility

Ocular apraxia (Cogan syndrome) (1231, 1245) is a congenital defect occurring primarily in boys. The patient is unable to bring a new object, e.g. the beginning of a new line during, reading, into the center of his visual field simply by a versive movement. He refocuses by turning the head quickly to the left, fixating on the target object on his macular and finally returning the head to its original position.

A progressive limitation of all voluntary movements is encountered after encephalitis of the brainstem or the basal ganglia, as well as in the degenerative syndrome, *progressive supranuclear palsy* (p. 109). Contrariwise, gaze is often retained with passive movement of the head to a particular point of fixation, with the eyeballs continuing to move relative to the orbits *(doll's eye phenomenon).* Following postencephalitic states and occasionally in midbrain tumors, *conjugate gaze spasms* may occur, consisting of convergence spasms and *oculogyric crises* (p. 106).

Irregular repetitive eye movements, called *opsoclonus* ("dancing eyes"), are a feature of paraneoplastic syndromes especially with neuroblastoma of childhood (748, 886). Opsoclonus is also observed in other situations, such as encephalitis and disturbances of the immune mechanisms (103). Corticosteroids may abolish it. *"Ocular bobbing"* is the term used to describe conjugate, spasmodic, arrhythmic downward movements of both eyeballs which return slowly to the neutral position. The condition is usually accompanied by complete failure of all horizontal gaze movements. Ocular bobbing is considered to be a clue to pontine damage, although the lesion may sometimes be in the cerebellum (154). *Seesaw nystagmus* (985) is the term used to describe an alternating, reciprocal vertical nystagmus of both eyeballs (upward movement of one coinciding with downward movement of the other). The responsible lesion appears to be situated in the midbrain, and parasellar lesions, syringobulbia, basal ganglia neoplasms, and vascular lesions may be responsible.

Differential diagnosis of bilateral eye movement disturbances: The differential diagnosis includes the supranuclear disturbances of eye movement described above. In a large group of patients (618) they constitute 25% of the acute cases. One also has to consider diffuse cranial nerve involvement, e.g. in basal meningitis, or a cranial polyradiculitis (p. 307), further a bilateral process at the cavernous sinus, a progressive dystrophy of the eye muscles, and myasthenia gravis.

Lesions of the Nerves to the External Ocular Muscle

These lesions always cause paralytic strabismus and double vision.

Oculomotor Palsy (Fig. 8.8 c)

Clinical aspects: The picture of complete oculomotor palsy includes ptosis, paralysis of the medial, inferior, and superior rectus muscles, as well as the inferior oblique, with a dilated pupil which fails to react to light or accommodation as evidence of an internal ophthalmoplegia. The paralyzed eye is deviated outward and downward, and as a result of paralysis of the superior rectus and inferior oblique muscles, it cannot be elevated above the horizontal plane. A progressive lesion of the oculomotor nerve after its passage through the dura usually causes a ptosis first, and later disturbances of ocular motility. In contrast, lesions of the oculomotor nucleus usually exhibit a reverse sequence of signs. An intact pupil in a peripheral oculomotor palsy usually indicates a peripheral ischemic lesion (1192); however, this picture may sometimes accompany oculomotor compression in the cavernous sinus or an intrinsic brainstem lesion (862). Exophthalmos in oculomotor palsy may be the result of a lack of retraction of the eyeball following paralysis of the rectus muscles with retention of slight anterior pull produced by an intact oblique muscle (893).

Most important causes: A complete oculomotor palsy follows lesions of the peripheral nerve due to the following:

Right-sided
Abducent Palsy (VI)

resting (= primary) position

greatest squint

compensatory head posture
(= smallest strabismus)

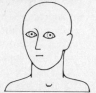

turning of the head to the side
of the paralyzed muscle

a

Right-sided
Trochlear Palsy (IV)

resting (= primary) position

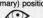

largest strabismus

compensatory head posture
(= smallest strabismus)

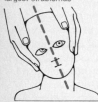

inclination of the head to the
side of the paralyzed muscle
b (Bielschowsky's phenomenon)

inclination of the head to the
normal side

Right-sided
Oculomotor Palsy (III)

resting (= primary) position

greatest strabismus

compensatory head posture

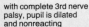

with complete 3rd nerve
palsy, pupil is dilated
c and nonreacting

not with ptosis, because
double vision is absent

Fig. 8.**8 a–c** Position of the
eyeball in paralyses of the
three nerves supplying the
external ocular muscles

- fractures of the skull base,
- traumatic avulsion of the nerve,
- tumors of the skull base,
- basal inflammatory lesions, e.g., tuberculous meningitis, syphilis, carcinomatous meningitis,
- aneurysms of the (infraclinoid) internal carotid or posterior communicating artery,
- arteriovenous fistula or septic thrombosis of a cavernous sinus;
- infection in the cavernous sinus, accompanied by signs of trochlear, abducent, and trigeminal involvement, with fever and periorbital congestion and exophthalmos – the so-called *cavernous sinus syndrome;*
- in vascular lesions of the brainstem, e.g., in the context of an arteritis,
- in diabetic neuropathy (sparing of the pupil, see below) or unilateral mydriatic pupillary paralysis caused by compression of the oculomotor nerves against the clivus due to raised intracranial pressure – the so-called clivus edge syndrome.

Specific forms: The superior *orbital fissure syndrome* may include paralysis of the trochlear and abducent nerves as well as oculomotor palsy and sensory loss in the distribution of the first division of the trigeminal nerve. The *orbital apex syndrome* is a paralysis of all three nerves supplying the external ocular muscles and a sensory deficit in the distribution of the first division of the trigeminal nerve, combined with an optic nerve lesion (peripheral visual field defects, central scotoma, optic atrophy, or papilledema).

Further causes of nuclear oculomotor palsy include multiple sclerosis. Paralysis of the oculomotor and other external ocular muscles may be the result of infection of the sphenoidal or ethmoidal sinuses. About 50% of cases of sphenoidal mucocele have external ocular palsies, occasionally accompanied by optic nerve involvement, frontofacial pain, and proptosis (389). Various forms of encephalitis, including Wernicke's syndrome and certain infectious diseases (diphtheria) and intoxications (botulism), may present clinically as an oculomotor palsy. If the oculomotor nucleus in the pontine tectum is affected, paralysis of the individual muscles innervated by the oculomotor nerve may no longer be complete; the involvement may be patchy. The various (vascular) brainstem syndromes that may commence as nuclear oculomotor palsy are listed in Table 1.**10** (Nothnagel's syndrome, Benedikt's paralysis, Weber's paralysis).

Trochlear Palsy (Fig. 8.**8 b**)

Clinical aspects: This lesion involves the superior oblique muscle; thus, outward and downward gaze is impaired. A characteristic posture, torticollis in *trochlear palsy,* is adopted by the patient, usually a child: in a right-sided paralysis, the head is tilted to the left, the face is turned to the left, and the chin is tucked in (Fig. 8.**8 b**).

Causes: Trochlear palsy may be an isolated finding, e.g., in multiple sclerosis. Usually other cranial nerves are involved, including those of the external ocular muscles, with accompanying brainstem damage or neoplastic or inflammatory lesions of the skull base or superior orbital fissure.

Abducent Palsy (Fig. 8.8 a)

Clinical aspects: This lesion involves the lateral rectus muscle; thus, outward gaze is impaired in the affected eye, with a corresponding horizontal diplopia. When the subject is looking straight ahead, a slightly adducted position of the affected eye, caused by overaction of the intact medial rectus muscle may be present.

Causes: Abducent palsy is the commonest type of external ocular palsy because the long intracranial course of the nerve trunk makes it prone to damage, e.g., by fractures of the skull base, brain tumors, basal meningitis or lesions of the cavernous sinus, superior orbital fissure, or paranasal sinuses. However, an abducent palsy may be a sign of increased intracranial pressure and then possesses no localizing significance. Occasionally it follows some days after a *lumbar puncture* and usually disappears within 6 weeks. In children, a *febrile infection* may lead to unilateral abducent palsy 1–3 weeks later; such lesions usually regress spontaneously after 1–3 months.

Specific forms: *Gradenigo's syndrome,* especially those cases caused by inflammatory lesions involving the apex of the petrous pyramid after otitis media, consists of abducent palsy, deafness, and sensory loss in the distribution of the first division of the trigeminal nerve. *Foville's syndrome* (abducent palsy and contralateral hemiplegia) is produced by brainstem lesions, particularly softening. *Bilateral abducent palsy* (604) is nearly as common as unilateral involvement and has the same causes, e.g., tumors, multiple sclerosis, trauma, subarachnoid hemorrhage, and polyradiculitis (cranial).

Further Causes and Differential Diagnosis of Disturbances of Ocular Motility

Space-Occupying Lesions of the Orbit

These lesions may interfere with normal eyeball motility for purely mechanical reasons. Dislocation of the eyeball invariably occurs, and sometimes proptosis is present. Proptosis due to retrobulbar varicocele may be aggravated by lowering the head. A pulsating exophthalmos accompanies arteriovenous fistula of the cavernous sinus. The combination of a variable degree of proptosis and disturbances of ocular movement may indicate the presence of *orbital pseudotumor,* i.e., an inflammatory reaction of the orbital soft tissues with myositis of the external ocular muscles.

Tolosa-Hunt Syndrome (515, 538, 678, 888)

This syndrome is a painful external ophthalmoplegia in which the first division of the trigeminal nerve is sometimes involved. It is caused by a granulomatous inflammation in the vicinity of the cavernous sinus, with the following **signs and symptoms** (515):

- affects men and women of any age,
- episodes of retrobulbar pain,

- pains occur days or weeks before or after it,
- paralysis of oculomotor, trochlear, first division of trigeminal and abducent nerves, rarely the facial nerve,
- intact pupillary function,
- episodes of pain last for weeks or months,
- one or many recurrences after months or years,
- rarely bilateral,
- carotid angiography shows a siphon of irregular caliber,
- orbital venogram shows stenosis of the superior orbital vein and absence of filling of the cavernous sinus,
- proptosis,
- raised ESR and temperature.

The prompt administration of corticosteroids serves both to control the lesion successfully and to confirm the diagnosis.

Myopathies and Nuclear Pareses of the Ocular Muscles

A *muscular dystrophic process* of the external ocular muscles is known, which impairs normal ocular movement in a very slowly progressive way and which may occasionally be associated with disturbances of swallowing. It is one of the commonest causes of acquired ptosis, occurring early and following a progressive course (p. 483). *Myasthenia gravis* often presents as an intermittent disturbance of eyeball motility (p. 487). *Hyperthyroidism* may be accompanied by paralysis of the eye muscles. *Möbius's syndrome* is a congenital paralysis of the eye muscles (usually an abducent palsy), combined with facial palsy and sometimes other deficits. Electromyographic and muscle-biopsy evidence of motor neuron, as well as peripheral nerve involvement, may be found. Congenital ptosis may be unilateral or bilateral; it is usually familial and occasionally accompanied by weakness of other external ocular muscles.

Anomalies of Innervation of the External Ocular Muscles

Various anomalies of innervation of the eye and other head muscles are described, caused partly by congenital absence of internuclear communication and partly to defective regeneration after a peripheral nerve lesion. They lead to abnormal associated movements.

Marcus Gunn Phenomenon

In this phenomenon, the so-called winking jaw, the patient exhibits a ptosis which disappears when he opens his mouth or moves his lower jaw.

Pseudo-Graefe's Sign

This sign – the eyelid rises when the patient drops his gaze – may appear during the recovery phase of an oculomotor palsy. The term is also applied to the lid lag on downward gaze exhibited by patients with myotonic syndromes.

Duane's Syndrome

This syndrome consists of a paralysis of the external rectus muscles of varying severity. In addition, retraction of the eyeball and narrowing of the palpebral fissure accompanies adduction of the affected eye. Electromyographically, simultaneous innervation of the internal and external rectus muscles can be confirmed.

Other Rarer Causes

Unilateral myokymia of the superior oblique muscle (529, 1172) is a benign syndrome of spontaneous onset and lasting for several years which may be self-limiting. It is accompanied by monocular nystagmus with episodes of double vision and oscillopsia. Fibrosis of the tendon of the superior oblique muscle and its pulley cause mechanical damage which hinders the movement of the eyeball upward and inward. It mimics a paralysis of the inferior oblique muscle and is called *Brown's syndrome*. It may be congenital or appear in adolescents or adults and disappear slowly and spontaneously (423). Fisher's syndrome, described on p. 298, is characterized by ophthalmoplegia, in addition to facial palsy, absent reflexes, and ataxia. The disturbances of ocular motility are believed to be at least partly caused by supranuclear damage, e.g., the effects of a brainstem encephalitis (24, 790, 793).

Pupillary Disturbances

Examination of the pupil: In the examination of the pupils, the following features should be described: shape (round or irregular), size (brightness of the environment to be noted!), whether they are symmetric in size, and whether they both react. The reaction to light is best tested by suddenly exposing one pupil to intense illumination (startle reaction to be avoided), while shielding the opposite eye from the light beam. Only in this way is it possible to evaluate the consensual reaction of the opposite pupil correctly. The convergence reaction is tested only if the pupil fails to respond to light. In doubtful cases, this is best performed with the patient recumbent and the examiner standing behind him. The patient is asked first to fix his gaze on the ceiling, then on the examiner's finger held 20 cm above the patient's nose. The "swinging flashlight test" may be used to demonstrate unilateral (or predominantly unilateral) optic nerve damage (792). The patient is tested in a dimly lit room with his vision fixed in the distance. Each pupil is examined separately with a well-focused beam of light, being illuminated for 5 s, then the beam is rapidly transferred to the opposite pupil. This movement is repeated with a regular rhythm so that each pupillary reaction can be compared and assessed. Only the illuminated pupil is evaluated. Under normal conditions, the light beam provokes an immediate contraction, then the pupil dilates to its final size. In lesions of the afferent loop (optic nerve), initial constriction fails to occur, and the degree of subsequent dilatation is more marked than that occurring during illumination of the healthy eye.

Anomalies of Pupillary Size and Shape

Pupillary ectopia is not rare. It is often associated with ectopia of the crystalline lens and other abnormalities of the eyeball; usually the ectopia is directed upward and outward. *Abnormalities of the shape of the pupil* (oval, square) may either complicate partial congenital aniridia (absent iris) or acquired posterior synechia, and may be associated with partial atrophy of the iris, e.g. in tabes dorsalis. Pupils of different size, *anisocoria,* may be a harmless congenital anomaly ("central anisocoria"). The difference between the two pupils is seldom greater than 1 mm; there is often variation between the sides and in the extent from hour to hour. It may be more marked in poor light, as in Horner's syndrome (p. 241). In individual cases, examination of the pupils in good light may reveal isocoria which upon light testing becomes anisocoria, the illuminated pupil contracting more than the other one.

This finding is not definitely abnormal. Anisocoria is present in ciliary ganglionitis (see below) and Horner's syndrome (p. 241). It may accompany compressive lesions of the oculomotor nerve (p. 343), it may be found in pupillotonia (p. 350), and it may be an early sign of CNS syphilis (p. 55). The pupillary asymmetry in oculomotor palsy, ciliary ganglionitis, and Adie's syndrome is more marked in bright light. Disturbances of pupillary motility may be investigated by locally or systemically administered drugs such as atropine, morphine, and pilocarpine (see Fig. 8.10).

Anomalies of the Pupillary Reaction

Local lesions (posterior synechia, glaucoma) should always first be excluded.

The *amaurotic pupil* possesses a normal diameter but fails to react to light. However, it reacts consensually to light stimulation of the opposite eye. Therefore, when both eyes are open both pupils appear to be normal.

In *oculomotor lesions,* the first sign may be a widely dilated pupil which fails to react to direct or consensual light or convergence stimulation; the eyeball movements may initially remain intact. The *Marcus Gunn pupillary sign* (530, 1245) identifies the reduced pupillary light reaction of one eye after retrobulbar neuritis. Upon covering the normal eye, the abnormal pupil becomes wider than that of the normal eye with reverse testing. *Argyll Robertson pupil* consists of contracted and often irregu-

lar pupils which react to convergence but fail to react to light stimulation. This sign usually indicates CNS syphilis, but a similar picture may be found in diabetes mellitus. *Adie's pupil* (pupillotonia) is usually unilateral: a dilated pupil reacting normally to convergence but only very slowly to light stimulation. The characteristic feature is the subsequent slow, tonic dilatation. Women are more often affected by this syndrome. Sometimes individual tendon reflexes may be absent. The syndrome may be caused by an inflammatory lesion of the midbrain. Another causative interpretation is a chronic lesion of the ciliary ganglion (see below) with defective reinnervation of the sphincter pupillae (714).

Mild chronic oculomotor palsy, e.g., accompanying an aneurysm or other slowly growing space-occupying or inflammatory lesion, may produce a clinical picture similar to Adie's syndrome.

Acute ciliary ganglionitis usually occurs a few days after an infection or an injury to the orbit. A widely dilated pupil is present which does not react to light or convergence stimulation. Initially, transient disturbances of accommodation may also be present and the patient has difficulty in reading print. Hence there is a pupillary anomaly without any accompanying disturbance of eyeball motility (differential diagnosis of oculomotor palsy). It is caused by a lesion of the ciliary ganglion.

Rarer causes: Widely dilated pupils failing to react to light stimulation should prompt suspicion of *drug ef-*

Table 8.5 Features of various pupillary disorders (right side abnormal) (see Fig. 8.9)

Syndrome	Special Features	Pupils at Rest	Direct Illumination	Contralateral Illumination	Convergence	Drugs
Amaurosis	Blind, papilla white	Right same size as left	Both pupils fail to react	Bilateral constriction	Bilateral constriction	Normal reaction to atropine and physostigmine
Oculomotor palsy	Vision intact. Disturbed mobility of right eye	Right much larger than left	Right unreactive to light, left reacts consensually	Right unreactive, left reacts	Right not constricted, left constricted	Constricts to miotics
Acute ciliary ganglionitis	Eye movements normal, otherwise identical with oculomotor palsy					
Synechiae	Eye movements normal, pupils of irregular shape	Right more contracted than left	Right unreactive to light, left reacts	Right unreactive, left reacts	Right not constricted, left constricted	Widens to mydriatics, synechiae then visible
Pupillotonia (Adie's pupil)	Usually unilateral (80%). Slow improvement of "visual sharpness" on testing close vision because of increasing accommodation	Right more widely dilated than left	Right virtually unreactive, constricts upon more prolonged and intense illumination, followed by slow (tonic) dilatation. Left reacts	Right unreactive, left reacts	Bilateral constriction, right (tonic) dilatation	Normal reaction to mydriatics
Argyll Robertson pupil	Usually bilaterally constricted pupils, often irregular	Right more or less equal with left	Bilaterally unreactive to light to greater or lesser degree	Bilaterally unreactive or reacts poorly to light	Definite constriction	Weaker mydriatics without effect. Physostigmine causes increased constriction, atropine causes mild dilatation
Atropine effect	Accommodation abolished. Lasts 10–14 days	Right far larger than left	Right unreactive, left reacts	Right unreactive to light, left reacts	Right not constricted, left constricted	No constriction with physostigmine

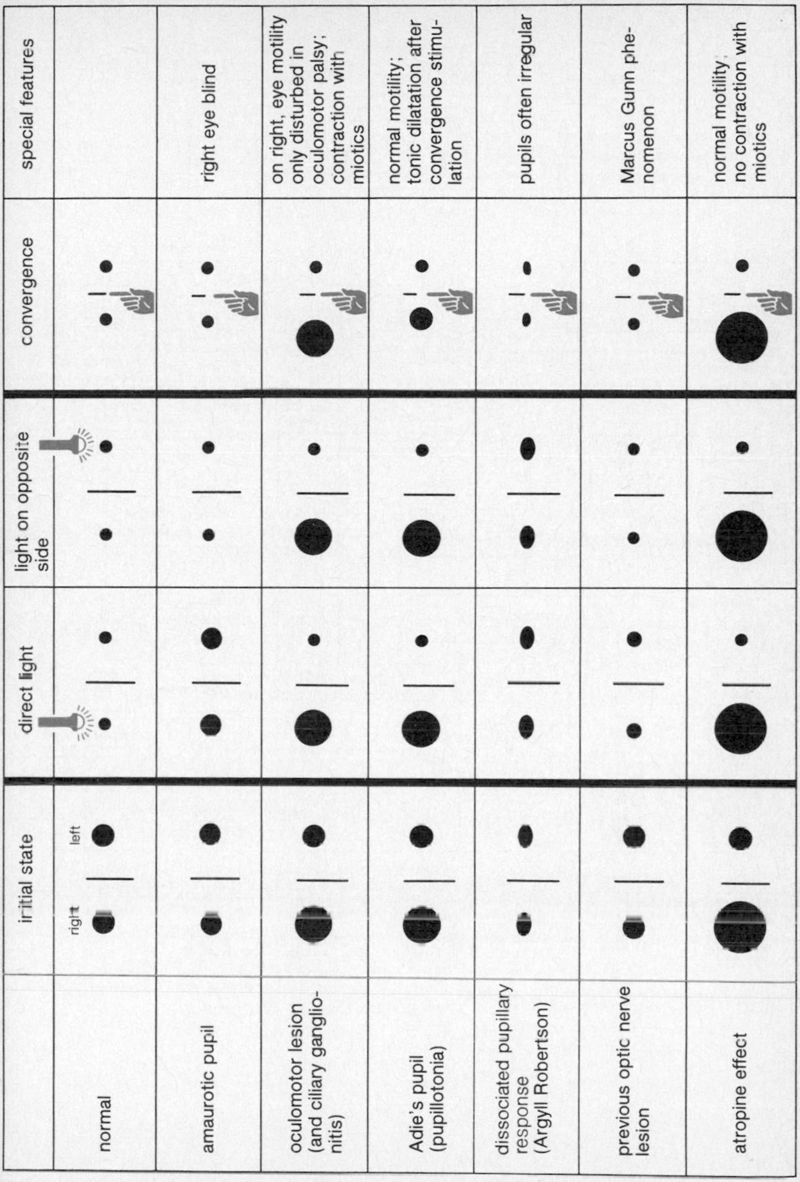

Fig. 8.9 Disturbances of pupillary reactions (right: pathologic)

	initial state	direct light	light on opposite side	convergence	special features
normal					
amaurotic pupil					right eye blind
oculomotor lesion (and ciliary ganglionitis)					on right, eye motility only disturbed in oculomotor palsy; contraction with miotics
Adie's pupil (pupillotonia)					normal motility; tonic dilatation after convergence stimulation
dissociated pupillary response (Argyll Robertson)					pupils often irregular
previous optic nerve lesion					Marcus Gunn phenomenon
atropine effect					normal motility; no contraction with miotics

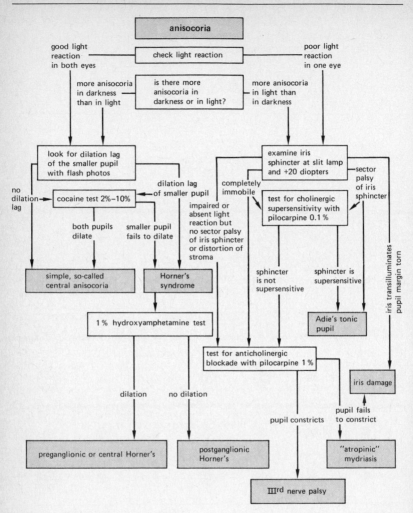

Fig. 8.**10**   Flow chart for evaluation of anisocoria (after *Thompson*)

fects (homatropine ointments) and toxic causes (botulism, diphtheria, Wernicke's syndrome, etc.). Transient unilateral pupillary dilatation may also occur in a *migraine attack* (840). Pupillary paralysis in acute pandysautonomia (55) (p. 233). Under normal conditions vigorous pinching of the upper borders of the trapezius muscles will dilate both pupils – the *ciliospinal reflex*. Absence of this reflex indicates dam-

age to the somatosensory afferents from the shoulder region, a brainstem lesion, or interruption of the descending sympathetic tract to the ciliospinal center.

Synopsis: Table 8.5 lists the most important pupillary abnormalities, which are graphically portrayed in Fig. 8.9. Figure 8.10 indicates the procedure for evaluating a case of pupillary inequality.

Trigeminal Disorders

Anatomy: The *sensory division of the trigeminal nerve* supplies the skin of half of the face from the forehead to the mandible with the exception of the mandibular angle (greater auricular nerve from the cervical plexus). The auriculotemporal division of the mandibular nerve (third division of trigeminal trunk) also supplies the tragus and the anterior part of the external auditory canal. The mucous membrane of the mouth, eye, and nose is also supplied. The *motor division of the trigeminal nerve* accompanies the mandibular division through the foramen ovale and supplies the masticatory and other muscles (temporalis, masseter, pterygoids, tensor tympani, tensor veli palatini, myohyoid, and anterior belly of the digastric muscle).

Examination technique: *Sensation* is tested by applying delicate touch stimuli and constantly comparing both sides, also by testing temperature sensation with a view to demonstrating a dissociated central disturbance as in lesions of the spinal trigeminal tract and nucleus descending as far as the C2 segment. Fibers from the ophthalmic (first) division reach farthest caudally; therefore,

under certain circumstances a local central dissociated sensory abnormality may arise. Objective examination involves the testing of various trigeminofacial reflexes. The *corneal reflex* is the easiest and most reliable since corneal sensitivity is reduced early in trigeminal lesions. The cornea is touched from the side (avoiding visually mediated blink and startle reactions, as well as contact with the conjunctiva or eyelashes), preferably either with a wisp of cotton or a facial tissue. A reduced or absent corneal reflex may indicate either a trigeminal or a facial nerve lesion. In the case of facial paralysis, the patient appreciates the touch stimulus subjectively and Bell's phenomenon (see below) occurs. In some patients the corneal reflex is normally very difficult to elicit.

The *motor fibers of the trigeminal nerve* are tested by examining the function of the masseter muscle. The examiner gently lays his fingers on both masseter muscles and asks the patient to clench his teeth. Paralysis of the pterygoid muscles manifests itself by deviation of the lower jaw to the paralyzed side with the mouth open. The masseter reflex is absent only if bilateral paralysis is present; however, it is not usually elicitable in normal subjects.

The *condition of the skin* may suffer in trigeminal palsy. Severe corneal atrophy in the form of a neuroparalytic keratitis may accompany trigeminal lesions.

Clinical aspects: *Unilateral nerve trunk lesions* may accompany fractures of the skull base, meningitis, tumors, or aneurysms. Rarer causes are *trigeminal neurofibroma* and other *tumors of the cerebellopontine angle. Cavernous sinus lesions,* e.g., thrombosis, may involve the first and second divisions and the nerves supplying the external ocular muscles; they usually cause proptosis and swelling of the eyelids. A rare cause of permanent damage of the alveolar nerve is the injection of *local anesthesia* prior to dental extraction. The mental nerve is often affected by *neoplastic metastases* in the vicinity of the mandible (numb chin sign) (405).

Lesions in the vicinity of the trigeminal nucleus and the central trigeminal tracts in the pons and medulla oblongata may be caused by *vascular damage, tumors, encephalitis, multiple sclerosis, syringomyelia* or *syringobulbia,* or *basilar impression* (677). The latter process may also be manifested by trismus.

Trigeminal paresthesias, usually occurring as part of a cranial polyneuritis (p.371), may be encountered in cases of poisoning with *trichlorethylene* or other chlorinated acetylenes (178). Often exhibiting painful features, they sometimes accompany the onset of a *peripheral facial palsy* (15) – a manifestation which may be explicable on the basis of a common blood supply to both nerve trunks (677). However, trigeminal paresthesias may occur without accompanying signs or symptoms, usually in the second or third divisions, and without pain or disturbed taste sensation or loss of muscular power. Recovery may occur within weeks, although some patients suffer permanent sensory loss. Lasting paresthesias and pains, which may be unilateral or bilateral and sometimes confined to two divisions of the nerve, may occur in certain collagen diseases, particularly *scleroderma* (61). A *burning tongue* may be present in many diseases, e.g., iron deficiency, vitamin B_{12} deficiency, or in colistin medication. It is also seen in elderly subjects, possibly as a result of brainstem circulatory disturbance.

Trigeminal neuralgia is by far the commonest facial pain and is discussed together with other facial neuralgias on p.459.

A *sensory trigeminal neuropathy* of undetermined etiology has been reported in one or more divisions of the nerve; in a few cases, both sides were involved. It may produce severe trophic changes (1140) and sensory defects, e.g., neuroparalytic keratitis (86, 1234). This lesion has a sudden onset and may last for days or months, occasionally for years. The patient experiences a numb sensation, paresthesia, or permanent pain, but he is not subjected to the short, sharp attacks of true trigeminal neuralgia. Sometimes taste sensation is disturbed in the anterior one-third of the tongue. Spontaneous healing is the rule. In several cases an underlying cause has subsequently come to light (613), e.g., multiple sclerosis, syringobulbia, a brainstem tumor, a cavernous sinus lesion, or scleroderma (352). A case is reported of a cervical cord lesion which was situated as low as C5, producing a trigeminal neuropathy or facial paresthesias (1316). In most cases the symptoms remain an isolated phenomenon, which might indeed reflect a viral ascending mononeuritis.

Facial Palsy

Anatomy: Efferent fibers to the glands in the region of the face travel with the trunk of the facial nerve and its branches (in addition to motor efferent fibers). Afferent fibers are present for the sensation of taste. Figure 8.11 provides a schematic review.

Signs of facial palsy: These can be deduced from Fig. 8.11. In *peripheral damage of the facial nerve* a picture of muscular paralysis, hyperacusis, reduced tear and salivary secretion, and an abnormal taste sensation over the anterior two-thirds of the tongue is present. The three last-named signs are caused by a lesion of the geniculate ganglion in the so-called intermediate part of the facial nerve. In complete facial palsy, all three divisions are affected to an equal degree and the patient is unable to shut his eye completely. In *central paralysis,* the forehead is always less severely affected than the mouth because the rostral part of the facial nucleus is bilaterally innervated; thus, the forehead muscles act synergistically with those on the "healthy" opposite side (Fig. 8.12). The patient can always shut his eyes in a central palsy, although normal muscular strength may be reduced.

Examination technique in facial palsy: *Motor functions* are tested in each division (wrinkling the forehead, closing the eyes, sniffing, whistling, showing the teeth, laughing, parting the lips). When the examiner is testing for wrinkling of the forehead, his finger should be pressed firmly to the patient's forehead in the midline to prevent contraction of the healthy side from being transmitted to the paralyzed side. The patient, in an attempt to shut a paralyzed eyelid, directs the eyeball upward (Bell's phenomenon). A subtle sign of mild facial palsy: the eyelashes remain more visible when the patient tries to shut his eyes tightly. When the chin is protruded and the teeth are exposed, asymmetric contraction of the platysma is visible.

Taste sensation in the anterior two-thirds of the tongue is tested by using a swab stick molded into a point and immersed in the test substances (20% glucose solution, 10% solution of table salt, 5% citric acid solution, 1% quinine solution). The patient must protrude his tongue for as long as it takes him to recognize the test substance – or fail to do so. He should be given a table listing the taste qualities of the four substances, sweet, sour, bitter, and salty,

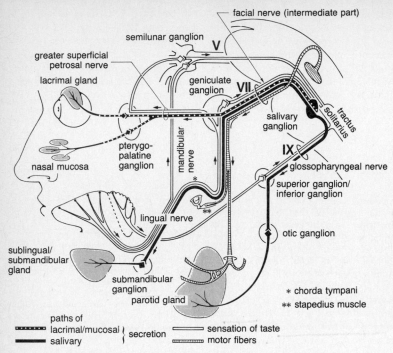

Fig. 8.11 Diagrammatic view of the facial nerve and its functions

and asked to indicate which taste he perceives. Comparison with the healthy contralateral side is always necessary, in view of the great individual variations in the capacity of normal subjects to differentiate between test substances.

Demonstration of a *disturbance of salivary secretion* is difficult – unlike the reduction in *lacrimal secretion,* which can be demonstrated by means of Schirmer's test: after preliminary anesthesia of the conjunctiva with 2 drops of a 0.4% solution of ambucaine in particularly sensitive persons, a 5 × 0.5 cm strip of filter paper is inserted into each conjunctival sac, the ends being folded over the lower lids. Normally within 5 min at least 3 cm of the filter paper has been moistened by the flow of tears. The results should be viewed as abnormal if less than 1.5 cm is moistened, i. e., when the difference with the normal side amounts to more than 30%.

Idiopathic Peripheral Facial Palsy (12, 13, 15)

Incidence and epidemiology: Of the peripheral palsies of the facial nerve, at least three-fourths are the "idiopathic" form (Bell's palsy) (12). Both sexes are affected as well as all

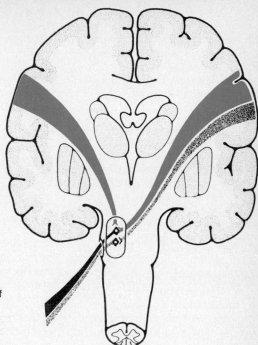

Fig. 8.**12** Bilateral cortico-bulbar innervation of the rostral area of the facial nucleus. In upper motor neuron palsy, the function of the upper branches of the facial nerve remain largely intact, because of the additional ipsilateral innervation

ages, but most patients are in their middle years. A familial incidence is also claimed.

Pathogenesis: Much evidence suggests that the disease is a cranial neuritis. The facial nerve is in the forefront, but not exclusively involved. The cause in most cases is assumed to be a viral infection (abnormal CSF cell count). The pathogenetic significance of the herpes simplex virus has been stressed (737). Analysis of an unusually large series of cases (15) has brought this primary etiology to the foreground.

In other cases a primary ischemia of the nerve trunk in the facial canal is thought to be responsible. An impressively high incidence of diabetics and prediabetics with abnormal glucose tolerance curves (66%) has been recorded in a large series of cases of facial palsy, and diabetes was commoner in the more elderly patients of the series (641). Peripheral facial palsy is also common in arterial hypertension: of 90 hypertensive adults it was present in 4%, and of 35 children with malignant hypertension in 20%. Observations made during the course of preoperative nerve stimulation support the theory of nerve compression within the facial canal. The conduction block appears to be located immediately distal to the entrance of the canal, therefore proximal to the geniculate ganglion (344, 364).

Clinical aspects: Usually within hours and only exceptionally over the course of 1-3 days, all the muscles supplied by one facial nerve become paralyzed. The degree of paralysis varies and need not be complete. Often the picture of complete paralysis is present when the patient awakes in the morning. No triggering cause can usually be identified. The *muscular weakness* has been described above. A disturbance of taste sensation should be looked for in the anterior two-thirds of the tongue (examination technique, see above). If carefully sought, discrete *signs of other cranial nerve involvement* can usually be found: In about one-half of patients, paresthesias, partly painful, are present in the trigeminal distribution and especially retroauricular pain on the affected side at the time of the paralysis or just before it (15, 679). Glossopharyngeal and vagus nerve involvement may also be present, less frequently of the cervical segments (12).

Recovery is complete in the most favorable cases within 4-6 weeks, while in others improvement may take 3-6 months to appear and leads only to partial recovery. At least 80% of cases show good recovery and only about 5%-8% a poor result with distressing residual signs and symptoms.

Residual signs: Advanced age, hyperacusis, and severe initial muscle weakness are prognostically unfavorable factors (1290). Careful examination will reveal residual signs in a significant proportion of patients: mild contracture of the facial muscles at rest, as well as synergistic mass innervation due to defective nerve regeneration. For example, when a patient shows his teeth, the ipsilateral eyelids shut. When he blows out his cheeks, the cheek on the affected side contracts along with the pursing of the lips, and appears less puffed out. The phenomenon of crocodile tears is rare, i.e., abnormal secretory fibers intended for the salivary glands but passing instead to the lacrimal gland. This misregeneration explains why the patient secretes tears during meals.

Recurrences as well as subsequent involvement of the contralateral nerve occur in about 10% of patients. Such patients show unusually severe electrophysiologic signs of denervation and have, therefore, perhaps a worse prognosis (756).

Treatment: This consists usually of prednisone medication. Provided another cause and the usual contraindications for prednisone treatment can be excluded, adults take 60 mg of prednisone on each of the first 4 days, then every 2 days 5 mg less (14). Some authors (1077, 1290) deny the success of this treatment, others recommend it (13, 14). Operative decompression by an otologic surgeon is advised after 3-4 weeks if no clinical recovery has occurred and if electromyography confirms total failure of electric stimulation.

Earlier operation has been recommended, but there is no absolute proof of the efficacy of surgery (344, 1077). In a comparative study of cases which presumably had a bad prognosis and which fulfilled the criteria for surgical treatment, no difference could be shown between patients operated within the first 2 weeks and those treated medically (784). The operation is no longer recommended in specialist clinics (14), and the author does not advise it.

Melkersson-Rosenthal Syndrome (22, 432)

Symptomatically, the facial palsy of this syndrome is identical to the idiopathic form described above. The syndrome is characterized by the triad

- facial palsy,
- swollen face, and
- plicated tongue (as in granulomatous cheilitis of Miescher).

Recurrences and bilateral facial palsies are particularly common. This condition, which is a multifocal granulomatous angiitis, involves other cranial nerves and presents with mono- and polyneuritides, plexus lesions, psychoses, and signs of encephalomyelitis (432). It exhibits a tendency to spontaneous recovery. Treatment consists of prednisone in the early stages.

Other Peripheral Facial Palsies

Craniocerebral trauma: In patients with skull fractures, about 3 per 1,000 are complicated by a delayed facial palsy, always associated with bleeding from the ear (973). In the context of *fractures of the base of the skull*, the facial palsy is present in about one-half of patients with oblique fractures of the petrous temporal bone, and 10%–30% of patients with longitudinal fractures. About 70% of cases of early paralysis, and about 90% of those with delayed paralysis, recover spontaneously. The prognosis of patients with oblique fractures is definitely worse. The best prognosis attaches to cases of delayed paralysis with longitudinal fractures, in whom the facial palsy only appears 1–20 days later, as a result of edema or hemorrhage. Cases of early paralysis caused by either oblique or longitudinal fractures should be submitted to operative decompression, as well as those cases of delayed paralysis caused by longitudinal fracture in which complete denervation is revealed by electromyography (973).

Postinfectious facial palsy: The commonest of these is a *herpes zoster oticus* palsy. This virus may be responsible for 15% of all peripheral facial palsies (12). Zoster vesicles are always visible around the ear. *The Ramsay-Hunt syndrome* is the combination with neuralgic pains following a zoster infection of the geniculate ganglion. A peripheral facial palsy may also follow *herpes zoster* in a cervical dermatome. Nuclear or peripheral facial palsies may accompany infectious diseases caused by other *neurotropic viruses* such as poliomyelitis, echo and Coxsackie infections, and in tick-borne radiculomyelomeningoencephalitis.

Other facial palsies: Middle ear diseases such as purulent otitis media or neoplasms, e.g., glomus tumors, may exhibit a facial palsy in addition to deafness and other local signs. Of *intracranial tumors,* cerebellopontine angle mass lesions sometimes cause a peripheral facial palsy. The Guillain-Barré type of polyradiculitis (p. 294) may often begin with bilateral facial palsies. In sarcoidosis unilateral or bilateral facial palsy may occur, together with parotid swelling and eye signs (Heerfordt's syndrome). Bacterial leukemic (p.163), or carcinomatous (p.203) meningitis may cause a facial palsy, together with involvement of other cranial nerves. Bilateral peripheral facial palsy – usually associated with trismus – has been repeatedly described in cases of *tetanus,* especially cerebral tetanus (755). Esmarch's bandage applied during anesthesia may lead to paralysis of the *marginal mandibular branch of the facial nerve,* causing weakness of the muscles of the mouth; sparing of the forehead and orbital branches of the nerve may lead to the mistaken diagnosis of an upper motor neuron (cerebral) lesion. In infants and neonates a lesion may be present which is visible only when the child cries; it is virtually confined to the left side of the face. This lesion is an isolated *congenital absence of the depressor anguli oris muscle,* which is viewed as a congenital aplasia (875). A congenital facial palsy forms part of Möbius's syndrome (p.347), in which numerous cases of bilateral congenital facial palsy (facial diplegia) have been described.

Hemifacial Spasm

Clinical aspects (66, 67, 546, 781): Hemifacial spasm is characterized by involuntary, synchronous, sudden tonic contractions of all the muscles of one side of the face supplied by the facial nerve. These tonic convulsive contractions last several seconds and recur irregularly every few minutes. An attack may be triggered by certain voluntary movements but usually no obvious external cause can be demonstrated. The disease as a rule begins after the age of 40 years and shows no tendency to spontaneous recovery. In

some cases, the disease persists stubbornly unchanged for months or years. *Continuous* hemifacial spasm is a feature of brainstem gliomas.

Pathogenesis: Occasionally the contractions start after a previous peripheral facial palsy. Causes that have been demonstrated in individual cases include an anomaly of the craniovertebral angle (p.20), an intracranial lesion involving the trunk of the facial nerve, and more frequently a vascular anomaly in the cerebellopontine angle (554). The posterior superior cerebellar artery is usually involved.

Treatment: In some cases a cure is achieved by operative exploration with a procedure such as packing a plug of muscle between the trunk of the nerve and the vascular anomaly, or by simple neurolysis. About 80% of operations are successful (554, 1057). Postoperative complications include the risk of unilateral deafness and an infected CSF fistula. Otologists prefer partial section of the extracranial trunk of the facial nerve, but this procedure – which should be abandoned – produces a partial paralysis of the facial muscles and relief of the spasm is only temporary. Injection of botulin toxin may be successful in relieving the condition.

Facial Myokymia

Clinical aspects: Facial myokymia is a condition in which individual muscles of one side of the face exhibit continuous wavelike contractions. **Causes** include multiple sclerosis (without accompanying facial weakness) or brain-stem tumors which may exhibit a facial palsy (977, 1228).

Facial Tics

This term denotes involuntary and sudden contractions of the facial muscles of variable location. They are present in neurotic or nervous individuals. A particular variety is *blepharospasm* (p. 127), which may be the oligosymptomatic manifestation of an extra pyramidal disturbance.

Progressive Hemifacial Atrophy

Clinical aspects: This term denotes a hereditary atrophy of the face which may present as a *"sclérodermie en coup* *de sabre"* in the midline of the face and forehead (22). The atrophic process involves bone and cartilage, as well as the brain itself. A unilateral Horner's syndrome and disturbances of external ocular movement often accompany the disease, as well as contralateral jacksonian seizures or generalized epilepsy. The **differential diagnosis** includes other facial asymmetries, e.g., caput obstipum musculare. *Bilateral facial atrophy* may be simulated by hypoplasia of the fat pad of Bichat in the cheek. True bilateral atrophy of the facial muscles caused by peripheral vasoconstriction has been described following beta-blocker medication and exposure of the face to cold (19).

Disturbances of the Vestibulocochlear Nerve (76)

Examination of the Sense of Hearing

Purpose of Examination

The neurologist, as a rule, should confine himself to determining whether partial or complete deafness is present, and he should differentiate between conduction and sensorineural deafness. Complete deafness is invariably a perceptive deafness caused by an inner ear lesion, and not a disease of the conducting apparatus (e.g., otitis media). CNS lesions, cortical or subcortical in location, because of the bilateral projection of the cochleocortical tracts, do not cause clinically significant disturbances of hearing.

The following three tests may be carried out by neurologists:

Auditory acuity: The hearing of whispered words and normal speech is first tested. For this purpose, the patient or an assistant places a finger in the opposite external auditory meatus and masks it by repeated firm pressure and release movements.

Weber's test: If a tuning fork is placed in the midline of the forehead, lateralization occurs toward the diseased ear in conduction deafness and toward the healthy ear in perceptive disorders.

Rinne test: This test is based on the fact that, in normal subjects, air conduction is better than bone conduction. A tuning fork is first placed on the mastoid and, as soon as it can no longer be heard, is held in front of the ear. Normally the fork should be heard twice as long in front of the ear as on the mastoid (Rinne test positive, i.e., normal). In conductive disorders the test is abnormal and the air conduction time is reduced or absent (Rinne test negative). In perceptive disorders, the Rinne test remains normal.

Features of Two Types of Hearing Loss

These may be summarized as follows:

In conduction deafness:

- hearing is diminished,
- the patient is not completely deaf,
- Weber's test lateralizes to the abnormal ear, and the
- Rinne test is abnormal (air conduction is reduced or absent).

In perceptive deafness:

- hearing is diminished, sometimes the patient is completely deaf,
- Weber's test is lateralized to the normal ear, and the
- Rinne test is positive, i.e., normal.

Recruitment Phenomenon

Fowler's recruitment phenomenon (measurement of binaural loudness balance) is especially useful in differentiating labyrinthine (i.e., cochlear) deafness caused by lesions such as acoustic trauma or Ménière's disease from retrolabyrinthine deafness due to trauma or a schwannoma of the eighth nerve. Damage to the organ of Corti affects the outer, more sensitive hair cells more severely. Sounds of equal intensity are less easily heard in the poorer ear than in the good one, the sound barrier being initially higher. With increasing intensities of sound, the undamaged inner hair cells begin to react (being "recruited") so that once a high intensity is reached, hearing is equal in both ears. Here recruitment is "positive." In conductive lesions of the auditory (vestibulocochlear nerve) this does not occur, recruitment is "negative."

Hearing Disturbances in a Neurologic Context

Unilateral or Bilateral Deafness of Sudden Onset

Causes: The commonest cause is an *infection,* frequently mumps (even without parotid swelling) and herpes zoster (even without obvious vesicular eruption). Less often a vascular lesion involving the labyrinthine (internal auditory) artery is responsible, which may lead to cochlear apoplexy (usually combined with labyrinthine failure). In cases of *rupture of the oval or round window,* immediate deafness is accompanied by tinnitus and sometimes dizziness. The usual cause is altitudinal trauma (air travel), craniocerebral trauma, or unusual exertion. Otosurgical treatment is indicated (382). Exceptionally, *multiple sclerosis* may present clinically as unilateral deafness. *Oblique fractures of the petrous pyramid* may involve the vestibulocochlear nerve. Only about 50% of cases of sudden deafness recover.

Progressive Loss of Hearing

Causes: Various neurologic diseases may present with increasing impairment of hearing. The first to consider are *tumors of the base of the skull* (e.g., see Garcin's syndrome, p.372) or the cerebellopontine angle syndrome (p.37), especially *acoustic neurilemmoma (schwannoma).* Usually the deafness is preceded by tinnitus. *Paget's disease of bone* involving the skull frequently causes progressive hearing loss before actual deafness, and occasionally also hemifacial spasm or trigeminal neuralgia. This is particularly likely in those cases leading to basilar impression, which are frequently also accompanied by pyramidal tract signs (244). *Glomus jugulare tumors* arising from the chemoreceptors of the vagus nerve (1135) cause, apart from a progressive loss of hearing with tinnitus, a homolateral murmur which is synchronous with the pulse, always heard by the patient and usually audible to the examiner. Signs of homolateral facial or other cranial nerve involvement appear later. In about 10% of cases signs of abnormally raised intracranial pressure are present. The swelling often reveals itself as a bluish mass on the eardrum on otoscopic examination. Treatment is surgical resection and/or embolization (511).

Progressive hearing loss may be a symptom of genetically determined *metabolic anomalies* such as Refsum's disease (p. 139), Niemann-Pick disease (p. 139), or other *systemic disorders*, e.g., Friedreich's ataxia (p. 224). Basal *meningitides* and *syphilis*, particularly congenital syphilis, may be followed by deafness. *Cogan's syndrome* (68, 75, 129, 233, 494) is viewed as a rare multisystemic disease, the signs affecting various organs. In about 50% of cases, the nervous system is involved. Apart from headache, mental changes, disturbances of consciousness, epileptic seizures, cerebral vascular accidents, and neuropathies, there may be increasing loss of hearing, vestibular lesions, and a nonsyphilitic interstitial keratitis. The disease affects young adults and bouts may persist for months or years. Prolonged follow-up has revealed a vasculitis in three-fourths of cases (233). About 10% show the most dangerous complication, namely involvement of the aortic valve. The topic of deafness is further discussed below *in the context of vestibular disorders*.

Tinnitus and Other Ear Noises
(75, 347, 686)

Tinnitus may be defined as a noise which is regular and persistent and which is confined to one ear or diffusely transmitted within the head. Patients make use of a variety of descriptive terms, such as pips, noise, murmur, etc.

Causes: In most cases, tinnitus is a benign, *self-contained disease entity* which is annoying but not dangerous, and which appears late in life. **Clinically,** tinnitus may accompany other diseases. It may be seen in *raised intracranial pressure* and is then abolished by the Valsalva maneuver or compression of both jugular veins (783). Tinnitus may also accompany a *cerebellopontine angle tumor*, as well as *Ménière's disease*. In these two last-named instances, the tinnitus is localized to one ear. An *ear murmur* synchronous with the *pulse* may be benign and harmless, but it should prompt suspicion of an *arterial stenosis* adjacent to the ear, *arteriovenous malformation*, e.g., extracranial occipital vessels, *arteriovenous fistula of the cavernous sinus*, or a *glomus tumor*.

Examination of Vestibular Function (1069)

Definition: Position and movements are controlled by the peripheral vestibular apparatus of the inner ear and its central nuclei and tracts. The stimuli arising here are directed centripetally to the brainstem where they are integrated with other afferent impulses (visual, proprioceptive), concerned with the maintenance of balance. A disturbance of the vestibular apparatus results in disturbances of balance

- subjectively (dizziness), and
- objectively (weakness and uncertainty of balance, ataxia).

Examination Technique

Nystagmus

Nystagmus is tested with the patient seated, first with distant vision and then with the patient moving his eye from side to side. If the nystagmus manifests itself only when the eyeballs reach extreme positions, the examiner should bring his finger back about 10°. It is important to remember that the nystagmus is significant only if it remains visible in that new position. Occasionally nystagmus will be first demonstrated when the patient shakes his head vigorously or repeatedly, or drops it backward or sideways. The following are differentiated:

- nystagmus grade I (present only if the patient looks in the direction of the nystagmus),
- grade II (in the primary position), and
- grade III (in all directions of gaze).

Positional Testing

This serves to detect an anomaly of the hair cells or cupulolithiasis (with benign paroxysmal positional nystagmus). The patient's head is tilted about 30° backward over the edge of the bed and simultaneously rotated about 30° to one side. After about 5 s a rotatory nystagmus appears in these entities, accompanied by an intense rotatory vertigo and nausea. If the head is rotated to the left side, these severe rotatory movements of the eyeballs occur in a clockwise direction; and if to the right, they are counterclockwise.

Basic Vestibular Testing

Vestibular testing by thermal and rotatory stimulation is usually carried out by an otologist. However, occasionally the neurologist will wish to verify for himself that the vestibular apparatus remains receptive to labyrinthine stimulation. This can be done most simply as follows: the patient is positioned so that his trunk (and head) are raised at an angle of 30° above the horizontal or he is seated erect with his head tilted backward 60°. After verifying the absence of tympanic perforation by prior otoscopic examination, the examiner irrigates the left external auditory canal with 100–200 ml of water at room temperature or 5–10 ml of iced water. This measure normally produces a horizontal nystagmus with the slow component to the left and the fast component to the right side. The patient points incorrectly to the left and shows a tendency to fall to the left. At the same time, ataxia and nausea appear. If these reactions are absent, it is because the vestibular apparatus can no longer be stimulated, i.e., connections between the labyrinth and brainstem have been interrupted.

Tests for Balance

In the context of the neurologic examination, the following tests possess particular importance in the presence of vertigo:

- *Romberg's sign:* The patient stands with his eyes shut, feet parallel and close together, and arms outstretched and supinated.

- *Straight line test (tandem gait):* The patient places one foot accurately in front of the other; the test should be carried out with the eyes first fixed on the ceiling and then shut. The healthy subject manages this maneuver quite easily, although sometimes difficulty is experienced with the eyes shut.
- *Unterberger gait test:* The patient performs a high-stepping gait while remaining on the spot with his eyes shut. After 50 steps, normal subjects may be expected to turn no more than 45°, usually to the left side.
- *Walking test (Babinski-Weil):* With his eyes shut, the patient takes two steps forward and then two steps backward. If a labyrinthine disturbance is present, he will turn gradually to the affected side.

Positional Test

The patient holds his arms up in a horizontal position with his eyes shut. If a labyrinthine disturbance is present, the arm on the side of the abnormality will deviate from this position.

Finger Test

The patient holds his arm in a raised position and aims at a precise point, such as the examiner's outstretched finger. If a labyrinthine abnormality is present, the patient with his eyes shut allows the arm to fall slowly and deviate to the side of the defect.

Vertigo and Nystagmus

Acute rotatory vertigo may accompany a variety of disorders (942). These include disorders of the *peripheral vestibular apparatus* and acute lesions in the neighborhood of the *vestibular nuclei* in the medulla oblongata.

Ménière's Disease (41, 942)

Clinical aspects: This disease is typified by attacks of rotatory vertigo which recur irregularly, appear explosively, last up to several hours, and then slowly recede over several more hours or rarely after some days. Most patients experience nausea or vomiting and are unable to stand up. Almost invariably the attacks are accompanied by tinnitus and mild deafness or at least a feeling of a blocked ear. Immediately after an attack, nystagmus is present, which shows the features of a peripheral vestibular disturbance, as defined in Table 8.6. Immediately after an attack, a unilaterally diminished excitability of the vestibular apparatus is also found; both signs later return to normal. Usually attacks of the disease begin between

Table 8.**6**   Features of peripheral forms of vestibular nystagmus (after *V. Henn* 1978)

- Direction of beat usually horizontal but with a torsion component. A vertical component is rare
- Slow phase toward the side of the lesion
- Reduced intensity through visual fixation (therefore increased with eyes shut)
- Increased by altering the position of the head or shaking it, or lying on the side of the affected labyrinth
- Amplitude of the slow phase of nystagmus increases if the eyes are turned away
- Sometimes unilaterally reduced caloric response
- Pursuit and saccadic eye movement normal

the ages of 20 and 50 years, affecting men and women equally. Only 10% of cases are bilateral. The initial attacks have no sequelae, but later an increasing loss of hearing develops, and an insensitivity of the vestibular apparatus which leads finally to complete labyrinthine failure and consequent cessation of the attacks. The cochlear site of the hearing disturbance may be proved by positive recruitment (see above).

Variants: One of these is *Lermoyez's syndrome (le vertige qui fait entendre)*. In this syndrome, a progressive unilateral hearing loss and tinnitus is followed some days later by an acute attack of vertigo which resembles Ménière's disease. Thereafter the patient's hearing improves. Another variant, the *Tullio phenomenon,* is a form of vertigo induced by noise.

Treatment (168): Treatment may be extremely difficult. During an attack, sedation with diazepam or phenobarbital is necessary. Cervical sympathetic blockade or infusion with procaine is recommended. Between attacks, reduced fluid and salt intake as well as diuretics are advised. Smoking and alcohol should be avoided. When conservative treatment fails and provided hearing is intact, selective saccotomy may be performed. Otherwise, labyrinthectomy or vestibular neurectomy may have to be carried out, leading to unilateral deafness.

Acute Isolated Vestibular Disturbance (Vestibular Neuronitis) (942, 988)

Clinical features: This is a type of rotatory vertigo of sudden onset which depends on the position of the head, and which may persist for several days before gradually subsiding. The patient vomits and may initially be confined to bed. (Not infrequently the first attack is experienced in the morning when the patient awakes.) Unlike Ménière's disease, no abnormal auditory sensation or loss of hearing is present. Initially nystagmus occurs and the vestibular apparatus shows a reduced caloric response.

Etiology: This is seldom established. Sometimes an infective lesion may be present, either generalized or localized to the skull.

Prognosis: In many cases, the disturbance is confined to a single unilateral episode. Other patients suffer recurrent attacks over many years. Following each acute attack, they may exhibit unsteadiness on walking or standing and especially after rapid head movements *(trigger labyrinth)*. Despite full clinical recovery, careful electronystagmographic tests are always abnormal, although the defect is seldom severe (998).

Variants: A similar picture is shown by the sequences of attacks occurring in the context of an *epidemic vertigo* (928). A similar picture may occur *after tick bite*. The term *benign paroxysmal vertigo of childhood* (201) is used to describe an acute recurrent rotatory vertigo appearing early in life: suddenly the child starts to hold on, can no longer walk unaided, and complains of feeling sick. On examination, he is pale, exhibits nystagmus, and may sometimes vomit. Each attack lasts only a few seconds or minutes. The attacks recur after an unpredictable interval, sometimes several within the same week. Vestibular testing is always abnormal. *Toxic effects of drugs* may also lead to vestibular disturbances with vertigo, e.g., streptomycin toxicity or barbiturate, or diphenylhydantoin intoxication.

Nystagmus of Benign Paroxysmal Type (487, 507, 844)

Clinical aspects: These patients complain of episodes of acute rotatory vertigo. In some, a severe attack of vertigo is precipitated only if the head is held in a specific and constant position – usually by turning over in bed to a particular side. The associated vagal stimulation may in some cases lead to syncope ("vestibular syncope") (845). The labyrinth shows a normal caloric response. However, positional testing (see above) may provoke an attack. The vertigo usually disappears spontaneously after one or more days, but it may recur.

Pathogenesis and etiology: This syndrome is caused by a unilateral disturbance of the peripheral otolith apparatus. Calcium is deposited in the sensory hairs of the cupular cells, resulting in an increased sensitivity of these cells to physiologic stimulation. In many cases, no cause can be identified, but craniocerebral trauma, vertebrobasilar circulatory insufficiency, labyrinthitis, middle ear disease, etc. may be present (487, 507).

Treatment: By the application of repeated, discrete stimuli, a central adaptation may be achieved which enables the patient to live a normal life, e.g., enabling him to turn round in bed without severe rotatory vertigo. He should be advised to avoid sudden movements of his head in order not to provoke attacks of vertigo.

Other neurologically relevant vertigo and nystagmus variants: Various diseases may be accompanied by vertigo or nystagmus (595), in addition to the abnormalities described above with the episodes of acute vestibular rotatory vertigo.

Congenital nystagmus is usually a pendular nystagmus, horizontal or rotatory. It is often part of a familial syndrome including strabismus, albinism, blindness, and color blindness; exceptionally it may be monocular. Fixation abolishes the nystagmus.

Latent nystagmus is also a congenital variety, appearing when one eye is covered although present in both eyes. It is always accompanied by a strabismus.

About 80% of young persons appear capable of producing a *voluntary nystagmus*. It is a pendular nystagmus of irregular frequency (1309).

Spasmus nutans (52, 377) is a separate disease entity, which is seen in infants aged 4–18 months, usually during the winter months. Its characteristic feature is a nystagmus which is horizontal, vertical, or rotatory, and unilateral or bilateral, and usually rapid and fine in character. Associated irregular, waggling movements of the head occur, in which the head may be turned to one side. No cause is known, and the signs and symptoms usually disappear within a few months. Tumors involving the third ventricle and optic chiasm may produce nystagmus or cause the child to incline his head to one side – and this may be mistaken for spasmus nutans (52).

"Autonomic" vertigo: Numerous patients with autonomic dystonia and hyperventilation tetany complain of nonspecific vertigo.

Vertigo is encountered in patients with cerebral arteriosclerosis or cardiovascular diseases producing intermittent *cerebral circulatory insufficiency,* especially vertebrobasilar insufficiency. These attacks may occur before the circulatory disease is complicated by syncope.

Spondylotic vertigo: Vertigo is far too often attributed to roentgenologically detectable cervical spondylosis, which is encountered every day by the practicing physician. Nonetheless, a true spondylotic vertigo exists (1235). It is particularly common after whiplash injuries of the cervical spine (1201) (p.378). Abnormal stimuli from the cervical intervertebral joints and soft tissues integrate with other afferent responses in the brainstem to provoke vertiginous symptoms.

Psychogenic vertigo is a diagnosis too often made. However, vertigo may sometimes be the external manifestation of a conflict situation, reflecting a "no longer in equilibrium" feeling or anxiety (977).

Bilateral destruction of the vestibular apparatus: **Clinically,** these lesions are indicated by the patient's inability, even with his eyes open, to walk on a soft mattress without falling over. In order to maintain balance correctly, at least two of the three external afferents (vestibular system, deep sensory modalities, visual connections) must be intact. In bilateral defects of the vestibular apparatus, the additional disorganization of the afferents from the joints and the skin of the soles of the feet is sufficient to impair balance seriously. **Causes** are usually postinfectious (mumps!) or toxic (streptomycin), and may sometimes follow traumatic damage.

Rarer causes: Repeated references are made to "dizziness" in the context of paraspastic or ataxic gait disturbances, abnormal proprioceptive afferents (e.g., posterior column lesions or polyneuropathies), epileptic absences, and also epileptic aura or true epileptic vertigo. Finally, visual disturbances such as double vision may be described by the patient as vertigo.

Glossopharyngeal and Vagal Disturbances

Anatomy: The nucleus ambiguus gives origin to nerve fibers that separate into various divisions to constitute the *glossopharyngeal* and *vagus* nerves, which innervate the muscles of the soft palate and the pharynx; the recurrent laryngeal nerve supplies the laryngeal muscles. The glossopharyngeal nerve provides sensory innervation for the soft palate, pharynx, tonsillar fossa, and middle ear. It also carries taste fibers from the posterior one-third of the tongue (see Fig.8.11). It supplies parasympathetic fibers to the parotis via the otic ganglion and the facial nerve. The vagus nerve carries sensory fibers from the external auditory canal and part of the external ear as well as from the posterior cranial fossa and efferent parasympathetic autonomic fibers to the thoracic and abdominal viscera.

Symptomatology: Paralysis of the vagus nerve (and glossopharyngeal nerve) may be demonstrated by inability to elicit the gag and palatal reflexes on the affected side. The patient volunteers that sensation is different on the two sides. The soft palate hangs down on the paralyzed side, and during retching or phonation ("aah") is displaced toward the healthy side: the posterior faucial wall is displaced horizontally toward the healthy side producing the stage curtain sign (see Fig. 1.**11**). Paralysis of the recurrent laryngeal nerve is initially evidenced as a hoarseness of the voice which within weeks becomes compensated. Occasionally, however, a disturbance of phonation may be demonstrated later on, when the patient sings. Glossopharyngeal neuralgia, see p. 461.

Causes: *Nuclear paralyses,* i.c., lesions of the nuclei of the ninth and tenth cranial nerves in the brainstem, may form part of a complex clinical picture in vascular disturbances, tumors, encephalitides, or demyelinating plaques of multiple sclerosis in the medulla oblongata (see Table 1.**10**).

Lesions of the nerve trunks may occur solitarily or combined with other lower cranial nerve deficits. They may form part of the syndrome of *basilar impression* or be caused by a neurofibroma or a *tumor of the skull base*, e.g., extracranial masses extending from the epipharynx. In *children* and adolescents, the association of *isolated unilateral glossopharyngeal and vagal palsy* with palatal paralysis and the stage curtain phenomenon is viewed as a separate clinical entity (65); it is interpreted as a cranial mononeuropathy (1004). These children, who are afebrile, suddenly exhibit nasal speech and a painless disturbance of swallowing; the CSF is usually normal including the protein content. The signs and symptoms almost always disappear completely within weeks or months. In patients with *fractures of the skull base* which extend into the jugular foramen, the cranial nerves traversing this foramen (9th, 10th, and 11th) may be paralyzed (Siebenmann's syndrome). Rarely, a similar clinical picture may occur in intracranial venous thrombosis or after torticollis; however, spontaneous recovery is the rule. A vascular mechanism is assumed in these benign and completely reversible palsies of the caudal cranial nerves (293). Tapia's syndrome (p. 76), i.e., involvement of the 9th, 10th, and 12th cranial nerves, may be caused by an *aneurysm* of the extracranial part of the internal carotid artery.

Differential diagnosis: This includes the palatal paralysis of diphtheria and pseudoparalytic myasthenia gravis.

Accessory Paralysis

Anatomy: The accessory nerve consists of two roots, internal and external. The *internal* root accompanies the posterior part of the vagus nerve – of which it is a part – in its intracranial course to the jugular foramen, innervating the larynx. The *external* (or spinal) root is the actual accessory nerve and runs a separate extracranial course. It innervates the sternomastoid muscle and the upper part of the trapezius muscle. The accessory nucleus is bilaterally innervated so that upper motor neuron lesions do not lead to significant functional deficits in either of these muscles.

Symptomatology and examination technique: Only motor deficits occur. If the lesion is situated in the lateral cervical triangle, only the *upper part of the trapezius muscle* is paralyzed. Examination reveals a dropped shoulder, a tilted scapula, and reduced muscle power on raising the shoulder. Nerve function is tested by the patient and examiner facing each other seated. The examiner places his hands on the patient's shoulders, using his thumb and index fingers to grasp the upper part of the trapezius muscles to demonstrate atrophy and to test active contraction. Muscular weakness can be satisfactorily evaluated by testing shoulder elevation against resistance. If the lesion involves the proximal part of the accessory trunk, additional weakness of the *sternomastoid muscle* is present. The sternomastoid rotates the head to the opposite side. Therefore, the right muscle is tested by checking the patient's ability to overcome resistance by rotating the head against the examiner's right hand, which is placed on the left side of the patient's face.

Causes: The commonest cause of isolated paralysis of the accessory nerve is iatrogenic trauma, usually as a result of *biopsy of lymph nodes on the posterior border of the sternomastoid muscle* (851, 1162). This is the cause in three-fourths of cases. Usually the patient notices the lesion some weeks after the biopsy when he starts to use his arm again and discovers specific muscular weakness or shoulder pain upon arm or shoulder movement. Typical findings are a dropped shoulder, a tilted scapula, and atrophy of the upper part of the trapezius muscle, without sensory deficit or involvement of the sternomastoid muscle. Paralysis of the accessory nerve may accompany anomalies of the craniovertebral junction, tumors of the foramen magnum, and the foramen jugulare syndrome. Additional neurologic signs are present in all of these conditions.

Hypoglossal Paralysis

Anatomy and examination technique: The 12th cranial nerve gains exit from the skull through the hypoglossal foramen in the occipital bone and supplies the tongue musculature. A lesion of the nerve presents as an atrophy of the tongue which, when protruded, deviates to the paralyzed side. Weakness of lateral movement to the opposite side may also be shown when the patient pushes his tongue against the inside of his cheek as the examiner palpates this movement with his fingers placed over the cheek.

Causes of tongue paralysis: An *upper motor neuron paralysis* may be present in acute stroke and be accompanied by other signs of *hemiplegia.* However, functional compensation is very rapid. Bilateral upper motor neuron paralysis – e. g., part of the picture of *pseudobulbar palsy* (p. 85) – is a marked handicap, producing severe disturbances of speech and swallowing. No atrophy occurs in such cases. *Buccolingual apraxia*

and oral diplegia in the *Foix-Chavany-Marie syndrome* have been discussed earlier (p. 69).

The commonest cause of a lower *motor neuron tongue paralysis* is *true bulbar palsy,* occurring as a feature of motor neuron disease (p. 221). Tongue paralysis associated with a crossed hemiparesis due to unilateral vascular damage of the medulla oblongata is the picture of so-called *Jackson's paralysis.*

Lesions of the *peripheral hypoglossal trunk* may complicate a *fracture of the skull base* involving the *posterior cranial fossa, basilar impression, tumors* of the base of the brain, *dissecting aneurysm of the carotid artery,* and extracranial tumors of the skull base. Occasionally, isolated and reversible attacks of paralysis are described following infection (16).

Multiple Lower Cranial Nerve Palsies

Cranial Polyradiculitis

Individual instances can be cited of cases in which, in addition to involvement of spinal nerves, lower cranial nerves were affected, especially the facial nerves. These cases are usually viewed as atypical examples of the Guillain-Barré syndrome (p. 294). Prolonged bouts of headache may herald these lesions, which tend to recover spontaneously. Recurrences months or years later are not uncommon. Granu-

lomatous inflammatory lesions of the perineural meninges are reported (1150). Mention should be made here of Fisher's syndrome (p. 298).

Recurrent Multiple Cranial Nerve Palsies

This picture may be the manifestation of sarcoidosis, a paraproteinemia, or a dysproteinemia (Bing-Neel syndrome). Multiple peripheral nerve palsies, which may sometimes start as an isolated cranial nerve deficit, may complicate vascular lesions such as periarteritis nodosa and are part of Cogan's syndrome (p.363) (68).

Progressive Paralysis of Multiple Cranial Nerves

This picture may indicate a chronic meningitis, meningeal carcinomatosis, or syphilis. Bilateral cranial nerve lesions have been described in cases of poorly controlled diabetes mellitus. Skeletal diseases such as those of Paget and Albers-Schönberg (marble bones) may be complicated by cranial nerve palsies. Trigeminal lesions and evidence of involvement of other cranial nerves have been described in trichlorethylene poisoning (pp.319 and 354).

Garcin's Syndrome

This syndrome, unilateral involvement of the lower cranial nerves, is usually caused by a tumor of the skull base.

Rarer Causes

A progressive deficit of the lower cranial nerves accompanied by signs of autonomic dysregulation – due to a lesion of the carotid sinus and sympathetic chain – many years after carotid angiography with Thorotrast may indicate the presence of a *thorotrastoma* (124). Lower cranial nerve palsies may accompany osteomyelitis of the skull base, as well as *malignant otitis externa.* An equally rare entity, the *stylokeratohyoid syndrome* (696), is a phylogenetically related anomaly of the hyoid bone which may lead to involvement of the 5th, 7th, 9th, and 10th cranial nerves, unilateral neck pain, disturbances of swallowing, and vertigo.

9. Spinal Radicular Syndromes (472, 851)

Symptomatology

Lesions of individual spinal nerve roots usually exhibit the following symptoms and signs:

- *Pains* in the territory of supply of the affected root (exceptionally in acute lesions pain may be absent).
- *Sensory loss* corresponding to the appropriate dermatome (see Fig. 2.1), which may be mapped out by testing the modality of cutaneous pain (but not that of superficial sensation or touch, which is not always diminished).
- *Paralysis of individual muscles* innervated by the particular nerve root. The muscles are listed in Table 9.1, and the characteristic features of lesions of individual roots are given in Table 9.2.
- *Muscular atrophy* is common but usually less impressive than the

atrophy seen in lesions of the peripheral nerves, and visible only about 3 weeks after the lesion.
- *Fasciculation* may sometimes accompany radicular lesions.
- *Tendon reflexes* may be diminished, corresponding to the affected nerve root (follow Tables 2.1 and 9.2).
- *Vertebral column signs and symptoms* may develop including pains, abnormal posture, or restricted movements, reflecting the intra- or paraspinous site of the lesion (tumor or disk prolapse).
- *Paravertebral sensory disturbances* may be present if the lesion involves the root proximal to the posterior ramus (i.e., not beyond the intervertebral foramen, e.g., disk herniation).

Disk Disease Causing Radicular Syndromes

Pathologic anatomy: The intervertebral disk consists of a fibrous ring, the anulus fibrosus, which confines the remaining soft contents of the disk within it. The central part consists of the gelatinous nucleus pulposus. Throughout life the disk slowly loses some of its

fluid content; consequently its elasticity diminishes. As a reaction to these changes, *spondylosis* deforms the edges of the adjacent vertebral bodies. In other cases, disk material may herniate through damaged fibers of the anulus fibrosus – a process which is called, ac-

Table 9.1 Radicular innervation of arm and leg muscles (from *Bing, R.:* Kompendium der topischen Gehirn- und Rückenmarksdiagnostik, Schwabe, Basle 1953)

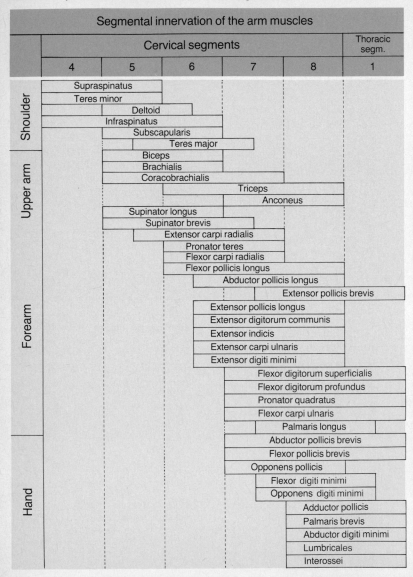

Segmental innervation of the arm muscles					
	Cervical segments				Thoracic segm.
	4	5	6	7	8	1

Shoulder: Supraspinatus; Teres minor; Deltoid; Infraspinatus; Subscapularis; Teres major

Upper arm: Biceps; Brachialis; Coracobrachialis; Triceps; Anconeus; Supinator longus; Supinator brevis; Extensor carpi radialis; Pronator teres

Forearm: Flexor carpi radialis; Flexor pollicis longus; Abductor pollicis longus; Extensor pollicis brevis; Extensor pollicis longus; Extensor digitorum communis; Extensor indicis; Extensor carpi ulnaris; Extensor digiti minimi; Flexor digitorum superficialis; Flexor digitorum profundus; Pronator quadratus; Flexor carpi ulnaris; Palmaris longus; Abductor pollicis brevis; Flexor pollicis brevis; Opponens pollicis; Flexor digiti minimi; Opponens digiti minimi

Hand: Adductor pollicis; Palmaris brevis; Abductor digiti minimi; Lumbricales; Interossei

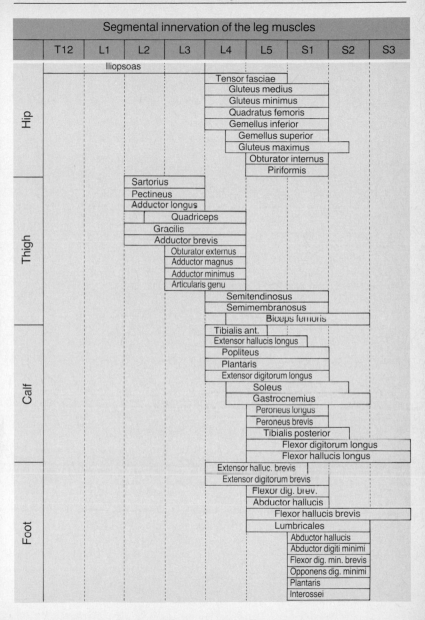

Segmental innervation of the leg muscles

	T12	L1	L2	L3	L4	L5	S1	S2	S3

Hip
- Iliopsoas
- Tensor fasciae
- Gluteus medius
- Gluteus minimus
- Quadratus femoris
- Gemellus inferior
- Gemellus superior
- Gluteus maximus
- Obturator internus
- Piriformis

Thigh
- Sartorius
- Pectineus
- Adductor longus
- Quadriceps
- Gracilis
- Adductor brevis
- Obturator externus
- Adductor magnus
- Adductor minimus
- Articularis genu
- Semitendinosus
- Semimembranosus
- Biceps femoris

Calf
- Tibialis ant.
- Extensor hallucis longus
- Popliteus
- Plantaris
- Extensor digitorum longus
- Soleus
- Gastrocnemius
- Peroneus longus
- Peroneus brevis
- Tibialis posterior
- Flexor digitorum longus
- Flexor hallucis longus

Foot
- Extensor halluc. brevis
- Extensor digitorum brevis
- Flexor dig. brev.
- Abductor hallucis
- Flexor hallucis brevis
- Lumbricales
- Abductor hallucis
- Abductor digiti minimi
- Flexor dig. min. brevis
- Opponens dig. minimi
- Plantaris
- Interossei

Table 9.2 Synopsis of radicular syndromes (851)

Segment	Sensation	Muscles Involved	Tendon Reflexes	Remarks
C3/4	Pain (hypalgesia) in shoulder region	Partial or total paralysis of diaphragm	No detectable changes	Partial diaphragmatic paralysis, C3 more ventral and C4 more dorsal
C5	Pain (hypalgesia) over lateral aspect of shoulder, covering deltoid muscle	Disturbance of innervation of deltoid and biceps brachii muscles	Diminished or absent biceps reflex	
C6	Dermatome on outer aspect of arm and forearm as far as the thumb	Paralysis of biceps brachii and brachioradialis muscles	Diminished or absent biceps reflex	This is useful to differentiate from the carpal tunnel syndrome
C7	Dermatome lateral and dorsal to C6 dermatome, including index to ring fingers	Paralysis of triceps brachii, pronator teres, and occasionally the finger flexors; often visible atrophy of the thenar eminence	Diminished or absent triceps reflex	Differential diagnosis of carpal tunnel syndrome: note the triceps reflex!
C8	Dermatome dorsal to C7, extending to include little finger	Small muscles of hand, visible atrophy especially of hypothenar eminence	Diminished triceps reflex	Differential diagnosis of ulnar nerve palsy: note the triceps reflex!
L3	Dermatome extending from greater trochanter over the extensor surface to the medial side of the thigh and knee	Paralysis of quadriceps femoris muscle	Diminished quadriceps reflex (knee jerk)	Differential diagnosis of femoral nerve palsy: area of saphenous nerve innervation remains intact

L4	Dermatome extending from lateral surface of the thigh across the knee to the anterior and medial quadrant of the leg, including the medial part of the sole	Paralysis of quadriceps femoris and tibialis anterior muscles	Diminished quadriceps reflex (knee jerk)	Differential diagnosis of femoral nerve palsy: involvement of tibialis anterior muscle
L5	Dermatome extending from above lateral condyle of femur, over the anterior and outer quadrant of the leg as far as the great toe	Paralysis and atrophy of extensor hallucis longus, often also extensor digitorum brevis muscles	Absent tibialis posterior reflex useful only if the opposite reflex can be clearly elicited	
S1	Dermatome extending from flexor surface of thigh to outer and posterior quadrant of leg, and over the lateral malleolus to the little toe	Paralysis of peroneal muscles, not infrequently also disturbances of innervation of the triceps surae (gastrocnemius-soleus) muscle	Absent triceps surae reflex (ankle jerk)	
Combined L4/5	L4 and L5 dermatomes	All extensor muscles of ankle; also disturbances of innervation of quadriceps femoris	Diminished quadriceps reflex. Absent tibialis posterior reflex	Differential diagnosis of peroneal nerve palsy: peroneal muscles escape. Note knee jerk and tibialis posterior reflex
Combined L5/S1	L5 and S1 dermatomes	Extensors of toes, peroneal muscles, occasionally also disturbances of innervation of triceps surae muscles	Absent tibialis posterior and triceps surae reflexes (ankle jerk)	Differential diagnosis of peroneal nerve palsy: tibialis anterior muscle escapes. Note the reflex findings

cording to its extent, *disk protrusion, herniation,* or *prolapse.* The herniating disk material may consist of fibrous material or of the soft gelatinous nucleus, *herniation of the nucleus pulposus.* This type of disk herniation may also luxate into the spinal canal and present as sequestrated material discontinuous with the original disk.

Disk material herniating into the spinal canal may compress the spinal cord or, if the herniation obliterates an intervertebral foramen, a *nerve root.* Such lesions may also result from the reactive spondylotic changes at the margins of the vertebral bodies.

Symptomatology of Disk Herniation:

- *Acute onset* of complaints, often but by no means always in association with excessive physical activity or a straining movement.
- *Intense pain,* initially usually spinal and restricting movements.
- Later, *pain radiating* into a territory corresponding more or less to the territory of the affected root.
- *Exacerbation* of the pain when specific movements are attempted, particularly straining, coughing, or sneezing.
- *Vertebral syndrome,* with rigidity of the spine at the level of the prolapsed disk and sometimes scoliotic deformity.
- *Pain on stretching* the corresponding root or the peripheral nerve trunk, e.g., a positive Lasègue's sign.
- *Neurologic signs* may be absent in the acute stage; thus, there may be no objective sensory loss, muscular weakness, or abnormal tendon jerks.
- *Subluxation* of a herniated disk

backward into the spinal canal above the level of L1 may give rise to the clinical picture of spinal cord compression, and below this level a picture of damage to several nerve roots – a cauda equina syndrome.

Disk Herniation and Spondylosis of the Cervical Spine

The **main symptoms and signs** are

- *neck pains,*
- episodes of acute *torticollis,* and
- radicular shoulder and arm pain.

Clinical picture (843): The complaints may arise with or without **causative factors** (neck trauma, intense muscular activity, whiplash injury of the cervical vertebrae). They may be **acute** or, more commonly, **subacute**, and make their appearance within a day or two. An acute *torticollis* develops with limitation of movement and a fixed position of the head, and depending on the level of the prolapsed disk, nerve root damage with *shoulder and arm pain* and *radicular signs.* The commonest spondylogenic root syndrome is a lesion of C7, followed by C6 and C8 involvement. The root affected often shows corresponding localized paresthesias. The characteristic features of individual root syndromes are identified in Table 9.**2**. Backward *stretching of the extended arm* at the shoulder joint may provoke pain. When the head is tilted to the side of the pain and then gently pressed in the axial direction, acute pain radiating down the arm is produced *(neck compression test).* True *spinal* *cord compression* is rare and usually presents as a chronic progressive lesion in the context of a myelopathy accompanying cervical spondylosis (p. 203). Exceptionally, it may have a subacute or even an acute onset in the form of an anterior spinal artery syndrome (p. 210). Spinal cord involvement is a neurosurgical emergency.

Treatment: In most patients, immobilization in a high cervical collar, applications of heat, and injections of local anesthetic and muscle relaxants may be useful. Chiropractic maneuvers are contraindicated because they may aggravate a disk prolapse or further compress a vertebral artery, thereby leading to spinal cord damage. The presence of acute medullary signs makes neurosurgical treatment a matter of urgency.

Differential diagnosis: The combination of long tract and radicular signs always prompts consideration of a *spinal cord tumor* (especially metastases). *Root tumors* such as the so-called hourglass neurofibroma cause radicular pains and neurologic signs in addition to roentgenographic evidence of enlargement of the appropriate intervertebral foramen (oblique projection). This may be particularly well demonstrated by CT scanning, (see Fig. 2.4). Such tumors and *lesions of the brachial plexus* cause radicular pains without a cervical syndrome. Other acute brachialgias accompany *neuralgic shoulder amyotrophy* (p. 409). The *carpal tunnel syndrome* may cause night pains which ascend to the neck.

Radicular Syndromes of the Thoracic Spine

These are rare and seldom caused by spondylosis. The differential diagnosis should include consideration of herpes zoster (p. 385), a hyperalgesic zone accompanying disease of an internal organ, and an intraspinal tumor.

Lumbar Disk Herniation
(328, 851)

Anatomy: The lumbar disks most often produce signs, and usually radicular involvement of a sciatic nerve. The topographic relationship of the nerve roots to the intervertebral disk explains why a particular disk herniation compresses the adjacent root. Thus, for example, prolapse of the L4–5 disk will compress the fifth root, which leaves the lumbar canal through the foramen between L5 and the sacrum.

Clinical history: In classic cases of lumbar disk herniation with low backache, the following should be carefully investigated:

   previous episodes of backache, acute lumbago, or sciatica are almost invariably present,
   precipitating factors of the present attack of pain,
- initial complaints concerning the *side of the back* involved, with limitation of movement of greater or lesser degree, and
- only subsequently, *radicular complaints,* particularly
   • cough pain,
   • pain radiating down the leg with specific distribution,

- *sensory deficits,* and
- *muscular weakness* affecting the foot or lower limb,
- evidence of damage to *additional roots* and of a cauda equina lesion,
  - side-to-side variation of the complains,
  - disturbances of urination.

Physical examination: In a patient with lumbar disk herniation, the following merit special attention:

- shape of the *vertebral column* and posture of the patient, particularly flattening of the lumbar lordosis and scoliotic deformity,
- *reduced mobility* of the vertebral column in the sagittal plane,
  - reduced Schober index (increase in the distance between the L5 spinous process and a point 10 cm above it initially measured with the patient erect, and then with the patient in maximal lumbar flexion, normal 10–15 cm),
  - increased finger to floor distance,
  - reduced spinal mobility upon extension backward with a tendency to tilt sideways.
- *Painful* lumbar vertebrae and paravertebral pressure points upon *percussion* and *palpation,*
- spontaneously increased *tonus* of truncal, erector muscles,
- position of the gluteal folds and tone of the *buttock muscles* (gluteus maximus paralysis in S1 syndrome),
- *trophic changes* in the lower extremities (calf circumference, later thigh circumference),

- *Lasègue's sign* ("reversed" Lasègue's sign in high lumbar disk lesions [547]). Also possibly – particularly in large disk disruption with subluxated protrusions – a "crossed" Lasègue's sign, i.e., pain down the back of the affected leg when the opposite leg is passively elevated (1275).
- *Neri's sign:* forward bending produces reflex flexion of the knee on the affected side,
- pain when pressure is exerted on the trunk of the sciatic nerve and its divisions as far distal as the Achilles tendon (Valleix's pressure points),
- *muscular weakness,* particularly of dorsiflexors of the great toe (also of the foot) in L5 lesions, of plantar flexion of the foot (hopping on one foot or standing on the ball of one foot in S1 lesions), of the quadriceps (standing up from a chair) in L4 (L3) lesions,
- *abnormal tendon jerks:* reduced or absent ankle jerk in S1 lesions, reduced (but not absent) knee jerk in L4 or L3 lesions,
- bandlike *sensory disturbances* (lateral border of foot in S1 lesions, dorsum of foot and great toe in L5 lesions, medial side of leg in L4 lesions) (see Fig. 2.1). For poorly understood reasons, some patients complain of a mild diffuse decrease of sensation in the entire leg, even with otherwise true monoradicular symptomatology.

Clinical Features of Common Disk Herniations

S1 Syndrome

The majority of cases are caused by a lesion of the L5-S1 disk. This level is the second commonest site of lumbar disk herniation. The radiating pain, paresthesias, and sensory deficits are projected to the lateral border of the foot. A positive Lasègue's sign is present, and sometimes positive Valleix's pressure points corresponding to the course of the sciatic nerve. A weak or absent ankle jerk is an early sign, also mild weakness of the gluteus maximus, with a lower position of the gluteal fold and reduced tone of the buttock muscles on maximal contraction of the affected side. Although not marked, there is weakness of the plantar flexors of the foot (difficulty in hopping on the affected foot or standing on tiptoe).

L5 Syndrome

Most cases are caused by lesions of the L4-5 disk, occasionally a lateral prolapse of the L5-S1 disk. In the latter instance, an additional lesion of the S1 root is often present (328). The L4-5 level is the commonest site of lumbar disk herniation. Sensory changes or deficits occur over the back of the foot and the lateral side of the calf. A positive Lasègue's sign and sometimes Valleix's pressure points are present. The posterior tibial reflex may be absent (normally, this reflex can only be inconstantly elicited, therefore important to compare with opposite side, see Table 2.1). Paralysis of the extensor hallucis longus muscle is to a greater or lesser extent a constant feature. If the tibialis anterior muscle is also paralyzed, a steppage gait occurs. Under such circumstances, suspicion arises of associated involvement of the L4 root ("vertebral peroneal palsy") (851).

L3 and L4 Syndromes
("high" lumbar disk herniation)

L3-4 and L2-3 disk herniation is far less frequent, the radiating pain and sensory disturbances being localized to the anterior part of the thigh and the lateral aspect of the calf. Lasègue's sign is usually absent but the femoral nerve is painful on stretching, and pain is felt in the leg on passive hyperextension of the hip joint with the knee flexed ("reverse" Lasègue's sign) (547). Pressure pain may be elicited over the formal trunk beneath the inguinal ligament. The knee jerk is always diminished but not completely absent. The quadriceps muscle is definitely weak (patient has difficulty in rising from a chair, or is unable to do so).

Ancillary Investigations

Conventional *lumbar spine roentgenograms* may show signs of a postural abnormality such as scoliosis, an asymmetric intervertebral space, or a narrowed one. Lumbar roentgenograms are usually necessary to rule out other lesions. If operative indications exist, the herniated disk must be demonstrated by *lumbar myelography* (radiculography) with a water-soluble contrast medium (Fig. 9.1). However, in 10%–25% of cases in which a herniated disk is anatomically confirmed, the lesion may not be visible in the myelo-

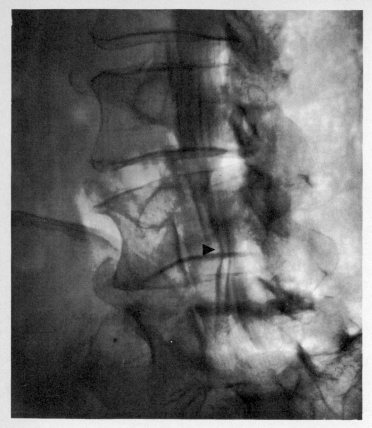

Fig. 9.**1**   Herniation of the L4–5 intervertebral disk to the left side, shown by a positive contrast myelogram. Note displacement of the L5 nerve root (arrow)

gram. In a further 10%, it gives a false-positive picture (328, 532). More recently, in those cases in which the level of the lesion can be confidently identified clinically, myelography is being replaced by *computed tomography* (Fig. 9.**2**). A laterally situated disk herniation will be revealed only by this method, not by myelography (328). Laterally si-

tuated disk herniations occur more commonly at higher spinal levels. *Electromyography* may contribute to the diagnosis by demonstrating denervation in a radicular pattern.

Differential Diagnosis

This includes the various pain syndromes in the region of the lumbar spine and pelvis (pp. 468 and 470),

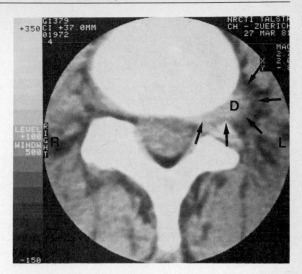

Fig.9.2 CT scan of spine demonstrating lateral herniation of a lumbar disk – left-sided L4–5 disk prolapse (D, arrows) (Courtesy of the Neuroradiological and Computed Tomographic Institute, 65 Talstrasse, Zurich, Dr. H. Spiess)

or other types of spinal root lesion (tumors, fractures), and causes of nonradicular paralysis, particularly lumbar plexus palsy and peripheral peroneal palsy. Those cases of paralysis beginning with pain, e.g., proximal asymmetric diabetic neuropathy (p.310) or paralysis in retroperitoneal hematomas (p.430) are unusually difficult to identify. Likewise, painful plexus lesions, such as those caused by tumors, are accompanied – like all other nonradicular peripheral lesions – by a disturbance of sweat secretion; this is not the case in lumbar disk damage (p.241). Sciatic neuritides may occur in the context of an arteritic lesion (798), and diffuse plexus damage with muscular weakness and atrophy is encountered in patients with arteriosclerosis.

Treatment

Conservative treatment is usually successful. It consists of bed rest, lying flat (boards under the mattress) or supine with hips and knees flexed at right angles with the calves resting on a well-padded surface. Initial applications of ice and later of heat, local anesthetic injections, muscle relaxants, analgesics, and anti-inflammatory preparations are used. Active gymnastic exercises should begin early.

The *indications for operation* are the following:

– massive disk prolapse with bilateral muscular weakness and/or sphincteric disturbances (absolute indication for emergency operation),

– acute onset of weakness of appropriate muscle groups,

– persistence of significant signs and symptoms for 2–4 weeks despite correctly applied conservative measures,

- frequent recurrences with significant complaints,
- very severe pain which fails to respond promptly or adequately to appropriate conservative measures, especially if objective signs of a root lesion are present,
- likewise, if clinical evidence of a large defect in the anulus fibrosus is present, i.e.,
  • if the sciatic syndrome in a previous attack or earlier in the same attack involved the opposite side,
  • if a crossed Lasègue's sign is present.

Operative technique: The classic operation is *diskectomy* with fenestration or hemilaminectomy providing extradural access to the disk. The operation may be carried out using microsurgical methods. *Chemonucleolysis* has also been applied (107, 333, 450). Injection of the enzyme chymopapain dissolves the binding between the glucosamine molecules in the nucleus pulposus. The procedure is carried out by percutaneous injection made under television control. This procedure is, however, not universally accepted. Diskectomy must always be recommended in cases of massive prolapse and sequestration, and in the presence of significant muscular weakness.

Prognosis

This is excellent in two-thirds of operated cases and unsatisfactory in 10%. Several factors appear to exert a negative influence on the results, namely lesions due to accidents at work, a history longer than 1 year before operation, and marked arthritic changes of the spine including anomalies of the lumbosacral junction (687). In completely removed disks, early recurrent disk herniation and postoperative adhesions may lead to an unfavorable outcome. About 1% of operated cases are complicated by an *intervertebral diskitis,* often "aseptic" (202). Days or weeks after the operation, the patient experiences lumbar backache upon movement and the ESR is found to be raised. Roentgenologic osteolysis of the epiphyseal plates of the vertebral bodies is evident 3–12 months later. The complaint regresses after several months of rest.

Space-Occupying Lesions of the Nerve Roots and Adjacent Structures

General symptomatology: These lesions lead either to increasing pain or other neurologic evidence of involvement of the affected root or to radicular signs – rarely, however, without pain, e.g., spinal neurofibroma. Spinal signs (local pain, deformity of the vertebral column, spontaneous fractures, and limitation of movement) may be present, depending on the site and nature of the tumor. Intraspinal extension leads to spinal cord (or cauda equina) compression.

A *radicular neurofibroma,* if an hourglass growth, may erode the intervertebral foramen (see Fig. 2.4) and give rise to spinal cord signs within the canal as well as a root syndrome and other extraspinal signs of compression.

Neurofibroma of the cauda equina occurs most frequently in young subjects. Backache and sciatica may develop over the course of years, before radicular signs and sphincteric disturbances occur. Conventional roentgenograms of the lumbar spine may reveal evidence of the tumor – enlargement of the vertebral canal, thinning of pedicles, or erosion of the posterior margin of a vertebral body. The lumbar CSF is always abnormal, showing a high protein level.

A *lumbosacral lipoma* is usually visible on the skin, but it may possess an intraspinal component (spina bifida occulta) and give rise to a cauda equina syndrome.

Meningeal sarcomatosis, which always involves a number of nerve roots, has been discussed on p. 203.

Ankylosing spondylitis: This rheumatologic affection may be responsible for a slowly progressive cauda equina syndrome. The likely cause appears to be arachnoid cysts which can be demonstrated by supine myelography (491).

Other Radicular Syndromes

Herpes Zoster

Etiology: This is a generalized infection of the body caused by a virus with markedly neurotropic properties.

Clinical aspects: Various local signs and symptoms may occur, which are not always preceded by *generalized manifestations* such as fatigue, joint pains, and fever. These features are followed by *nervous system involvement,* especially of the spinal ganglia. Pains occur which are unilateral and initially vague in nature, followed 3–5 days later by the typical vesicular *cutaneous eruption* localized to the corresponding dermatome. The pain has a sharp, circumscribed, and radicular character. Associated motor nerve lesions may also be present, e.g., brachial palsy in herpes zoster of the neck, facial palsy in cervical herpes zoster, and especially otic herpes zoster (p. 359), polyradiculitis, monoradicular palsy, and rarely myelitic paraplegia. *Cerebral involvement* may follow viral invasion in the form of an encephalitis (562). Reports indicate that many cases of ophthalmic herpes zoster are followed by (homolateral) ischemic brain lesions attributed to an arteritis, presumably resulting from viral invasion of the arterial wall (311, 512). The CSF shows lymphocytic pleocytosis up to 50 cells with a normal protein content.

Late effects and their treatment: The acute manifestations are sometimes followed by a most obstinate and painful syndrome, *herpes zoster neuralgia.* This severely painful complication, which affects mainly elderly subjects following the infection, is very difficult to treat. Benefit may sometimes be gained from the antiepileptic carbamazepine or high doses of tricyclic antidepressants (70–150 mg a day) (292). Local vibration massage and compression bandages sometimes give relief. Not infrequently patients resort to posterior column stimulation. Postherpetic facial pains may respond to electrocoagulation of the homolateral descending (spinal) tract of the trigeminal nerve.

Symptomatic herpes zoster: The lesion lies in the vicinity of the spinal ganglion and facilitates the viral infection. The clinical deficit may prompt the suspicion of a tumor or granuloma, especially in elderly subjects.

Differential Diagnosis of the Radicular Syndromes

This includes lesions in the vicinity of the *plexus* or the *peripheral nerves.* Therefore, a brachial plexus lesion (p. 395) must be differentiated from C8 root damage, or a carpal tunnel syndrome (p. 416) from a C6 root lesion. Lumbar plexus lesions are characterized by a disturbance of sweat secretion (see above), which is absent in lumbar radicular sydromes (p. 241). Specific *pain syndromes* may exhibit a pseudoradicular character (p. 464).

10. Lesions of Peripheral Nerves

The following brief account of this clinically important subject in neurology provides no more than a review, and specialized works should be consulted (279, 322, 493, 639, 851, 1067, 1170).

General Clinical Features

The diagnosis of a peripheral nerve lesion rests on the following elements:

- Pure *motor,* pure *sensory,* or more frequently mixed *paralysis* is present, depending on the function of the nerve affected.
- The paralyzed muscles exhibit *atrophy,* which starts to be visible within 3 weeks of the lesion.
- *Fasciculations* are only exceptionally present in the paralyzed muscles and more often indicate an anterior horn cell lesion.
- *Electromyographically,* the signs of a neurogenic paralysis are present, and occasionally a disturbance of the conduction velocity in the peripheral nerve trunk occurs (see below).
- A *topographic diagnosis* is possible from careful analysis of the individual paralyzed muscles and identification of the peripheral nerves (or roots, plexus components) supplying them (see Tables 9.1 and 9.2).
- *Reflexes* may be absent, depending on the nerve or nerve root affected (see Table 2.1).
- *Sensation* is abnormal in the dermatomes affected (see Fig. 2.1). All modalities are equally severely affected and their marginal zones are sharply defined.
- *Paresthesias and pains* are frequently present. Topographic diagnosis depends on the distribution of paresthesias, which correspond to the extent of the dermatomes. The pains are more diffuse. For example, the pains accompanying distal lesions may affect the entire extremity, as in the carpal tunnel syndrome (p. 416).
- Since sudomotor fibers accompany and divide with the sensory nerve fibers, *disturbances of sweat secretion* may be observed.
- The case history or physical ex-

amination may provide evidence of a *local cause* of the lesion (trauma, fracture, chronic external pressure damage, anatomic steno-

sis, swelling, etc.). Almost every mononeuropathy has a mechanical origin.

Ancillary Investigations

While painstaking clinical examination will yield the correct diagnosis in the majority of cases, ancillary investigations sometimes give precision to localizing the site of the lesion and the extent of the damage, document signs of regeneration, and explain the cause.

Electromyography

Concentric *bibpolar needle electrodes* are most often used to evaluate peripheral nerve lesions. Each electrode consists of a platinum wire isolated within a steel cannula, the diameter corresponding to a 14 gauge injection needle. Using the *multielectrode,* in which several electrodes are inserted in the cannula but isolated from the wall of the needle, the territory of an entire motor unit may be examined. The electric current flowing from the muscle is amplified and displayed on the screen of a

cathode ray oscilloscope. By coupling a loudspeaker in parallel, it is possible to record the current acoustically. Needle electrode examination registers a single action potential of a motor unit, which is the summation of potentials of all its individual fibers. Normal and abnormal potential curves are shown in Fig. 10.1.

An *entire motor unit* is affected by a lesion of the peripheral motor neuron in which a ganglion cell or the axon leading from it are damaged. With increasingly active innervation, fewer motor units than usual can be mobilized, and it proves impossible to obtain a complete interference pattern by means of maximal innervation (Fig. 10.2). Under normal conditions, minimal voluntary innervation will result in individual potentials being recorded, stronger innervation will result in additional participation of potentials of the adjacent

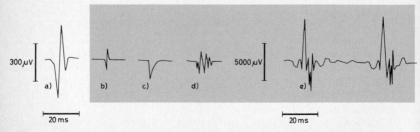

Fig. 10.**1a–e** Various potentials in electromyography **a** Normal potential of a motor unit **b** Fibrillation potential with complete denervation **c** Positive sharp wave denervation potential **d** Small polyphasic potential, as may be seen with reinnervation **e** Giant unit with chronic anterior horn lesion

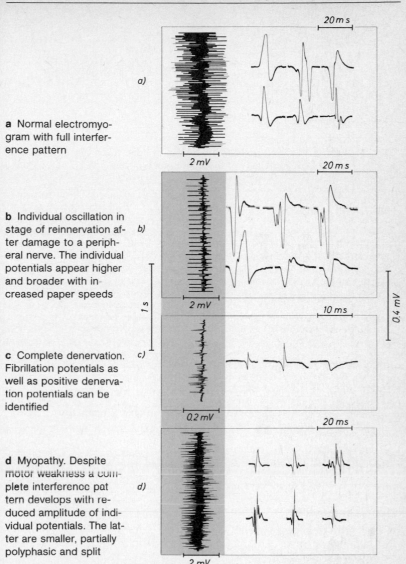

a Normal electromyogram with full interference pattern

b Individual oscillation in stage of reinnervation after damage to a peripheral nerve. The individual potentials appear higher and broader with increased paper speeds

c Complete denervation. Fibrillation potentials as well as positive denervation potentials can be identified

d Myopathy. Despite motor weakness a complete interference pattern develops with reduced amplitude of individual potentials. The latter are smaller, partially polyphasic and split

Fig. 10.**2a–d** Electromyographic recording. In the left half of the picture from above downward are the muscle potentials recorded continuously at a relatively slow paper speed, in the right half isolated extracts of the recording made 20–40 times faster

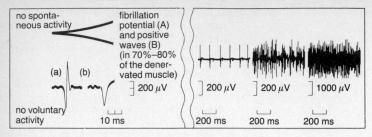

Fig. 10.**3** Results of electromyographic testing in denervation and reinnervation muscle. The increasing intensity of the interference picture can be noted during reinnervation

motor units, and maximal innervation will produce a picture in which separation of the individual action potentials is impossible – the baseline (complete interference picture, Fig. 10.**2a**) is obscured by gross superimposition of individual potentials. In a myopathy, in which only individual fibers of different units are affected by the dystrophic process, the number of motor units as such is not reduced and the interference pattern is unchanged. However, the form of the individual action potentials is altered, each being of shorter duration and smaller (Fig. 10.**2d**), because of loss of single muscle fibers from the motor unit. Following reinnervation of a previously completely denervated muscle, the electrical signs are observed up to 6 weeks before the clinical improvement. Figure 10.**3** summarizes the characteristic electromyographic findings in the course of reinnervation.

Electroneurography

Motor Nerve Conduction Time

The motor conduction time is measured by stimulating a nerve trunk with a square-wave impulse of supramaximal intensity. The delay between the time of application of the stimulus and the appearance of action potentials in the muscles is measured. The speed with which the stimulus passes distally along the nerve can thus be calculated, on the basis of the distance between the stimulation site and the reacting muscle. If several sites on a nerve trunk are stimulated, the rate of conduction can be estimated along individual segments of the trunk, irrespective of delay at the neuromuscular junction. For example, in compression syndromes it is possible to confirm isolated delay in a defined segment of a nerve trunk, or to observe a globally slowed conduction time in diffuse lesions such as polyneuropathies.

Sensory Nerve Conduction

Orthodromic and antidromic sensory conduction can be determined by stimulating a sensory or mixed peripheral nerve and by recording from the nerve itself. In the case of compression of a mixed peripheral nerve, the sensory conduction time provides more accurate information about conduction disturbances than the measurement of motor conduction.

Sweat Tests

Reference was made on p. 237 to the anatomic innervation of the sweat glands. A lesion of a nerve trunk can be proved, in the presence of a corresponding secretory abnormality, by means of special sweat tests (1078). For example, the spontaneous sweat secretion may be observed and documented by the *ninhydrin test*. The patient washes his hands in soapy water and dries them carefully. He then places his hands, or each of the fingers separately, on a sheet of white paper and presses gently. The outline of the fingers and hand may be traced with a pencil. Both hands should be tested. The examiner should avoid touching the sheet of paper, which is then passed several times through a 1% ninhydrin solution in acetone, to which has been added a drop of glacial acetic acid. The sheet is heat-dried in an incubator at 110 °C or in a hot air sterilizer. After drying for 2 more days in the atmosphere, the sheet is fixed with the following solution:

Copper sulfate	1.0 g
Distilled water	5.0 g
Methanol	95.0 g
Nitric acid	gtt V

By this test, individual sweat points may be demonstrated. Fixation enables the record to be retained permanently. The test can also be carried out on the soles of the feet.

Classification of Lesions of Peripheral Nerves

The severity of the damage to a peripheral nerve depends on the nature and intensity of the lesion, and these factors determine prognosis and treatment. A fully reversible functional disturbance without anatomic interruption of the nerve (neuropraxia) contrasts with the following two lesions: first, axonal interruption but retained nerve sheath (axonotmesis), in which there is a good chance of regeneration; and second, a macroscopic discontinuity of both axons and nerve sheaths (neurotmesis), in which surgical repair is essential.

Neurapraxia

This term is used to describe a situation in which the function of a peripheral nerve is disturbed without interruption of the continuity of any of its components; complete recovery within days is possible. Sensation remains intact, or it may be disturbed only in the sense of dysesthesia being present. No muscular atrophy occurs and no fibrillation potentials are visible in the electromyogram. Conventional electric testing confirms that the muscle can be stimulated by applying a galvanic current to the nerve trunk. An example of this condition is pressure paralysis.

Axonotmesis

This is a lesion of the nerve in which the axons are interrupted but the sheaths remain intact, leading to the clinical picture of peripheral nerve palsy with atrophy and degeneration. Under optimal anatomic conditions, the process of regeneration runs its normal course, provided that prolonged chronic compression has not led to irreversible fibrosis of the perineural structures. An example of axonotmesis is the carpal tunnel syndrome (p. 416).

Neurotmesis

This term describes interruption of both axons and nerve sheaths. The regenerating axon is deprived of a suitable linking structure and a neuroma develops (see below). Such lesions accompany severe plexus injuries as well as severance or disruption of peripheral nerves. Surgical treatment by means of nerve suturing or grafting is indicated.

Quantification of Grades of Paralysis

Only a painstakingly precise description of the quantitative aspects of the findings will enable a confident opinion to be expressed at a later stage concerning the presence or absence of reinnervation. Upon this opinion rests the indication for possible operative treatment. The power of each individually tested muscle is best recorded according to the classification recommended by the British Medical Research Council:

0 = no activity,
1 = visible contraction without motor effect,
2 = movement (through full range of motion) with force of gravity eliminated,
3 = movement against force of gravity,
4 = movement against resistance,
5 = normal.

Regeneration of Peripheral Nerves

After traumatic nerve damage without loss of continuity, or after surgical suturing of a torn peripheral nerve, axons grow toward the periphery. The speed of regeneration is about 1 mm a day, i.e., 3 cm a month. The course of regeneration should be followed up by means of clinical examination, electromyography, and testing for the *Hoffmann-Tinel sign*. This test consists of tapping the trunk of the sutured nerve with the forefinger. This provokes paresthesias in the peripheral distribution of the nerve, when the blow is applied at the point that the sprouting axons have reached. While this test may sometimes be positive in cases in which no significant clinical reinnervation subsequently occurs, it is an extremely useful indication of peripheral nerve regeneration.

Pain Syndromes Following Lesions of Peripheral Nerves (843)

Neuroma Pains

This is the most frequent pain syndrome encountered after interruption of the continuity of a peripheral nerve. The lesion is caused by the disorganized overgrowth of regenerating axons at the site of injury. The pain is usually confined to the site of the neuroma and is provoked by pressure or a blow. Small post-traumatic neuromas of peripheral nerves such as digital branches of the median nerve may cause severe, proximally radiating pains *(algie diffusante)* in addition to intense local pains, and the entire nerve trunk may be tender to pressure. The term *pseudoneuroma* is applied to enlargement of the nerve trunk (often painless) caused by hypertrophy of the endoneurial tissues at the site of chronic external pressure, as in the groove of the ulnar nerve at the elbow. Of course, such dilatations must not be resected.

Phantom Pains

This phenomenon may appear spontaneously or secondarily to external stimuli after limb amputation. The pains are projected to the absent part of the limb. Neuroma pain may sometimes be abolished by resecting the neuroma and burying the proximal stump in the soft tissues. In other cases, peripheral nerve stimulation by means of surface or implanted electrodes may bring relief (210).

Causalgia (843)

This term is used to describe a pain syndrome of unusual intensity, in which external stimuli provoke burning sensations of increasing and diminishing severity. Initially the attacks are provoked by tactile stimuli, but later auditory or visual stimuli provoke the pain. Compresses may bring relief. Severe autonomic and trophic disturbances may occur, and the patient's attitude and personality may be influenced by the intense pain. Causalgia is usually the result of direct (partial) traumatic nerve damage, presenting either immediately or within a few hours of the injury. Most cases are war casualties, the median and peroneal nerves being the most frequently damaged. Peripheral operative intervention is valueless, but sympathetic blocking or resection is often successful.

Brachial Plexus Palsy

Anatomy and general remarks: The brachial plexus is reproduced diagrammatically in Fig. 10.4. Its topographic relationships to adjacent structures may be briefly sketched as follows: the brachial plexus on its course from the cervical vertebral column to the upper arm occupies a space shaped like an hourglass, the narrowest part being the segment between the clavicle and the first rib. The ventral branches participating in the plexus lie, first between the anterior and posterior intertransverse muscles, then posterior to the vertebral artery, vein, and nerve, and finally in the scalene groove, the space

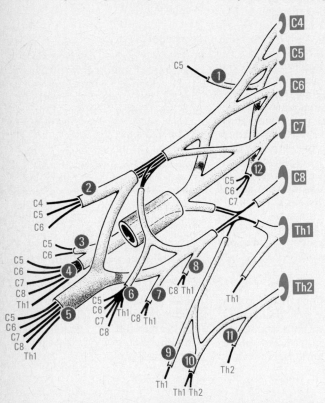

Fig. 10.4 Diagrammatic representation of the brachial plexus. Distribution of the individual nerve root axons into the peripheral nerves
1 = dorsal scapular nerve, 2 = musculocutaneous nerve, 3 = axillary nerve, 4 = radial nerve, 5 = median nerve, 6 = pectoral nerves, 7 = ulnar nerves, 8 = medial antebrachial cutaneous nerve, 9 = medial brachial cutaneous nerve, 10 and 11 = intercostobrachial nerve, 12 = long thoracic nerve

bounded by the first rib and the scalenus anterior and medius muscles. The anterior root of T1 reaches this space along the posterior surface of the pleural cap, which is strengthened by the costopleural ligament. The subclavian artery occupies the most anterior position in the scalene space, lying directly in contact with the first rib. The scalene space may be the seat of typical anatomic variations. Thus, cervical ribs are present in 0.5%-1% of subjects. While short cervical ribs involve only the anterior root of C7, long cervical ribs may compromise the space from below. The subclavian artery and brachial plexus invariably pass over a cervical rib. The costoclavicular space is narrowed by downward or backward traction on the shoulder, and pressure may be exerted on the brachial plexus or the subclavian artery. On the other hand, if the arm is held aloft, the infraclavicular part of the brachial plexus forms an angle in relation to the supraclavicular part so that it may be compressed against either the subclavius muscle or the insertion of the pectoralis minor muscle.

Lesions of the cervicobrachial plexus: These lesions are not infrequent, in view of their peculiar topographic relationship to the highly mobile structures of the shoulder girdle. Experience indicates that specific topographic localization of the lesion is not always easy, in view of the complicated structure of the brachial plexus. The numerous interconnections between the nerve fibers arising from the individual roots of C5-T1 (C4-T2) ensure that the individual muscles of the shoulder girdle and upper limb are plurisegmentally innervated, and they may be severely or less severely involved, depending on the site of the particular lesion. Table 10.1 lists the signs

and symptoms arising from various lesions of the brachial plexus and the peripheral nerves of the upper extremities.

Traumatic Brachial Plexus Palsy (322, 490, 851)

Traumatic brachial plexus palsy is the commonest lesion of the brachial plexus.

Causative mechanisms: Most cases are caused by a direct blow to the shoulder, to which motorcyclists are especially vulnerable. The actual mechanism consists in a sudden, severe tearing of the plexus. Dislocation of the shoulder joint with direct pressure on the plexus is not an invariable feature. A severe pull on the arm, e.g., if the hand is caught in a conveyor belt, may produce a plexus injury. The subclavian artery also may be damaged, even in a closed plexus injury (see below).

Lesion of the Upper Brachial Plexus

This lesion, known as Erb-Duchenne paralysis, involving C5 and sometimes C6, is the commonest form. It consists of paralysis of the abductor and external rotator muscles of the shoulder, the upper arm flexors, and the underlying supinator muscle, as well as partial involvement of the extensors of the elbow, dorsal extensors of the hand, and several scapular muscles. Sometimes a patch of diminished sensation is present over the shoulder and the outer part of the upper arm, as well as over the radial aspect of the forearm; however, sensation may be undisturbed (Fig. 10.5).

Table 10.1   Review of lesions of the brachial plexus and peripheral nerves of the upper extremities [778]

Nerve	Muscles Affected	Sensory Deficit	Function	Specific Test	Etiology	Remarks	Differential Diagnosis
Upper brachial plexus C5–C6							
Dorsal scapular C4–C5	Rhomboid major Rhomboid minor		Adduction of scapula toward vertebral column	Standing, hand on hip, elbow backward			
Supra-scapular C5–C6	Supraspinatus Infraspinatus		Adduction and external rotation of shoulder	First 15° of shoulder abduction			
(Axillary nerve, see below)					Trauma (with or without dislocation of the shoulder)	Motorcyclists at risk	
(Long thoracic nerve, see below)			Movements most commonly disturbed in upper brachial plexus palsy are:		Backpack paralysis, pressure on shoulder when carrying weights	Long thoracic nerve commonly involved	
(Musculo-cutaneous nerve, see below)							Root lesion (spondylosis, disk herniation), familial proximal spinal muscular atrophy

(Radial nerve, see below)	Abduction of shoulder flexion of elbow, supination of forearm (sometimes, external rotation of shoulder)	Neuralgic shoulder amyotrophy, serogenic neuritis	Bilateral in ¼ of cases	Venous thrombosis of the arm
		Tumor infiltration		Amyotrophic lateral sclerosis
Lower brachial plexus (C8) T1				
Medial brachial cutaneous C8–T1	Adduction and abduction of the fingers, flexion of the interphalangeal joints (flexion of the wrists)	Trauma, birth injury	Sometimes with Horner's syndrome	Root lesions, peripheral ulnar palsy, amyotrophic lateral sclerosis, myopathy with distal muscular atrophy (e.g., dystrophia myotonica), syringomyelia
Antebrachial cutaneous C8–T1		Scalenus anticus syndrome (with and without cervical rib), costoclavicular syndrome, Pancoast's tumor of the lung apex, lymphoma infiltration	Sometimes with symptoms of subclavian artery involvement	
(Median nerve, see below)			Early pain and Horner's syndrome	
(Ulnar nerve, see below)				

Medial antebrachial cutaneous nerve

Table 10.1   (Continued)

Nerve	Muscles Affected	Sensory Deficit	Function	Specific Test	Etiology	Remarks	Differential Diagnosis
Long thoracic C5–C7	Serratus anterior		Scapula drawn laterally and anteriorly, tip rotated	Pushing the outstretched arms against a wall (scapulae stand out like wings)	Operations on the axilla, lifting heavy weights, backpack paralysis, "inflammatory-allergic"	Part of syndrome of neuralgic shoulder amyotrophy	Scapular involvement in (shoulder girdle type of) progressive muscular dystrophy
Axillary C5–C6	Deltoid		Abduction of shoulder	External rotation and elevation of the arms beyond 15°	Trauma (often with shoulder dislocation)		Muscular dystrophy
	Teres minor		External rotation of shoulder				
Musculo-cutaneous C5–C7	Coraco-brachialis		Supporting the shoulder joint (flexion and adduction of upper arm)		Traumatic		
	Biceps brachii		Flexion of upper and forearm, supination of forearm				

Radial C5–C8 (T1)				
Brachialis (partly supplied by radial nerve)	Flexion of the upper arm	Flexion of the elbow with the forearm supinated	Rarely isolated without trauma	
Triceps brachii and anconeus	Extension of elbow			Sparing of triceps brachii muscle
Brachioradialis	Flexion of elbow			Spontaneous recovery
Brachialis (and musculocutaneous)	Flexion of elbow	In midposition between pronation and supination		Often purely motor involvement
Extensor carpi radialis brevis and longus	Flexion (and radial abduction) of wrist	With digits flexed	Fracture of the humerus	
Supinator	Supination of forearm and hand	With elbow extended	"Alcoholic palsy" of the upper arm	
Extensor digitorum communis	Extension of metacarpophalangeal joints	Flexion of interphalangeal joints of fingers	"Lead neuritis"	
Extensor carpi ulnaris	Flexion (and ulnar abduction) of wrist	Flexion of fingers	Isolated paralysis of the deep branch at level of the supinator	

1 Axillary nerve
2 Lateral antebrachial cutaneous nerve (from musculocutaneous nerve)
3 Superficial branch of radial nerve

Table 10.**1** (Continued)

Nerve	Muscles Affected	Sensory Deficit	Function	Specific Test	Etiology	Remarks	Differential Diagnosis
	Extensor digiti minimi		Extension of little finger				
	Abductor pollicis longus		Abduction of proximal phalanx of thumb		Pressure lesions of the sensory nerves of the thumb (cheiralgia paresthetica)		
						Rupture of extensor tendon	
	Extensor pollicis longus		Extension of distal phalanx of thumb	Distal phalanx flexed			
	Extensor pollicis brevis		Extension of proximal phalanx of thumb				
	Extensor indicis		Extension of index finger	Other fingers flexed			
Median C5–T1	Pronator teres and pronator quadratus		Pronation of forearm				
	Flexor carpi radialis		Palmar flexion and radial abduction of wrist		Trauma, e.g., supracondylar fracture of humerus	If proximal paralysis "preacher's hand"	

N. medianus

Muscle	Function	Test sign	Cause	Note	Association
Palmaris longus	Palmar flexion of wrist only				
Flexor digitorum sublimis	Flexion of middle phalanx of finger		"Alcoholic palsy" of upper arm	Good prognosis	Volkmann's ischemic contracture
Flexor digitorum profundus II et III	Flexion of terminal phalanges of middle and ring fingers		Supracondylar process of humerus		(Lower) plexus lesions
Flexor pollicis longus	Flexion of distal phalanx of thumb		Cut by wound at wrist		
Flexor pollicis brevis (superficial head)	Flexion of proximal phalanx of thumb		Carpal tunnel syndrome	Brachialgia paresthetica nocturna	
Abductor pollicis brevis	Abduction of metacarpal of thumb	Abducts the thumb in grasping an object ("bottle sign")	(Occupational) pressure at the wrist	Often purely motor involvement	Amyotrophic lateral sclerosis
Opponens pollicis	Rotation of thumb				
Lumbrical muscles I and II	Flexion of metacarpophalangeal and extension of interphalangeal joints of index and middle fingers	Touching the base of the little finger with the tip of the thumb			

Table 10.**1**   (Continued)

Nerve	Muscles Affected	Sensory Deficit	Function	Specific Test	Etiology	Remarks	Differential Diagnosis
Ulnar C8–T1	Flexor carpi ulnaris		Palmar and ulnar flexion of wrist	Abducting the little finger			
	Flexor digitorum profundus IV and V		Flexion of terminal interphalangeal joints of ring and little finger		Pressure lesion at elbow	Occupational, confinement to bed	C8 root lesion
	Palmaris brevis		"Skin muscle" of hypothenar eminence	Puckering of skin of hypothenar eminence on abduction of the little finger	Nerve damage at elbow, e.g., fractures	With or without additional trauma, bilaterally	
	Abductor digiti quinti	Ulnar nerve	Abduction of little finger				
	Opponens digiti quinti		Opponens action of little finger		Trauma, elbow fractures	Especially medial epicondyle	Medial epicondylitis ("tennis elbow")
	Flexor digiti quinti brevis		Flexion of metacarpophalangeal joint of little finger		Late paralysis after old elbow fracture	Especially lateral epicondyle	Muscular dystrophy with distal atrophy

Lumbrical muscles III and IV	Flexion of metacarpophalangeal and extension of interphalangeal joints of middle and ring fingers	Paralysis accompanying degenerative disease of elbow joint	Sometimes bilateral	(Dupuytren's contracture) Amyotrophic lateral sclerosis
Interosseous muscles	Adduction and abduction	Lateral movements of middle finger	Pressure lesion at wrist	Usually purely motor involvement
Adductor pollicis	Adduction of thumb	Froment's sign (p.419)	Abnormally frequent flexion and extension at elbow	e.g., drilling machines
Flexor pollicis brevis (deep head)	Flexion of metacarpophalangeal joint of thumb			

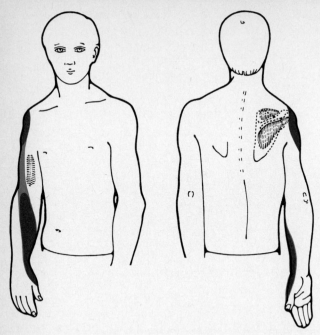

Fig. 10.**5**   Position of arm and area of sensory deficit in right upper brachial plexus palsy

Lesion of the Lower Brachial Plexus

This form, known as Dejerine-Klumpcke paralysis, involving T1 and sometimes C8, is less common. All the intrinsic muscles of the hand are involved, sometimes also the long flexors of the fingers and occasionally the wrist flexors. The triceps muscle is usually spared. Some cases may show a lesion of the cervical sympathetic chain with a *Horner's syndrome* (narrowing of the palpebral fissure, constricted pupil, enophthalmos, and sometimes conjunctival hyperemia), which indi-

cates damage of the T1 root proximal to the origin of the white ramus communicans to the sympathetic trunk (p. 237). The difference in the palpebral fissures in Horner's syndrome disappears on upward gaze, while that in oculomotor palsy is accentuated. Sensation is always disturbed in lower plexus lesions, a deficit being present on the ulnar side of the forearm and hand (Fig. 10.**6**).

C7 Paralysis

This is rare and involves particularly the area of distribution of the radial

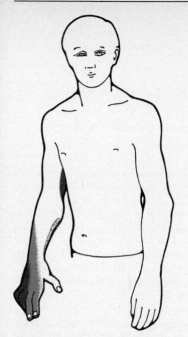

Fig. 10.6 Position of arm and area of sensory deficit in right lower brachial plexus palsy

Total Brachial Plexus Palsy

All plexus components are involved. Many cases of traumatic brachial palsy present initially with total paralysis, which in the course of time recedes to become an upper or a lower plexus palsy.

Birth Injury of Brachial Plexus
(420, 1023)

Birth trauma to the brachial plexus may be produced in the course of spontaneous delivery in a normal fetal position, if disproportion exists between the infant's shoulder and the maternal pelvis. Usually it is a complication of forceps delivery, being caused by direct pressure of a blade of the forceps on the brachial plexus. Delivery of the aftercoming head in a breech presentation may inflict direct damage by pressure of the operator's fingers on the brachial plexus. An upper plexus injury is the most frequent.

Prognosis

The prognosis of upper brachial palsy is better than that involving the lower brachial plexus, and more than one-half of patients with an upper plexus lesion recover completely. An unfavorable prognostic sign is unusually severe trauma (high speeds), complete paralysis from the start, additional bony injury, Horner's syndrome, involvement of the muscles of the scapula and thoracic cage, and pain. In particular, pain is a prognostically unfavorable *sign of an avulsed nerve root*. Blood-tinged CSF in the acute stage also suggests this possibility, which later is confirmed by signs of spinal

nerve; the brachioradialis muscle is spared as a result of its additional nerve supply from C5 and C6.

Fascicular Paralysis

Three types of fascicular paralysis are encountered:

- dorsal type affecting the axillary and radial nerves,
- lateral type affecting the musculocutaneous nerve and lateral trunk of the median nerve, and
- medial type affecting the ulnar nerve and medial trunk of the median nerve.

cord involvement. The presence of Horner's syndrome indicates merely damage to the C8 and T1 nerves proximal to the origin of the white rami communicantes; it is not specific or conclusive evidence of an avulsed root. Myelography may reveal the presence of empty root sleeves or arachnoid cysts. Intracutaneous injection of histamine into analgesic areas provokes a red halo in the skin (positive axon reflex) if the communication between the spinal nerve ganglion and the site of injection is preserved, while the halo does not occur if the damage is peripheral. Electroneurography reveals that, despite evidence of analgesia, the peripheral sensory conduction time remains normal – proving that continuity is retained between the spinal ganglion and the peripheral nerve and that an avulsed nerve root is present (519, 724).

Treatment

The first aim of treatment is to prevent shoulder contractures. Immediate measures include positional splinting with an abduction splint, passive exercises, and, later, active exercises. Operative treatment by nerve suturing can be considered only in uncomplicated lesions of the upper components of the brachial plexus. Surgical treatment is being attempted with increasing frequency in patients who fail to recover function or if a nerve root avulsion is confirmed (see above), and autotransplants have been inserted. As a general rule, no useful improvement can be expected in totally denervated muscles after the passage of 12–18 months, and any further improvement in upper limb function requires orthopedic corrective measures.

Other Causes of Brachial Plexus Palsy

Chronic External Pressure

Untrained military recruits may suffer from backpack (rucksack) palsy, a condition involving the upper brachial plexus and particularly the long thoracic nerve. A similar clinical picture may be produced by *carrying a heavy weight* on one shoulder. Female patients who are held by *shoulder supports in Trendelenburg's position* on the operating table for gynecologic operations may subsequently present with a brachial palsy. All these lesions caused by external pressure carry a good prognosis, although recovery may take many months.

Anatomic Relationships of Compression Syndromes

Peculiar anatomic relationships in the upper thoracic outlet, especially its distal part, may lead to a brachial palsy, with or without additional external factors. Since the precise mechanism may not be demonstrable, the global term *thoracic outlet syndrome* is used (322, 851).

Scalene Syndrome and Cervical Rib Syndrome

Pressure may be exerted on the nerve trunks of the brachial plexus and sometimes also on the subclavian artery in the region of the scalene groove, where these structures pass through the opening between the scalenus anterior and scalenus medius muscles. A lesion is far more likely to occur in the presence of an anomaly of the scalene insertion, and especially if a *cervical rib* is present. This rudimentary structure may consist of a fibrous band, rather than a bony anomaly; thus, it may not be visible in roentgenograms. However, it is important to point out that cervical ribs seldom cause clinical trouble and only exceptionally require operative removal.

Costoclavicular Syndrome

Asthenic individuals with sloping shoulders are particularly prone to develop this syndrome, which occurs if the space between the clavicle and first rib, the costoclavicular space, is abnormally narrow. A brachial plexus palsy may result, although nerve compression is far less frequently encountered than is generally believed, and cases of unexplained shoulder pain are too often attributed to it. For the diagnosis, objective signs of a brachial plexus lesion (usually lower) should be present, or else definite evidence of subclavian artery compression. In genuine cases, the signs and symptoms are often provoked by carrying heavy weights. Certain movements, e.g., backward inclination of the head with simultaneous rotation of the chin to the affected side (Adson's maneuver), may provoke signs such as obliteration of the radial pulse. The latter sign will also be produced in about 50% of normal subjects by a forceful downward pull on the shoulder. In a genuine case of subclavian artery compres-

sion, auscultation may reveal the presence of a murmur due to poststenotic aneurysmal dilatation of the artery. Thrombosis and consequent embolization may provoke Raynaud-like phenomena in the fingers (p. 467).

Hyperabduction Syndrome

This is a rare condition caused by compression of arteries and nerves against the coracoid process of the scapula and the pectoralis minor muscle during hyperabduction of the arm.

Treatment of compression syndromes: In the absence of objective motor or sensory abnormalities, treatment consists merely in gymnastic exercises to strengthen the shoulder girdle muscles and to prevent specific aggravating external factors. Surgical excision of the scalenus anterior muscle and removal of a cervical rib or partial resection of a first rib in cases of costoclavicular compression are justified only in the presence of objective clinical deficits. However, such cases are accompanied by roentgenologic signs of an anomaly or pathologic operative findings (681). For this reason, some surgeons favor the supraclavicular approach, which provides a better view of the relevant anatomic structures than the easier axillary approach.

Apical Lung Tumor (Pancoast Tumor)

This lesion is a particular cause of brachial plexus palsy that is often missed in the early stages. Other tumors, e.g., sarcoma or lymphoma, may produce identical signs and symptoms. **Clinically,** severe pain in the distribution of the C8 and T1 dermatomes is the usual presenting symptom, radiating to the ulnar side of the hand and followed by a lower brachial plexus palsy; later a total paralysis may develop. Damage to the cervical sympathetic trunk causes Horner's syndrome and disturbances of sweat secretion in the corresponding region of the body in three-fourths of patients. Occasionally the tumor erodes vertebrae and extends into the vertebral canal, causing signs of spinal cord compression. Careful examination of the lung apices is indicated in every case of brachialgia. The *roentgenographic appearance* is characteristic. **Treatment** is unsatisfactory, although in many cases X-irradiation may temporarily abolish the pain.

Radiation Damage to the Brachial Plexus

X-irradiation may be followed after a latent interval of one or more years by a progressive brachial plexus palsy (322, 642, 846, 851, 1138). Usually, although not invariably, the lesion complicates the therapeutic or prophylactic X-irradiation of regional lymph nodes in cases of breast cancer. **Clinically,** the lesion may be heralded by severe pain, which is a prominent feature in about 15% of patients. It may be confined to the upper part or the lower part, or involve the whole brachial plexus. The prognosis in relation to the pain and paralysis is poor: spontaneous recovery of paralysis does not occur and only rarely do the pains disappear spontaneously. The differential diagnosis between postirradiation palsy and tumor recurrence may not be easy. Comparison between 78 patients with a neoplastic brachial palsy (of whom 34 also underwent X-irradiation) and 22 patients with radiation-induced brachial palsy revealed the following differences: very severe pain was present in four-fifths of the tumor cases but it was a prominent feature in only one-fifth of the radiation cases. Three-fourths of the tumor cases showed signs of a lower palsy, while three-fourths of the radiation cases showed an upper palsy. Horner's syndrome was correspondingly more common in the tumor cases, lymphedema in the radiation cases. If the signs and symptoms appeared within 1 year of the radiation treatment, the radiation damage was associated with doses above 6,000 rad (60 Gy), and the tumor cases with smaller doses (642). **Pathogenetically,** animal experiments have shown that, apart from direct damage, the brachial plexus is subjected to strangulation by tough indurated connective tissue (1138). Ischemic brachial palsies of sudden onset may also follow X-irradiation, being similar to lesions seen after vascular damage due to other causes.

Treatment: Operative neurolysis has yielded disappointing results. It might be applied in exceptional cases to lessen pain but has no effect on the paralysis.

houlder Amyotrophy ...euritis") (320, 851)

...etically, this condition may ...ned as an inflammatory or ...gic lesion of the brachial plex-... A clinically identical form may follow serum injections (p.320), although the latter association is rare.

Clinically, most patients are young adults, males appear to be more often affected than females. The *onset* is acute, without obvious cause, and occurs only rarely in association with other unusual infections or exposure of the shoulder region to cold. Clinical examination reveals no systemic abnormalities, as a rule there is no fever. The presenting symptom is *intense shoulder pain,* often occurring at night, which is usually racking in nature, and sometimes radiates to the upper arm or beyond. Usually the pain is followed some hours later by *weakness* of individual muscles of the shoulder and upper arm. In other cases, a few days may elapse before definite muscular weakness is present. In some cases, the pain is so severe that the patient is prevented from using the arm; thus, the time of onset of the muscular weakness is uncertain. The pain usually subsides after a few days and is relieved by the paralysis, but it may remain present in a mild form for weeks or even months, being provoked afresh by movements of the arm. Bilateral cases are exceptional.

Physical examination: Paralysis of individual muscles of the shoulder girdle and upper arm is present, all these muscles usually being inner-vated by the upper brachial plexus. Exceptionally a distal palsy may be present, e.g., the picture of a radial palsy. The right side is more often affected. Only about one-fourth of patients show sensory changes, usually on the outer surface of the shoulder and upper arm. Diaphragmatic paralysis may also occur, which prompts the question of how many cases of isolated diaphragmatic palsy should be attributed to brachial plexus neuritis, if a mechanical C3-4 lesion is not present. The CSF is always normal.

Prognosis: This is usually good. In one-half of the patients the pain disappears within weeks, at the latest after 3 months. The muscular weakness may only begin to recede after 9-12 months, and recovery of motor function may take as long as 2 years. Residual pains may last many months, exceptionally a residual paralysis may be permanent. Recurrences are rare including recurrent familial cases.

Treatment: In the acute stage, anti-inflammatory preparations including cortisone are used, later local applications of heat and physiotherapy.

Differential Diagnosis of Brachial Plexus Lesions

This includes paralysis of individual muscles and nerve roots of the upper extremities, as well as central lesions that show a predilection for distal paralysis. Certain specific pain syndromes involving the upper extremities (p.464) should be considered.

Long Thoracic Nerve

Anatomically, the long thoracic nerve receives its fibers from the C5-7 roots. It possesses no sensory fibers and innervates the serratus anterior muscle.

Clinically, a lesion of the nerve paralyzes the serratus anterior muscle. The medial border of the scapula lifts from the thoracic wall to produce the picture of a winged scapula, which is most prominent when the arm is lifted forward or when the patient pushes the outstretched arm against a wall.

Several mechanical or other factors may be involved. Because of its long course, the long thoracic nerve is not infrequently damaged – sometimes in isolation, e.g., transport workers or in backpack injuries. Other factors must be responsible for the nerve being involved with special severity in cases of neuralgic shoulder amyotrophy and after certain infectious diseases.

Axillary Nerve

Anatomically, a lesion of the axillary nerve (C5-6) is characterized by paralysis of the deltoid and teres minor muscles. Sensation is lost over a small area of the proximal arm.

Clinically, forward elevation and abduction of the arm is limited, and paralysis of the teres minor muscle prevents external rotation of the shoulder joint. Atrophy of the deltoid muscle on its lateral aspect is usually impressive.

Causes: The most frequent cause of axillary palsy is anterior dislocation of the shoulder joint. The diagnosis of axillary nerve involvement may be delayed by the initial limitation of movement of the shoulder due to pain (importance of testing sensation before reducing the dislocation!).

Prognosis: Usually good.

Differential diagnosis: This includes arthrogenic causes of deltoid atrophy, painful humeroscapular periarthritis, a torn rotator cuff, and muscular dystrophy (bilateral!).

Suprascapular Nerve

Anatomically, this nerve (C4-6), which innervates the supraspinatus and infraspinatus muscles, reaches these muscles by passage through the scapular groove.

Clinically, paralysis of these muscles results in limited abduction of the shoulder joint and external rotation of the upper arm. Sensation is not affected, but chronic irritation of the suprascapular nerve may produce pain.

Causes: Trauma (dislocation of the shoulder joint), or chronic pressure in the scapular groove, e.g., ganglion, may be responsible. In the latter case, neurolysis may be indicated.

Musculocutaneous Nerve

Anatomically, a lesion of the musculocutaneous nerve (C5-7) provides motor branches to the biceps brachii and coracobrachialis muscles and part of the brachial muscle. The musculocutaneous nerve has a terminal sensory branch, the lateral antebrachial cutaneous nerve.

Clinically, an isolated lesion of this nerve is rare, causing weakness of elbow flexion and supination of the forearm. A discrete sensory disturbance is present on the radial side of the forearm.

Causes: Although usually traumatic, an isolated musculocutaneous palsy may occur without injury or other cause being detected. The nerve is usually involved in an upper brachial plexus palsy.

Differential diagnosis: The important condition to differentiate from a musculocutaneous palsy is rupture of the long tendon of the biceps brachii muscle.

Radial Nerve

Anatomy: The radial nerve receives fibers from the C5-8 roots. Before the nerve enters the radial groove in close apposition to the bone to pass around the humeral shaft, it supplies a motor branch to the triceps muscle, as well as one or more sensory branches, the posterior brachial cutaneous branch, and sometimes an antebrachial cutaneous branch. Distal to the level of the elbow joint, where the radial nerve supplies the brachioradialis, extensor carpi radialis longus, and lateral head of the brachialis muscles, it divides on the anterior surface of the lateral humeral condyle into a superficial sensory divi-

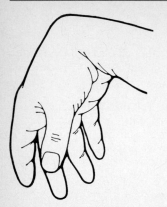

Fig. 10.7 Typical position of right hand in radial palsy

sion and a deep motor division. The sensory division innervates the skin on the radial side of the dorsum of the hand over the first interosseous space. The deep motor branch traverses the supinator muscle, and not infrequently it is damaged at this level (see below).

Clinical picture: This depends on the site of the lesion. The most typical picture is a *wrist drop* in which the ability to extend both the wrist and the metacarpal joints is lost (Fig. 10.7). Not infrequently a cushion of edematous tissue (Gubler's swelling) is present on the back of the hand. If the lesion is more proximal, the triceps muscle (extensor of the elbow joint) also is paralyzed. However, in injuries of the upper arm – the commonest site of all radial nerve lesions – it is not involved. Sensation is impaired over only a small area of skin, dorsally over the first interosseous space. Particular care is required to demonstrate this specific deficit.

Causes of Radial Paralysis

Traumatic

Not infrequently, radial palsy forms part of the picture of a *traumatic brachial plexus injury.* Radial paralysis following *fractures of the humeral shaft* is by far the commonest peripheral nerve lesion accompanying extremity fractures. The signs and symptoms of this injury are a wrist drop, paralysis of the brachioradialis muscle, and the typical sensory deficit on the back of the hand. If complete or partial paralysis appears at the time of the fracture, the patient's clinical course will indicate whether the continuity of the nerve or nerve fibers has been interrupted. The commonest injury by far is a simple nerve contusion, and spontaneous recovery is the rule. Failure of recovery of an initial radial palsy presents a difficult decision concerning operative revision. Electromyographic studies may be helpful: if no signs of reinnervation have appeared in the brachioradialis or extensor carpi radialis longus muscles after 5-6 months, surgical exploration of the fracture site is always justified. Earlier exploration may be indicated in individual cases, depending upon the severity of the injury, the degree of initial displacement of the bone fragments, etc. Complete rupture of the nerve is very rare. The prognosis after neurolysis is good. If the radial palsy first appears only 3-4 weeks after the fracture, or if an incomplete paralysis deepens during this period, it must be assumed that the nerve has become embedded in fibrous tissue or bony callus, and operative neurolysis is therefore indicated.

Pressure Palsy

Chronic pressure exerted in the axilla, e.g., *crutch palsy,* causes wrist drop and paralysis of the triceps brachii muscle. The commonest type of radial palsy is *pressure palsy in the midupper arm,* which is exerted on the nerve as it winds around the humeral shaft. The nerve is closely applied to the bone in this part of its course so that local pressure – usually applied during sleep or after alcohol intake – may damage it. The patient awakes with a typical wrist drop and shows – at least initially – a sensory deficit on the dorsum of the hand over the first interosseous space. Corresponding with the usual cause, this injury is referred to as "park bench paralysis" or "Saturday night palsy." The prognosis is always good: recovery may start within a few days and it may be complete without treatment within weeks. An isolated patch of sensory loss over the lateral surface of the terminal digits of the thumb is referred to a *cheiralgia paresthetica.* This loss of sensation occurs with damage to the superficial division of the radial nerve, usually its lateral terminal rami. The lesion is caused by pressure damage, e.g., prolonged use of scissors, a painter's palette, etc. The condition is harmless and always disappears spontaneously.

Compression Syndromes

The radial nerve in its passage *through the supinator muscle* may adhere to the surrounding tissues, and the nerve is susceptible to mechanical damage in this part of its course which affects the deep motor division. Gradually over the course of weeks or months, the innervated muscles become weak and paralyzed. Initially only the extensor muscles of the ring and little fingers are involved, but later the complete picture of wrist drop develops. The extensor carpi radialis longus muscle may be spared, the brachioradialis muscle is always normal. This picture may be caused by a lipoma or neurofibroma, or perhaps merely by chronic mechanical damage to the nerve at the level of its passage through the supinator muscle; indeed, the term "supinator tunnel syndrome" is used. Surgical exploration is indicated.

Differential Diagnosis

In the differential diagnosis of radial palsy, a *central (cerebral) paralysis of the distal arm* must be excluded. In such cases, the weakness of the dorsal extensor muscles is always accompanied by other motor deficits and abnormal reflexes. If in "central wrist drop" the flexor muscles are powerfully contracted (gripping an object, clenching the first), a reflex mechanism activates the extensor muscles as well so that the hand assumes a position of extension. Wrist drop caused by to *lead poisoning* is discussed on p. 147. Tendon rupture may cause paralysis of the extensor pollicis longus muscle *("drummer's palsy").* In the presence of severe ulnar deviation of the digits relative to the corresponding metacarpal bones, e.g., chronic rheumatoid arthritis, the *long extensor tendons are displaced sideways* from the finger axis. During finger flexion, therefore, they may slide laterally and ventrally and come to lie beneath the axis of movement of the metacarpophalangeal joints.

When the extensors are contracted, an additional flexion movement is produced. This deformity may mimic a radial palsy.

Median Nerve

Anatomy: The median nerve (C5–T1) arises from the medial and lateral fasciculi of the brachial plexus. It divides first at the level of the elbow, innervating the flexor muscles of the forearm (pronator teres, flexor carpi radialis, palmaris longus, and flexor digitorum superficialis). After passage through the pronator teres muscle, the nerve also supplies branches to the flexor pollicis longus, flexor digitorum profundus (radial division), and pronator quadratus muscles. It then passes under the transverse carpal ligament in the carpal tunnel, together with the tendons of the long flexors of the fingers, into the palm of the hand. Here it supplies motor branches to the abductor pollicis brevis, opponens pollicis, and the superficial head of the flexor pollicis brevis muscles. Terminal sensory branches pass to the skin of the radial half of the palm, the palmar aspect of the thumb, index, and middle fingers and the radial side of the index finger, and the dorsal aspect of the two distal phalanges of the index and middle fingers and the radial side of the ring finger (see Fig. 2.1).

A high lesion of the median nerve prevents the patient from making a fist and allows him to flex only the fingers supplied by the ulnar nerve. The so-called preacher's hand position results (Fig. 10.8). However, if the median nerve is damaged beyond the level of the forearm, only the hand muscles supplied by it are

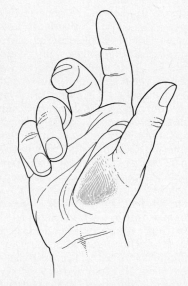

Fig. 10.8 "Preacher's hand" in right median nerve palsy with thenar atrophy

paralyzed, and a different clinical picture results. The patient is unable to abduct his thumb completely so that, if he is asked to grasp a large tumbler or a bottle in his hand, a gap will separate the object from the web between the thumb and index finger – the so-called bottle sign (Fig. 10.9). Attempts to approximate the thumb to the little finger result in inadequate pronation of the

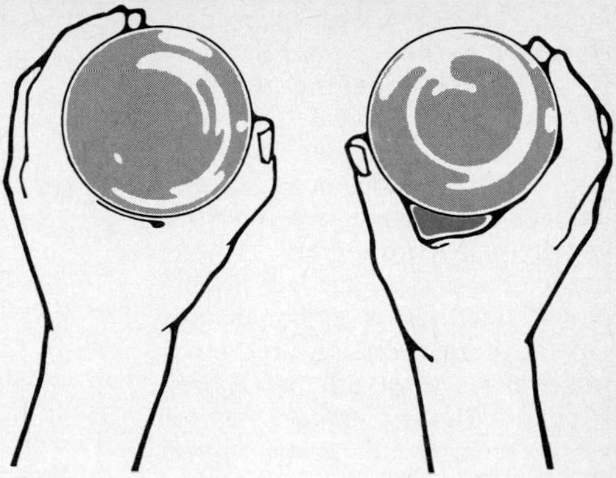

Fig. 10.**9** Inadequate abduction of the right thumb in median nerve palsy. The subject is unable to grip a round object (bottle sign) and the thumb is not sufficiently rotated

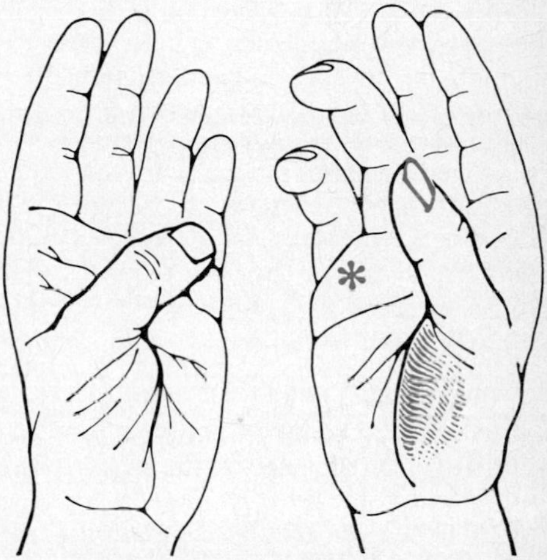

Fig. 10.**10** Right median nerve palsy. Poor approximation of thumb and little finger. The paralysis prevents the thumb from rotating, so that the thumbnail is viewed tangentially and not seen from its dorsal surface

thumb so that its side, rather than its tip, is brought into contact with the palm of the hand or the tip of the little finger. The thumbnail is seen only partially from the side (Fig. 10.**10**). Atrophy of the lateral aspect of the thenar eminence is typical.

Causes of Median Palsy

Traumatic

The median nerve may participate in traumatic lesions of the upper arm, elbow, and back of the wrist. A rare cause is damage of the nerve trunk in the upper arm due to fracture of the humeral shaft. A supracondylar humeral fracture of the extension type with dislocation occasionally may lead to a median nerve palsy. In such cases, the occurrence of *Volkmann's ischemic contracture* of the finger and hand flexors is more to be feared than mechanical damage to the median nerve, which usually recovers spontaneously. Actual damage to the median nerve in elbow fractures is extremely rare. Operative revision, as in cases of humeral fracture with radial palsy, is confined to individual cases possessing specific indications. A median nerve lesion accompanying fractures of the distal forearm bones also is rare. The presence of an incised wound of the wrist, however superficial it may appear, should always prompt a careful search for signs of median (and ulnar) nerve damage. Because the pain of the wound limits movement, the diagnosis is often more easily made by demonstrating an area of sensory loss than by confirming the presence of paralysis.

Damage from External Pressure

Pressure damage may be caused by the weight of the head of the sleeping partner *("lover's paralysis")* or by ischemia caused by a *pressure cuff* (Esmarch bandage). Both have a good prognosis. Occupational chronic pressure damage to the median nerve at the wrist may lead to a purely motor median palsy with thenar atrophy. This lesion may be difficult to differentiate from spinal muscular atrophy. The same is true of median nerve injury occurring after prolonged cycling (p. 421).

Carpal Tunnel Syndrome

Anatomically, the site of damage is the carpal tunnel. The median nerve passes beneath the flexor retinaculum (transverse carpal ligament) together with the tendons of the long finger flexors and their sheaths.

Pathogenesis: Chronic compression of the nerve is the decisive factor (279). In individual cases, the syndrome may follow a healed fracture or arthritis of the carpal bones. Sometimes hypothyroidism, amyloidosis, gout, or diabetes mellitus is present. In "palindromic rheumatism," a relapsing form of rheumatoid arthritis involving the wrist joint, a symptomatic form of carpal tunnel syndrome may occur. Usually the signs and symptoms appear without any additional local factor being present.

Clinical picture (115, 279, 851): Women are more often affected than men, often at the menopause and sometimes during or immediately after a pregnancy. A sudden severe increase in weight accounts for individual cases. Initially the disturbances are purely *subjective,* and in many patients objective signs may never occur or only after an interval of years. The classic clinical picture is that of a nocturnal *brachialgia paresthetica*. While this syndrome is by no means pathognomonic of chronic pressure damage to the median nerve in the carpal canal, the vast majority of such cases can be attributed to it. Typically the patient awakens at night after a brief period of sleep to find that one or both hands are numb and feel swollen. Finger movements are difficult and clumsy, and the whole limb may be painful; sometimes the pains extend proximally into the shoulder and neck. Shaking and massage of the hands produces relief, but the patient is awakened again by the complaint after a further brief interval so that her sleep is interrupted. In the morning, the first functions of the day are often made difficult by clumsy and stiff fingers. Although less common in the course of the day, similar isolated episodes may disturb the patient. Sometimes, but not invariably, careful questioning will reveal preferential involvement of the thumb and adjacent three fingers. Particularly strenuous physical exercise, e.g., washing clothes or housework, may aggravate the symptom. Both the brachialgia and the objective deficits usually begin in the dominant hand, but sooner or later are bilateral.

Physical examination: This is usually negative in the early stages of the syndrome, although occasionally there may be pain upon pressure on the median nerve trunk in the carpal canal. Several years of constant compression of the nerve trunk may be necessary before paralysis and atrophy of the thenar muscles occur, with or without sensory loss. Sensory changes alone may sometimes be present. Abduction weakness of the thumb and a positive bottle sign (see Fig. 10.6) can usually be detected. A *provocative test,* forced dorsal extension or palmar flexion of the wrist for about 1 min (Phalen's test) may elicit the typical subjective complaints in the course of the examination.

Electroneurographically, a prolonged distal motor latency can be demonstrated, as well as a disturbance of the distal motor and the orthodromic or antidromic sensory conduction velocity.

Treatment: During the stage of *nocturnal brachialgia paresthetica* without striking objective physical signs, the condition is usually satisfactorily treated by resting the wrist at night on a smooth palmar splint. If this measure fails or if significant sensory loss or muscular weakness occurs, operative section of the transverse carpal ligament is the method of choice. Progressive thenar atrophy is not usually reversible, but the sensory loss and particularly the nocturnal pains may be dramatically abolished. In uncomplicated cases, a local injection of a crystalline suspension of corticosteroid into the carpal canal is recommended (758). This measure abolishes the symptoms in about two-thirds of patients, but only one-fourth remain cured after one year.

Other Compression Syndromes

Supracondylar Process of the Humerus

The trunk of the median nerve lies in close proximity to this process, a phylogenetically determined spur of bone projecting from the anteromedial surface of the humeral shaft about a hand's breadth above the medial epicondyle, present in about 1% of human subjects. Occasionally the spur gives rise to median nerve signs.

Pronator Teres Muscle Syndrome

The median nerve, at the level of its passage through this muscle, is liable to chronic mechanical damage, especially with the arm held in the extended position. Thus, one may speak of a pronator teres syndrome. Such patients exhibit paresthesias in the radial fingers as well as tenderness to pressure over the pronator teres muscle.

Anterior Interosseous Nerve Syndrome (Kiloh-Nevin Syndrome)

Anatomically, the pure motor branch of the median nerve in the forearm innervates the flexor pollicis longus, the flexor digitorum profundus muscles of the index and middle fingers, and the pronator teres.

Pathogenetically, a lesion may follow a forearm fracture, but more commonly it is associated with another local cause, and at least one-half of cases are "spontaneous." Some of the latter cases may result from compression by a fibrous band. **Clinically,** the patient is unable to flex the distal joints of his thumb and index fingers, and thus form an "O"

with these two fingers. **Treatment** consists in operative exploration of the posttraumatic and rapidly progressive cases. Other cases sometimes heal spontaneously.

Rarer causes: Uremic subjects in whom an arteriovenous shunt has been fashioned in the forearm to facilitate dialysis may experience an ischemic neuropathy of the median nerve distal to the shunft (150).

Differential diagnosis: This includes a (lower) brachial plexus palsy and C8–T1 root damage, which may also be heralded by thenar atrophy. The sensory loss, if present, usually permits a distinction to be made. A central disturbance of stereognosis (in lesions of the cerebral cortex or cervical spinal cord) may initially mimic a peripheral sensory loss involving the thumb and the index and middle fingers.

Ulnar Nerve

Anatomy: The ulnar nerve arises from the lower brachial plexus, the C8 and T1 roots. The first muscular rami of the ulnar nerve arise distal to the elbow joint and supply the flexor carpi ulnaris and the ulnar part of the flexor digitorum profundus. The next division of the nerve – into muscular rami and the superficial sensory ramus to the ulnar side of the palm of the hand and fingers – occurs at the wrist; between the elbow and the hand, only the dorsal ramus emerges, which supplies the skin of the ulnar side of the back of the hand. The function of the flexor carpi ulnaris muscle can be tested by observing and palpating its tendon during palmar and ulnar flexion of the hand. The

ulnar part of the flexor digitorum profundus muscle, also supplied by the ulnar nerve, is the only flexor of the distal interphalangeal joint of the little finger. The palmaris brevis muscle (which causes retraction of the skin over the proximal part of the hypothenar eminence during abduction of the little finger) is the only muscle supplied by the superficial palmar branch, the otherwise sensory terminal branch of the ulnar nerve (see Fig. 2.1 a). The purely motor terminal branch (ramus profundus) supplies all of the interosseous and lumbrical muscles on the ulnar side. These are the most important muscles responsible for fine movements of the fingers.

Clinical picture: The clinical picture of ulnar palsy is dominated by paralysis of the interosseous muscles. Interosseous palsy leads to hyperextension of the metacarpophalangeal joints of the fingers, especially the ring and little fingers, and slight flexion of the interphalangeal joints ("claw hand") (Fig. 10.11). The ring and especially the little finger are abducted from their neighbors. Abduction and adduction movements of the fingers remain possible, incomplete, through the action of the long extensor and long flexor muscles, respectively. An important diagnostic sign accompanies paralysis of the adductor pollicis muscle: if a flat object, such as a card, is gripped firmly between the thumb and index finger, the distal phalanx of the thumb needs to be strongly flexed, with the aid of the flexor pollicis longus muscle (median nerve). The involuntary contraction of flexor pollicis longus is called Froment's sign (Fig. 10.12). The limit of sensory loss can invariably be found in the midline of the ring finger. Muscular atrophy is most obvious on the dorsal surface of the hand between the thumb and the index finger.

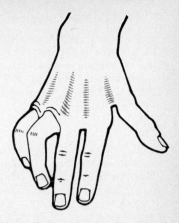

Fig. 10.**11** Typical claw hand in right ulnar palsy. Atrophy of the interosseous muscles. Hyperextension of the metacarpophalangeal joints and flexion of the interphalangeal joints, particularly those of the ring and little fingers. Hyperextension of the metacarpophalangeal joint of the thumb *(signe de Jeanne)*

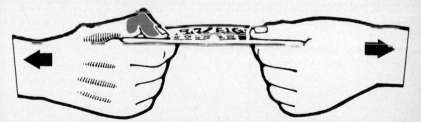

Fig. 10.**12** Right ulnar palsy. The newspaper between the thumb and index finger is held by contraction of the flexor pollicis longus (median nerve) since the adductor pollicis muscle is paralyzed (Froment's sign)

Causes of Ulnar Palsy

Ulnar palsy is the commonest peripheral nerve lesion, both as a traumatic complication and as a nontraumatic event. The most frequent site is the elbow, the second commonest the wrist.

Trauma

Direct trauma, e.g., following a blow or a knife wound, presents no etiologic problem. In the *elbow region* a primary ulnar palsy following a fracture is relatively rare – usually after a fracture of the medial condyle. At the *wrist,* the ulnar nerve may be damaged by direct trauma, e.g., fragments of glass.

Late Paralysis

A *tardy ulnar palsy* may appear months or years after an elbow injury (fracture, dislocation, etc.). The patient is usually an adult, and the ulnar palsy develops insidiously. Questioning will usually elicit a history of elbow fracture in youth or early life – a history going back for years or even decades. Often, but not invariably, a healed lateral condylar fracture may be present, and examination of the elbow reveals a valgus deformity. The physical findings on palpation of the sulcus may be typical: it is possible with practice to palpate the abnormally fixed, thickened, and sometimes painful ulnar nerve in its course behind the medial epicondyle, although the nerve may be incorporated in a mass of connective tissue which prevents it from being readily defined. The forearm muscles are far less severely affected than the hand muscles, but atrophy of the first interosseous muscle is usually marked; the sensory loss is often very slight.

Chronic Pressure Damage in the Sulcus Region

Often misunderstood are a group of lesions which are not directly traumatic in origin. In about 80% of these cases, the ulnar nerve is damaged at the *elbow joint* where it lies in direct contact with the humerus, therefore relatively exposed to injury. *Pressure paralysis* is particularly common following prolonged resting of the elbow upon a hard surface. Very careful questioning may be necessary to elicit the actual moment of damage. Most injuries of this type involve occupations in which the elbows usually rest on a surface, e.g., telephone operators, precision grinders, or else they are due to habitual postures which the patient adopts. Even the light pressure of the elbows on the bedclothes may lead to ulnar nerve palsy in *bedridden patients;* in these, the lesion may come on suddenly and is not always confined to thin or severely ill patients. Such lesions may unjustifiably be attributed to some operative or other therapeutic maneuver. The palsy occurs more commonly on the side nearer to the patient's bedside table. The **prognosis** of patients with pure pressure palsy is usually good. Treatment consists solely in preventing further nerve damage. Anterior transposition of the ulnar nerve is seldom indicated.

Anomalies in the Sulcus Region

Dislocation of Ulnar Nerve from the Sulcus

This lesion, which is virtually always a congenital anomaly, is found in 5% of individuals and always bilateral. During flexion movements of the elbow, the nerve is displaced from its bed to ride on the tip of the medial epicondyle or glide over it in an anterior direction. Sometimes the nerve is visible, it is always palpable with careful examination. The examiner sits opposite the patient and uses the index and middle fingers of his right hand to palpate the right sulcus during extension and flexion of the elbow joint. Even without additional factors, the flexion and extension movements of the elbow themselves may damage the nerve trunk repeatedly as it glides back and forth. Apart from objective signs of ulnar nerve involvement, subjective complaints such as paresthesias and local and radiating pains may occur. The pains, often localized to the medial side of the elbow, may be mistakenly diagnosed as "tennis elbow."

Excessive Movements of the Elbow Joint

Even without dislocation, excessive movements of the joint may lead to chronic microtrauma to the ulnar nerve in its passage between bones, ligaments, and the medial head of the triceps muscle. Painful paresthesias and weakness may thus be provoked, as is seen in workers operating drilling and stamping machines. The prevention of painful movements, including perhaps a change of occupation, and deliberate avoidance of elbow flexion, combined with local measures such as support and soft padding applied to the medial aspect of the elbow joint, usually lead to recovery. Operative measures are not justified.

Arthroses of the Elbow Joint

These lesions, either posttraumatic or degenerative, may lead to chronic damage to the ulnar nerve. The clinical picture corresponds to a delayed paralysis, described above. The same is true of chondromatosis in which, apart from the roentgenologic appearances and the clinically obvious joint disturbances, palpation of the sulcus yields typical findings. A *ganglion* of the elbow joint may produce a similar appearance in the presence of a normal roentgenogram. The treatment of choice is surgical operation in cases of chronic ulnar nerve damage caused by abnormal joint changes or perineural thickening in the sulcus. The ulnar nerve should be transposed as soon as possible to the anterior surface of the elbow joint beneath the origin of the ulnar flexor muscles. When this procedure is carried out in cases of chondromatosis, it is not necessary to remove loose bodies from the joint cavity. The prognosis is usually good, provided that the operation is performed early.

Chronic Pressure Damage of the Wrist

Clinically, chronic pressure palsy at the level of the wrist joint sometimes does not involve the superficial palmar (sensory) ramus of the nerve. This type of weakness, which often also spares the ramus of supply to the hypothenar muscles, may give rise to differential diagnostic difficulties. The presence of a pure motor lesion with atrophy of the intrinsic hand muscles always prompts the suspicion of spinal muscular atrophy. The importance of the preserved function of the palmaris brevis muscle has already been pointed out. If the hypothenar muscles are spared, the little finger is held in an abducted position. In advanced cases, the important diagnostic feature is the contrast between the severely atrophied first dorsal interosseous muscle (between the thumb and index finger) and the hypothenar muscles, which are virtually intact.

Causes: Chronic pressure damage to the ulnar nerve at the wrist is an occupational hazard in laborers using knives, carpentry tools, sledge hammers, pneumatic equipment, etc. Likewise cyclist's palsy is caused by pressure on the ulnar nerve at the wrist level, sometimes accompanied by a median nerve lesion. Occasionally an ulnar palsy may be a late complication, appearing after a long symptom-free interval, caused by scarring in a wound of the hypothenar soft tissues or after an inflammatory lesion of the palmar aponeurosis. Other causes are a wrist ganglion or a gouty tophus. In rare cases, a chronic lesion of the ulnar nerve may be observed, unaccompanied by any detectable external factor, as it passes between the pisiform bone and the hook of the hamate bone, the so-called *loge de Guyon*.

Treatment: This depends upon the cause of the lesion, and it is directed either exclusively at the prevention of further tissue pressure damage or, exceptionally, at operative exploration to perform neurolysis or remove a ganglion.

Differential Diagnosis

The differential diagnosis of ulnar palsy includes lower brachial plexus palsy, a lesion of the medial fasciculus of the plexus, and damage to the C8 and T1 roots. The distal, purely motor involvement caused by damage to the deep branch (ramus profundus) may be incorrectly attributed to spinal muscular atrophy. In Dupuytren's contracture, a flexed position of the ring and little fingers is always accompanied by characteristic thickening of the palmar aponeurosis and skin changes; the hyperextended metacarpophalangeal joint, which is always present in paralysis of the interosseous muscles, is absent. A striking number of cases of Dupuytren's contracture are associated with, and possibly caused by, subluxation of the ulnar nerve at the elbow joint. The same is true of two other rare congenital deformities of the little finger, campodactyly and clinodactyly. Occasionally paralysis may be mimicked if the finger joints are locked in specific positions by a purely mechanical cause, such as a lesion of the lateral attachment of the extensor apparatus on the posterior surface of the metacarpophalangeal or interphalangeal joints, which results in the extensor tendon slipping past the lateral side of the joint and coming to rest in the flexed position, ventral to its axis of movement. This situation arises in the rheumatic diseases but also in the presence of abnormal connective tissue laxity. Any request made to the patient to extend the joint results only in increased flexion, sometimes with an associated dystonic finger position.

Lumbosacral Plexus

Anatomy: This plexus is comprised of the L1–S3 roots. It lies well protected from external damage in the retroperitoneal space. The plexus gives rise to the following:

- the superior gluteal nerve exiting from the suprapiriform foramen,
- the inferior gluteal nerve, and
- the sciatic nerve, which both exit through the infrapiriform foramen,
- obturator nerve passing out of the pelvis through the obturator foramen, and
- femoral nerve passing out between muscles beneath the inguinal ligament.

Clinically, the pictures of paralysis vary greatly, depending on the particular part of the lumbosacral plexus involved (851). Table 10.2 shows the principal clinical features of the commonest peripheral nerve lesions of the pelvic girdle and lower extremities.

Causes of paralysis (851, 941) are usually retroperitoneal space-occupying lesions (neoplastic metastases, lymphoma, local malignancy especially of the rectum, urogenital system, and female sex organs), hematomas (see below), or aneurysms. Damage due to X-irradiation and intra-arterial chemotherapy (941) are also factors. Diagnostic ultrasound and abdominal CT are helpful.

Genitofemoral and Ilioinguinal Nerves

Anatomy: Both nerves arise from the L1–2 segments. Both are largely sensory nerves and their cutaneous distribution in the inguinal and genital regions is shown in Fig. 2.1.

Clinical picture: Lesions of the genitofemoral nerve and the ilioinguinal nerve lead to *sensory loss* in the cutaneous distribution of these nerves in the groin, the upper medial aspect of the thigh, and the scrotum or labium majus. The cremasteric reflex is absent. A partial paralysis of the abdominal muscles is present which may not be perceptible clinically. *Pain syndromes* may be prominent: genitofemoral nerve lesions give rise to intense *spermatic neuralgia*. Ilioinguinal lesions cause obstinate groin pains when the patient is erect; when recumbent, he assumes a position of slight flexion and

Table 10.2 Review of lesions of the lumbar plexus and peripheral nerves in the lower extremities [778]

Nerve	Muscles Affected	Sensory Deficit	Function	Specific Test	Etiology	Remarks	Differential Diagnosis
Lumbar plexus L1–L4	Especially hip flexors (rotators of hip joint) and adductors, also flexors of knee	1 Iliohypogastric 2 Posterior femoral cutaneous 3 Lateral femoral cutaneous 4 Obturator 5 Iliohypogastric	See individual muscles		Traumatic, retroperitoneal processes (tumors, hematomas), squatting position, diabetes mellitus		

Sacral plexus L5–S3	Especially gluteal and ischiocrural muscles, and dorsi- and plantar flexors of the foot and toes	See individual muscles		Multiple root lesions, cauda equina syndrome, occlusions of the pelvic arteries
Femoral L2–L4	Iliacus and pectineus	Flexion and internal rotation of hip	Testing with patient seated and legs dangling	High lumbar disk herniation, progressive muscular dystrophy (isolated involvement of thigh), muscular atrophy due to knee joint disease, femoral form of diabetic neuropathy
	Sartorius	Flexion, adduction, and external rotation of hip		
	Quadriceps femoris	Extension of knee (and flexion of hip)	Operations, injuries, hyperextension of the hip, hemophilia	
Obturator L2–L4	Obturator externus, pectineus and adductor brevis	Adduction and external rotation of hip		
	Adductor longus Adductor magnus	Adduction of hip		

6 Saphenous
7 Anterior cutaneous branch of femoral nerve

Table 10.2 (continued)

Nerve	Muscles Affected	Sensory Deficit	Function	Specific Test	Etiology	Remarks	Differential Diagnosis
	Gracilis		Adduction and medial rotation of hip and flexion of knee				
Lateral femoral cutaneous L2–L3			Purely sensory involvement	Pressure just medial to anterior inferior iliac spine is painful, hyperextending hip causes more pain	Chronic mechanical damage at point of emergence in inguinal ligament	Meralgia paresthetica	High lumbar disk herniation
Ilioinguinal L1(–L2)			Mainly sensory involvement	Overextension of hip joint	Chronic mechanical damage at point of emergence in muscles of abdominal wall		Lesions of hip joint
Superior gluteal L4–S1	Gluteus medius Gluteus minimus		Internal rotation of hip in light flexion	Abducting the straightened leg with patient lying on opposite side, downward tilting of pelvis on opposite side upon walking	Traumatic, including paralysis due to faulty intramuscular injection		Pelvic girdle form of progressive muscular dystrophy

Inferior gluteal L5–S2	Tensor fasciae latae	Abduction of hip	(positive Trendelenburg's sign)	Muscular dystrophy
	Gluteus maximus	Extension of hip	Patient prone, knee flexed to 90°; lifting the thigh from the examination couch	
Tibial L4–S3	Gastrocnemius	} Plantar flexion of foot (and knee flexion)	First 15° of knee flexion	Trauma in popliteal fossa; isolated lesion may present as partial sciatic nerve damage	L5–S1 disk herniation
	Plantaris			
	Soleus			
	Popliteus	Flexion of knee joint	Knee flexed to 90°	

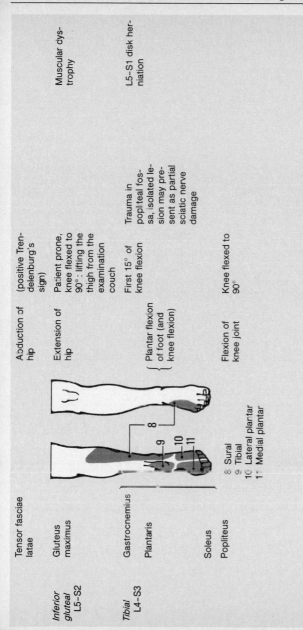

8 Sural
9 Tibial
10 Lateral plantar
11 Medial plantar

Table 10.**2** (continued)

Nerve	Muscles Affected	Sensory Deficit	Function	Specific Test	Etiology	Remarks	Differential Diagnosis
	Tibialis posterior		Supination and plantar flexion of foot	Toe flexors should not be activated			
	Flexor digitorum longus		Flexion of terminal phalanges of toes				
	Flexor hallucis longus						
	Flexor digitorum brevis		Flexion of middle phalanges of toes				
	Flexor hallucis brevis						
	Abductor hallucis						
	Abductor digiti minimi						
	Adductor hallucis						
	Quadratus plantaris						
	Lumbrical muscles						
	Interosseous muscles						

		Dorsiflexion of foot		Direct trauma Fractures of fibula		L4–L5 disk herniation, other root lesions, polyneuropathies, muscular dystrophy, distal muscular atrophy in myopathies, anterior tibial (artery) syndrome
Lateral popliteal (common peroneal) L4–S2	Tibialis anterior		Walking on heels Steppage gait			
	Extensor digitorum longus	Extension of terminal phalanges of toes and extension of foot				
	Extensor hallucis longus					
Anterior tibial (deep peroneal)	Peroneus tertius	Extension of metatarso-phalangeal joints		Pressure palsy	Good prognosis	
	Extensor digitorum brevis					
	Extensor hallucis brevis					
Musculocutaneous (superficial peroneal)	Peroneus longus	Eversion and plantar flexion		Serogenic paralysis	Rare	
	Peroneus brevis					

12 Lateral popliteal
13 Musculocutaneous
14 Sural
15 Anterior tibial

medial rotation of the hip *(ilioinguinal syndrome).*

Causes: These syndromes are usually caused by operative damage to the genitofemoral or ilioinguinal nerve, either through direct trauma or by being incorporated in the operative scar, e.g., herniotomies, and the ilioinguinal nerve in nephrectomies and retrocecal appendectomies. The latter nerve may also be compromised spontaneously at the site of its passage through the muscles of the abdominal wall. Treatment consists of neurolysis or resection of the nerve proximal to the site of compression.

Femoral Nerve

Anatomy: This nerve arises from the L2-L4 roots, traverses the lumbar plexus, and passes with the iliac and psoas muscles, which it supplies. It passes from the pelvis to the thigh beneath the inguinal ligament in the company of the psoas muscle. In the thigh, the femoral nerve supplies the quadriceps femoris muscle and contains sensory rami for the anterior surface of the thigh and the medial surface of the leg (saphenous nerve).

Clinical picture: Lesions of the femoral nerve cause *paralysis* of the extensor muscles of the knee (climbing stairs!) and reduce or abolish the knee jerk. Hip flexion is reduced since a portion of the quadriceps muscle is a hip flexor; this sign is more marked after intrapelvic lesions involving the iliopsoas muscle. *Cutaneous sensory loss* involves the anterior aspect of the thigh and the anteromedial surface of the leg (saphenous nerve).

Causes: The femoral nerve may be damaged in its intra-abdominal course beneath the inguinal ligament by a *psoas hematoma* or by *operative interference* (appendectomy, herniotomy, hysterectomy). Cases have been described of damage to the femoral nerve by sudden hyperextension of the hip joint, a lesion carrying a poor prognosis. Femoral nerve palsy is a strikingly common peripheral nerve lesion in the hemorrhagic diatheses. The *saphenous nerve* may be damaged in the course of its *passage through the crural fascia,* causing pain over the anterior and medial aspects of the leg and a corresponding sensory loss. Neuropathia patellae, see p. 471.

Differential diagnosis: This includes quadriceps paralysis caused by lesions of the L3 or L4 roots, usually secondary to prolapse of the L2-3 or L3-4 intervertebral disks, in which the vertebral syndrome is already present, and the simultaneous presence of other motor root signs, radicular sensory loss, and sometimes roentgenologic changes in the vertebral column enable a differential diagnosis to be made. Isolated (bilateral) atrophy and pure motor deficit in the thigh muscles of elderly subjects may indicate a myopathy, but this is rare. Diabetic neuropathy may be responsible for (unilateral) acute femoral paralysis. Inactivity and knee joint lesions may cause a so-called arthritic muscular atrophy of the thigh muscles. In infants, repeated injections into the quadriceps muscle may produce a contracture of the knee extensors necessitating quadriceps tenotomy (736). Apart from muscular atrophy, changes occur in the subcutaneous fatty tissues of the thigh. A lipoid atrophy develops in diabetics who receive insulin injections. Horizontal bands of atrophy of the subcutaneous tissues traditionally were encountered in washerwomen (lipoatrophia semicircularis), and are nowadays found in persons whose work brings them in frequent contact with protruding objects such as the edges of furniture (443).

Lateral Femoral Cutaneous Nerve (Meralgia Paresthetica)

Anatomy: The lateral femoral cutaneous nerve (L2-3) is a pure sensory nerve. It leaves the pelvis close to the medial side of the anterior superior iliac spine and traverses the fibers of the inguinal ligament, i.e., the thickened lower margin of the aponeurosis of the external oblique muscle of the abdominal wall. At this point, it is tightly surrounded by the tendinous fibers of the inguinal ligament and makes a right-angled bend to change direction from its horizontal course in the pelvis to a vertical course in the thigh. This angle is related phylogenetically to the erect posture assumed by man.

Clinical picture: An acute lesion of this nerve leads to cutaneous sensory loss over the anterior and lateral aspect of the thigh. More common is a chronic lesion, the so-called *meralgia paresthetica* (279, 851). The patient complains of paresthesias and shooting or burning pains over the anterior and outer surfaces of the thigh. The complaints are always aggravated by extension of the hip and may be partly or completely abolished by flexion, e.g., if the foot is placed on a raised platform. Men are three times more often affected than women. In about 10% of cases the complaint is bilateral. Often the stage of paresthesias leads to permanent hypesthesia or anesthesia and analgesia in the area of distribution of the nerve (see Fig. 2.1). An intermittent variety may occur. Apart from the typical sensory disturbance, three-fourths of cases have a tender spot over the inguinal ligament 2 fingerbreadths medial to the anterior superior iliac spine. The symptoms may be aggravated by stretching the nerve through hip extension ("reversed" Lasègue's sign). Only about one-fourth of patients recover spontaneously.

Causes: The lateral femoral cutaneous nerve may be damaged by *direct trauma* in the course of its passage through the inguinal ligament or iatrogenically following hip operations. Far more common is chronic mechanical damage, a compression syndrome of the inguinal ligament itself. This lesion occurs as a result of the anatomic factors mentioned above, or sometimes combined with the effects of other factors, e.g., constricting garments or girdles, an abnormal increase in weight (paunch), increased demand on the abdominal muscles attached to the inguinal ligament (pregnancy, marching, strenuous physical activity, disturbances of normal smooth gait in diseases of the locomotor apparatus, etc.), also in unusually prolonged extended positions of the hip joint, where the patient is lying supine (bedridden patients, sleeping on a bare surface, etc.). All these factors may lead to the syndrome of meralgia paresthetica described above.

Treatment: In most cases of meralgia paresthetica, the symptoms are only mild and it is exceptional for the pain to be so severe that active treatment is essential. Apart from preventing the trigger factors mentioned above, hydrocortisone injections or operative neurolysis of the nerve at its point of passage through the inguinal ligament must be undertaken.

Differential diagnosis: This is concerned chiefly with prolapse of a high lumbar disk. Diagnostic mistakes are usually prevented by the presence of symptoms and signs referable to the spine, as well as a different cutaneous distribution of the sensory loss and muscular weakness.

Obturator Nerve

Anatomy: This nerve arises from the L2-4 roots and leaves the pelvis through the obturator foramen. It supplies the adductor muscles and contains sensory cutaneous rami from the distal medial part of the thigh.

Clinically, a lesion of the obturator nerve causes weakness of thigh adduction and sensory loss on the medial side of the lower thigh and the

knee joint. If the lesion amounts only to irritation of the obturator nerve, pains are present on the medial side of the knee *(Howship-Romberg phenomenon)*. This lesion must be differentiated from an intrinsic disturbance of the knee joint.

Causes: Fracture of the pelvis, neoplasm, or obturator hernia.

Gluteal Nerves

Anatomy: The *superior gluteal nerve* arises from the L4–S1 roots. It supplies the hip abductors, i.e., gluteus medius and gluteus minimus, as well as the tensor fasciae latae muscles. It leaves the pelvis through the suprapiriform foramen. The *inferior gluteal nerve* (L5–S2) supplies the gluteus maximus muscle, the most powerful hip extensor. It leaves the pelvis dorsal to the sciatic nerve through the infrapiriform foramen.

Clinically, paralysis of the hip abductors results in the pelvis tilting toward the side of the raised leg (Trendelenburg's sign) during walking. If the paralysis is only partial, the patient attempts to overcome the pelvic tilt by tilting his head and trunk to the affected side (Duchenne's gait) (Fig. 10.**13**). Paralysis of the gluteus maximus produces weakness of hip extension, e.g., inability to rise from a chair or mount stairs.

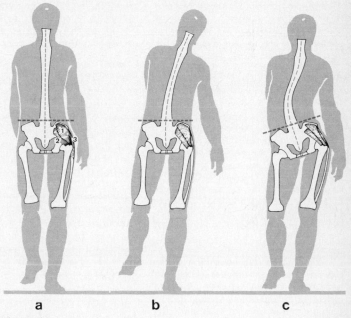

a   b   c

1 = gluteus medius muscle
2 = gluteus minimus muscle
3 = tensor fasciae latae muscle

Fig. 10.**13a–c** Gait abnormality caused by weakness of right hip abductors **a** Normal **b** With slight weakness, the trunk prevents a tilt of the pelvis to the healthy side by slight sideways arching to the pathologic side (Duchenne's sign) **c** With severe weakness, the pelvis tilts to the side of the healthy leg (Trendelenburg's sign)

Causes: Direct trauma, parturition, unskilled intragluteal injections (injection paralysis, see below).

Differential diagnosis: In the case of lesions of these nerves, other causes of a radicular lesion must be considered. For example, a partial gluteus maximus palsy may accompany a lumbosacral disk herniation with an S1 syndrome. Involvement of the pelvic girdle muscles in progressive muscular atrophy (dystrophy) (bilateral!) must also be considered, as well as the waddling gait of (congenital) dislocation of the hip.

Sciatic Nerve

Anatomy: The sciatic nerve, arising from the L4–S3 roots, is the largest and longest peripheral nerve in the body. It comprises all parts of the lumbosacral plexus and leaves the pelvis through the infrapiriform foramen. The nerve divides at a varying level in the thigh, but always before it passes into the popliteal fossa, into its two divisions, the lateral popliteal (common peroneal) and medial popliteal (posterior tibial) nerves. However, the nerve fibers for the two divisions are already grouped far proximal to the point of separation of the trunk; indeed, a definite morphologic subdivision can be clearly detected at the level of the infrapiriform foramen. The medial popliteal *(posterior tibial)* nerve supplies the semitendinosus, semimembranosus, long head of the biceps femoris, and part of the adductor magnus muscles. The lateral popliteal (common peroneal) nerve supplies muscular branches to the short head of the biceps femoris muscle and articular branches to the knee joint. The sciatic nerve *supplies,* in addition to the ischiocrural muscles, all the muscles of the leg and foot. In contains sensory fibers from the greater part of the skin on the lateral and dorsal surfaces of the leg and the skin of the foot, with the exception of the region of the medial malleolus and a narrow strip on the medial side of the foot, which is supplied by the saphenous nerve.

Clinical aspects: The signs and symptoms of a sciatic lesion amount to a combination of a peroneal palsy and a posterior tibial lesion (see below). More proximal lesions may also involve the articular rami to the knee flexors with muscular paralysis and absent or diminished reflexes (see Table 2.**1**).

Causes: The commonest cause is direct *trauma* (e.g., gunshot or stab wound), *fracture of the pelvis,* (especially fracture dislocation involving the acetabulum), or dislocation of the hip joint. *Pressure paralysis* at the buttock may occur in unconscious patients who are incorrectly positioned. An *ischemic* sciatic lesion may be part of the picture of an arteritis (798). The iatrogenic lesion produced by intragluteal injection will be described below.

Lateral Popliteal (Common Peroneal) Nerve

Anatomy: This nerve, arising from the L4–S2 roots, winds itself out of the popliteal fossa, emerging just distal to the head of the fibula on its lateral side. The nerve lies in direct contact with the fibula at this level and separates into superficial and deep divisions. The musculocutaneous (superficial peroneal) nerve supplies the peroneal muscles and intrinsic damage to the nerve produces a sensory loss over the lateral surface of the calf and most of the dorsum of the foot, and the patient is unable to elevate the lateral side of his foot. The anterior tibial (deep peroneal) nerve supplies the dorsiflexors of the foot and toes and the skin overlying the first interosseous space.

Clinical picture: Paralysis of the common peroneal nerve is one of the commonest peripheral nerve palsies. The typical clinical picture of peroneal palsy (deep division, i.e., anterior tibial nerve) is a *steppage gait,* in which the patient has to lift his leg high with each step in order to prevent his toes from dragging on the ground during the forward swing. If the superficial division is also involved, the lateral border of the foot drops with each step, a sign particularly noticeable from behind.

Causes of Peroneal Palsy

Trauma

Fractures of the head of the fibula are sometimes complicated by peroneal palsy. *Dislocation of the knee joint* may occasionally involve the peroneal nerve. A *fall leading to a sprained ankle* may result in a peroneal palsy due to sudden stretching of the nerve.

Pressure Palsy

The commonest cause of isolated peroneal palsy is damage to the nerve trunk in the vicinity of the *head of the fibula.* A pressure palsy may be produced by simple crossing of the legs, unsatisfactory positioning of the limbs of an unconscious or paralyzed patient, a too tight plaster cast, or specific activities involving a kneeling position. Thin individuals are particularly at risk. The prognosis of patients with this type of pressure palsy is always good. A *ganglion* in the vicinity of the tibiofibular joint may produce chronic nerve damage. On several occasions the author has encountered pressure damage of the distal cutaneous divisions of the common peroneal nerve on the *dorsum of the foot* caused by a tight-fitting shoe, usually hiking or ski boots, in which dysesthesias and hypesthesias are present. Loss of sensation of the medial surface of the *distal phalanx of the big toe* may also be caused by shoe pressure, especially in the presence of osteophytosis of the distal interphalangeal joint or hallux valgus. A pain syndrome of the sciatic nerve, the piriformis syndrome, is described on p. 470.

Injection Paralysis (1162)

Causes: Injection paralysis may follow injections made into or in the vicinity of the sciatic nerve. However, most cases of paralysis involve damage to the common peroneal division of the sciatic trunk. This statement requires further elaboration. Injection paralysis depends chiefly upon the site of the injection, see below. The nature of the injection solution is unimportant, compared with the site; damage has been recorded from a wide variety of substances.

Pathologic anatomy: An intense foreign body reaction develops around the sciatic nerve, which leads to dense fibrosis, some of which may penetrate between the bundles of nerve fibers.

Clinical picture: In about two-thirds of cases, the onset of weakness follows immediately upon the injection; only one-sixth of patients experience immediate pain. In about 10% of cases, the paralysis develops only after a free interval of hours or even days. The picture is dominated, apart from the paralysis which is maximal 24–48 h after its onset, by a pain syndrome which may become causalgic in type.

Prevention and treatment: Intragluteal injections should be made only into the upper and outer quadrant of the buttock, in a direction at right angles to the body surface (and not inframedially, caudally, or medially). If an injection paralysis occurs, prompt surgical exploration is indicated to remove all pockets of injection fluid from the nerve trunk and its vicinity and to free all adhesions.

Differential Diagnosis of Peroneal Palsy

General Differential Diagnosis

Numerous causes may produce a clinical picture that resembles a lesion of the peripheral peroneal nerve. The first of these is prolapse of the L4–5 disk with damage to the L5 root, which leads to marked weakness of the extensor muscles of the big toe and sometimes sensory loss over the dorsum of the foot ("vertebral peroneal palsy"). This sensory loss extends proximally in the corresponding dermatome. The presence of backache and a radicular distribution of the sensory loss point to the correct diagnosis. Many polyneuropathies start distally in the lower extremity and may produce the picture of a peroneal palsy with a steppage gait. The late stages of the Charcot-Marie-Tooth type of peroneal muscular atrophy (p. 303) may show, apart from the signs of peroneal palsy, atrophy and paralysis of the calf muscles, absent ankle jerks, and rarely a distal sensory loss. An invariable finding in these familial lesions is a club foot. The Curschmann-Steinert type of myotonic dystrophy may show atrophy and paralysis of distal muscles, but other signs of this dominant hereditary disease are usually present.

Anterior Tibial (Tibial Compartment) Syndrome (851)

This syndrome, caused by ischemia of the foot and toe extensors in the tibial compartment, is often confused with a peripheral peroneal palsy.

Pathology: The pathologic lesion is an ischemic necrosis of the muscles in the tibial compartment (tibialis anterior, extensor hallucis longus, and extensor digitorum longus muscles). The compartment is sealed on all sides by bony and connective tissue walls so that none of its contents can expand. If edema occurs within it as a result of an ischemic process, e.g., thrombosis, embolism, or occlusion of a proximal artery, a vicious circle is created through compression of capillaries, which in turn provokes more edema. A similar vicious circle may arise if the pressure is increased by a tibial fracture or a traumatic or postoperative hematoma within the compartment itself. Swelling of the soft tissues may also be produced by excessive physical demands upon the leg muscles (marching, football, etc.).

Clinical aspects: The clinical picture consists of intense pain with swelling and redness of the pretibial region. At the same time, dorsiflexion of the foot and toes becomes painful, and within the space of hours a complete paralysis may be present. Since the anterior tibial nerve (deep division of the peroneal nerve), which also traverses the tibial compartment, may be damaged by ischemia, the extensor digitorum brevis and extensor hallucis brevis muscles on the dorsal surface of the foot may be paralyzed, and an area of sensory loss is present over the first interosseous space. In some cases, the ischemic damage also involves the musculocutaneous nerve (superficial division of the peroneal nerve), which receives a nutrient twig from the anterior tibial artery. If this occurs, an additional (neurogenic) paralysis of the peroneal muscles and corresponding sensory loss are present. In the early stages, the picture of paralysis is identical to that of a common peroneal nerve palsy, but a differential diagnosis is usually possible on the basis of the initial clinical features – viz. intense pain in the tibial compartment and a frequently absent pulse of the dorsalis pedis artery (although an absent pulse is not necessary for the diagnosis).

Recovery: Usually only the neurogenic part of the paralysis recovers; without operation the muscles in the tibial compartment undergo fibrosis and retraction. In the later stages, palpation reveals them to be as hard as wood, the ankle joint cannot be plantar-flexed beyond 90°, and the big toe assumes a hammer toe deformity due to shortening of the extensor hallucis longus muscle.

Electromyographically, the necrotic muscles show no activity ("silent EMG"). The extensor digitorum brevis and peroneal muscles, on the other hand, may show the picture of a neurogenic palsy.

Treatment: Early diagnosis is essential since operative splitting of the anterior crural fascia must be carried out within the first few hours, if irreversible ischemic necrosis of the muscles is to be prevented.

Posterior Tibial (Medial Popliteal) Nerve

Anatomy: The posterior tibial nerve arises from the L4–S3 roots, its fibers lying on the medial side of the sciatic trunk. It supplies all the plantar flexor muscles of the foot and toes as well as all the small foot muscles with the exception of the extensores breves on the dorsum of the foot. Cutaneous sensory rami supply the skin of the heel and sole. The posterior tibial nerve is particularly rich in autonomic fibers.

Clinical aspects: A lesion of the posterior tibial nerve causes paralysis of all flexor muscles of the foot and toes. Even a partial paralysis prevents the patient from walking on his toes, and the ankle jerk is diminished. In complete paralysis, the foot assumes a valgus position due to predominance of the peroneal muscles. The toes can no longer be spread or flexed maximally. The ankle jerk is absent. Sensation over the sole of the foot is absent.

Causes: The posterior tibial nerve is well protected in the popliteal fossa and damage at this level is rare, e.g., gunshot wounds. The sciatic trunk or one of its terminal divisions may be damaged in supracondylar femoral fractures. In subluxation of the knee joint, the posterior tibial nerve is far less frequently involved than the common peroneal. In fractures of the tibial platform or proximal half of the shaft with dorsal angulation or dislocation, the trunk of the posterior tibial nerve may be damaged, and primary operative exploration is justified in such cases. In other patients, sensory changes in the sole of the foot and paralysis may only appear in the course of fracture healing, prompting the suspicion of perineural scar tissue formation and justifying operative neurolysis. The same applies to fractures through the distal one-third of the tibia. Subjects in certain occupations who perform tasks that demand continuous peddling movements, e.g., potters, are likely to cause chronic mechanical damage to both posterior tibial and common peroneal nerves leading to paralysis, because of their anatomic relations to the muscles around the knee joint.

Tarsal Tunnel Syndrome

This term is used to describe a chronic lesion of the posterior tibial nerve in the vicinity of the medial malleolus under the flexor retinaculum, complicating a Pott's fracture with or without displacement of the fragments, a sprain of the ankle, or presenting spontaneously (rare). Compression of the posterior tibial nerve or of its two divisions, the lateral and medial plantar nerves, leads to painful sensory disturbances in the sole of the foot which are aggravated by walking. Physical examination confirms these sensory changes in the distribution of the plantar nerves, as well as reduced or absent sweat secretion over the sole of the foot, and paralysis of the small muscles of the sole. Often the course of the posterior tibial nerve is tender to palpation. Apart from those cases in which demonstrable neurologic deficits are present, the syndrome may present merely as painful sensations occurring in the sole of the foot upon walking. This complaint can be abolished by *anesthetic blocking of the posterior tibial nerve* behind the medial malleolus – a maneuver used as a diagnostic test. The diagnosis may be confirmed *electromyographically.*

Treatment consists of operative freeing of the nerve trunk under the flexor retinaculum. A florid pannus-like tissue reaction is present; sometimes a pseudoneuroma formation of the nerve trunk is found.

Metatarsalgia (Morton's Toe)

This condition is caused by a fusiform pseudoneuroma of a digital nerve. It is usually situated in the third or fourth interdigital space, just proximal to the division of the nerve. **Clinically,** the patient complains of neuralgic and often burning pains in the sole of the foot, usually in the vicinity of the head of the third or fourth metatarsal bone and in the corresponding toes. The pain first appears during walking, but in time becomes continuous and may then radiate proximally. The pains are often incorrectly attributed to "splayfoot (valgus) deformity." Physical examination shows that intense pain can be provoked by pressure on the sole of the foot or displacement of a head of one metatarsal bone by pressing it against an adjoining one. The diagnosis may be confirmed by infiltration of local anesthetic of the plantar nerves at their site of division in the third interdigital space (using an approach from the dorsum of the foot), a maneuver which causes the pain to disappear abruptly.

Treatment in mild cases consists in wearing special shoes or foot supports within the shoes, which sustain the foot arch just behind the metatarsal heads. If the unpleasant neuralgic pain persists, the neuroma must be excised.

11. Headache and Facial Pain

(85, 508, 670, 1132, 1291)

Headache may be an accompanying feature of another definable disease, or a disease entity in itself. This latter category in particular will be dealt with in the following section.

General Considerations

Structures Sensitive to Pain in the Head and Face

The brain itself is insensitive to pain. On the other hand, pain receptors are present in all the extracranial soft tissues and in certain parts of the intracranial space such as the basal dura and pia mater, the venous sinuses and their immediate tributaries, arteries of the circle of Willis, and nerves with sensory afferents. In essence, pain can be provoked in the head or face by pressure or tension on any of the above-mentioned pain-sensitive intracranial structures and especially the extracerebral arteries, or by phenomena involving the extracranial tissues.

Case history of the headache patient: Precise analysis of the nature of the head pain often permits the physician to reach the correct etiologic diagnosis. The following questions should be systematically asked:

- *Family* history of headache (and its nature) or epilepsy?
- *How long* have headaches been present?
- *Nature* of headaches,
  - time of onset each day,
  - speed of onset ("attack"),
  - site,
  - nature of the pain,
  - triggering and alleviating factors,
  - relationship between the intensity of the pain and the time of day,
  - duration of the headache, and
  - accompanying signs occurring during or before the attacks, particularly eye signs, paresthesias, redness of the face, lacrimation, pallor, nausea, vomiting, urinary frequency.
- *Frequency.*
- *Previous treatment* and other measures and their efficacy. Analgesic abuse?
- *Effects* on work capacity and daily life?
- *Generalized symptoms* apart from the attacks of headache,
  - memory disturbances,
  - neurologic signs,

- weight loss,
- fatigue,
- cardiac and circulatory complaints,
- renal diseases,
- epileptic attacks.
- *Personality* and lifestyle of the patient,
  - character,
  - occupational stress,
  - conflicts,
  - living habits,
  - toxic substances and medications.

Physical examination of the headache patient: Although in the majority of cases no abnormal findings are present, physical examination must be careful and complete:

- General medical status with particular attention to
  - blood pressure,
  - circulatory functions,
  - renal functions,
  - infections,

- meningitis,
- evidence of malignancy,
- ORL diseases.
- Neurologic status, particularly
  - signs of raised intracranial pressure,
  - focal deficits,
  - meningism,
  - cranial nerve palsies.
- Mental status, including
  - organic mental syndrome,
  - neuropsychologic deficit,
  - disturbances of consciousness,
  - depression,
  - neurotic disturbances,
  - conflict situations.

Classification of Head and Face Pain

In anticipation of a systematic discussion, Table 11.1 provides a useful classification **based on etiologic factors.** Table 11.2 deals with the differential diagnosis of headache according to phenomenologic factors.

Table 11.1 Etiologic classification of the most important causes of headache and facial pain. Abbreviated classification following the proposal of the Headache classification committee of the International Headache Society (Cephalalgia 1988; 8 [suppl. 7]: 1–96)

1. Migraine
   1.1 Migraine without aura
   1.2 Migraine with aura
      1.2.1 Migraine with typical aura
      1.2.2 Migraine with prolonged aura
      1.2.3 Familial hemiplegic migraine
      1.2.4 Basilar migraine
      1.2.5 Migraine aura without headache
   1.3 Ophthalmoplegic migraine
   1.4 Retinal migraine
   1.5 Childhood periodic syndromes that may be precursors to or associated with migraine
      1.5.1 Benign paroxysmal vertigo of childhood
      1.5.2 Alternating hemiplegia of childhood

Table 11.**1**   (Continued)

1. Migraine
   1.6 Complications of migraine
   1.7 Migrainous disorder not fulfilling above criteria

2. Tension-type headache
   2.1 Episodic tension-type headache
   2.2 Chronic tension-type headache
   2.3 Headache of the tension type not fulfilling above criteria

3. Cluster headache and chronic paroxysmal hemicrania
   3.1 Cluster headache
      3.1.1 Cluster headache periodicity undetermined
      3.1.2 Episodic cluster headache
      3.1.3 Chronic cluster headache
   3.2 Chronic paroxysmal hemicrania
   3.3 Cluster headache-like disorder not fulfilling above criteria

4. Miscellaneous headaches unassociated with structural lesion
   4.1 Idiopathic stabbing headache
   4.2 External compression headache
   4.3 Cold stimulus headache
   4.4 Benign cough headache
   4.5 Benign exertional headache
   4.6 Headache associated with sexual activity

5. Headache associated with head trauma
   5.1 Acute post-traumatic headache
   5.2 Chronic post-traumatic headache

6. Headache associated with vascular disorders
   6.1 Acute ischemic cerebrovascular disease
   6.2 Intracranial hematoma
   6.3 Subarachnoid hemorrhage
   6.4 Unruptured vascular malformation
   6.5 Arteritis
   6.6 Carotid or vertebral artery pain
      6.6.1 Carotid or vertebral dissection
      6.6.2 Carotidynia (idiopathic)
      6.6.3 Post endarterectomy headache
   6.7 Venous thrombosis
   6.8 Arterial hypertension
   6.9 Headache associated with other vascular disorder

7. Headache associated with non-vascular intracranial disorder
   7.1 High cerebrospinal fluid pressure
      7.1.1 Benign intracranial hypertension
      7.1.2 High pressure hydrocephalus
   7.2 Low cerebrospinal fluid pressure
   7.3 Intracranial infection
   7.4 Intracranial sarcoidosis and other noninfectious inflammatory diseases
   7.5 Headache related to intrathecal injections
   7.6 Intracranial neoplasm
   7.7 Headache associated with other intracranial disorder

Table 11.1   (Continued)

8. *Headache associated with substances or their withdrawal*
   8.1 Headache induced by acute substance use or exposure
   8.2 Headache induced by chronic substance use or exposure
   8.3 Headache from substance withdrawal (acute use)
   8.4 Headache from substance withdrawal (chronic use)
   8.5 Headache associated with substances but with uncertain mechanism

9. *Headache associated with non-cephalic infection*

10. *Headache associated with metabolic disorder*
   10.1 Hypoxia
   10.2 Hypercapnia
   10.3 Mixed hypoxia and hypercapnia
   10.4 Hypoglycemia
   10.5 Dialysis
   10.6 Headache related to other metabolic abnormality

11. *Headache or facial pain associated with disorder of cranium, neck, eyes, ears, nose, sinuses, teeth, mouth or other facial or cranial structures*
   11.1 Cranial bone
   11.2 Neck
   11.3 Eyes
   11.4 Ears
   11.5 Nose and sinuses
   11.6 Teeth, jaws and related structures
   11.7 Temporomandibular joint disease

12. *Cranial neuralgias, nerve trunk pain and deafferentation pain*
   12.1 Persistent (in contrast to tic-like) pain of cranial nerve origin
      12.1.1 Compression or distortion of cranial nerves and second or third cervical roots
      12.1.2 Demyelination of cranial nerves
      12.1.3 Infarction of cranial nerves
      12.1.4 Inflammation of cranial nerves
      12.1.5 Tolosa-Hunt syndrome
      12.1.6 Neck-tongue syndrome
      12.1.7 Other causes of persistent pain of cranial nerve origin
   12.2 Trigeminal neuralgia
      12.2.1 Idiopathic trigeminal neuralgia
      12.2.2 Symptomatic trigeminal neuralgia
   12.3 Glossopharyngeal neuralgia
   12.4 Nervus intermedius neuralgia
   12.5 Superior laryngeal neuralgia
   12.6 Occipital neuralgia
   12.7 Central causes of head and facial pain other than tic douloureux
      12.7.1 Anaesthesia dolorosa
      12.7.2 Thalamic pain
   12.8 Facial pain not fulfilling criteria in groups 11 or 12

13. *Headache not classifiable*

Table 11.2 Differential diagnosis of types of head and facial pain

Features	Diagnosis	Localization	Duration	Onset and Trigger Factors	Accompanying Features	Findings	Remarks
Repeated attacks (acute) of headache	Migraine	Often unilateral, head and temples. Side variable	Hours to days	Weather, tension, menses	Vomiting, visual aura, perhaps focal symptoms	Neurologic examination normal. EEG may be abnormal	Sometimes increase after oral contraceptives
	Cluster headache	Eye and temples. Always unilateral and on the same side	30 min to several hours	Frequently "on schedule", often at night	Reddening of face, lacrimation, and vomiting	Normal	Differential diagnosis: nasociliary neuralgia
	Hypertensive crises	Diffuse	Minutes to hours	Irregular	Sometimes vomiting and confusion	Hypertension, fundal changes, and vascular insults	Consider pheochromocytoma
Repeated attacks of intense facial pain	Trigeminal neuralgia	2nd and 3rd divisions of trigeminal nerve, always on the same side	Seconds	Trigger zones (touching, chewing, speaking)	Contortion of the face	Normal	
	Auriculotemporal neuralgia	Preauricular	Minutes	Chewing	Local sweating and reddening of the skin	Normal	Often follows parotid disorders

	Location	Duration	Precipitating factors	Accompanying symptoms	Findings	Remarks
Nasociliary neuralgia	Inner angle of the eye	Minutes to hours	Local pressure, chewing	Conjunctivitis, lacrimation	Normal	Sometimes permanent pain. Differential diagnosis: Sluder's neuralgia or cluster headache
Sluder's neuralgia	Inner angle of the eye	Minutes		Sneezing	Occasionally sinusitis	Differential diagnosis: nasociliary neuralgia
Glossopharyngeal neuralgia	Base of tongue and tonsillar fossa	Seconds	Deglutition, trigger zone		Normal	
Geniculate ganglion neuralgia	Auditory canal and roof of palate	Seconds	Often after otic herpes	Sense of taste and flow of saliva	Normal	
Atypical facial pain	Half of the face, diffuse	Unrelenting pain of lesser or greater severity	May follow dental treatment	Occasionally redness of face and sweating	Normal	Often burning in character, very resistant to therapy
Subarachnoid hemorrhage	Diffuse (rarely occipital or unilateral)	Days	Straining	Sometimes disturbances of consciousness, vomiting	Meningism, sometimes focal symptoms	Lumbar puncture, CAT scanning
Intracerebral hemorrhage	Unilateral	Days		Sometimes vomiting	Focal symptoms	
Disturbances of CSF flow, intermittent	Diffuse (sometimes unilateral)	Minutes or hours	Sometimes suddenly on changing body position	Vomiting, confusion, drowsiness	Sometimes meningism	Sometimes disappears on changing body position

Head pain of sudden onset (grouping: Subarachnoid hemorrhage, Intracerebral hemorrhage, Disturbances of CSF flow, intermittent)

Table 11.**2** (Continued)

Features	Diagnosis	Localization	Duration	Onset and Trigger Factors	Accompanying Features	Findings	Remarks
Chronic head pain, usually diffuse	Cough headache	Diffuse		Coughing, straining		Rarely lesions of the posterior cranial fossa	Sometimes after trauma
	Vasomotor headache	Diffuse	Hours to days	Tension, alcohol			Sometimes post-traumatic
	Headache in hypertension	Diffuse	Hours to days	Most severe in the morning	Sometimes intermittent neurologic signs	Hypertension	
	Headaches in intracranial space-occupying lesions	Diffuse, seldom localized	Unrelenting headache		Sometimes vomiting and signs of raised intracranial pressure	Sometimes focal signs and papilledema	
	Posttraumatic headache	Diffuse	Days	Aggravated by alcohol, exposure to sunlight, or repeated shaking		Usually Normal	Case history

Generalized diseases, toxic or due to drugs, psychogenic or depressive	Diffuse	Virtually continuous	According to the cause		Carbon monoxide, lead, oral contraceptives, bromide
Subacute headache pain, usually long-lasting and diffuse					
Meningitis, encephalitis	Diffuse	Virtually continuous	According to the basic cause	Meningism, sometimes focal symptoms	
Cerebral circulatory disturbances	Diffuse	Hours to days	Sometimes vomiting or disturbances of consciousness	Sometimes focal symptoms	
Postinfectious headache	Diffuse	Days to months			
Low CSF pressure	Diffuse	Hours	On sitting or standing	Sometimes vomiting	Disappears on lying down or with pressure on jugular veins. Lumbar puncture pressure measurement: fluid sometimes needs aspiration. CSF protein high

Table 11.2 (Continued)

Features	Diagnosis	Localization	Duration	Onset and Trigger Factors	Accompanying Features	Findings	Remarks
Chronic localized head pain	Headache in cervical spondylosis	Occipital, sometimes unilateral, radiating forward	Hours to days	Holding head in the same position for prolonged periods, e.g., reading, bed rest	Neck pain, sometimes brachialgia	Painful occipital spots, sometimes cervical radicular lesions	Usually older patients, sometimes after cervical whiplash injury
	Cranial arteritis	Often temporal	Long-lasting			Painful temporal artery, elevated ESR	Usually older subjects
	Eye affections	Frontotemporal	Hours to days	After reading, particularly in the evening	According to the basic cause		
	Ear, throat, and nose affections	According to the cause	Often in the morning				
	Headache of dental origin	Face, temporal region	Virtually continuous	Act of chewing, effect of cold or hot		e.g., Costen's syndrome	

Headaches due to Vasomotor Disturbances

Pathogenesis

Three factors appear to play a pathogenetic part in vasomotor headache, particularly migraine.

Vasomotor-humoral factors: These are evident. Phase 1 consists of a vasoconstriction which causes signs of focal ischemic lesions of the cerebral cortex (1291). This phase explains the neurologic deficits of *migraine accompagnée,* although recent intracranial blood flow techniques have cast doubt on this explanation. Phase 2 consists of a vasodilation, in which expansion of the larger extracranial branches produces pulsating pain, often unilateral. Since the capillaries do not dilate, the patient has a pale complexion. Only in cluster headache (Horton's neuralgia) (p. 454) do the capillaries dilate and give the patient a ruddy complexion. Phase 3 consists of edematous permeation of the periarterial tissues, and this phase is accompanied by a continuous dull ache. These changes in the circulatory system are partly mediated or accompanied by humoral changes in which serotonin plays an important part (1291). For reasons that are not clear and partly exogenous in origin, serotonin is released at the outset of an attack from depots in the intestinal wall, brain, and especially the platelets and mast cells. A high serum serotonin level in phase 1 is responsible for the initial intracranial vasoconstriction. However, serotonin – together with histamine, which is also released from the mast cells – increases capillary permeability. This effect favors the transudation of a plasmakinin, neurokinin, and this substance lowers the pain threshold. The outpouring of serotonin and the consequent fall in the serum serotonin level cause further dilation of the arterial walls and provoke the sensation of pain. Serotonin is broken down by monoamine oxidases and excreted in the urine as 5-hydroxyindoleacetic acid. Other authors (508) attribute the onset of migrainous symptoms to the opening up of special arteriovenous anastomoses. It is assumed that these blood channels enjoy a preferential blood flow and that the capillary bed distal to the anastomoses consequently is no longer irrigated.

Thrombocytes: In patients with migraine, a disturbance of the aggregation properties of the platelets appears to be present (649). This finding has therapeutic implications.

CNS factors: These factors have again come to the fore in recent years (670). Impulses arising from the midbrain may be responsible for the attack-like qualities, the accompanying autonomic phenomena, the epilepsy-like EEG changes, and the unilaterality of migraine headache.

Vasomotor Headache (508, 670, 1132, 1291)

Terminology: This is the "common headache" or "common migraine" and is referred to under certain conditions as "tension headache."

Clinical aspects: Vasomotor headache is the commonest type of chronic headache. It is a diffuse *pain* which may be maximal over the forehead, temple, or vertex and has a dull or pulsating character. It is aggravated by bending or pushing. The headache tends to appear at unspecified times of the day, although in adults it is especially prone to occur in the morning upon awakening or soon after rising. As a rule, there are no accompanying symptoms. Various transitional forms with migraine occur (see below). Young or middle-aged subjects are most often affected and both sexes with equal severity, although women are subjectively worse. Trigger factors may be a change in the weather, sleep deprivation, alcohol abuse ("hangover headache"), and mental stress. Ordinary *posttraumatic headache* that follows craniocerebral trauma has the same features as vasomotor headaches. It is aggravated by the patient bending down or shaking his head, and the precipitating influence, alcohol and sunbathing, is especially striking. Other forms of headache also may follow craniocerebral trauma. **Physical examination** of the patient with an ordinary vasomotor headache usually reveals normal neurologic features, although autonomic disturbances, constipation, and sometimes tetanic spasms may be present.

Treatment consists in persuading the patient to lead a rational life, and to eliminate external and internal causes of tension. Drug treatment consists in the use of ergot alkaloids and sedatives.

Migraine (85, 508, 670, 1022, 1132, 1291)

Pathogenesis: This is discussed on p. 449.

Epidemiology: The incidence of migraine in schoolchildren is said to average about 5%, especially in older girls. In adults, epidemiologic surveys yield an unexpectedly high incidence – about 25% in women and 17% in men (1250). More than one-half of the patients with migraine have relatives suffering from headaches, but not all have typical migraine. Women are more often affected – or at least, women seek medical aid more often than men.

Classification

Migraine is characterized either by the typical attack of headache (classic migraine) or by the wide range of accompanying signs which may dominate the clinical picture. Table 11.3 presents a possible classification.

Classic Migraine

Clinical aspects: The only symptom is the headache, which is the characteristic feature in about 50% of migraine cases. In about 65% the headache is "hemicranial" in type. It usually starts in the frontotemporal region and spreads to involve the entire one-half of the head. It is often boring, deep-seated, throbbing, and aggravated by external stimuli such as light and noise. The pain reaches its maximum within a few hours and leads to nausea and vomiting in about 60% of cases. In many patients, the same side of the head is

Table 11.3   Classification of migraine

Simple (common) migraine

Complicated migraine
- Ophthalmic migraine
- *Migraine accompagnée* with
  - Sensory signs
  - Motor signs
  - Aphasia
- Migraine with jacksonian seizure
- Migraine with vertigo (vestibular migraine)
- With ataxia ("cerebellar" migraine)
- Ophthalmoplegic migraine
- Basilar migraine
- Dysphrenic migraine
- Abdominal migraine
- Cardiac migraine
- *Migraine meningée*

Cluster headache (Carotodynia)

often repeatedly affected, although constant involvement of one side should always prompt the suspicion of a symptomatic form of migraine. Not infrequently, autonomic signs are present such as sweating, abdominal colic, diarrhea, tachycardia, dryness of the mouth, oliguria, and urinary frequency after the attack. As a rule, the attacks last many hours and their frequency may vary from one a year to one a day.

Factors provoking attacks include atmospheric influences, photic effects, menstruation, exercise, and prolonged periods of bed rest (Sunday migraine, holiday migraine), as well as mental stress (responsibilities, preoccupations, work stress, etc.). The use of oral contraceptives frequently provokes migrainous headaches which are accompanied by specific EEG abnormalities. Since the EEG changes persist after the

contraceptive is withdrawn, a predisposition to migraine has been suggested. Occasionally attacks of migraine may be caused by the pressor substance tyramine, which is present in certain types of cheese and which may provoke hypertensive crises during treatment with monoamineoxidase inhibitors (dietetic migraine).

Neurologic examination: The neurologic status in classic migraine is normal. The *EEG* is normal in only one-half of patients with migraine. The remainder show nonspecific dysrhythmic features or focal signs (usually with signs of paralysis). About 16% exhibit paroxysmal hypersynchronous changes with theta waves and scattered sharp waves similar to the picture in clinical epilepsy. The term hypersynchronous headache is applied to this form of migraine.

Treatment is the same as in vasomotor headache. Infrequent attacks are best treated by an analgesic or, at the very start of an attack, an ergotamine combination preparation as a suppository or tablets. Rarely, an analgesic will have to be combined with dihydroergotamine 0.5-1 mg i.v. In order to reduce the frequency of attacks, one of the following may be used over several weeks: dihydroergotamine 2.5 mg $3 \times /d$, or hydergine 10–25 drops $3 \times /d$, or propranolol (Inderal) 3–4×20 mg up to 3×60 mg or clonidine, one $3 \times /d$, or the MAO inhibitor phenelzine sulfate (Nardil) 15 mg $3 \times /d$. A calcium channel blocker in the evening may be effective. Aggregation inhibitors such as acetylsalicylic acid 0.5 g 2 × /d may be given. If tension is a prominent symptom, thymoleptic drugs are advisable. In chronic cases a prostaglandin synthesis inhibitor may be given. In patients in whom hypersynchronous EEG features are present – and not only in these – antiepileptic medication such as phenytoin 50 mg 3 × /d is recommended. The patient should avoid tension-building drugs such as coffee and other excitants, and follow a calm lifestyle including adequate exercise.

Complicated Migraine

The great majority of migraine sufferers at one or other time in their lives exhibit additional signs which accompany their attacks. These signs comprise mostly impressive neurologic deficits, and this whole group of patients may be classified as cases of complicated migraine. The accompanying signs may sometimes be the only manifestation of an attack – so-called *migraine sans migraine.* Trigger factors similar to those seen in classic migraine are present in complicated migraine. If signs of complicated migraine first appear in women taking oral contraceptives, or if the signs worsen, the oral contraceptive should be withdrawn. An above-average proportion of migraine sufferers have epilepsy, particularly temporal lobe epilepsy. The treatment of complicated migraine is the same as in classic migraine.

Ophthalmic Migraine

This is the commonest form and is characterized by the fact that the attack of headache is preceded by visual symptoms. This is the case in about one-third of migraine cases. A typical feature is the *scintillation scotoma,* a phenomenon consisting of colored flashes of light with jagged outlines which radiate progressively outward from the center of a homonymous field defect (fortification spectra). Within 5–15 min, these flashes reach the periphery of the field, leaving a transient central scotoma in their wake. Less commonly, horizontal visual field defects may be present; these are caused by retinal ischemia. The scintillation scotoma is followed by a typical attack of headache on the side opposite to or on the same side as the homonymous field defect, as already described. Rarely, the scotoma remains the only manifestation of the attack, i.e., it is unaccompanied by headache or other signs. Amaurosis fugax (pp. 72–3) may probably also be a manifestation of headache-less migraine. In this context, the optic nerve may be permanently damaged.

Ophthalmoplegic Migraine

This form consists of an external ocular palsy, usually oculomotor paralysis, on the same side as the headache. The palsy disappears over the course of weeks or months. This particular picture may conceal various intracranial lesions which produce symptomatic headache, e.g., aneurysms of the posterior communicating artery (p. 91) or a lesion of the cavernous sinus. Sometimes a dilated pupil on one side or the other will be present (840).

Migraine Accompagnée

This form is a type of hemicrania, which is preceded by signs of cerebral irritation or neurologic deficit, other than those described above. Thus, paresthesias may be found, usually of the upper extremities but also of the face, which may move from side to side in the course of an attack or be present contemporaneously on both sides; monoplegias or hemiplegias may occur ("hemiplegic migraine"); aphasia; homonymous visual field defects; sensory disturbances; and jacksonian attacks. As a rule, the attack of headache follows immediately upon these signs and symptoms, thus permitting a confident diagnosis to be made. Sometimes the headache precedes the neurologic deficits. The headache may be contralateral or homolateral to the neurologic signs. This form of migraine is particularly common in children and is the first manifestation in at least one-half of migraine cases (1022). The neurologic deficits usually disappear within an hour or less but occasionally they may last much longer; exceptionally, they may be permanent. The EEG after an attack of *migraine accompagnée* shows a large abnormal focus which may remain present for several days. Attacks of *migraine accompagnée* are sometimes accompanied by CSF pleocytosis (89, 1024).

Basilar Migraine

This term is used to describe those cases in which the accompanying vasospastic signs involve the vertebrobasilar territory; often the headaches are occipital. Some cases of ophthalmic migraine or bilateral visual loss may be grouped here; other cases show vertigo, gait ataxia, dysarthria, or tinnitus. It is possible that patients with bilateral paresthesias of the hands, head, and tongue should also be included. This migraine form affects a disproportionately large number of young women. Loss of consciousness may accompany these attacks, and typical epileptic potentials may be present in the EEG made during an attack. Basilar migraine responds particularly well to antiepileptics.

Alternating Hemiplegia of Infancy (644)

This entity may be a particular form of basilar migraine. It usually appears in the 1st year of life as a case of progressive psychomotor retardation. Attacks of hemiplegia affecting either side occur, which last from 15 min to several days, accompanied by dystonic attacks, choreoathetotic movements, tonic crises, nystagmus, and irritability. Naloxone is useful in treatment, as well as a calcium antagonist (217).

Specific Forms of Complicated Migraine

Among other forms of migraine to be mentioned are *abdominal crises,* which are not uncommon in children, and the associated mental signs such as abnormal fluctuations in mood (anxiety, depression), disturbed thought processes, and confusional and anxiety states. The latter may lead to a true "migraine psychosis" *(dysphrenic migraine).* Apart from jacksonian seizures already mentioned and the attacks of migraine, these patients may exhibit true epileptic manifestations such as grand mal attacks with surprising frequency – in 5%–6% of cases. *Cardiac migraine* describes a particular form in which attacks of precordial pain occur in migraine sufferers, with or without simultaneous attacks of headache, and nonspecific T-wave changes in the ECG during the attack. Both heart and head pains respond to treatment with beta-blockers (695).

Cluster Headache (Histamine Headache, Erythroprosopalgia, Horton's Neuralgia) (651, 747, 785)

This hemicranial form of vasomotor headache has many similarities to migraine, as well as several typical features.

Characteristics of headache attacks: These are diagnostically decisive. The headache attacks have a very sudden onset, reach their maximal severity in about 20 min, and disappear completely within 1–2 h. The pain is intense, stabbing in nature, and strictly confined to the orbital and supraorbital regions. It recurs constantly on the same side. Sometimes there is photophobia and nausea. In about one-third the attacks awaken the patients from sleep, usually at a specific hour of the night, and the majority experience one to three attacks within 24 h. Periods of one or more weeks of frequent attacks (so-called clusters) alternate with symptom-free intervals lasting months or years.

Physical findings during an attack: Typical findings are redness of the eye, lacrimation and nasal obstruction, and redness of the face, all homolateral to the pain.

Transitional forms with typical migraine are not rare so that attacks of cluster headache and classic migraine may follow each other in one and the same patient (747, 785), or in one patient the attack characteristics of both types are mixed.

In 20% of patients, there is a family history of attacks of headache.

Chronic cluster headache: Attacks of cluster headache may sometimes occur without symptom-free intervals so that one speaks paradoxically of chronic cluster headache (970). This form responds well to indomethacin.

Treatment consists, apart from ergot derivatives and pizotifen (see above), of serotonin inhibitors, e.g., methysergide (Sansert) 1 tablet $3 \times /d$ for 1–2 months. The hazard of prolonged medication, viz. retroperitoneal fibrosis, should be borne in mind. Other patients respond to oxygen inhalation or to a course of corticosteroids. Indomethacin and lithium are useful in the chronic form of cluster headache.

Differential diagnosis: The clinical picture must be distinguished from certain other types of facial pain, namely trigeminal neuralgia (p.460), nasociliary neuralgia (p.461), and Sluder's neuralgia (p.461).

Rarer Forms of Vasomotor Headache

Carotodynia (905, 979)

This form possesses specific analogies to cluster headache; women are almost exclusively affected, the headache occurs always on the same side, it affects chiefly the side of the neck, and only rarely the maxillary or periorbital region. Superimposed on a continuous dull ache are acute attacks lasting minutes or hours and occurring repeatedly throughout the day. During such attacks, the ipsilateral carotid artery is painful and pulsates vigorously, and the periarterial tissues appear to be swollen. The pain is abolished by the same preparations that are beneficial in migraine and cluster headache. Indomethacin is particularly useful, singly or in combination with a tricyclic antidepressant (905).

Ice-Cream Headache

This is a particular form of vasomotor headache. Cold stimulation of the gums triggers an intense headache within 20–30 s, usually localized to the temporal region. The attack of pain passes off after about 20 s.

Cough Headache

This form is provoked by coughing, and sometimes by straining or bending down. It lasts only a few seconds and may be harmless, although in other patients cough headache may indicate a space-occupying lesion or arachnoiditis in the posterior cranial fossa. Headache in the presence of raised intracranial pressure may be aggravated by coughing.

Postcoital Headache

This form of headache occurs during coitus, as well as in other circumstances of suddenly raised intracranial pressure. The pain is stroke-like and intense, and lasts from minutes to hours (1055). Meningism is absent and the pain passes over more rapidly than in subarachnoid hemorrhage. However, pending the demonstration of a clear CSF by lumbar puncture, some patients with postcoital headache resemble cases of acute subarachnoid hemorrhage (669). A meningeal form of migraine is discussed (1055).

Headaches in Organic Vascular Diseases

Cranial Arterial Occlusion

Headaches only occasionally accompany *intracranial arterial occlusions*. In the case of *carotid occlusion*, they are localized to the orbital region, in cases of *basilar occlusion* they are diffuse or encircle the head. Spontaneous dissecting aneurysms of the internal carotid artery are accompanied by intense pain of the homolateral face (142) (p. 93).

Arterial Hypertension

It is not certain if hypertensive patients without hypertensive crises suffer more headaches than normotensive subjects. However, when headaches are present, they cannot be distinguished from those caused by vasomotor disturbances. Hypertensive headache commonly commences in the early morning when the patient awakes; it is diffuse and remains present throughout the day. Essential for the diagnosis is measurement of the arterial blood pressure and full neurologic and general physical examination. The presence of papilledema in cases of hypertension necessitates differentiation from a brain tumor headache.

Pheochromocytoma

Headaches arise abruptly in this condition. The attacks, lasting from a few minutes to 1 h at most, are accompanied by sweating, palpitations, and pallor. They are often triggered by bending, turning, exertion, or excitement.

Temporal Arteritis (Cranial Arteritis, Horton's Syndrome)
(842)

Pathogenesis: Temporal arteritis is one of the manifestations of a giant-cell arteritis. The disease is an autoimmune process and is characterized by typical changes in the media and internal elastic layers of the large and medium-sized arteries. It involves exclusively the branches of the external carotid artery, occasionally other large arteries of the trunk, and only very exceptionally the branches of the internal carotid artery.

Clinical aspects: The patients are invariably over 50 years of age. *Headache* is often the first symptom. It is very severe, usually localized to the temple or the forehead, and frequently bilateral. It is a throbbing and continuous ache or a jaw pain occurring during mastication ("intermittent claudication of the jaw"). Often the superficial temporal artery may be palpated as a thick, tortuous, and painful tube, and pulsation may be absent. Exceptionally, the superficial temporal artery is normal to palpation and pulsates. Sometimes the headaches are localized elsewhere than to the temple. Since giant-cell arteritis is a generalized disease, **other signs and symptoms** may be present apart from headache, notably optic nerve involvement, retinal artery occlusion, external ocular palsies, polyneuropathies, etc. Cases of granulomatous giant-cell arteritis involving the CNS may be associated with temporal arteritis. **Generalized signs and symptoms** include fatigue, loss of appetite, loss of weight, night sweats, and low-grade fever. They may be accompanied by another manifestation of giant-cell arteritis, polymyalgia rheumatica, occurring as pains in the large joints. The most dreaded complication is sudden blindness caused by occlusion of the posterior long ciliary artery.

Ancillary investigations: The ESR with very few exceptions (1029) is markedly elevated, reaching levels of over 50 mm in the first hour. The diagnosis is established by a biopsy of the superficial temporal artery, which is justified upon clinical suspicion of the condition even if a normal pulsation is present. Histologic sections at various levels of the artery are required.

Differential diagnosis: On the one hand, this includes other causes of unusual headache in elderly individuals. On the other hand, the superficial temporal artery can be thickened and appear pulsating when it is a collateral to an occluded internal carotid artery (847). Lastly, in rare instances in young patients, one finds a painful swelling of the temporal artery, with marked eosinophilia. This process can involve other organs and is called juvenile arteritis of the temporal artery with eosinophilia (149).

Treatment: Corticosteroids, e.g., prednisone 1–2 mg/kg body weight/day is required until the ESR has returned to normal. Decreasing doses of cortisone are then advisable for many months, even years. A further rise of the ESR indicates reactivation of the process, which is usually "burnt out" only after several years. Because of the risk of blindness, the start of treatment should never be postponed until the results of the biopsy are known.

Spondylotic Headache and Cervical Migraine

Pathogenesis: Pathologic changes in the upper cervical vertebrae may produce pains radiating in a cranial direction. In view of the great frequency of roentgenologic evidence of such changes, the diagnosis of spondylotic headache is probably made too often. The following features should be present:

- simultaneous presence of other local, radicular, or autonomic signs of cervical spondylosis (p. 378);
- or a whiplash injury of the cervical spine, e.g., following an automobile accident (p. 378); or,
- at the least, typical headache (see below).

Clinical aspects: The typical spondylotic headache is usually unilateral and either confined to the neck or radiates from the occiput forward; the patient describes the sensation with the gesture of "removing a helmet." The pain may reach the face. The headache is often associated with certain movements or postures of the head (prolonged reading) or an unfavorable sleeping position at night. The case history often reveals the presence of an acute torticollis. Physical examination in these patients, who are mostly elderly, will reveal tenderness to palpation of the cervical spinous processes and the paravertebral neck muscles, as well as limited movements. Roentgenologic signs of spondylosis or spondylarthrosis are present, as well as deformity of the lateral aspects of the vertebral bodies.

Treatment: This is difficult. In acute cases and especially if accompanied by torticollis, extension treatment is required. The immediate effect of manual extension may be utilized in the differential diagnosis. Subsequently and in chronic cases, immobilization of the cervical spine in a felt or plastic collar, correct positioning of the head at night, local warmth, muscle relaxants, and anti-inflammatory preparations are indicated.

Other (Symptomatic) Forms of Headache

Headache in Intracranial Space-Occupying Lesions

Headache is an early or presenting symptom in about one-half of all brain tumor patients, and more commonly with posterior fossa tumors. In supratentorial tumors, the headache usually occurs on the side of the tumor. Other methods of examination will reveal the etiologic diagnosis. In children with cerebellar tumors, headache may be the only symptom for a long time.

Headache in Intermittent Disturbances of CSF Drainage
(pp. 36 and 38)

The pain is usually lancinating, very intense, and accompanied by nausea, vomiting, and sometimes brief loss of consciousness. Occasionally opisthotonus occurs. The attack may last seconds or minutes, seldom longer, and then disappears less rapidly than it started. Any lesion which can lead to intermittent obstruction of the normal flow of CSF may provoke attacks. Typical examples are *colloid cyst of the third ventricle* and other intraventricular tumors. Such lesions may also cause drop attacks, in which the patient loses the power of his limbs and collapses to the ground, without suffering headache or loss consciousness.

Spontaneous Aliquorrhea (Hypoliquorrhea, Acute Pseudomeningitis)

The term aliquorrhea is applied to a CSF low-pressure syndrome which may arise after acute craniocerebral trauma, subdural hematoma or hygroma, or spontaneously (190). Spontaneous low-pressure syndromes occur particularly often in women. A typical feature is the intense headache which occurs when the patient is erect and which disappears when she lies down or when pressure is applied to the jugular veins. Drowsiness and vomiting may occur, as well as marked meningism, in the presence of normal neurologic findings. Lumbar puncture with the patient recumbent reveals a CSF pressure under 5 cm of water. Sometimes the pressure is so low that the fluid fails to drip out of the needle spontaneously. The CSF is often xanthochromic, and the protein level may exceed 1 g/ 100 ml. Treatment consists of bedrest, plenty of fluids, and an infusion of 0.5% saline. The same type of headache may appear after lumbar puncture.

Headache Due to Ophthalmic Causes

Headache accompanies anomalies of refraction, especially the childhood heterophorias. The headache worsens in the course of the day and disappears when appropriate corrective measures are taken. In acute cases of glaucoma, an intense frontal headache may be accompanied by vomiting, bradycardia, and visual disturbances.

Headache in ENT Lesions

Sinus infections may cause obstinate headaches which are often well localized. The same applies to chronic otitis media and ENT space-occupying lesions. A supraorbital neuralgia may cause localized forehead pains and result either from frontal sinusitis or a mechanical cause. A particular form of supraorbital neuralgia is goggle headache, which is caused by wearing underwater goggles that are too tight (550).

Headache in Generalized Diseases

Headache may be particular severe in certain infectious diseases, such as Q fever. They may outlast the duration of the acute infection. Chronic iron deficiency, e.g., blood loss anemia may begin with by persistent headaches. The Morgagni-Morel syndrome, an etiologically ill-defined entity affecting elderly women, consists of adiposity, hirsutism, frontal internal hyperostosis, disturbances of carbohydrate metabolism including diabetes mellitus, disturbances of sleep and balance, and headaches.

Psychogenic Headache

Not every headache occurring in stressed individuals or accompanying personal conflict situations is a psychogenic headache. Nowadays this diagnosis is made too often. Psychogenic factors play an important part in so-called *tension headache* (1291). This term is used to denote various entities, mostly occipital in distribution, which show, as a common feature, spastic contraction of the neck muscles of varying intensity during states of mental stress. Differentiation from true *occipital neuralgia* is not always easy, and the latter condition is all too frequently diagnosed. Operative section of the greater occipital nerve is seldom successful (508). Headache may indicate an *incipient psychosis*.

Facial Neuralgias

General features: Neuralgias are pains which occur in the distribution of a specific peripheral nerve and usually possess a cutting or boring character. In the face, neuralgic pains are often intense and prolonged. They may be provoked by touching specific peripheral "trigger zones" or by certain actions such as speaking, swallowing, or chewing. Apart from the most common cases, in which no obvious cause can be found, symptomatic varieties of facial neuralgia are encountered, which may be the only sign of a lesion such as a neoplasm or infection in the vicinity of a peripheral sensory nerve. In the latter cases only (and not invariably), the pain syndrome is accompanied by demonstrable neurologic signs; in the remainder, the diagnosis rests upon a meticulous case history.

Trigeminal Neuralgia (391)

Pathophysiology: It is assumed that stimuli skip from tactile to pain fibers (ephaptic transmission) because of a lesion of the myelin sheaths. These lesions are attributed to mechanical factors associated with the aging process or to the effect of pulsating arterial loops adjacent to the facial nerve in the cerebellopontine angle (994). Other mechanical factors are responsible in the symptomatic cases caused by organic lesions in the vicinity of the trigeminal nerve.

Clinical Aspects

Idiopathic (Essential) Trigeminal Neuralgia

This condition only affects patients over the age of 50 years. The pain is usually localized in the second (maxillary) or third (mandibular) divisions of the trigeminal nerve. The latter condition is called mandibular neuralgia. Because of this localization, patients often first seek advice from a dentist. Initially, the pain is unilateral and always confined to the same zone. It has a shooting or lightning character, usually lasts only a few seconds, and has an intensity that is scarcely bearable. It may recur every few minutes, up to 100 times a day. Many patients are on the brink of suicide. While the patient may be completely symp-

tom-free at first between attacks, a persistent dull interval ache develops when the disease becomes chronic and the attacks last longer. Often the pains are provoked by chewing, talking, or touching specific areas of the face or mouth (trigger zones). Some patients are too frightened to touch their mouths, refuse to eat, and will not speak. In these idiopathic cases, no abnormal neurologic deficit is present. Some patients, after frequent bouts of pain, may become spontaneously symptom-free for months or years. Neuralgia recurs in the same or a different division of the trigeminal nerve, and in about 3% of cases it has a bilateral distribution.

Symptomatic Forms

These forms occur in association with multiple sclerosis (p. 243) or mass lesions in the vicinity of the trigeminal nerve, and often show specific features. These include: young age of the patient, bilateral involvement, chronicity, and demonstrable neurologic deficits. However, symptomatic forms may exhibit an attack-like character similar to the idiopathic form of the disease.

Treatment: In the symptomatic forms, treatment must be applied to the underlying cause. In the idiopathic forms, *medical treatment* is begun with carbamazepine slowly increasing to 200 mg 3-5 × /d, or a slow release preparation. If the pain is unbearable, carbamazepine may be combined with another antiepileptic (clonazepam) up to 2 mg 4 × /d or phenytoin 100 mg 2-3 × /d. Baclofen may be effective, either instead of or combined with carbamazepine (390). The failure of conservative treatment is an indication for a *neurosurgical procedure*. These previously included infiltration of the gasserian (semilunar) ganglion, electrocoagulation (Kirschner), or retroganglionic neurotomy (Spiller-Frazier). Today, differential thermocoagulation of the gasserian ganglion is the method of choice (1179). In view of the causative role claimed for a tortuous arterial loop situated adjacent to the intracranial course of the nerve trunk, exploration is recommended, as in hemifacial spasm (554, 994, 1057).

Auriculotemporal Neuralgia

In this rare form, the neuralgia is localized to the preauricular and temporal regions. Usually it occurs days or months after a disease of the parotid gland, and sometimes in its absence as well. The cause is assumed to be failure of regeneration of parotid parasympathetic fibers after damage to sensory rami reaching the skin and salivary glands. Gustatory stimuli from acidic or spiced food or the act of chewing may provoke burning pains, redness of the skin, and profuse sweating in the distribution of the auriculotemporal nerve (gustatory sweating), particularly in the preauricular region. Since the intensity of the pain is aggravated by chewing, the condition may be easily confused with mandibular neuralgia (see above) and Costen's syndrome (p. 462).

Nasociliary Neuralgia

This form is also uncommon. The pain, which is assumed to be caused by a lesion of the ciliary ganglion, is either episodic or prolonged and affects the na-

sal region, the inner canthus of the eye, and the eyeball; there is redness of the forehead, congestion of the nasal mucous membranes, conjunctivitis, and lacrimation. The pains may by provoked by contact with trigger zones, e. g., the inner canthus of the eye, or by chewing so that an incorrect diagnosis of trigeminal neuralgia may be made. The pain syndrome may sometimes accompany carotid aneurysms. Local application of a 5% solution of cocaine to the nasal mucosa may immediately interrupt an attack, and thus aid diagnosis. Since local inflammatory lesions may occasionally be responsible, a therapeutic course of antibiotics and cortisone is justified.

Sluder's Neuralgia

This is a pain syndrome, similar to the one described above, caused by a lesion of the pterygopalatine ganglion. Paranasal sinus infections are occasionally responsible. Characteristic attacks of sneezing occur in many cases.

Glossopharyngeal Neuralgia
(1037)

This is an uncommon type. It affects elderly subjects most often but may occur at any age. It is typified by attacks of intense pain of sudden onset, less frequently by prolonged pain. These attacks are unilateral and confined to the tongue, tonsillar region, and hypopharynx. Sometimes the pain may radiate to the ear so that the picture mimics an auriculotemporal neuralgia. Swallowing, particularly of cold liquids, may provoke severe pain, as may talking or protruding the tongue. Trigger zones are present in the tonsillar and pharyngeal regions. Rarely the pain may be bilateral and in about 10% of cases combined with trigeminal neuralgia. Exceptionally, it may be associated with attacks of syncope (845). Spontaneous recovery is not infrequent. Medical treatment is the same as for trigeminal neuralgia. Surgical management by resection of the glossopharyngeal nerve and the upper roots of the vagus is nearly always successful (1037).

Neuralgia of the Geniculate Ganglion

This form was originally described as the result of herpetic infection of the geniculate ganglion, with the typical cutaneous blisters involving the tragus and mastoid region, and accompanied by a peripheral facial palsy *(Ramsay Hunt syndrome)*. However, geniculate neuralgia sometimes occurs in the absence of herpetic manifestations or facial paralysis. The pains are confined to the preauricular region and the external auditory meatus, the roof of the palate, the maxilla, and the retroauricular mastoid region. They are lancinating in type and may be accompanied by abnormal taste sensations in the anterior half of the tongue and excessive salivation.

Other Facial Neuralgias

Neuralgia of the Superior Laryngeal Nerve

This rare form provokes attacks of severe unilateral pain in the thyrohyoid membrane.

Neuralgia of the Auricular Division of the Vagus Nerve

This form provokes suboccipital and shoulder pain and acute retroauricular pain that can be elicited by local pressure.

Suboccipital Neuralgia

This diagnosis is too frequently made in the presence of occipital or neck pain.

Neuralgia of the Temporomandibular Joint (Costen's Syndrome)

Pathogenesis: This form of neuralgia is caused by a functional disturbance of the temporomandibular joint (TMJ), usually the result of a maloccluded jaw. Occasionally a primary disease of the TMJ or its muscles is present but the more usual cause is a premature contact between the teeth which leads to compensatory adaptation of the surrounding muscles and an altered position and mechanism of the joint.

Clinical aspects: Young and middle-aged women are most often affected. Initially the patients complain of *preauricular pains* which are aggravated by chewing. About one-half also complain of facial pain or headache, the intensity of which may be maximal in the preauricular region, and radiating to the forehead, mandible, and occiput. These symptoms are unilateral in most patients. The act of chewing may sometimes trigger the pain or aggravate it. Less often, associated features such as dizziness, tinnitus or mild deafness, scintillations in the visual field, buccofacial dystonias, toothache, or disturbances of swallowing are present. **Physical examination** reveals a tender TMJ, the patient has difficulty in opening and closing his mouth, and the teeth are maloccluded. The author believes that the diagnosis of this syndrome is made too often.

Treatment: Radical odontologic correction is indicated. Injections of local anesthetic and cortisone into the TMJ may provide symptomatic relief. Habitual bruxism (grinding of teeth) may also cause facial muscular pain.

Atypical Facial Neuralgia (421)

This term is applied to a diffuse syndrome of pain possessing a burning character which distresses the patient. Some cases have no obvious cause, others may follow small and uncomplicated dental procedures. The pain is prolonged, unilateral, of variable intensity and particularly affects middle-aged women. As a rule, no abnormal physical features can be found. The distressing nature of the pain drives the patient to seek relief, and the trail from physician to physician often escalates into dental and maxillofacial surgery. Occasionally facial flushing, Horner's syndrome, and tenderness of the carotid artery are present, so-called sympathalgia. Sometimes these signs and symptoms conceal a carotodynia (p. 455). Ergotamine tartrate and serotonin inhibitors, indomethacin, and tricyclic antidepressants are used, but usually the signs and symptoms defy all treatment.

12. Various Pain Syndromes of the Trunk and Extremities

While pain is often neurogenic, the neurologist has to interpret pain syndromes in a wider context. He is obliged to consider pains that are not primarily neurogenic in nature.

The most important of the latter pain syndromes and their differential diagnosis are described in this section.

Shoulder Arm Syndrome (Cervicobrachialgia)
(843, 848, 851)

Cervical Disk Prolapse and Cervical Spondylosis

These common causes of a brachial pain syndrome are indicated by the presence of torticollis, neck pain, local pain on coughing, a radicular distribution of paresthesias or sensory loss, and a segmental distribution of muscular and reflex abnormalities.

Thoracic Outlet Syndrome

The *scalenus syndrome with or without cervical rib* (p. 406) gives signs of lower brachial plexus palsy as well as compression of the subclavian artery. Tumors of the *apex of the lung (Pancoast's tumor)* (p. 407) are typified by the most intense pain, signs of progressive lower brachial plexus palsy, and involvement of the cervical sympathetic chain.

Neuralgic Shoulder Amyotrophy
(p. 409)

This syndrome is typified by acute shoulder pains occurring at night, combined with weakness of the shoulder muscles.

Brachialgia Paresthetica Nocturna

This is the most frequent brachialgia encountered in neurologic practice. In its most typical form, it is almost invariably caused by a *carpal tunnel syndrome* (p. 416). The patient is waked by the unpleasant sensation of swelling and stiffness of his hand. Objective signs, viz. median nerve damage in the carpal tunnel, may take years to appear.

Causalgia

This pain syndrome, with its characteristic burning sensation, is most frequently seen after traumatic median nerve lesions (p. 415).

Intramedullary Lesions

These lesions, particularly *syringomyelia of the cervical cord,* may be accompanied by intense shoulder and arm pains.

Scapulohumeral Periarthritis

This condition is the commonest cause of shoulder pain. It is usually produced by a "tendinitis," i.e., degenerative changes in the tendons of the short rotator muscles of the shoulder joint, particularly the supraspinatus muscle. Sometimes calcium deposits within the tendons irritate the subdeltoid bursa and cause a chronic bursitis. Fewer than one-half of cases show roentgenographic evidence of calcification. The symptoms tend to occur in middle-aged and elderly subjects. Scapulohumeral periarthritis is an unusually frequent accompaniment of coronary artery disease, in which the local pain may sometimes start acutely. The latter is provoked by active abduction, a movement which brings the painful area of the diseased tendon into contact with the coracoacromial roof of the shoulder joint. However, if the arm is passively elevated by the examiner with the shoulder girdle muscles relaxed, the head of the humerus drops forward and the movement is almost free from pain. A local point of tenderness may be found over the diseased tendon and the joint capsule.

Shoulder Hand Syndrome (Frozen Shoulder)

Etiologically, this condition sometimes follows a rotator cuff injury, and in other cases myocardial infarction or shoulder trauma. Often a period of immobility of the shoulder is followed by the syndrome. It may also be provoked bilaterally by phenobarbital medication (133).

Clinically, the condition develops gradually, causing a painful limitation of movement of the shoulder joint over a long period. Definite degenerative changes may be demonstrable in the joint, as well as a tenosynovitis of the long head of the biceps muscle. The lesion usually affects subjects aged 40–60 years, particularly women with cardiovascular disease. While the pain gradually subsides, the limitation of movement increases. Often simultaneous trophic changes are present.

Sudeck's Dystrophy of the Hand

This condition not infrequently accompanies the frozen shoulder syndrome described above. It may develop after one or more episodes of trauma with or without fracture. The signs are edema of the soft tissues; smooth and cold, often cyanotic skin; restricted movements of the finger joints; patchy osteoporosis of the bones; and intense burning pains. Treatment with guanethidine sulfate 20–30 mg a day is often successful (1181).

Lateral Humeral Epicondylitis (Tennis Elbow)

This lesion is typified by a painful origin of the long extensor muscles of the hand and fingers on the lateral side of the elbow, caused by overstraining of these muscles at work or during sports. A similar mechanism underlies *radial styloiditis.*

Attacks of Gout

These may cause intense and localized hand pains, by no means always localized to the base of the thumb *(cheiragra or cheiralgia).*

Snapping Scapula

This condition, caused by limitation of the free mobility of the scapula in relation to the wall of the thorax, may produce severe pain in the dorsal shoulder region. Grinding, which is palpable and sometimes audible, accompanies scapular movements. The lesion is usually a local disturbance of the subscapular space, e.g., a bursa, anterior angulation of the superior scapular angle, thickening of the angle (Luschka's tubercle), an accessory bone (os omovertebrale), or neoplasm.

Fibrositis ("Muscular Rheumatism", "Tenomyalgia," Pseudoradicular Complaints)

These various **terms** describe a pain syndrome characterized by a pain-dominated limitation of muscular activity. It is encountered in situations in which the joint capsule for various reasons becomes painful. Often spasm and other functional changes occur in the muscles moving such joints. The pains are solely related to movement, and one may speak of "muscular rheumatism." **Clinically,** pain is not the only symptom of this arthrogenic muscular lesion, a wide variety of recurrent and typical reflex changes may be present in the muscles, which may be described together as "tenomyalgia." These changes include a dull, boring sensation in the muscles themselves, rapid fatigue, painful contractures with fasciculation, and a rigor-like increase in tone. Various factors trigger this condition apart from the changes in the joint capsule mentioned above, local trauma and functional overstraining of the muscles may be responsible. If a pain syndrome of this type occurs in an upper extremity, a brachialgia results. Because of the radiating nature of the pain, one speaks of *pseudoradicular complaints* (184). **Treatment** should be aimed at eradicating trigger factors, e.g., correction of occupational postural defects and overstraining, and in treating the painful joint capsule by procaine or hydrocortisone injections.

Scapulocostal Syndrome

This syndrome is probably no more than a special variety of "muscular rheumatism." It is **caused** by a disturbed functional relationship between the scapula and the thoracic cage. It may result from a lesion of the shoulder region (secondary type), paralysis or amputation of the upper extremity (static type), or positional defects, e.g., overtaxing the muscles of one shoulder girdle (primary type). The latter is the commonest type. **Clinically,** the syndrome affects subjects aged 35-60 years. Unilateral as a rule, it affects patients in occupations involving certain postures (chauffeurs, tailors, stenographers, etc.). The pain has a gradual onset, first in the shoulder region and then radiating distally in a pseudoradicular pattern. Pains may be present in the neck and occipital region, the upper arm, and deltoid region, as well as the anterior thorax; occasionally they radiate into the hand. Although the complaints may last for years, they may suddenly grow worse in the course of a few days. Palpation may reveal a well-localized painful zone along the medial margin of the scapula: it may be more obvious if the patient places his hand on the opposite shoulder, thereby abducting the scapula. The pain and its radiation may be reproduced by an injection of distilled water into the zone. **Treatment** includes injections of novocaine. Physiotherapy to the shoulder girdle muscles may be helpful, but sometimes a change of occupation is necessary.

Arteriopathies

Occlusion of the *subclavian artery,* e.g., as part of an aortic arch syndrome or in cervical rib, may cause arm pain during physical exercise – a genuine *intermittent claudication* of the arm. In the subclavian steal syndrome, the exercise-related arm pains are accompanied by complaints of vertigo (p. 79).

Vasomotor Disturbances

Raynaud's syndrome (148), with the typical blanching of individual fingers *(doigts morts)*, and with subsequent reddening and occasional ulceration of the fingertip, may be accompanied by paresthesias, a feeling of stiffness, and dragging pain in the fingers themselves. Young women are most often affected. Apart from the *idiopathic form (Raynaud's disease)*, *symptomatic forms* may occur. In men a collagen disease, particularly scleroderma, should always be considered.

Venous Thrombosis

The *Paget-Schrötter syndrome* is **caused** by compression or complete thrombosis of the axillary or subclavian vein. The most likely trigger factor is unusually strenuous use of the arm, but occasionally no obvious cause of venous thrombosis can be demonstrated. A rare cause is a bilateral *sternocostoclavicular hyperostosis* resulting from a hyperostotic spongiosclerosis: it begins with local pain and swelling of the clavicular region (628). **Clinically,** men are by far more commonly affected than women, the right side more than the left. The patients are usually young subjects aged 20 30 years. The onset is acute, usually within 1 h, and the course is progressive for several days. In addition to shoulder pain and a feeling of tension in the arm, swelling occurs and sometimes discoloration. The veins may be prominent, sometimes paresthesias and weakness are present, and the thrombotic and painful veins may be palpable in the axilla. The circulation time following injection of a test substance into the veins of the affected arm is very delayed. Venography is essential in the diagnosis. *Treatment* is not always necessary since the acute signs and symptoms disappear spontaneously in the course of days or weeks. Patients diagnosed in the acute stage are treated with anticoagulants. Operation is seldom necessary.

Glomus Tumors

These small nodules arise from the *glomus bodies of the skin*. They appear as arteriovenous anastomoses in intimate relationship with the fibers of the autonomic nervous system. Glomus organs are particularly numerous in the distal extremities such as the fingers and toes. The tumors developing in these sites are invariably benign and produce a typical clinical picture. Initially, the tumor nodule, which is often situated beneath the fingernail, may be visible through it as a bluish spot. It gives rise to pains which radiate throughout the extremity. Spontaneous pains also occur, and if the arm is held in the hanging position, dull abnormal sensations are produced which involve the distal part of the extremity for varying periods. Local autonomic disturbances may also accompany these tumors. **Treatment** consists in surgical excision.

Referred Pain

Pains associated with disease of the internal organs may radiate to the shoulder and upper extremity. Chest pain radiating to the arm in *angina pectoris* is not always immediately recognizable when it arises during sleep, as in Prinzmetal's angina (774). The pain of a *gallbladder lesion* radiates to the right shoulder.

Pain Syndromes of the Trunk and Back

Pain syndromes of the trunk are usually the manifestation of a medical or surgical disease of the internal organs. In addition, several disease pictures with characteristic features, partly rheumatologic and orthopedic, will be discussed in this section.

Girdle Pain

Girdle pain always prompts the suspicion of an *intraspinal lesion* such as a tumor or disk prolapse causing unilateral or bilateral irritation of a thoracic root. Characteristically the patient describes the picture by using both hands to indicate how the pain radiates forward around his chest wall or trunk. *Herpes zoster* may be recognized by the typical cutaneous eruption. Chronic postherpetic pains, which have been described on p.385, are unusually obstinate and occasionally require tricyclic antidepressants.

Abnormal Mobility of the Tenth (or Ninth) Rib (138)

Injury to the chest wall may cause a stubborn pain syndrome in the region of the costal arch. It occurs more frequently on the right side than the left, and affects women more often than men. Specific movements such as bending or lifting heavy objects provoke it. More unusually, a dull persistent pain may be present which is often burning in type. Dysesthesias or hypesthesias may be found in the ninth thoracic dermatome. The costal cartilage of the tenth rib along the costal arch between the parasternal notch and the lateral axillary line is not fixed to the costal arch, instead it is freely mobile. Acute pain can be elicited during examination by forcibly manipulating the free end of the rib, and the infiltration of a local anesthetic agent abolishes it, thus confirming the diagnosis. Resection of the free end of the rib brings a cure.

Syndrome of Rectus Abdominis Muscle

These pains may be provoked acutely by *hemorrhage into the rectus abdominis muscle* in the course of certain exercises. A *compression syndrome of the ventral rami* of the dorsal thoracic spinal nerves leads to a syndrome of movement-dependent pains which may be accompanied by coin-sized sensory deficits. The pain may be abolished by the infiltration of a local anesthetic agent (635). Pains in the lateral and posterior part of the abdominal wall may be part of the clinical picture of a *Spiegel hernia* (128). This hernia is commonly covered by the intact aponeurosis of the external oblique muscle of the abdomen, and may be undiagnosable clinically.

Ankylosing Spondylitis (Bekhterev's Disease)

This is an autosomal dominant disease with incomplete penetrance affecting mainly young adult males. The sacroiliac as well as the apophyseal and costovertebral joints are usually first affected, giving rise to severe and increasing lumbar pain. This pain occurs at night in bed, sometimes radiating in a sciatic distribution. Less frequently, thoracic pain, heel pain, and pain in proximal joints are present. The diagnosis is confirmed by the presence of other features of the disease such as iritis, a raised ESR, and especially roentgenologic findings in the sacroiliac joints and later in the vertebral column. Cauda equina syndrome in ankylosing spondylitis, see p.385.

Spondylolisthesis

Pathogenetically, the interarticular part of the vertebra is elongated or its continuity is interrupted (spondylolysis). The body of the fixed vertebra and its superior articular facet slip forward, while the vertebral arch and inferior articular facets remain in situ: 80% of cases involve the L5 vertebra, and the remainder the L4 or L3 vertebra. If the displacement exceeds the width of the vertebral body, the term *spondyloptosis* is used. Spondylolisthesis is present in a small percentage of the population; the relatively frequent presence of abnormal roentgenologic findings in subjects who are asymptomatic confirms that the majority remain permanently free from symptoms. Only about 10% of patients with positive roentgenologic findings exhibit physical signs and symptoms. Although both sexes are affected with equal frequency, clinical complaints are twice as common in men as in women. This statistic indicates that the development of pain in spondylolisthesis is connected with physical activity.

Symptoms: These appear more commonly after the end of the growth period than before it, and they may initially be vague - nonspecific pain and a feeling of weakness in the lumbosacral region, which tends to appear after being seated for long periods or carrying heavy weights. *Physical examination* shows that the range of movements remains unrestricted. In thin subjects a dimple is palpable in the midline of the back and may be visible. Radicular signs are sometimes present, but true sciatica is rare.

Treatment should be considered, according to the severity of the complaints, by means of a surgical support or a chip arthrodesis.

Interspinous Osteoarthritis (Baastrup's Disease)

In this condition, the opposing surfaces of adjacent lumbar spinous processes exhibit a profuse sclerosis. It does not represent an independent disease entity, being merely the visible manifestations of a variety of degenerative changes in the lumbar vertebrae (Baastrup's phenomenon). Resection of a single spinous process - an operation that is too often carried out - is justified only if pain is present on hyperextension of the lumbar spine and if the spinous processes are tender to palpation, if the appropriate roentgenologic findings are present, if the pain can be alleviated by infiltration with local anesthesia, and if other causes of the pain (which are more common) can be excluded.

Sacroiliac Strain

This is a state of tenderness of the sacroiliac ligamentous apparatus, in which the pain both occurs locally and radiates to the lumbosacral region and down the back of both legs. The clinical picture may be precipitated by violent torsion movement; the pain is usually produced by lifting a weight while bending forward, and then attempting to straighten up. Physical examination reveals local tenderness, and the pain can be provoked by forced extension of the sacroiliac joints, i.e., Mennell's maneuver; the patient lies on his healthy side with the ipsilateral knee and hip joints flexed, and the examiner then forcibly extends the outstretched leg on the affected side. The diagnosis is confirmed if the patient obtains relief from pain by wearing a hip belt.

Coccygodynia

This lesion causes troublesome dragging and burning pains in the vicinity of the tip of the sacrum. It is a complication of sacral injuries, certain operations, abnormal root pouches, and arachnoid cysts (1312), and especially of repeated microtrauma (prolonged sitting on a hard surface, so-called television bottom). There is usually no neurologic deficit. Pain can be provoked upon rectal examination by digital movement of the coccyx. Inflammatory and neoplastic changes in the genital and anal regions should be excluded.

Compression Syndrome of Spinal Nerve Rami

Specific cases of lower lumbar pain are attributed to irritation of the dorsal rami of the spinal nerves at the level where the rami lie in direct contact with the capsule of the facet joints. Pressure pain is present, not only over the articular facets but also on the iliac crest (752). The dorsal rami of the spinal nerves after supplying the paravertebral spinal muscles penetrate the tendinous insertion and the overlying fascia. Persistent local pain syndromes which are posture-related may result from mechanical damage to the rami in their course (995). The term *notalgia paraesthetica* (957) is used to describe local paravertebral pains caused by compression of the endings of the thoracic sensory rami. These small terminal branches undergo mechanical damage at their point of passage through the spinal fascia. Sometimes a local injury acts as a trigger factor. A coin-sized area of related sensory loss between the scapula and the midline may be found.

Pelvic and Leg Pains (851, 857)

Hypogastric Pains

In women these may be caused by varicosities of the pelvic veins, which can be shown by transuterine venography (95).

Inguinal Pains

The *ilioinguinal syndrome* causing inguinal pain and a flexed and internally rotated position of the hip joint is discussed on p. 430. The *snapping iliopsoas tendon* may be audible, but only seldom produces much pain. The tendon clicks as it slides over the iliopectineal eminence during slow extension of the hip joint from the flexed position with simultaneous contraction of the iliopsoas muscle (733). The presence of inguinal pain should always prompt a search for *hernia*.

Piriform Syndrome

This syndrome is a condition of intense local pain in the gluteal region, usually caused by injury to the buttock. The pain may radiate to the sacrum, hip joint, and sometimes down the leg; it is aggravated by bending or by lifting weights. Physical examination reveals a well-localized area of tenderness in the region of the sciatic notch, and forced flexion and internal rotation of the hip may cause diffuse pain throughout the buttock region.

Gluteal Pain

In addition to the piriform syndrome, gluteal pains may be caused by irritation of the sciatic bursa which lies between the gluteus maximus muscle and the ischial tuberosity. This irritation is the cause of an occupational lesion associated with prolonged sitting – so-called tailor's bottom.

Hip Joint Pain

In coxarthrosis, the initial pain is typical. It may be pseudoradicular in type, radiating down the lateral side of the leg ("general staff stripe"). The patient walks with his hip held stiff, and rotational movements are particularly restricted (tested by seating the patient on the edge of the bed). Three of the numerous *bursae around the hip joint* may become painful through overstraining of adjacent tendons and joints (283): the trochanteric bursa between the greater trochanter and the tendinous attachment of the gluteus maximus muscle; the iliopectineal bursa between the iliopsoas muscle and the iliopubic eminence (iliopectineal); and the sciatic bursa (see above). Periarthropathy of the hip is mostly encountered in elderly individuals. Intense pain with movement and local tenderness of the hip region are in the foreground, while hip mobility and the X ray are normal. Rarely, the latter may show periarticular calcifications later on.

Algodystrophy of the Hip (298)

This condition affects middle-aged men. Local pain associated with weight-bearing in the region of the hip joint becomes sufficiently severe within a few weeks to cause a limp. Usually no cause can be identified, only rarely is a local predisposing abnormality present, and exceptionally the condition may follow aortic bifurcation surgery (241). Hip movements remain normal. Roentgenologic signs of osteopenia of the femoral head occur after a delay of 1–2 months, but the articular surface remains preserved. The signs and symptoms disappear within a few months, and roentgenologic improvement follows clinical recovery.

Knee Joint Pain

Apart from the common local causes of orthopedic and rheumatologic nature (283), rarer lesions occur, e.g., *neuropathia patellae*. This lesion is caused by compression of the infrapatellar ramus of the saphenous nerve as it penetrates the fascia. Pains are experienced beneath the patella. Pains on the medial side of the knee joint may be produced by irritation of the obturator nerve at the level of the obturator foramen *(Howship-Romberg phenomenon)* (p. 432).

Leg Pain

The intense pains on the anterior aspect of the leg occurring in ischemic necrosis of the foot and toe extensors, the *anterior tibial compartment syndrome*, has been discussed on p. 436. *Nocturnal cramps* of the calf muscles, although harmless, are a painful nuisance. Usually in the early hours of the morning, the patient is awakened by attacks of intense pain in the calf muscles. The foot is held in a position of plantar flexion by the muscular contractions, and the act of dorsiflexion is impossible. Passive stretching of the calf muscles by standing or walking on the affected leg brings immediate relief. Body cooling tends to precipitate an attack. Subjects of all ages are affected. The cause is not known. Attacks may sometimes be prevented by warmly covering the legs or by pressing a pillow under the affected knee. *Symptomatic* calf cramps associated with fasciculation are found in motor neuron disease (p. 221), and after myelitis (359). The cramps usually respond to quinine 200–400 mg, chloroquine phosphate 250 mg, tocopherol 100 units 3 × /d (also effective in the restless legs syndrome), or diphenhydramine 25–75 mg/day.

Foot Pain

A *calcaneal spur,* which causes local heel pain on walking, will be visible in a roentgenogram. *Plantar fasciitis,* an inflammation of the plantar fascia, may be diagnosed by eliciting pain on pressure palpation of the heel and its fascia. The condition may be confused with the tarsal tunnel syndrome. The *tarsal tunnel syndrome,* a lesion usually complicating distortion of the foot, is caused by chronic compression of the posterior tibial nerve beneath the flexor retinaculum behind the medial malleolus. It causes foot pains during walking. The diagnosis is confirmed by demonstrating sensory changes on the sole of the foot and paralysis of spreading of the toes (p. 438). Pain provoked by walking is also a feature of Morton's metatarsalgia (p. 439).

Burning Leg and Foot Pains

This group of lesions encompasses several syndromes, in which the autonomic nervous system appears to play a part. *Erythromelalgia* (erythermalgia) affects men as well as women in middle age. The patient complains of burning and often painful sensations of the feet and hands, particularly on walking, but also in bed under the bedclothes. Warmth aggravates the pain. The painful parts often appear red or cyanotic and the skin is warm to palpation. The local application of cold compresses or elevation of the extremity may bring relief. Treatment with the tricyclic antidepressant clomipramine is successful (126). Apart from idiopathic primary forms, symptomatic cases are encountered following heavy metal poisoning, hypertension, and polycythemia. Almost indistinguishable from erythromelalgia is the *burning feet syndrome,* a phenomenon encountered in various polyneuropathies as well as in hereditary sensory neuropathy (321). Slight axonal degeneration of peripheral nerves causes a *syndrome of muscular pains and fasciculation* (245, 534). The clinical picture consists of muscular pains, cramps, burning sensations, and even paresthesias of the legs, and occasionally also the limb girdles and arms. Physical exercise aggravates the picture and rest relieves it. Benign fasciculation is almost always present in the calf muscles. Occasionally the ankle jerk is diminished. The clinical picture remains unchanged over the course of years.

Restless Legs and Toes

The commonest of this group is the *restless legs syndrome* (anxietas tibiarum). This condition is more often encountered in women, and in about one-third of cases it appears to be inherited as an autosomal dominant (141). The patient complains of unpleasant sensations which are often difficult to define, involving the lower extremities between the midpoint of the thigh and the midpoint of the calf. They are always bilateral. These sensations are not actually painful and they are unaccompanied by paresthesias. They usually appear toward the evening or at night and are definitely associated with sitting or reclining in a soft chair such as an upholstered theater or first-class airplane seat. Temperature has no definite effect. Typically, the patient has an irresistible urge to exercise his legs and restlessly walks up and down. Occasionally the syndrome is announced by myoclonic contractions of the leg muscles (141). No objective neurologic deficit or circulatory disturbances can be demonstrated. The attacks are separated by symptom-free intervals. Treatment consists in a combination of vasodilator drugs and phenobarbital. *Restless toes* is a separate syndrome, in which associated leg pains also may occur. Cases are described which have been triggered by trauma (1089) or form part of the picture of a polyneuropathy (867). The cause of this disturbance is presumed to lie in the afferent fibers of the posterior roots and to be responsible for spontaneous discharge and stimulation of posterior root fibers producing reflex movements in the dependent muscles (872). Disturbances of sleep rhythm not infrequently form part of the clinical picture. Injection of the lumbar

sympathetic chain brings transient relief; resection of the chain is only briefly successful (1139).

Intermittent Claudication

The ischemic pains associated with organic disturbances of arterial perfusion are always exercise-related. *True intermittent claudication* may affect the calf muscles only, or the hip and thigh muscles as well, depending on the site of arterial occlusion. Even amputation stumps may be affected. Pain brings the patient to a standstill ("shopwindow disease"). After a brief rest, the patient can go a little further. This history and the vascular findings (palpation, auscultation, Ratschow's test, i.e., pain produced by foot movements executed with the leg elevated, oscillometry, and Doppler ultrasonography) provide the diagnosis. Occasionally, muscular atrophy may be present. The customary finding is arteriosclerosis of the blood vessels. An abnormal course of the popliteal artery medial to the medial head of the gastrocnemius muscle behind the knee may be responsible for exercise-related intermittent claudication in young subjects and may be corrected operatively (46). *Intermittent claudication of the cauda equina* in spinal stenosis may cause bilateral sciatic pains and absent reflexes on exercise. In this condition, pain is not usually abolished when the patient simply stands still: he is obliged actively to alter the position of his vertebral column to obtain relief, e.g., by sitting down, stooping, or squatting.

13. Myopathies (9, 125, 569, 1247)

General Remarks

Definition: A myopathy is defined as a disease in which the muscle itself is affected by a pathologic process. Muscular involvement may be the main feature of the disease, e.g., progressive muscular dystrophy, or merely one symptom of a generalized disease, e.g., the myopathy accompanying malignant neoplasms.

Elements of Diagnosis:

- usually but not invariably, there is *bilateral* involvement of muscles;
- pure *motor* involvement is present (flaccid paralysis) without sensory disturbance;
- *atrophy* is often visible but it may be absent, e.g., myasthenia gravis, or when muscles is replaced by fatty tissue;
- *reflexes* are diminished in proportion to the degree of paralysis, or they may be absent;
- *pains* are occasionally present, e.g., in paroxysmal myoglobinuria, ischemic muscular necrosis, or myositis;
- *fasciculation* is absent, in contrast to the picture with chronic involvement of anterior horn cells;
- the onset and progression of the paralysis are either insidious or *slowly progressive:* only rarely is the course rapid, e.g., dyskalemias;
- in specific cases, a *familial incidence* may be observed;
- the **ancillary investigations** most useful in diagnosis are
  - muscle biopsy (9, 125),
  - electromyography (519, 724),
  - serum enzyme estimation,
  - immunologic examination,
  - electrolyte examination,
  - testing with cholinesterase inhibitors,
  - CSF (negative),
  - general medical and laboratory tests (endocrinologic, metabolic, etc.).

Classification

An attempt is made in Table 13.1 to group these muscular diseases according to etiology and pathogenesis, while at the same time taking into account their chief clinical characteristics. Since the actual pathogenetic defect in many myopathies is unknown, further progress in research is likely to outdate this classification.

Table 13.1 Proposed classification of myopathies

1. *Dystrophic myopathies*
   a) Progressive muscular dystrophy
      - Type I (facioscapulohumeral form)
      - Type II (pelvic girdle form)
      - Type III (X-chromosomal sex-linked form)
         • Malignant Duchenne's type
         • Benign Becker's type
   b) Myotonic dystrophy (Curschmann-Steinert disease)
   c) Other dystrophic muscular lesions
      - Ocular muscle dystrophy
      - Congenital muscular dystrophy
      - Distal forms
2. *Syndromes with abnormal relaxation of muscle fibers*
   a) Myotonia congenita (Thomsen's disease)
   b) Paramyotonia congenita (Eulenburg's disease)
   c) Neuromyotonia and syndrome of continuous muscle-fiber activity
   d) Stiff man syndrome
3. *Myasthenia gravis*
4. *Myositides*
   a) Polymyositis and dermatomyositis
      - Primary form
      - With collagen diseases
      - With malignancies
      - With other conditions
         • Sarcoidosis
   b) Infectious myositides
5. *Muscular involvement in metabolic disorders (with known metabolic anomaly)*
   a) Muscular signs and symptoms in recognizable enzyme defects
      - Glycogenoses
      - Acid maltase deficiency
      - Muscle phosphorylase deficiency (McArdle's disease)
      - Carnitine deficiency
   b) Muscular signs and symptoms in disturbances of potassium metabolism
      - (Familial) periodic paralysis, or paroxysmal hypokalemic paralysis
      - Hereditary episodic adynamia, or hyperkalemic paralysis
      - Normokalemic paralysis
      - Symptomatic hypokalemias
   c) Rhabdomyolysis (paroxysmal myoglobinuria)

Table 13.**1**   (Continued)

6. *Muscular involvement due to other causes (mechanism unknown)*
   a) Muscular signs and symptoms in endocrine diseases
      - Disturbances of thyroid function
        • Hyperthyroidism
        • Hypothyroidism
      - Cushing's disease
      - Acromegaly
      - Hyperparathyroidism
   b) In malignant diseases
   c) In collagen diseases
   d) In infectious diseases
      • Botulism
      • Tetanus
   e) Malnutrition

7. *Muscular involvement in exogenous poisons*
   a) Alcohol
   b) Drugs
   c) Other toxic substances

8. *Other muscular diseases and symptoms*

Dystrophic Myopathies

Progressive Muscular Dystrophy (568, 569, 829, 1247)

Epidemiology and pathogenesis: Progressive muscular dystrophy is by far the best known hereditary disease of muscle. It is also the commonest myopathy, affecting about 0.2–0.3 per 1,000 of the population. The muscle fibers, on the basis of a genetically determined defect of structure or metabolism, show a functional disturbance which is clinically progressive and leads to morphologic metaplasia of the muscles. The statement "no muscle disease" frequently recorded under the heading of family history in the case notes should always be treated with reservation, and should not be accepted without further investigation. The pathogenesis of the disease is still not clearly understood (568); neurogenic, vascular, and primary myogenic causes have been postulated.

Characteristics of the muscular abnormality: Typical of the disease is the *slow onset* and very slowly progressive weakness of specific muscle groups. The point at which the muscular disturbance manifests itself depends on the progress of the disease, its severity, the physical activity of the individual, and other variable factors. Marked progress may sometimes be observed only over the course of months or years. Almost invariably, the first muscles to be affected are those nearer the trunk, namely the shoulder girdle and upper arm muscles, the buttocks, hip flexors, and especially the knee extensors. Later in the course of the disease, other muscle groups also are gradually involved. The distribution of the lesions is fairly *symmetric*. No pain or sensory disturbances occur, nor does the disease affect the patient's general state of health. Progressive deterioration of the diseased fibers in the affected muscles leads to wasting, i.e., *muscular atrophy*. Sometimes the diminishing muscle bulk is replaced by an increase in fatty and connective tissues, particularly in certain childhood forms of the disease, so that the muscle masses appear to be normal in size or even enlarged *(pseudohypertrophy of the calves)*, despite pronounced weakness. Only parts of the muscle may be affected, other parts retaining a normal contractility – the so-called *boules musculaires* of French authors. The involvement of specific muscles leads to *characteristic postural abnormalities and disturbances of movement*, which will immediately suggest the diagnosis to an experienced observer. Involvement of the facial muscles leads to a snoutlike protrusion of the lips ("pseudohypertrophy of the lips"). Paralysis of the shoulder girdle muscles produces a winged scapula. An infant or child with the disease, if lifted with the examiner's hands in the axillae, will tend to slip through ("loose shoulders"). Involvement of the abdominal and spinal muscles leads to the so-called wasp-tail deformity, which obliges the patient to walk with an arched back. Paralysis of the buttock muscles causes a waddling gait and Trendelenburg's sign or Duchenne's gait (p.433 and Fig.10.**13**). Paralysis of the knee extensor muscles obliges the patient when rising from the floor to use his arms as well, which he places on his thighs (Gowers' sign).

Involvement or other organs: While overshadowed by the muscular lesions, these abnormalities can always be demonstrated on careful search. Thus, the myocardium is frequently involved, although cardiac insufficiency is rare. Acute dilatation of the stomach has been described. Children with progressive muscular dystrophy often exhibit intellectual defects.

Ancillary investigations: *Electromyography* reveals a picture which is conclusive for diagnosis (p.214). *Muscle biopsy* (9, 125) also reveals a pathognomonic appearance. The specimen for examination should be removed from a clinically diseased muscle which is definitely but not maximally involved, i.e., not atrophic or paralyzed. The biopsy, usually performed after infiltration of a local anesthetic agent (without adrenalin) should yield a specimen $1 \times 1 \times 2$ cm in size and contain a parallel bundle of muscle fibers. After brief fixation, the specimen should be correctly positioned so that precise cross sections and longitudinal sections can later be prepared for histologic study. Conventional staining methods are used, see p.216. Histochemi-

Table 13.2 Classification of progressive muscular dystrophies according to inheritance, clinical features, and prognosis (After H. Moser, 1985 [758])

Type	Inheritance	Incidence	Age of Onset	Clinical Features	Prognosis
I Facioscapulo-humeral form	Autosomal dominant	4 per million	2nd and 3rd decades	Starts in face and shoulder girdle	Slowly progressive
II Limb girdle form a) Ascending b) Descending	Autosomal recessive sporadic	38 per million	Very variable, 1st and 2nd (up to 4th) decades	Starts in pelvic or shoulder girdle, variable facial involvement	Variable, work capacity definitely restricted
III X-chromosomal pelvic girdle form a) Duchenne (malignant)	Sex-linked recessive	279 boys per 1 million male births	Walking age	Starts in pelvic girdle. Pseudohypertrophy of calves	a) Rapidly progressive, death usually before 20th year
b) Becker (benign)		5 times less common than malignant form	1st and 2nd		b) Slowly progressive, benign course
IV Congenital form a) De Lange (malignant)	Autosomal recessive		Before birth	Atrophy and contractures, some present at birth	a) Rapid deterioration, death often in infancy
b) Batten-Turner (benign)					b) Benign stationary or slowly progressive
V Distal forms	Autosomal dominant		Variable, 1st to 4th decades	Distal limb muscles first involved	
VI Ocular forms	Autosomal dominant		Variable	External ocular muscles, sometimes also facial and shoulder girdle muscles	Usually benign, slowly progressive
VII Oculopharyngeal form	Autosomal dominant		3rd to 4th decades	Progressive ptosis, ophthalmoplegia and dysphagia	

cal examination enables the two fiber types to be differentiated (type I and type II) and the loss of the normal mosaic pattern to be observed. Muscle phosphorylase is absent in McArdle's disease (p. 496). Blood *serum* examination reveals an elevated creatine kinase level, sometimes above 100 units. Increased levels of this enzyme may also be seen in the polymyositides, as well as in a variety of other situations, e.g., physical activity, muscular trauma, epileptic attacks, acute alcoholic intoxication, hypothyroidism, arterial emboli, cardiac infarction, specific medications such as clofibrate etc. (230).

Individual Forms of Muscular Dystrophy

Progressive muscular dystrophy may be classified, from genetic and clinical points of view, into three genetic forms and five subgroups (125, 569, 829, 1247), the appearances of which are given in Table 13.2.

Facioscapulohumeral Form (Type I)

This form is *inherited* as an autosomal dominant. Since the expressivity is extremely variable, superficial evaluation and inadequate study may suggest the occurrence of apparently isolated and recessive cases. About 4 cases per million births are encountered. The disease manifests itself in the 2nd and 3rd decades of life, and the facial and shoulder girdle muscles are first affected. The serum creatine kinase level is only slightly elevated. The *course* of the disease is unusually prolonged so that the individual

may retain his work capacity up to an advanced age. The pelvic girdle muscles are affected later and usually only mildly so that mobility is preserved and the patient's life expectancy remains undiminished.

Limb Girdle Form (Type II)

This form is *inherited* as an autosomal recessive (38 cases per million births). Sporadic cases also occur (27 cases per million). The *onset of the disease* is extremely variable, occurring at any time between the 1st and 4th decades, usually in the 1st and 2nd. In *patients with facial involvement,* the signs and symptoms appear earlier and the pelvic girdle muscles are not infrequently first involved, in contrast to type I. In the *patients without facial involvement,* the muscles first affected are as often the pelvic girdle as the shoulder girdle; thus, the clinical pattern may be either ascending or descending. The *clinical progress* and pattern of muscular involvement also are extremely variable. The deltoid muscle is often spared, unlike spinal muscular atrophy and the polymyositides. Contractures and hypertrophy of the calf muscles occur. Occasionally a young woman with this form of the disease may present clinically as a case of Duchenne dystrophy (see below). The serum creatine kinase level is usually elevated, but not as markedly as in the Duchenne form. The course of the disease is very slow: severe disability usually takes many years to develop, leading to difficulty in walking and working and shortening of life expectancy. Certain rare and isolated cases of thigh muscle dystrophy may be atypical varieties of this form.

Malignant Form of Duchenne Dystrophy (Type III a)

This form is *inherited* as a sex-linked recessive and affects only boys. It is the commonest form of muscular dystrophy, occurring in 279 boys in every one million live male births, i.e., 4–5 times more frequent than the benign form.

Clinical features: This form of the disease usually presents between the ages of 2 and 6 years, although congenital forms also occur. The pelvic girdle muscles are first affected and a marked hypertrophy of the calf muscles is usually present. Typical features are a marked lordosis of the back and a marked Gowers' sign (see above). The disease is rapidly progressive, involving in turn the remaining pelvic girdle and extremity muscles, and leading within a few years to total incapacity. Cardiac involvement is not unusual (269). Impaired intellectual function may be present and parallels the severity of the muscular disability: It appears to result from a genetically determined congenital defect of brain development (1020). The serum creatine kinase level is very high initially (several hundred, sometimes over 1,000 units), but later it returns to normal (856). Few patients survive beyond the age of 20 years. *Carriers* of Duchenne form of progressive muscular dystrophy, may now be identified by determining their DNA polymorphism.

Female Carriers of Duchenne Dystrophy

The *female carrier* rarely shows clinical signs of the disease (830), although she may experience cramps of her calf muscles on exertion and have weak lower limbs. Not infrequently her calf muscles are hypertrophied. The resting serum creatine kinase level may be elevated but it returns to normal at about the age of 20 (856). The diagnosis can be made, even in symptom-free carriers, by estimation of the serum creatine kinase level after physical exertion, and by muscle biopsy, electromyography (1064), muscle ultrasound examination (1027), MR scanning, and ECG evidence of cardiomyopathy. The form apparently observed in *girls* can be shown upon closer analysis to be either another myopathy (e.g., autosomal recessive limb girdle form) or a nonmyopathic muscular atrophy, rather than a case of the Duchenne form (932).

Benign Form of Duchenne's Dystrophy (Becker) (97)

This form is about 5 times as rare as the malignant form. The disease rarely commences before the end of the 1st decade and the patient is not disabled until the 3rd decade; most die aged 40–60 years. The serum creatine kinase levels are a little higher than in the shoulder girdle forms but definitely lower than in the malignant form.

Treatment of progressive muscular dystrophies: No curative therapy is known. Proper nursing, physiotherapy, and orthopedic correction are the most important measures. Anabolic steroids, nucleoside-nucleotide mixtures, vitamin E, etc. are sometimes prescribed. In cases of Duchenne dystrophy, prednisone 2 mg/kg a day has been recommended, and at least transient beneficial effect has been claimed in a series of patients followed for 2 years (312). However, unequivocal proof of the benefit of any such treatment is still lacking (855).

Myotonic Dystrophy (Curschmann-Steinert) (125, 569)

Pathogenesis and epidemiology: This entity is the second commonest hereditary disease of muscle and is transmitted as an autosomal dominant. Penetration of the disease in male heterozygotes amounts to 100%, in female heterozygotes to 60%. In Switzerland, affected subjects account for 50 cases per million of the population. Men appear to be somewhat more commonly affected than women.

Characteristics of the muscular abnormality: The signs and symptoms usually present for the first time – in contrast to myotonia congenita (Thomsen's disease) (see below) – between the ages of 20 and 30 years, but they may occasionally appear much earlier, even in infancy. The main characteristics of the disease are summarized in Table 13.3. The *dystrophic muscular signs* are the most prominent feature. The atrophy first appears distally in the legs, forearms, and hands, causing corresponding difficulty with walking

Table 13.**3**   Most important characteristics of myotonic dystrophy (Curschmann-Steinert)

- Second commonest disease of muscle (50 per one million population)
- Inherited (autosomal dominant)
- Usually appears in 3rd decade of life
- Atrophy and weakness begin in distal muscles
- Myotonic reaction of muscles (tongue!)
- Myopathic facies with ptosis
- Baldness
- Cataract, blepharoconjunctivitis
- Testicular atrophy (menstrual disturbances)
- Affects work capacity in 4th and 5th decades (life expectancy shortened)

and grasping objects. Later the proximal muscles are also affected. The facial muscles show very early atrophic changes, particularly the temporalis, orbiculares oculi et oris, sternomastoid, and swallowing muscles. The sunken temple, ptosis, and vacuous facial expression, the so-called *facies myopathica,* has been described as the "misery expression." In addition, the muscles in certain patients show a *myotonic reaction* which is less marked than in myotonia congenita and which will be described in connection with the latter disease (p. 484). It does not disturb the patient. Sometimes propranolol may provoke this phenomenon for the first time. General anesthesia in patients with myotonic dystrophy may lead to a prolonged disturbance of muscle function (1226).

Involvement of other organs: Numerous *other clinical manifestations* may be present apart from the muscle lesions, since myotonic dystrophy is an extensive generalized dystrophic disease. The *eyes,* apart from ptosis, may exhibit lid lag, convergence spasm, and occasionally a pseudo-Graefe's sign (p. 347). Slit lamp examination almost invariably reveals the presence of cataract. Keratitis also may be present, as well as atrophy of the ciliary body and reduced intraocular pressure. *Partial hearing loss* for high frequencies and *endocrinologic disturbances* are found, especially testicular atrophy. Female patients may experience menstrual irregularities. Although clinical evidence of *heart* lesions is rare, ECG changes are frequent (prolonged PR interval or widened QRS complex). The *gastrointestinal tract* shows disturbed contractility of the esophagus and stomach, and an elongated sigmoid colon has been described, confirming the involvement of smooth muscle in the dystrophic process. Signs may of a *midbrain lesion* also be present, as well as *psychopathologic* changes, e.g. acute psychotic episodes or a diffuse organic mental syndrome.

Ancillary investigations: *Muscle biopsy* (9, 125) confirms the muscular lesion; apart from the generalized dystrophic appearance, the picture is dominated by a marked increase in central nuclei, ring fibrils, and sarcoplasmic masses. Type I fiber atrophy is characteristic. The *blood serum* creatine kinase level is usually moderately elevated. *Electromyography* shows signs of myopathy, with the typical myotonic discharge ("dive bomber noise" through loud-speaker). *Electrophysiologic* evidence of peripheral nerve involvement is present (914). The EEG shows abnormalities including delayed cerebral electrical activity. *Cranial CT scanning* reveals a gradual increase in the size of the cerebral ventricles.

Prognosis and treatment: Most patients are disabled by the 4th and 5th decades and their work capacity is restricted. Life expectancy is reduced. No treatment directed at the cause is known. Orthopedic measures (splints to improve the stepping gait, operations to correct foot deformities) and physiotherapy are the most important measures. Occasionally the myotonic components of the disease (see below) require treatment.

Myotonic Dysembryoplasia (892)

This entity is a dystrophic disease of muscle which is present at birth. Usually, but not always, it is inherited from the maternal line. Boys as well as girls are affected. It is characterized by difficulty in drinking and swallowing, the baby's face is paretic and masklike, and a high palate is always present. Muscular tone is reduced and motor development is retarded. The sternomastoid and temporalis muscles are atrophic. Occasionally clinical evidence and usually electromyographic signs of myotonia are present. Congenital anomalies are common (foot deformities, scoliosis, micrognathia, etc.).

Other Muscular Dystrophies

Ocular Myopathies

Isolated (900) or familial *dystrophy of the external ocular muscles* (92, 541) leads to a progressive reduction in the range of movement of the eyeballs, as well as ptosis. In an ophthalmologic series of cases, this cause accounted for one-third of the patients with acquired ptosis (572). In cases of levator palsy with relatively well-retained lid retraction, a permanently retracted upper lid may be present. The intrinsic ocular muscles are unaffected. Such cases previously were described as *progressive nuclear ophthalmoplegia* (Graefe's disease).

Mitochondrial myopathies

Definition: These are conditions which affect primarily, but not exclusively, the muscles and in which the mitochondria show morphological abnormalities (regarding size, the cristae, inclusions of the crystalline structures, fat, and myelin bodies). They are based on a biochemical defect which sometimes can be indentified and allows classification. The clinical symptoms are nonspecific and very variable. They usually consist in proximal muscle weakness which is progressive and often associated with ptosis and a disturbance of eye movements. Muscle pains from exhaustion are frequent, and occasionally also myoglobinuria.

As an example, the Kearns-Sayre syndrome will be mentioned here (111). Initially, a progressive disturbance of eye movements associated with ptosis is in the foreground. In some patients, more careful examination may reveal other clinical signs of muscular dystrophy, particularly involving the neck and shoulder muscles which may be confirmed by biopsy. Muscle fibers with very irregular outlines ("ragged red fibers"), abnormal mitochondria, and fat-

containing vacuoles (900), are often present. These findings are often familial (541). Occasionally difficulties with swallowing are also present ("oculopharyngeal dystrophy"). Hearing difficulty, ataxia, and an increased CSF protein level (441) as evidence of an accompanying radiculopathy are also described. Important diagnostic criteria are the presence of retinal pigmentary disturbances and abnormal conduction times in the ECG (92, 900). This disease picture presents before the age of 20 years as a sporadic occurrence and leads, during the 2nd and 3rd decades, to heart block and death unless a pacemaker is implanted. For the differential diagnosis of disturbances of ocular motility, see p. 346.

Distal Myopathies

Hereditary Late Distal Myopathy (Welander's Disease)

This rare disease affects adults of any age. It is an inherited autosomal dominant lesion, which presents with paralysis and atrophy of the forearm and lower leg muscles, as well as the small muscles of the foot and hand. The disease progresses very slowly. Twenty years may elapse before work capacity is significantly reduced. The myopathic nature of the disease may be confirmed by electromyography and muscle biopsy.

Hereditary Distal Myopathy in Childhood

These cases are clinically similar. Differentiation from peroneal muscular atrophy (Charcot-Marie-Tooth disease) (p. 303), which may produce a purely motor lesion and occasionally also presents a myopathic picture on muscle biopsy, is essential (841). Likewise, myotonic dystrophy, which begins peripherally, must be distinguished.

Congenital Muscular Dystrophy

This entity is described as a hereditary autosomal recessive disease in which muscular weakness is present at birth and which runs a fairly rapid course. Clinically and by biopsy, this disease cannot be distinguished from progressive muscular dystrophy.

Syndromes with Abnormal Relaxation of Muscle Fibers

Myotonia Congenita (Thomsen's Disease)

Transmission and pathophysiology: This is an autosomal dominant disease, with a high degree of penetration, which is genetically unrelated to Steinert's form of myotonic dystrophy. Isolated (recessive) cases are also described. The myotonia is presumably the result of an abnormal property of the muscle fiber itself since it can survive blocking or degeneration of the peripheral nerve as well as curarization. Becker described a form of recessively transmitted generalized myotonia.

Clinical features: The disease may appear very early, sometimes "in the cradle." The characteristic feature is the *myotonic reaction,* which affects all skeletal muscles of the body. The muscles relax abnormally slowly after actively contracting, and this defect can be demonstrated by electric or mechanical stimulation. Any firmly grasped object cannot be promptly released, a clenched fist cannot be suddenly reopened. Tapping the tongue with the side of a tongueblade or a hard tap on the thenar muscles produces a prolonged local contraction. Electric stimulation with very low currents causes an immediate simple tetanic (cathode closure) contraction. The patient is unable to carry out sudden movements, although repetitive acts are possible. Eye movements may be disturbed by myotonic spasms of the external ocular muscles and therefore a pseudo-Graefe's sign may be elicited (p.347). Exposure to cold may aggravate the myotonic reaction strikingly. No actual paralysis or muscular atrophy is present: many subjects possess particularly well-developed musculature and an athletic habitus. The intensity of the symptoms diminishes over the years. As a rule the patients are able to carry out most occupations. Life expectancy is not reduced.

Ancillary investigations: *Electromyography* reveals highly characteristic features of the disease. High-frequency small potentials are discharged over several seconds following a voluntary contraction, and produce a "dive bomber noise" through the loudspeaker. *Muscle biopsy* may yield no significant diagnostic information, but histochemical examination shows a deficiency of type IIb fibers (258).

Treatment: If treatment becomes necessary, certain new derivatives of local anesthetics may be utilized to facilitate the fast passage of sodium through the muscle fibers. These include the antiarrhythmic agent tocainide hydrochloride, xylocaine, or mexiletine hydrochloride.

Differential diagnosis: This includes diseases with a myotonic abnormality of the contraction mechanism as well as diseases exhibiting muscular hypertrophy. *Myotonic dystrophy* shows a later onset of clinical features, dystrophic muscular signs, cataract, and other specific features. Paramyotonia (see below) must be considered, as well as *adynamia episodica hereditaria* (p. 500) with its disturbance of potassium metabolism. *Myxedema* may lead to muscular hypertrophy and prolonged muscular relaxation after eliciting reflexes, as well as cramps. Thyroid extract is indicated in such cases. *Myxedematous muscular enlargement (Kocher-Debré-Semelaigne syndrome)* is a childhood abnormality combining signs of hypothyroidism with hypertrophy of the limb muscles, which may be strong or weak. The *Schwartz-Jampel syndrome,* a disease inherited as an autosomal recessive, is a myotonia characterized by generalized muscular rigidity, a small mouth, puffy cheeks, deep-set eyes, a high-pitched voice, and a Perthes-like dysplasia of the femoral heads (944). The calf-muscle hypertrophy of the *Duchenne form of progressive muscular dystrophy* may be easily differentiated by the associated weakness of other muscle groups; similarly, *pseudo-myopathic spinal muscular atrophy (Kugelberg-Welander syndrome),* may begin with hypertrophy of the calf muscles. *True muscular hypertrophy* may have a unilateral distribution and be isolated; usually it appears in childhood or adolescence and is slowly progressive. Some patients exhibit myotonic phenomena, pains, and hyperhidrosis. Cornelia de Lange described a syndrome of *congenital muscular hypertrophy* with extrapyramidal rigidity, debility, and disturbed dentition. The *stiff man syndrome* and *neuromyotonia* (see below) may be recognized by the presence of prolonged electrical activity in the muscles.

Paramyotonia Congenita (Eulenburg's Syndrome)

Transmission: This disease is inherited as an autosomal dominant with virtually complete penetrance.

Clinical features: The patient exhibits an active myotonia at birth, which is markedly aggravated by exposure to cold, and attacks of flaccid paralysis affecting chiefly the proximal muscles. These attacks are unrelated to cold and may last from minutes to hours. Sometimes a so-called myotonia paradoxa occurs (increasing stiffness with repetitive use of a muscle). The muscles are neither atrophied nor hypertrophied, and no cataract or endocrine disturbances are present. The signs of the disease tend to diminish over the years.

Treatment: See myotonia congenita, above.

Differential diagnosis: Since the signs and symptoms of myotonia may not be obvious – they are sometimes only visible in the tongue or elicited by exposure to cold – and since the paralytic episodes may be present without accompanying myotonic signs at all, this condition may be difficult to differentiate from hereditary episodic adynamia (p. 500).

Neuromyotonia (Syndrome of Prolonged Muscular Activity)

Definition: This is a hereditary anomaly of muscle function characterized by stiffness of the musculature, spontaneous fine muscular twitching (myokymias), and electromyographic evidence of prolonged activity. Various descriptions such as pseudomyotonia and pseudotetany have appeared in the literature.

Pathogenesis: The basis of this hereditary disease appears to be a discrete polyneuropathy detectable only by electrophysiologic methods (1221). A dominant hereditary form is described (60).

Clinical features (245, 545, 732, 1221): The syndrome appears suddenly and runs an episodic course. A state of permanent contraction is present in all skeletal muscles, which appear to be hardened so that movements are halting and can take place only by overcoming the resistance of the antagonists. In the later stages, contractures occur. However, there is no muscular atrophy or paralysis, and no myotonic reaction occurs on mechanical stimulation. A permanent fine muscular twitching may be observed. Electromyography reveals the typical feature, a continuous activity of potentials of variable duration, even with the pa-

tient relaxed, which is maintained after nerve block but abolished by curarization, rather than being retained, as in myotonia.

Prognosis: A review made 14 years after the original cases had been described (545) showed that a spontaneous complete recovery had occurred.

Treatment: Antiepileptic drugs, particularly diphenylhydantoin, also carbamazepine bring prompt relief.

Differential diagnosis: This syndrome must be distinguished from tetanus, the myotonic syndromes, and the stiff man syndrome (see below) (1221). Continuous muscle fiber activity has been described in connection with gold therapy (438). In the syndrome of muscular pains and fasciculation described on p. 473, which may be associated with an underlying polyneuropathy, pain is a prominent feature and no electromyographic evidence of continuous muscle fiber activity is present.

Stiff Man Syndrome

Pathogenesis: Apart from an exceptional familial form, all cases are isolated. The syndrome may be caused by a disturbance of the inhibitory action of Renshaw cells in the spinal cord. Pharmacologic studies reveal excretion of the noradrenalin metabolite 3-methoxy-4-hydroxyphenyl glycol in the urine, which parallels the severity of the clinical picture (1085). This suggests the existence of a central adrenergic system stimulating the motor neuron, which is increased by L-dopa and beneficially influenced by diazepam. Phenomenologically, similar cases have been described after encephalitis with a CSF lymphocytosis and inflammatory infiltration of the spinal cord and brainstem (1268). Symptomatic exogenous myotonia, see p.485.

Clinical features (1221): This curious disease entity usually begins in middle age and affects men more commonly than women. The syndrome consists of progressive and permanent stiffness of the muscles, starting in the back and neck and spreading to involve the proximal muscles of the extremities in the later stages. The patient is unable to bend down, and experiences intense and painful muscle spasms. Sensation is intact, the muscle stretch reflexes are brisk, and pyramidal signs are absent or equivocal. Exceptionally, external stimulation may provoke myoclonic spasms, then described as the *jerking stiff man syndrome* (23).

Ancillary investigations: Individual cases show reducing substances in the urine. Muscle biopsy is normal or shows a nonspecific appearance. Most (but not all) patients exhibit electromyographic evidence of a continuous discharge of normal action potentials from individual motor units. As in tetanus, this activity is not prevented by the active innervation of antagonists. The stiffness of the muscles can be abolished by spinal anesthesia or regional anesthesia of the peripheral nerves.

Prognosis: Uncertain.

Treatment: Diazepam is beneficial, as is baclofen (812).

Differential diagnosis: The syndrome must be differentiated from neuromyotonia (1221) and tetanus.

Myasthenia Gravis (Erb-Goldflam Disease)
(337, 340, 504, 850, 904)

Main features: The diagnosis of myasthenia gravis depends on the following characteristics:

- increasing fatigue of individual muscles upon increasing exercise; thus, clinical evidence of the disease is more pronounced toward evening;
- recovery on resting, starting within minutes or within the hour;
- involvement of muscles not supplied by the same peripheral nerves;
- frequent onset with paralysis of the eye, soft palate, and throat muscles;

- varying intensity of clinical signs, occasionally an episodic course;
- absence of sensory disturbances, pain, fasciculation, or atrophy;
- immediate improvement or disappearance of the paralysis following injection of a cholinesterase inhibitor (p.490), e.g., edrophonium chloride;
- myasthenic reaction with progressive reduction in the amplitude of the potentials on repeated stimulation, which can be well demonstrated electromyographically (Fig.13.1).

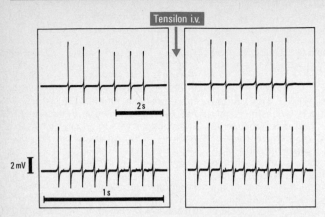

Fig. 13.1 Effect of repeated stimulation of the ulnar nerve on contraction of the abductor digiti minimi in a patient with myasthenia gravis. Before injection of edrophonium chloride, definite reduction in amplitude, particularly with stimulation frequency of 50/s. After injection of 10 mg of edrophonium chloride, return to normal

Pathophysiology (44, 123, 850): Changes occur in the molecular structure of the neuromuscular junction, particularly in the postsynaptic membrane, on the basis of autoimmune mechanisms; however, they may be reversible. Cell groups in the germinal centers of the thymus produce IgG globulins to which the muscle antibodies also belong, and which may be found in about 40% of myasthenics. Apparently the thymus gland also produces immunocompetent small lymphocytes, carriers of the cellular immune reaction. It seems likely that mutations of the proliferating thymus cells produce these "forbidden clones" which lead to the production of autoantibodies, in disregard of the immunotolerance to endogenous tissue. These mutating clones lead to a situation in which an immunologic reaction is provoked in the thymus, as if they were directed against a foreign tissue. On the basis of the antigenic association among the thymus, thyroid, and muscle tissues, the autoimmune reaction thus provoked may be directed against the two last-named tissues as well, and eventually lead to myasthenia gravis. The part bound to serum gamma globulin, the substance which mediates the immune process, can cross the placenta to the fetus and produce a reversible myasthenia gravis. This substance is demonstrable by animal experiments (106). The active serum fraction, which provokes clinical and electrophysiologic myasthenia in mice as well as a reduction in acetylcholine receptors, can be identified as IgG (1206). The change in the anatomic substrate of the neuromuscular junction appear to be a reduction in the number of acetylcholine receptors (351). Young women with myasthenia commonly show the HLA B-8, Dw3-Drw3 Haplo type.

Epidemiology: The prevalence of myasthenia gravis is said to be 3 cases per 100,000 population. Before the age of 40 years, women are more commonly affected; myasthenia in the elderly affects mostly males. Familial cases are rare, but other autoimmune diseases are found in the relatives of myasthenics.

Clinical features: The disease may appear *at any age,* although the first signs usually develop between the 20th and 40th years. Of the children born to a myasthenic mother, 10%–15% show a myasthenia which rapidly disappears (922); a true persisting congenital myasthenia is very rare. *Subjectively,* the patient first notices abnormal fatigability of individual muscles, which on continuous use become weak and paralyzed and then with rest recover within minutes or within the hour. These symptoms either appear in the course of the day or are aggravated toward evening. The muscles most likely to be involved are those supporting the head and neck and those with small motor units (eyelid elevator, soft palate, and eye muscles including the superior rectus). Thus, the **early signs** comprise ptosis, double vision, nasal speech, disturbances of swallowing, and inability to hold the head up or move it satisfactorily. Pure ocular forms also occur. The trunk and extremity muscles become paralyzed later: only exceptionally are they involved at

the onset or before the head muscles. A diagnostic feature, apart from the very variable intensity of the muscular weakness, is the fact that the affected muscles are innervated by different peripheral nerves. The deficits are not necessarily symmetric. During **clinical examination** it is usually possible only to establish the above-mentioned functional disturbances of individual muscle groups, i.e., prompt and definite reduction in power following repetitive muscular movements. In the ocular forms, irregular eyeball movements may be seen which resemble nystagmus, in addition to muscular exhaustion on prolonged gaze to one side or upward. Ptosis may be accentuated by repeated forced closing and opening of the eyes or by repeated or prolonged upward gaze (Simpson's test) (430). About 10% of patients exhibit muscular atrophy in the course of the disease. Associated autoimmune diseases are described, notably thyroiditis and lupus erythematosus.

Ancillary Investigations

Electrophysiologic Examinations

Electromyography shows a fall in the amplitude of the muscle potentials in the affected muscle on repeated nerve stimulation, and this fall can be prevented by the injection of a cholinesterase inhibitor (Fig. 13.1). This phenomenon may not invariably be observed in clinically unaffected muscles. Refined electrodiagnostic methods are available, e.g., observing an initial *posttetanic facilitation* (519) showing the absence of a positive *"staircase phenomenon"*

(519, 724) in myasthenics, or demonstrating an abnormal *"jitter phenomenon"* (1144). This consists of an asynchrony in the transmission of the stimulus from the axon to two muscle fibers belonging to the same motor unit. In the quantitative evaluation of induced optokinetic nystagmus, myasthenics exhibit a definite increase after edrophonium chloride, which is not seen in healthy subjects or in cases of external ocular palsy of other causes (1136).

Test Injection of a Cholinesterase Inhibitor

This test may be carried out at the bedside. Edrophonium chloride (Tensilon) is administered intravenously in increments to a total dose of 10 mg (1 ml) within 15 s. The effect begins after 30 s and lasts only about 3 min. A previously present ptosis will disappear promptly within 1-2 min, but in ocular myasthenia the effect on the external ocular muscles is less dramatic. Atropine sulfate should be available as an antidote (1 mg intravenously, possibly repeated), and ECG monitoring is advisable. If the Tensilon test is applied in a patient who has already been treated with a cholinesterase inhibitor in order to evaluate the usefulness of a higher dose, it is customary to inject 2 mg (or 0.2 ml) intravenously 1 h after the oral dose. The decision can then be made, depending on the effect, as to whether an increase in dose is necessary or whether the weakness represents a cholinergic effect. The myasthenic patient may show great sensitivity to curare (danger of using muscle relaxants during general anesthesia!).

Immunologic Tests

Of the greatest importance is the demonstration of *antibodies to acetylcholine receptors* in the serum (393, 708, 823). These are specific for myasthenia gravis and can be demonstrated in slightly more than 80% of cases. In patients with the ocular form, the titer is lower (absent in 50%), but even 17% of the generalized forms are antibody-negative (1128). In patients with thymomas it is higher (708). A higher titer is observed in the more severe cases and correlates with the presence of HLA-B8 antigens (607). Corticosteroid treatment and also thymectomy reduce the titer. Clinical improvement correlates well with titer in many cases, although these two parameters are not always parallel.

Serologic and immunofluorescence testing may reveal the presence of *antimuscle antibodies* in the serum of myasthenics. Immunochemical techniques and immune electron microscopy show the presence of *immune complexes (IgG and C3) on the motor end plates of myasthenics.* These substances are less abundant in patients with severe myasthenia because they retain fewer acetylcholine receptors (340). About one-half of myasthenic patients will show *blocking antibodies,* which prevent binding of alpha-bungarotoxin to the end plate receptors (123). The titer does not correlate well with clinical severity.

Spontaneous Course

This varies greatly. About one-fourth of patients show spontaneous remissions lasting an average of

4½ years, but as long as 15 years. The mortality rate is highest in the first 2 years, then declines markedly and averages about 15%–20% of all cases.

Treatment

- cholinesterase inhibitors,
- corticosteroids,
- immunosuppressants,
- plasmapheresis,
- thymectomy,
- support measures.

Cholinesterase inhibitors: These substances are given in appropriate divided doses during the day. Pyridostigmine (Mestinon) and less frequently neostigmine (Prostigmine) are prescribed. Spironolactone may serve as an adjuvant. The myasthenic patient can tolerate very high doses of these drugs, except the elderly patient. Daily doses of 600 mg of pyridostigmine may be reached.

Overdosage leads to a *cholinergic crisis*. Because of the therapeutic consequences (reduction or temporary withdrawal of drugs, atropine administration), this condition must be distinguished from a *myasthenic crisis*. In the cholinergic crisis, acetylcholine accumulates in the body and sometimes provokes specific and dramatic effects. The nicotinic effect of acetylcholine manifests itself as depolarization blocking of motor endplates with muscular weakness which cannot be distinguished from myasthenic weakness. Involuntary muscular contractions, fasciculation, and painful cramps may also occur. The muscarinic ef-

fect is manifested by sweating, nausea, a feeling of epigastric pressure, abdominal cramps, increased intestinal motility, and dyspnea. Mental symptoms include agitation, anxiety, and irritability. An intravenous injection of Tensilon 1–2 mg rarely provides the answer when the muscular weakness is convincingly abolished.

Corticosteroids: Prednisone may be given from the start of treatment in high doses – either 100 mg every 2nd day or gradually increasing doses beginning with 20 mg/d. Other authors recommend methylprednisolone 60 mg intramuscularly daily for 10 days (187). If a definite improvement occurs, the patient should be given a maintenance dose of 50–70 mg every 2nd day. This regimen can be repeated if necessary. The effect appears to be better after thymectomy. Initially the symptoms are frequently aggravated; therefore, treatment should always be started with continuously available supervision and respiratory aid. Cases of ocular myasthenia, which is known to fail to respond satisfactorily to cholinesterase inhibitors, can be successfully treated with corticosteroids (367). A beneficial effect may sometimes appear only after a latent period of up to 3 weeks. ACTH treatment, previously very popular, is now no longer used.

Immunosuppressives: Immunosuppressive agents are used in elderly subjects, also as support therapy in patients showing an unsatisfactory response to corticosteroids. They include 6-mercaptopurine 50–75 mg a day, or azathioprine 100 mg a day. A beneficial effect may take several weeks to appear. In myasthenics, the use of benzodiazepine and certain other pharmacologic agents (p. 504) is contraindicated.

Plasmapheresis: This is recommended in patients in whom the disease is worsening or in cases being prepared for thymectomy. It is also used as a therapeutic umbrella for exchange transfusions to combat the myasthenic reaction of the neonate in myasthenic mothers (919).

Thymectomy: Thymectomy is today, with specific reservations, the treatment of choice. The results are particularly impressive in women under 40 years of age who have suffered from the disease for less than 2 years. In such patients, thymectomy convincingly improves the prognosis, and surgical exploration is always indicated. The prognosis in non-neoplastic thymic lesions is the better, the more germinal centers are found to be present in the extirpated gland (1056). In patients over 60 years of age, no macroscopic evidence of thymic tissue exists and no germinal centers are present; therefore, on a theoretical basis no effect can be expected from thymectomy in the elderly (899). The effect is better if thymectomy is followed by prednisone treatment. The operative mortality in a large case series amounted only to about 3%. Operation should be offered to patients with roentgenologically visible thymic hyperplasia or a thymoma, as well as patients in whom no ab-

normal thymic tissue can be detected. The technique of partial extirpation during mediastinoscopy has been abandoned in favor of conventional sternotomy for thymectomy, in view of the technical dangers and the risk of leaving behind thymic rests. The author believes that combined thymectomy and corticosteroid treatment should be offered to all myasthenics except those in whom formal contraindications exist. The beneficial effects, which may appear only after a latent period as long as 2 years, can be expected in 70% or more (496).

Differential Diagnosis

Myasthenic Reaction on Other Muscle Diseases

Muscular weakness with severe fluctuation in the degree of weakness, depending on the activity of the muscle, is a feature of certain myositides, e.g., Sjögren's syndrome, cases of hypothyroidism (p. 502), and individual patients with amyotrophic lateral sclerosis (p. 221).

Eaton-Lambert Syndrome

This is a myasthenic syndrome which in 50% of the cases is etiologically based on bronchogenic carcinoma. In all these paraneoplastic cases, the cancer of the lung declared itself at the latest two years following the onset of myasthenia-like symptoms. If these syndromes last longer than five years, it is practically never on the basis of the carcinoma of the lung (903). *Clinically,* the presenting signs are usually weakness and easy fatigability of the muscles of the pelvic girdle and proximal lower limbs. The tendon jerks are diminished or absent. On activity, power increases transiently for a few seconds (facilitation). Half of the patients show a slight ptosis, and many complain of dryness of the mouth. In contrast to myasthenia, the antibodies against acetylcholine receptors are not increased (881, 903, 1165).

Electromyographically, on repeated stimulation the muscle action potentials initially are small, but increase with more frequent stimulation. The amplitude also increases, and maximal active muscular contraction is achieved after a few seconds of repetitive stimulation. There is no response to cholinesterase inhibitor but curare alters the conduction rate – a reaction with an autoimmune etiology (673). **Therapeutically,** prednisone is useful (1165), as are immunosuppressives and plasmapheresis (881).

Drugs

Certain substances may provoke marked myasthenic reactions (585, 967), notably *penicillamine* (194, 1098), which is used to treat rheumatoid arthritis. Its effects and symptomatology are indistinguishable from true myasthenia gravis. Even the antibodies to acetylcholine receptors may be present. Ocular myasthenic forms occur particularly often (1098). The myasthenic signs and symptoms usually disappear after withdrawal of the penicillamine but reappear if treatment is resumed. On rare occasions, the signs persist despite withdrawal of treatment (194). Myasthenic complications also may follow epilepsy treatment with *phenytoin* and trimethadione. Similarly, chloroquine and resorcin, as well as D-, L-carnitine (243) may cause myasthenia-like signs in normal subjects or aggravate the situation in myasthenics. Magnesium salts, lithium salts, chlorpromazine, and benzodiazepine exert similar unfavorable effects in myasthenics.

Rare causes are malnutrition (p. 505) and specific poisons (p. 504).

Myositides

This heading includes true muscle infections with identifiable pathogens, as well as other muscular diseases with the histologic characteristics of inflammation in which no pathogenic organism is found.

Polymyositis and Dermatomyositis (9, 83, 146, 185, 499, 533, 910, 1247)

Definition and pathogenesis: This is a generalized and symmetric, progressive disease of muscle with the histologic picture of tissue inflammation. The following subgroups have a specific disease pattern:

- without detectable associated disease (true polymyositis),
- with cutaneous involvement (dermatomyositis),
- with malignant disease (83),
- with collagen disorders,
- in childhood.

The basis of all these lesions is an immunopathologic disorder.

Clinical features: At the time of onset most patients are over the age of 30 years, but the disease is found in adults and children. Women are twice as often affected as men. The initial picture may consist of joint pains, general malaise, and fever, but soon muscular involvement becomes evident. This is greatest close to the trunk and has a symmetric pattern with corresponding muscular weakness; sometimes local muscular pain may be present. Cutaneous changes, usually a patchy lividity, may accompany the muscular disorder (dermatomyositis). The skin changes may show a butterfly distribution across the root of the nose and cheeks, but may be localized to the hands or the nail beds. A localized lipodystrophy is also described (910). Children with dermatomyositis very often have calcified deposits (calcinosis) in the subcutaneous soft tissues (185). The lesion may be rapidly progressive or chronic and insidious, and it is necessary to differentiate the latter variety from a dystrophic myopathy. In the symptomatic forms, which may show the picture of a true myositis or dermatomyositis, evidence of the primary lesion (neoplasm, collagenosis) will be present. The rare Shulman syndrome (835) is a fasciitis with scleroderma-like skin changes, elevated erythrocyte sedimentation rate, eosinophilia, and mild fever. Aside from inflammatory infiltration of the fascia, not infrequently a concomitant myositis is found. It responds promptly to steroids.

Ancillary investigations: The *blood* shows an increased ESR and a raised serum globulin level. The serum creatine kinase level often is raised, in acute cases above 1000 units. *Electromyography* shows changes which, although typical, are not pathognomonic: short polyphasic potentials, fibrillation potentials, and pseudomyotonic repetitive discharges. Muscle biopsy shows a typical picture. Some fibers show severe degeneration, others abundant regeneration, and still others none at all. Inflammatory cells are present, and occasionally an increase in the connective tissue content.

Treatment (499): The success of treatment with corticosteroids depends upon a prompt start and a high initial dose. It is likely to beneficial if begun within the first 24 months after the onset of the weakness. Initially prednisone 1 mg/kg body weight per day is given for 1 month. If treatment starts later, progression of the disease can be halted and a partial recovery achieved. If corticosteroids have no effect, immunosuppressants may be used, e.g., methotrexate or cyclophosphamide (264). In acute cases not responding and in children (169), plasmapheresis has a role.

Prognosis: About one-fourth of patients die. About one-half of those receiving an optimal therapeutic regimen (see above) are cured or significantly improved (499).

Other Myositides

Acute Benign Myositis Following (Viral) Infection

This entity was originally described in children (51). Usually it appears 1-2 days after an influenza-like illness with signs of upper respiratory tract involvement: it is an intense pain syndrome of the thigh and calf muscles in particular and less commonly the back and arm muscles. No striking muscular weakness is present, but movements are limited by pain. The serum creatine kinase level is markedly elevated. Histologic examination has confirmed myopathic changes in muscles (157). Most signs and symptoms disappear within 1-2 weeks. A similar picture is seen in adults.

Giant-Cell Polymyositis

This is a rare syndrome, in which the polymyositis is associated with thymoma, myocarditis, and occasionally signs and symptoms of myasthenia with thyroid abnormalities (869).

Menopausal Myopathy

Also called "menopausal muscular dystrophy," this condition should perhaps be viewed as a polymyositis.

Ocular Muscle Myositis

This is part of a nonbacterial inflammatory lesion of the orbital contents (p. 347).

Specific Infectious Myositides

True purulent myositides are found in the Tropics, which appear to be confined to a single muscle. Even in the northern hemisphere, myositis may be part of the picture of *toxoplasmosis or trichinosis* (calcification!).

Myositis in Sarcoidosis

See p. 503.

Muscular Involvement as a Metabolic Disturbance (with Anomaly Known)

Muscular Signs and Symptoms with Known Enzyme Defect

Glycogen Storage Diseases

General features: At least four forms of muscular involvement are known in the diseases of glycogen metabolism. The cardiomuscular form of the disease in children and adolescents appears in about 50% of cases as a muscular abnormality. These children, who are physically retarded but usually normal mentally, show cardiac enlargement and an abnormally large tongue. The skeletal muscles are weak and may be hypotonic. The tendon jerks may be completely absent. The glycogen content of skeletal muscle, which normally amounts to about 0.5 g%, is increased four- to eightfold. This increase may be confirmed by muscle biopsy, e.g., by the use of Best's carmine stain, which reveals vacuolation of the muscle fibers and displacement of the fibrils by deposits of glycogen.

Glycogenosis Type II (Pompe's Disease)

This form is characterized by a deficiency of acid maltase which hydrolyzes glycogen to glucose. This defect of glycogenesis is inherited as an autosomal recessive lesion. It may lead to progressive muscular weakness and may not manifest until adulthood (62, 1153, 1208). In individual adult cases, clinical and even biopsy differentiation of this form from spinal muscular atrophy may be difficult (964). Biopsy reveals numerous vacuoles in both types of muscle fiber. Ultrastructural and cell culture studies show that the membrane-bound vacuoles are filled with glycogen granules. The patient may develop respiratory distress on a muscular basis. When it is treated, e.g. with intermittent positive alveolar pressure, the patient may be able to return to work (1208).

Glycogenosis Type III (Defect of Debrancher Enzyme) and Type IV (Deficiency of Brancher Enzyme)

These forms show hepatomegaly and sometimes muscle signs and symptoms.

McArdle's Disease

Also known as *glycogenosis type V,* this form is an inherited disease, often recessive, caused by a congenital deficiency of myophosphorylase. This deficiency renders impossible the production of glucose-1-phosphate from muscle glycogen. The patient gives a history of painful cramps after exertion present from childhood, especially affecting the calf muscles. Myoglobinuria is present. Some patients with advancing age develop permanent paralysis and shortening of muscles, possibly as a result of the muscle necrosis which frequently accompanies the myoglobinuria. During an attack of paralysis, a silent electromyographic tracing is obtained. Venous blood taken from an extremity under ischemic conditions after muscular activity shows no increase in lactic acid. The phosphorylase deficiency can be demonstrated by biochemical and histochemical methods. Phosphorylase

appears to be present in other organs: e.g., glucagon or adrenalin administration causes a normal rise in the blood sugar, due to mobilization of liver glycogen.

Lipid Storage Myopathy (1016)

This rare disease, often present at birth, is **clinically** static or runs a course which is only slowly progressive. Various *biochemical defects* lead to a histologic picture of lipid storage myopathy, which explains the variable course of the disease, from stationary to intermittent or progressive (339). **Therapeutically,** specific forms with carnitine deficiency respond to carnitine supplements (296), others to cortisone (338).

Myoglobinurias

Myoglobinuria is the clinical manifestation of muscle fiber destruction. Numerous causes are responsible. The two main types are:

- *genetically determined cases*
  - with known, and
  - with unknown enzyme defect,
- *sporadic cases,* e.g.,
  - excessive muscular activity,
  - physically determined muscular disturbance, e.g., crush injury,
  - ischemic muscular necrosis,
  - drug-induced or
  - exogenous toxin, e.g., Haff disease, and
  - metabolic toxin.

Myoglobinuria with Known Enzyme Defect

To this group belong the diseases with known deficiency of myophosphorylase, as well as some with carnitine palmityl transferase and lactate dehydrogenase deficiency.

Myoglobinuria in Inherited Enzyme Defect (as yet Unknown) Malignant Hyperthermia
(118, 694, 1092)

This appears to be a muscular abnormality *inherited* as an autosomal dominant which usually remains clinically silent. *Biopsy* shows specific myopathic features including histochemical abnormalities, and the blood *serum* of patients contains high level of creatine kinase. The life-threatening *disease picture* develops in children (694) and young adults in the course of *general anesthesia*, particularly when powerful inhalation agents such as halothane and muscle relaxants such as succinylcholine or curare are used. The clinical picture includes difficulty with intubation, tachycardia, arrhythmia and sometimes cardiac arrest, hyperventilation, muscular rigidity, and especially a sudden and alarming hyperthermia. **Pathogenetically**, the disease picture is caused by an inherited anomaly of ATPase distribution at the membrane level. Abnormally structured membranes release calcium ions. An unexplained elevation in creatine kinase level prior to anesthesia should serve as a warning signal. *Therapeutically,* dantrolene 2.5 mg/kg should be rapidly infused in the acute stage.

Rhabdomyolysis (Paroxysmal Myoglobinuria)

The *biochemical defect* responsible for this (inherited) form remains unknown. **Clinically**, muscular weakness, particularly of the proximal groups, is accompanied by pain, fever, and leukocytosis. Usually no cause is apparent, but sometimes a history of physical exertion or infection may precede the bout of illness. Two-thirds of the patients are under 20 years at the onset and men are 4 times more frequently affected than women. There is acute destruction of the striated muscle fibers, the contents of which – glycogen, myoglobin, creatine, muscle enzymes, and potassium – are passed into the circulation. The myoglobin may be observed as a reddish-brown color in the urine within 3–5 days. The serum creatine kinase level is greatly elevated. Renal function may be impaired by blockage of tubular function. The patient may start to recover after 1–2 weeks, and continue over several months. *Histologically,* apart from necrosis of muscle fibers and an abundant inflammatory reaction, reparative changes and abundant regeneration may be ovserved within a few days.

Muscular Signs and Symptoms in Disturbances of Potassium Metabolism
(397, 523, 801)

General features: This group of myopathies, mostly inherited, is characterized by severe muscular weakness or paralysis which appears suddenly without a sensory deficit. It is accompanied by an abnormal level of serum potassium – either reduced (familial periodic paralysis) or increased (hyperkalemic periodic paralysis). The ECG shows corresponding changes. Details of the dyskalemic paralyses are given in Table 13.**4**. Muscular disturbances also arise from symptomatic, exogenous disturbances of the metabolism of potassium.

Periodic Paralysis (Familial Paroxysmal Hypokalemic Paralysis) (397, 801)

This lesion is typified **clinically** by attacks of paralysis, with or without a family history. The disturbance may occur after a bout of particularly strenuous exercise following a rest period, after cooling off, or after a large carbohydrate meal. The pa-

Table 13.4 Dyskalemic familial paralyses (After *Martens, H. G.*, 1985 [736])

	Hypokalemic Paralysis "Paroxysmal Paralysis"	Hyperkalemic Paralysis Hereditary Episodic Adynamia	Normokalemic Paralysis and Periodic Paramyotonic Adynamia
Inheritance	Autosomal dominant	Autosomal dominant	Autosomal dominant
Sex predominance	Men more often affected	Men more often affected	Men and women equally affected
Onset of disease	2nd decade	1st decade	1st decade
Frequency of paralysis	Every 1–3 months	Daily or weekly	Every 1–3 months
Length of paralysis	ca. 8–24 h (–4 days)	ca. 1–4 h	2–20 days (–60 days)
Time of day	During sleep	Over the whole day, mostly in the morning	During sleep
Clinical picture	Generalized paralysis usually sparing facial and respiratory muscles	Lower limbs	Usually generalized
Electrolytes before attack starts	Na and K retention	K elimination	–
Electrolytes when attack subsides	Na elimination	–	–
Serum K^+ during attack	Reduced (as low as 1.8 mval/l)	Raised (up to 7.3 mval/l)	Normal or rising (up to 2.5 mval/l)
ECG during attack	Reduced amplitude, negative T waves, U waves, and depressed ST segment	High peaked T waves, isoelectric ST segment	–

	$H_2O\uparrow$, $Na^+\uparrow$ ($K\downarrow$) vacuoles	$K^+\downarrow$ ($H_2O\uparrow$, $Na^+\uparrow$) vacuoles	Vacuoles
Muscles during attack			
Aldosterone during attack	Increased	Reduced	–
Primary disturbance	Na^+ flow to muscles	Disturbed reabsorption K^+	
Secondary disturbance	Aldosterone excretion	–	–
Membrane potential	Normal ($\downarrow$)	Reduced	Reduced
Provocation	Night-time sleep Na^+ intake increased Adrenocortical hormone Muscular activity after adrenaline injection Large increase in carbohydrate intake, insulin	Rest after labor K^+ increased Blockade of adrenal cortex Alcohol, fasting, damp weather	Rest after labor K^+ increased Alcohol, cold
Prevention of attack	Light muscular activity Na^+ withdrawal Spironolactone Aldosterone blockade Acetazolamide (250 mg q 6 h)	Light muscular activity Large increase in Na^+ Aldosterone Acetazolamide	Light muscular activity Large increase in Na^+ Fluorhydrocortisone Acetazolamide
Treatment during attack	Potassium 10–20 g KCl 120 mval K^+	Ca^{++}, glucose, NaCl, carbohydrate	NaCl

ralysis usually ascends from the lower extremities, and within hours a flaccid quadriparesis or quadriplegia is present, including diminished or absent muscle stretch reflexes. Sometimes the quadriparesis is asymmetric. Often it is accompanied by paresthesias. Sensation is usually intact. The diaphragm and muscles of the face and head are spared. Sphincteric function remains intact and consciousness is preserved. In the course of an attack, the muscles have an increased circumference. Of the **ancillary investigations,** biopsy reveals vacuolated muscle fibers, reflecting an expansion of the endoplasmic reticulum. Electromyography reveals fibrillation potentials, signs of denervation, and an absence of electrical activity at the height of the attack. The ECG shows typical changes (ST segment depressed, T wave widened, QT interval prolonged). A constant feature is the low plasma potassium level which is present during an attack. The **course** is usually toward spontaneous recovery, and the signs and symptoms disappear in reverse order and over the same period of time as they appeared. Dramatic recovery follows the administration of potassium. Without treatment, the patient may perish. In the familial cases, further attacks of paralysis remain a constant possibility, which may eventually lead to permanent muscular changes and paralysis.

Adynamia Episodica Hereditaria (Gamstorp's Disease, Hyperkalemic Periodic Paralysis) (397, 523)

This autosomal dominant disease with virtually complete penetrance appears to occur particularly frequently in Sweden. **Clinically,** many similarities exist with the entity described above, periodic paralysis, but in this condition each attack is heralded by a *hyperkalemia.* The initial attacks occur in childhood. They are frequent, several a week, and each attack is brief, lasting less than 60 min. The patient in the course of his life may become free from attacks. Precipitating factors include physical exercise, exposure to cold, and fasting. In each attack, the paralysis ascends from the lower extremities but, in contrast to hypokalemic periodic paralysis, the bulbar and facial muscles may also be involved. The tendon jerks are diminished or absent. Associated but not invariable signs of myotonia may be present so that the condition must be distinguished from paramyotonia. Paresthesias are common. The plasma potassium level is high at the onset of an attack, and small therapeutic amounts of potassium may provoke it. The **prognosis** is always good. **Long-term treatment** may be undertaken with carbonic anhydrase inhibitors, e.g., acetazolamide 250 mg in the morning and 125 mg or less later on. Equally good results have been obtained with dichlorphenamide 50 mg and 25 mg/d or less.

Periodic Paralysis with Normokalemia

This is a rare, autosomal dominant disease with variable penetrance. The **attacks** are longer and more severe in type: they may last for 3 weeks and recur repeatedly in the course of a year. **Treatment** consists of sodium chloride administration in large doses.

Symptomatic Hypokalemias

Etiologically, many cases of hypokalemia are symptomatic, due to renal disturbances, diuretics, potassium loss from the intestine, potassium loss from exchange resins, primary aldosteronism (Conn's syndrome), and drug intoxication secondary to excessive intake of desoxycorticosterone or extract of licorice. The triggering role of hyperthyroidism should be mentioned. **Therapy** consists in combining the emergency administration of potassium with measures to combat the underlying disease.

Muscular Involvement due to Other Causes (Mechanism Unknown)

Muscular Signs and Symptoms in Endocrine Disorders

Hyperthyroidism (833)

Chronic Thyrotoxic Myopathy

In this myopathy, the weakness affects mainly the proximal muscle groups, especially the pelvic girdle. The patient experiences difficulty in rising from a squatting position or from a very low chair or foot-stool *(signe du tabouret).* About one-half of the patients with hyperthyroidism show this sign. Less commonly, an atrophy of the peripheral muscles is also present. Fasciculation has also been described (833) so that the syndrome requires differentiation from amyotrophic lateral sclerosis. The reflexes are increased. Pyramidal signs have been described, as well as other evidence of involvement of the CNS – Basedow's paraplegia (353). Muscle biopsy shows a lymphocytic infiltrate.

Complete recovery accompanies correction of the metabolic disturbance.

Acute Fatal Thyrotoxic Myopathy

This form is very rare and is accompanied by signs and symptoms of bulbar involvement.

Other Effects of Hyperthyroidism

Thyrotoxicosis is frequently present in *myasthenics.* The hypermetabolic state of the patient aggravates the myasthenic disturbance. A small proportion of patients with *periodic paralysis* (less than 10%) suffer from thyrotoxicosis, and its elimination abolishes the attacks of weakness. The hyperthyroidism appears to activate a latent disturbance of potassium metabolism.

Exophthalmic Ophthalmoplegia

In this form, which not infrequently is unilateral, the abnormalities of external ocular movement – usually paralysis of the superior rectus muscle – parallel the exophthalmos. The condition may appear after thyroidectomy and is relatively resistant to treatment.

Hypothyroidism

Apart from signs of CNS involvement (p. 153) and a carpal tunnel syndrome (p. 416), disturbances of muscular function are also attributed to thyroid hypofunction. The commonest of these is *proximal muscle weakness* in the pelvic and shoulder girdles. The muscle stretch reflexes, particularly the ankle jerk, show an abnormally slow relaxation phase. Direct tapping of a muscle provokes a contraction which relaxes very slowly (myoedema). Signs and symptoms like those of myasthenia may appear (1184). Histologic evidence of a subsarcolemmal mucoid substance is present. Muscular hyperplasia in congenital myxedema has already been mentioned (p. 153). These features regress completely if the thyroid deficiency is compensated.

Muscular Signs and Symptoms in Cushing's Disease

These are not rare. Usually a proximal weakness of the leg and pelvic girdle muscles is present, occasionally also atrophy. The gluteal muscles are least frequently involved. Electromyography reveals myopathic patterns. Muscle biopsy shows structural changes in individual fibers, also groups of atrophic fibers.

Acromegaly (617, 948)

Most patients with acromegaly eventually develop a carpal tunnel syndrome (p. 416). They may also exhibit weakness of proximal muscle groups, the electromyogram revealing myopathic features. However, the serum enzyme levels and muscle biopsy remain normal. Hypophysectomy leads to prompt improvement of the carpal tunnel syndrome and slow improvement of the myopathy (948).

Addison's Disease

Occasionally muscle contractures, affecting especially the muscles of the lower extremities and the abdomen, accompany this disease. These contractures appear suddenly, are heralded by pain, and regress only very slowly (208).

Hyperparathyroidism

The muscular signs and symptoms of this disease have been described on p. 155.

Muscular Involvement in Collagen Diseases

The myopathies referred to in this section belong in the group of myositides with known etiology.

Wegener's Granulomatosis

Patients with this disease may exhibit diffuse muscular weakness, in addition to CNS and peripheral neurologic signs and symptoms (p. 158). Biopsy reveals myopathic changes including inflammatory infiltrate, vacuolation, and fibrillary necrosis.

Lupus Erythematosus

Apart from the CNS complications of this disease (p.157), diffuse and very severe myalgic pains occur, and the muscles themselves are tender to palpation. Although the muscles are weak, none is usually paralyzed. If paralysis does occur, proximal groups are affected. Electromyography shows a picture resembling polymyositis. Biopsy reveals a myositis with cellular infiltrate, perivascular in distribution, and resembling periarteritis nodosa. Individual fibers show structural changes a vacuole formation. Vacuolation is also described as the typical *effect on muscle of chloroquin,* a drug sometimes used in the treatment of lupus erythematosus. Cases of combined simultaneous lupus erythematosus and myasthenia gravis have been observed.

Sjögren's Syndrome

This also appears to be an autoimmune disease. A slowly progressive myopathy my occur (25), in which the proximal muscle groups are affected and may atrophy. Electromyography and muscle biopsy reveal the picture of a myositis.

Rarer Collagen Disorders

Scleroderma shows muscle signs and symptoms similar to those of Sjögren's syndrome. A relatively benign collagen disease, *mixed connective tissue disease* (Sharp's syndrome), is characterized by joint pains and Raynaud's syndrome, in addition to myositis (1102). Behçet's disease (p.252) may be accompanied by myopathy.

Muscular Involvement in Malignant Diseases

Myositis with Malignant Tumors (500)

Together with the CNS features (p.156) and the polyneuropathies (p.322), the myositides form part of the paraneoplastic syndrome. This syndrome is caused by metabolic or immunologic effects and is unrelated to local tumor growth. Clinically, it is composed of elderly patients who exhibit paraneoplastic myositis, with slowly progressive weakness and atrophy of proximal muscles. A malignant tumor is present in 70% of men and 25% of women who present this clinical picture after the age of 50 years. Bronchogenic carcinoma is the commonest, but malignant tumors in other sites should also be sought. The muscular signs and symptoms may precede other clinical manifestations of the tumor by 2 or more years. Electromyography and muscle biopsy reveal the presence of polymyositis (p.493). Occasionally the muscular symptoms regress after radical resection of the primary tumor.

Lambert-Eaton Syndrome

This syndrome, myasthenic muscular involvement in bronchial and other malignant tumors, has been discussed on p.492.

Myopathy in Sarcoidosis (579)

Incidence: Biopsy or autopsy reveals typical granulomas in the muscles in about 60% of all patients with sarcoidosis.

Clinically, a myopathy may be caused by granulomas in the muscles, although these may be asymptomatic. Muscular involvement is usually bilateral and symmetric, with weakness and atrophy of the proximal groups. Occasionally the affected muscles ar slightly painful. The tendon jerks may be diminished or absent. Sensation is intact. Muscular involvement may be accompanied by evidence of involvement of other organs, or it may be an isolated finding without other clinical evidence of sarcoidosis being present. The other signs and symptoms of CNS sarcoidosis have been described on p.53.

Ancillary investigations: Electromyography indicates a myopathy. The diagnosis is made on the basis of involvement of other organs in the disease (hilar lymphadenopathy, ocular manifestations, parotid swelling, skin changes, negative tuberculin test, etc.) and particularly muscle biopsy, which reveals the typical granuloma with epitheloid cells and Langhans' giant cells.

Course: Either slowly progressive or characterized by stuttering bouts of deterioration alternating with intervals of complete remission.

Muscular Involvement in Exogenous Poisons

Chronic Alcoholism

Acute Alcoholic Myopathy

This impressive manifestation in chronic alcoholics includes pain, weakness, and necrosis of muscles. The serum creatine kinase level is raised, and the normally occurring increase in the lactic acid level upon muscular activity is reduced, as in McArdle's disease (p. 496). The signs are nearly always accompanied by other features of chronic alcoholism (pp. 152 and 317). The condition is slowly reversible following abstinence from alcohol.

Subacute or Chronic Myopathy

This appears in the course of weeks or months as weakness and atrophy of the trunk muscles. The condition is usually reversed by alcohol abstinence, but certain deficits may be permanent.

Hypokalemic Myopathy in Alcoholics (1035)

This condition may produce an independent disease picture. Within a few days a rapidly progressive weakness develops, but the muscles are not painful or swollen, and there is no myoglobinuria. An accompanying hypokalemia is present which may be corrected by the administration of potassium.

Therapeutic Drugs (585, 672, 967)

Certain therapeutic *drugs lowering the cholesterol level* such as diazacholesterol may produce typical symptomatic myotonia which is detectable clinically and electromyographically. An associated muscular weakness occurs, and damage to the muscle fibers may be confirmed by histologic examination. The signs and symptoms disappear if the drug is withdrawn. Propranolol may provoke myotonia in patients with myotonic dystrophy (135). Chloroquine (and colchicine) treatment may cause a vacuolation myopathy already described on p. 502. *Penicillamine* and other pharmaceuticals may produce myasthenic signs and symptoms (p.493). During beta-blockade a proximal myopathy has been described (378). *Treatment with steroids,* especially fluorohydrocortisone, may be complicated by weakness of the girdle and proximal extremity muscles. Electromyography reveals myopathic changes, and the serum levels of individual muscle enzymes are elevated. Muscle biopsy shows signs of a primary myopathy. The clinical signs and symptoms disappear rapidly and completely upon cortisone withdrawal.

Muscular Involvement in Other Diseases

Undernutrition

Under circumstances of prolonged *undernutrition*, e.g., prisoner of war camps, a myasthenic weakness may occur which is accompanied by ptosis and fatigability of the neck muscles (Japanese, *kubisagari:* "The one who hangs his head"). In cases of *vitamin E deficiency,* a severe myopathy similar to that shown in animal experiments, may

be expected. Apart from other clinical signs and symptoms (p. 316), muscular weakness has been described (1253). In children with chronic cholestasis, vitamin E deficiency may lead to a chronic progressive myopathy, which may be successfully treated with alpha-tocopherol (444).

Dialysis

Proximal muscular weakness is described in dialysis patients in whom the presence of HLA-A3, B7 and B14 antigens is combined with hemochromatosis (165). Biopsy reveals evidence of iron deposition in the muscle fibers and macrophages.

In uremic patients treated by dialysis, proximal muscular weakness may indicate secondary hyperparathyroidism with osteodystrophy, which may be controlled by parathyroidectomy (683).

Other Muscular Diseases and Symptoms

Congenital Nonprogressive Myopathies

This heading includes some muscular diseases, some of which can be identified histologically and others of which are inherited congenital lesions. They have a static or only mildly progressive course. They were previously – and remain – designated by the unsatisfactory title of myatonia congenita (Oppenheim's disease, floppy baby).

Central Core Disease

This is viewed as a hereditary congenital anomaly of muscle caused by a disturbance of synthesis and function of the central fibrils of individual muscle fibers. The child is hypotonic and

shows weakness of proximal muscles. Walking is delayed, but in most cases the disease is not progressive. The tendon jerks are present, sensation is intact, and the muscle masses, although poorly developed, show no atrophy. Muscle biopsy reveals a characteristic picture: the centers of many fibers contain one or more groups of abnormal fibrils which can be identified by their particular staining characteristics. They are more eosinophilic than the surrounding fibrils and their cross-striations are well preserved in longitudinal sections. Their appearance contrasts with that of the surrounding normal fibrils, in that the individual periodic elements appear to have lost their regular arrangement. The presence of cross-striations, the absence of a third intermediate zone between center and periphery, and the absence of other signs of denervation distinguish these changes in the central fibrils from the "target fibers" seen in denervation.

Nemaline Myopathy

This is a similar hereditary, nonprogressive myopathy. Muscle biopsy reveals rodlike structures in the muscle fibers, consisting of protein molecules which are either irregular or arranged in a palisade pattern. Segmental structures resembling fibrils are also present. The combination of central core disease and nemaline myopathy may be encountered in the same patient. The question arises if nemaline myopathy, a rare biopsy finding, is a separate specific disease entity or a single morphologic endproduct of several genetically determined anomalies.

Megaconial and Pleoconial Myopathy

Under these headings cases are described in which electron-microscopic examination reveals large mitochondria with inclusion bodies. They probably do not denote a disease entity, but rather a reaction of muscle fibers to different metabolic disturbances.

Myotubular Myopathy (125)

This is an anomaly in which the muscle fibers partially retain their embryonal appearance, the nuclei of many fibers being central (centronuclear myopathy). The anomaly is a congenital myopathy, and clinically cases run a nonprogressive course.

Congenital Muscular Dystrophy

This progressive myopathy (684) has been described on p. 484.

Other Muscular Abnormalities

Many cases of nonprogressive congenital myopathy have an uncertain etiology. It is possible that *generalized muscular hyperplasia* (Krabbe's form) belongs to this group. A rare anomaly of muscle is the so-called *hypertrophic branchial myopathy* (757), which is characterized by a progressive hypertrophy of the masseter, temporal, and pterygoid muscles with myopathic changes of these muscles confirmed by biopsy. *Myosclerosis* (161) is probably caused by several etiologic factors. The muscles are hard and show contractures. Biopsy reveals a profuse proliferation of connective tissue and other changes, e.g., inflammatory reaction. Familial changes have been described. Treatment with D-penicillamine, up to 750 mg/d, has been successful.

Differential Diagnosis of Myopathies

Childhood

It is necessary to exclude cases of progressive nonmyopathic muscular weakness of childhood, including spinal muscular atrophy (Werdnig-Hoffmann disease) and sometimes even hypotonic cerebral palsy. *Agenesis of individual muscles,* most commonly the pectoralis major, is easy to recognize by its isolated and unilateral character and the absence of progression. *Arthrogryposis multiplex* (460), a condition producing congenital deformities and limitation of joint movements and contracture of muscles, may be the complication of an early myopathy (313) or of other causes of immobilization in utero. *Calcinosis universalis,* which is far more frequent in young women and girls than in boys, is heralded by weakness followed by muscular pains, and finally the widespread deposition of calcium in the subfascial planes of muscles and by generalized ill-health.

Adulthood

Here also *spinal muscular atrophy* must be considered. *Diabetic amyotrophy* (p. 310) also must be distinguished from a chronic myopathy. *Progressive lipodystrophy* (Morgagni-Barraquer-Simons' disease) is a rare disease characterized by progressive and symmetric shrinkage of the subcutaneous fatty layers of the upper half of the body, with simultaneous increase in the dependent parts form the level of the navel downward. The disease affects mainly women and appears in the 1st or 2nd decades of life. It begins with a loss of fatty tissue from the face, giving the patient a death-mask appearance, and the process then spreads caudad over the course of months or years. The etiology is unknown; some authors implicate a midbrain disturbance. *Progressive ossifying myositis* is a hereditary disease in which numerous foci of true new bone are deposited in the muscles. In a variety of CNS lesions, such as brain trauma, focal deposits of bone may be laid down within the space of a few weeks in the vicinity of the large joints (hip, shoulder, elbow, and knee); the term *myositis ossificans neurotica* or *heterotopic ossification* is applied to this appearance. *Arthrogenic muscular atrophy* occurs in the muscles adjacent to the diseased joint, particularly the quadriceps femoris in disturbances of the knee joint. Pure motor forms of *polyradiculitis* (Guillain-Barré syndrome) (p. 294) may at first be mistaken for an acute myopathy.

References

1 Aarli, J. A.: Nervous complications of measles: clinical manifestations and prognosis. Europ. Neurol. 12: 79-93, 1974

2 Aaslid, R., T. Markwalder, H. Nornes: Noninvasive transcranial Doppler ultrasound recording of flow velocity in basal cerebral arteries. J. Neurosurg. 57: 769-774, 1982

3 Aaslid, R., H. Nornes: Musical murmurs in human cerebral arteries after subarachnoid hemorrhage. J. Neurosurg. 60: 32-36, 1984

4 Achari, A. N., M. S. Anderson: Serum creatine phosphokinase in amyotrophic lateral sclerosis: correlation with sex, duration, and skeletal muscle biopsy. Neurology 24: 834-837, 1974

5 Acker, W., E. J. Aps, S. K. Majumdar et al.: The relationship between brain and liver damage in chronic alcoholic patients. J. Neurol. Neurosurg. Psychiat. 45: 984-987, 1982

6 Ackermann, R.: Erythema chronicum migrans und durch Zecken übertragene Meningopolyneuritis (Garin-Bujadoux-Bannwarth): Borrelien-Infektionen? Dtsch. Med. Wschr. 108: 577-580, 1983

7 Adams, A. E.: Thalamische Funktionen und Syndrome. Dtsch. Med. Wschr. 99: 2117-2121, 1974

8 Adams, H. P., N. F. Kassel, J. C. Torner, A. L. Sahs: CT and clinical correlations in recent aneurysmal subarachnoid hemorrhage: a preliminary report of the cooperative aneurysm study. Neurology 33: 981-988, 1983

9 Adams, R. D.: Diseases of Muscle: a Study in Pathology, 3rd ed. Harper & Row, New York 1975

10 Adams, R. D., M. Victor: Principles of Neurology, 3rd ed. McGraw-Hill, New York 1985

11 Adams, R. D., G. Lyon: Neurology of Hereditary Metabolic Diseases of Children. Hemisphere, Washington, D. C. 1982

12 Adour, K. K.: Current concepts in neurology: diagnosis and management of facial paralysis. New Engl. J. Med. 307: 348-351, 1982

13 Adour, K. K., J. Wingerd: Idiopathic facial paralysis (Bell's palsy): factors affecting severity and outcome in 446 patients. Neurology 24: 1112-1116, 1974

14 Adour, K. K. et al.: Prednisone treatment of idiopathic facial paralysis (Bell's palsy). New Engl. J. Med. 287: 1268-1272, 1972

15 Adour, K. K. et al.: The true nature of Bell's palsy: analysis of 1000 consecutive patients. Laryngoscope 88: 787-801, 1978

16 Afifi, A. K., Z. H. Rifai, K. B. Faris: Isolated, reversible, hypoglossal nerve palsy. Arch. Neurol. 41: 1218, 1984

17 Aggerbeck, L. P. et al.: Hypobetalipoproteinemia: clinical and biochemical description of a new kindred with Friedreich's ataxia. Neurology 24: 1051-1063, 1974

18 Aguayo, A. J. et al.: Peripheral nerve abnormalities in the Riley-Day syndrome: findings in a sural nerve biopsy. Arch. Neurol. 24: 106-116, 1971

19 Aho, K., K. Haapa: Facial atrophy during sotalol treatment. J. Neurol. Neurosurg. Psychiat. 45: 179, 1982

20 Aicardi, J., J. J. Chevrie: Atypical benign partial epilepsy of childhood. Develop. Med. Child Neurol. 24: 281-292, 1982

21 Aicher, F.: Die Phänomenologie des nach Klüver und Bucy benannten Syndroms beim Menschen. Fortschr. Neurol. Psychiat. 52: 375-397, 1984

22 Aita, J. A.: Neurocutaneous Diseases. Thomas, Springfield/Ill. 1966

23 Alberca, R., M. Romero, J. Chaparro: Jerking stiff-man syndrome. J. Neurol. Neurosurg. Psychiat. 45: 1159-1160, 1982

24 Al-Din, A. N., Anderson Milne, E. R. Bickerstaff: Brainstem encephalitis and the syndrome of Miller Fisher: a clinical study. Brain 105: 481-495, 1982

25 Alexander, G. E., T. T. Provost, M. B. Stevens, E. L. Alexander: Sjögren syndrome: central nervous system manifestations. Neurology 31: 1391-1396, 1981

26 Allen, C. M. C.: Predicting the outcome of acute stroke: a prognostic score. J. Neurol. Neurosurg. Psychiat. 47: 475-480, 1984

27 Alpert, J. N. et al.: Glossopharyngeal neuralgia, asystole and seizures. Arch. Neurol. 34: 233-235, 1977

28 Alter, M.: The digiti quinti sign of mild hemiparesis. Neurology 23: 503-505, 1973

29 Alvord, E. C. et al.: Subarachnoid hemorrhage due to ruptured aneurysms. Arch. Neurol. 27: 273-284, 1972

30 Ambrose, J. et al.: An assessment of the ac-

curacy of computerized transverse axial scanning (EMI-Scanner) in the diagnosis of intracranial tumour: a review of 366 patients. Brain 98: 569–582, 1975

31   Aminoff, M. J.: Acanthocytosis and neurological disease. Brain 95: 749–760, 1972

32   Aminoff, M. J.: Treatment of unruptured cerebral arteriovenous malformations. Neurology 37: 815–819, 1987

33   Anderson, D. C., S. Bundlie, G. L. Rockswold: Multimodality evoked potentials in closed head trauma. Arch. Neurol. 41: 369–374, 1984

34   Anderson, F. M.: Occult spinal dysraphism: a series of 73 cases. Pediatrics 55: 826–835, 1975

35   Anderson, F. H., J. R. Lehrich: Lhermitte sign following head injury. Arch. Neurol. 29: 437–438, 1973

36   Anderson, L. T. et al.: The effect of L-5-hydroxytryptophan on self-mutilation in Lesch-Nyhan disease: a negative report. Neuropädiatrie 7: 439–442, 1976

37   Annegers, J. F. et al.: Seizures after head trauma: a population study. Neurology 30: 683–689, 1980

38   Anon.: Cooperative study. Am. J. Neurosurg. 25, 321–368, 1966

39   Anon.: Encephalopathy and fatty infiltration of viscera in children [editorial]. Lancet ii: 473–474, 1969

40   Anon.: Diabetic neuropathy: a preventable complication [editorial]. Lancet ii, 583–584, 1972

41   Anon.: Le vertige de Menière [editorial]. Nouv. Presse Méd. 2: 857, 1973

42   Anon.: Carotid endarterectomy and TIAs [editorial]. Lancet i: 51–52, 1974

43   Anon.: Glycerol in acute cerebral infarction [editorial]. Lancet ii: 1246–1247, 1975

44   Anon.: Myasthenia gravis [editorial]. Lancet i: 1227–1228, 1975

45   Anon.: Extracranial-intracranial anastomosis [editorial]. Lancet i, 1384–1385, 1979

46   Anon.: Vascular troubles in the popliteal fossa [editorial]. Lancet i: 347–348, 1980

47   Anon.: Bingswanger's encephalopathy [editorial]. Lancet i: 923, 1981

48   Anon.: Proposal for revised seizure classification [editorial]. Epilepsia 22: 493–495, 1981

49   Anon.: Neuroleptic malignant syndrome [editorial]. Lancet i: 545–547, 1984

50   Anon.: Drugs for epilepsy. Med. Lett. Drugs Ther. 28: 1–4, 1989

51   Antony, J. H. et al.: Benign acute childhood myositis. Neurology 29: 1068–1071, 1979

52   Antony, J. H. et al.: Spasmus nutans – a mistaken identity. Arch. Neurol. 37: 373–375, 1980

53   Appenzeller, O.: The autonomic nervous system: an introduction to basic and clinical concepts. 3rd ed. Elsevier, Amsterdam 1982

54   Appenzeller, O., M. Kornfeld: Indifference to pain: a chronic peripheral neuropathy with mosaic Schwann cells. Arch. Neurol. 27: 322–339, 1972

55   Appenzeller, O., M. Kornfeld: Acute pandysautonomia. Arch. Neurol. 29: 335–339, 1973

56   Arieff, A. I., R. Guisado: Effects on the central nervous system of hypernatremic and hyponatremic states. Kidney Int. 10: 104–116, 1976

57   Asbury, A. K.: Proximal diabetic neuropathy. Ann. Neurol. 2: 179–180, 1977

58   Asbury, A. K. et al.: Oculomotor palsy in diabetes mellitus: a clinicopathological study. Brain 93: 555–566, 1970

59   Aschoff, J. C.: Reconsideration of the oculomotor pathway. In: Neurosciences, Third Study Program, ed. by F. O. Schmitt, F. G. Worden. MIT Press, Cambridge/Mass. 1974, pp. 305–310

60   Ashizawa, T., I. H. Butler, Y. Harati, S. Roongata: A dominantly inherited syndrome with continuous motor neuron discharges. Ann. Neurol. 13: 285–290, 1983

61   Ashworth, B., G. B. W. Tait: Trigeminal neuropathy in connective tissue disease. Neurology 21: 609–614, 1971

62   Askanas, V. et al.: Adult-onset acid maltase deficiency: morphologic and biochemical abnormalities reproduced in cultured muscle. New Engl. J. Med. 294: 573–578, 1976

63   Assal, G., E. Perentes, J.-P. Deruaz: Crossed aphasia in a right-handed patient: postmortem findings. Arch. Neurol. 38: 445–458, 1981

64   Asselman, P. et al.: Visual evoked responses in the diagnosis and management of patients suspected of multiple sclerosis. Brain 98: 261–282, 1975

65   Auberge, C., G. Ponsot, P. Gayraud et al.: Les hémiparalysies vélopalatines isolées et acquises chez l'enfant. Arch. Franç. Pédiat. 36: 283–286, 1979

66   Auger, R. G.: Hemifacial spasm: clinical and electrophysiologic observations. Neurology 29: 1261–1272, 1979

67   Auger, R. G., D. G. Piepgras, E. R. Laws et al.: Microvascular decompression of the facial nerve for hemifacial spasm: clinical and electrophysiologic observations. Neurology 31: 346–350, 1981

68   Aupy, M., J. M. Orgogozo, P. Loiseau et al.: Atteinte multiple des nerfs crâniens révélant une périartérite noueuse: relation avec le syndrome de Cogan. Rev. Neurol. 136: 59–65, 1980

69   Azorin, J. M., M. Bouchacourt, T. Lavergne, S. Giudicelli: Syndrome malin des neuroleptiques: efficacité de la bromocriptine. Presse Méd. 13: 1702, 1984

70   Azzarelli, B., U. Roessmann: Diffuse "anoxic" myelopathy. Neurology 27: 1049–1052, 1977

71   Babb, R. R., P. B. Eckman: Abdominal epilepsy. J. Amer. Med. Ass. 222: 65–66, 1972

72   Baier, W. K.: The "startle disease" in brain-

damaged patients: report of case. Neuropädiatrie 11: 72–75, 1980
73   Baier, W. K., U. Beck, H. Doose et al.: Cerebellar atrophy following diphenylhydantoin intoxication. Neuropediatrics 15: 76–81, 1984
74   Ballard, P. A., J. W. Tetrud, J. W. Langston: Permanent human parkinsonism due to 1-methyl-4-phenyl-1,2,3,6-tetra-hydropyridine (MPTP): seven cases. Neurology 35: 949–956, 1985
75   Baloh, R. W.: Dizziness, Hearing Loss and Tinnitus: the Essentials of Neurology. Davis, Philadelphia 1984
76   Bancaud, J., A. Bonis, S. Trottier et al.: L'épilepsie partielle continue: syndrome et maladie. Rev. Neurol. 138: 803–814, 1982
77   Banerji, N. K., L. J. Hurwitz: Neurological manifestations in adult steatorrhoea (probable gluten enteropathy). J. Neurol. Sci. 14: 125–141, 1971
78   Banerji, N. K., J. H. D. Millar: Paraplegia associated with cystinuria. J. Neurol. Sci. 12: 101–104, 1971
79   Bank, W. J., G. Morrow: A familial spinal cord disorder with hyperglycinemia. Arch. Neurol. 27: 136–144, 1972
80   Bannister, R.: Autonomic Failure: a Textbook of Clinical Disorders of the Autonomic Nervous System. Oxford University Press, Oxford 1983
81   Bannister, R.: Brain's Clinical Neurology, 6th ed. Oxford University Press, Oxford 1985
82   Barbeau, A.: Six years of high-level levodopa therapy in severely akinetic parkinsonian patients. Arch. Neurol. 33: 333–338, 1976
83   Barnes, B. E.: Dermatomyositis and malignancy: a review of the literature. Ann. Intern. Med. 84: 68–76, 1976
84   Barnett, H. J. M. et al.: Cerebral ischemic events associated with prolapsing mitral valve. Arch. Neurol. 33: 777–778, 1976
85   Barolin, G. S.: Kopfschmerz – Headache. Spatz, München 1977
86   Barraquer-Bordas, L. et al.: Neuropathie sensitive du trijumeau, pure, bilatérale, avec troubles trophiques oculaires: apport d'une observation et révision du problème. Rev. Neurol. 129: 222–226, 1973
87   Barrios, R. R. et al.: The study of ocular motility in the comatose patient. J. Neurol. Sci. 3: 183–206, 1966
88   Bartels, M., B. Riffel, M. Stöhr: Tardive Dystonie: Eine seltene Nebenwirkung nach Neuroleptika-Langzeitbehandlung. Nervenarzt 53: 674–676, 1982
89   Bartleson, J. D., J. W. Swanson, J. P. Whisnant: A migrainous syndrome with cerebrospinal fluid pleocytosis. Neurology 31: 1257–1262, 1981
90   Barua, A. R. et al.: Tetanus myopathy. Indian J. Med. Res. 64: 673–679, 1976
91   Barza, M., S. G. Pauker: The decision to biopsy, treat, or wait in suspected herpes encephalitis. Ann. Int. Med. 92: 641–649, 1980

92   Bastiaensen, L. A. K. et al.: Ocular myopathy: a case history with elektron microscopy, biochemistry and review of literature. Ophthalmologica 168: 325–347, 1974
93   Bauer, H.: Multiple Sklerose: Grundlagen und Hypothese der modernen Ursachenforschung. Z. Neurol. 198: 5–32, 1970
94   Baughman, F. A. et al.: Sex chromosome anomalies and essential tremor. Neurology 23: 623–625, 1973
95   Beard, R. W., S. Pearce, J. H. Highman, P. W. Reginald: Diagnosis of pelvic varicosities in women with chronic pelvic pain. Lancet ii: 946–949, 1984
96   Bebbington, E., C. Hopton, H. T. Lockett, R. J. Madeley: Epidemic syncope in jazz bands: logistic aspects of an investigation. Community Med. 2: 302–306, 1980
97   Becker, P. E.: Humangenetik, Vol. III/1. Thieme, Stuttgart 1964
98   Beer, G., R. B. Schwartz: Subakute Myelo-Optiko-Neuropathie (SMON) bei Thalliumintoxikation. Nervenarzt 53: 451–455, 1982
99   Behan, P. O., I. Bone: Hereditary chorea without dementia. J. Neurol. Neurosurg. Psychiat. 40: 687–691, 1977
100 Behse, F., F. Buchthal: Alcoholic neuropathy: clinical, electrophysiological and biopsy findings. Ann. Neurol. 2: 95–110, 1977
101 Bell, E. J., R. A. McCartney, M. H. Riding: Coxsackie B viruses and myalgic encephalomyelitis. J. Royal Soc. Med. 81: 329–331, 1988
102 Bell, J. A., H. J. F. Hodgson: Coma after cardiac arrest. Brain 97: 361–372, 1974
103 Bellur, S. N.: Opsoclonus: its clinical value. Neurology 25: 502–507, 1975
104 Bellur, S. N., V. Chandra, I. W. McDonald: Association of meningiomas with extraneural primary malignancy. Neurology 29: 1165–1168, 1979
105 Ben Amor, M. et al.: Hérédoataxie cérébelleuse de Pierre Marie. Nouv. Presse Méd. 1: 177–180, 1972
106 Bender, A. N. et al.: Myasthenia gravis: a serum factor blocking acetylcholine receptors of the human neuromuscular junction. Lancet i: 607–609, 1975
107 Benoist, M., A. Deburge, J. Busson: La chimionucléolyse dans le traitement des sciatiques par hernie discale. Presse Méd. 13: 733–736, 1984
108 Benos, J.: Die neuropsychiatrische Symptomatik des Heroinismus. Fortschr. Neurol. Psychiat. 47: 499–519, 1979
109 Bentson, J. et al.: Steroids and apparent cerebral atrophy on computed tomography scans. J. Comput. Ass. Tomograph. 2: 16–23, 1978
110 Berciano, J.: Olivopontocerebellar atrophy: a review of 117 cases. J. Neurol. Sci. 53: 253–272, 1982

111 Berenberg, R. A. et al.: Lumping or splitting? "Ophthalmoplegia-plus" or Kearns-Sayre syndrome? Ann. Neurol. 1: 37–54, 1977

112 Berger, G., W. Sprügel, W. Seyferth: Diagnostik extrakranieller Carotiserkrankungen. Dtsch. Med. Wschr. 108: 86–93, 1983

113 Berger, J. R., W. A. Sheremata, E. Melamed: Paroxysmal dystonia as the initial manifestation of multiple sclerosis. Arch. Neurol. 41: 747–750, 1984

114 Berguer, R., R. B. Bauer: Vertebrobasilar Arterial Occlusive Disease: Medical and Surgical Management. Raven Press, New York 1984

115 Beringer, U.: Das Carpaltunnelsyndrom. Analyse von 231 Fällen mit Hinweisen auf die operativen Behandlungsergebnisse. Schweiz. Med. Wschr. 102: 52–58, 1972

116 Berman, M., S. Feldmann, M. Alter et al.: Acute transverse myelitis: incidence and etiologic considerations. Neurology 31: 966–971, 1981

117 Bernat, J. L., R. W. Hunter: The benign lateral medullary syndrome. Arch. Neurol. 35: 112–113, 1978

118 Bernhardt, D., H. Schiller: Maligne Hyperthermie in Allgemeinanaesthesie. Abnorme histochemische und elektronoptische Muskelbefunde in Kombination mit pathologischen Serum-CPK-Werten als Beweis für das Vorliegen einer primären Myopathie. Anaesthesist 22: 367–372, 1973

119 Bernoulli, C., J. Siegfried, G. Baumgartner et al.: Danger of accidental person-to-person transmission of Creutzfeldt-Jakob disease by surgery. Lancet i: 478–479, 1977

120 Bernsmeier, A., A. Schrader, A. Struppler: Differentialdiagnose neurologischer Krankheitsbilder (Bodechtel), 4th ed. Thieme, Stuttgart 1984 (cf. 140)

121 Berry M. P., R. D. T. Jenkin, C. W. Keen et al.: Radiation treatment for medulloblastoma. J. Neurosurg. 55: 43–51, 1981

122 Berthier, M., S. Starkstein, R. Leiguarda: Asymbolia for pain: a sensory-limbic disconnection syndrome. Ann. Neurol. 24: 41–49, 1988

123 Besinger, U. A., K. V. Toyka, M. Hömberg et al.: Myasthenia gravis: Long-term correlation of binding and bungarotoxin blocking antibodies against acetylcholine receptors with changes in disease severity. Neurology 33: 1316–1321, 1983

124 Beth, H., H. Matiar-Vahar: Bulbäre Syndrome bei cervicalen Thorotrastomen. Nervenarzt 41: 226–232, 1970

125 Bethlem, J.: Myopathies. North-Holland, Amsterdam 1977

126 Beylot, J., B. Bioulac, C. Beylot et al.: Résultat favorable de la clomipramine dans un cas d'érithromélalgie rebelle: tentative d'approche physiopathol. Ann. Méd. 223–226, 1980

127 Bhandari, Y. S., B. S. Narendra Sakari: Subdural empyema: a review of 37 cases. J. Neurosurg. 32: 35–39, 1970

128 Biaggi, J., K. Küpfer, H. Stirnemann: Die Spiegeli'sche Hernie. Schweiz. Med. Wschr. 107: 119–121, 1977

129 Bicknell, J. M., J. V. Holland: Neurologic manifestations of Cogan syndrome. Neurology 28: 278–281, 1978

130 Bird, T. D., D. Lagunoff: Neurological manifestations of Fabry disease in female carriers. Ann. Neurol. 4: 537–540, 1978

131 Birdsong, J. H., A. S. McKinney: Long-range motor performance changes in levodopa-treated patients with Parkinson's disease. Neurology 24: 107–115, 1974

132 Bischoff, A.: Die alkoholische Polyneuropathie. Klinische, ultrastrukturelle und pathogenetische Aspekte. Dtsch. Med. Wschr. 96: 317–322, 1971

133 Blanquart, F., G. Houdent, P. Deshayes: L'ago-dystrophie iatrogène gardénalique. Sem. Hôp. Paris 50: 499–503, 1974

134 Blau, I., I. Casson, A. Liebermann, E. Weiss: The not-so-benign Miller Fisher syndrome - a variant of the Guillain-Barré syndrome. Arch. Neurol. 37: 384–385, 1980

135 Blessing, W., J. C. Walsh: Myotonia precipitated by propranolol therapy. Lancet i: 73–74, 1977

136 Bobath, B.: Abnorme Haltungsreflexe bei Gehirnschäden, 2nd ed. Thieme, Stuttgart 1976; 3rd ed. 1984

137 Bochkov, N. P., Y. M. Lopukhin, N. P. Kuleshov et al.: Chromosomenbrüchigkeit bei Ataxia teleangiectasia - erhöhte Neoplasieanfälligkeit. Humangenetik 24: 115–128, 1974

138 Bockman, J. M., D. T. Kingsbury, M. P. McKinley et al.: Creutzfeldt-Jakob disease prion proteins in human brains. New Engl. J. Med. 312: 73–78, 1985

139 Boddie, H. G. et al.: Benign intracranial hypertension: a survey of the clinical and radiological features, and long-term prognosis. Brain 97: 313–326, 1974

140 Bodechtel, G.: Differentialdiagnose neurologischer Krankheitsbilder, 3rd ed. Thieme, Stuttgart 1974; 4th ed. 1984 (cf. 120)

141 Boghen, D., J.-M. Peyronnard: Myoclonus in familial restless legs syndrome. Arch. Neurol. 33: 368–370, 1976

142 Bogousslavsky, J., F. Regli, P. A. Despland: Anévrysmes disséquants spontanés de l'artère carotide interne: évaluation prospective du pronostic et de la reperméabilisation artérielle dans 14 cas. Rev. Neurol. 140: 625–636, 1984

143 Bogousslavsky, J., P.-A. Despand, F. Regli: Spontaneous carotid dissection with acute stroke. Arch. Neurol. 44: 137–140, 1987

144 Bogousslavsky, J., P. C. Gates, A. J. Fox, H. J. M. Barnett: Bilateral occlusion of vertebral artery: clinical patterns and long-term prognosis. Neurology 36: 1309–1315, 1986

145 Bogousslavsky, J., J. Miklossy, J. P. Deruaz

et al.: Unilateral left paramedian infarction of thalamus and midbrain: a clinico-pathological study. J. Neurol. Neurosurg. Psychiat. 49: 686–694, 1986

146 Bohan, A., J. B. Peter: Polymyositis and dermatomyositis. New Engl. J. Med. 292: 344–347, 403–407, 1975

147 Boller, F. et al.: Optic ataxia: clinical-radiological correlations with the EMI-scan. J. Neurol. Neurosurg. Psychiat. 38: 954–958, 1975

148 Bollinger, A., P. Butti: Primäres und sekundäres Raynaud-Syndrom. Schweiz. Med. Wschr. 106: 415–421, 1976

149 Bollinger, A., H.-J. Leu, U. Brunner: Juvenile temporal arteritis with hypereosinophilia. Klin. Wschr. 64, 526–529, 1986

150 Bolton, C. F. et al.: Ischaemic neuropathy in uraemic patients caused by bovine arteriovenous shunt. J. Neurol. Neurosurg. Psychiat. 42: 810–814, 1979

151 Bonduelle, M. et al.: Etude clinique et évolutive de cent vingt cinq cas de sclérose latérale amyotrophique: limites nosographiques et associations morbides. Presse Méd. 78: 827–832, 1970

152 Bonduelle, M., P. Bouygues, C. F. Degos et al.: Les formes bénignes de la sclérose en plaques. Rev. Neurol. 135: 593–604, 1979

153 Boothby, J. A. et al.: Reversible forms of motor neuron disease: lead neuritis. Arch. Neurol. 31: 18–23, 1974

154 Bosch, E. P. et al.: Ocular bobbing: the myth of its localizing value. Neurology 25: 949–953, 1975

155 Botterell, E. H. et al.: Hypothermia, and interruption of carotid, or carotid and vertebral circulation, in the surgical management of intracranial aneurysms. J. Neurosurg. 13: 1–42, 1956

156 Bousser, M. G., E. Eschwege, M. Haguenau et al.: Essai coopératif contrôle "A. I. C. L. A.". Prévention secondaire des accidents ischémiques cérébraux liés à athérosclérose par l'aspirine et le dipyridamole. Rev. Neurol. 139: 335–348, 1983

157 Bove, K. E., P. K. Hilton, J. Partin, M. K. Farrel: Morphology of acute myopathy associated with influenza B infection. Pediat. Pathol. 1: 51–66, 1983

158 Boyle, R. S., R. A. Shakir, A. I. Weir et al.: Inverted knee jerk: a neglected localising sign in spinal cord disease. J. Neurol. Neurosurg. Psychiat. 42: 1005–1007, 1979

159 Bradley, W. G.: Proximal chronic inflammatory polyneuropathy with multifunctional conduction block. Arch. Neurol. 45: 451–455, 1988

160 Bradley, W. G., F. Krasin: A new hypothesis of the etiology of amyotrophic lateral sclerosis: the DNA hypothesis. Arch. Neurol. 39: 677–680, 1982

161 Bradley, W. G. et al.: The syndrome of myosclerosis. J. Neurol. Neurosurg. Psychiat. 36: 651–660, 1973

162 Brainin, M., M. Omasits, A. Seiser: Angiome des Hirnstammes mit jahrelangem klinischen Verlauf. Nervenarzt 55: 659–664, 1984

163 Brandt, S. et al.: Encephalopathia myoclonica infantilis (Kinsbourne) and neuroblastoma in children: a report of three cases. Develop. Med. Child Neurol. 16: 286–294, 1974

164 Bray, P. F., J. F. Bale, R. E. Anderson, E. R. Kern: Progressive neurological disease associated with chronic cytomegalovirus infection. Ann. Neurol. 9: 499–502, 1981

165 Bregman, H., M. C. Gelfand, J. F. Winchester et al.: Iron-overload-associated myopathy in patients on maintenance haemodialysis: a histocompatibility-linked disorder. Lancet ii: 876–879, 1980

166 Brennan, R. W., R. M. Bergland: Acute cerebellar hemorrhage: analysis of clinical findings and outcome in 12 cases. Neurology 27: 527–532, 1977

167 Brenneis, M., G. Harrer, H. Selzer: Zur Temperaturempfindlichkeit von Multiple Sklerose-Kranken. Fortschr. Neurol. Psychiat. 47: 320–325, 1979

168 Breuninger, H.: Behandlung des Morbus-Menière. Dtsch. Med. Wschr. 96: 1506–1507, 1971

169 Brewer, E. J., E. H. Giannini, B. D. Rossen et al.: Plasma exchange therapy of a childhood onset dermatomyositis patient. Arthr. and Rheum. 23: 509–513, 1980

170 Brewer, N. S. et al.: Brain abscess: a review of recent experience. Ann. Intern. Med. 82: 571–576, 1975

171 Brin, F., R. E. Gregg, T. A. Pedley et al.: Vitamin E deficiency and neurologic disease: clinical and electrophysiologic evaluation in 24 patients. J. Neurol. 232 (suppl.) 180, 1985

172 Brinkmann, K., H. Schaefer: Der Elektrounfall. Springer, Berlin 1982

173 Brodaty, D., O. Bical, J. Bachet et al.: Les paralysies phréniques induites par le froid en chirurgie cardiaque. Nouv. Presse Méd. 10: 3137–3140, 1981

174 Brody, J. A., R. Detels: Subacute sclerosing panencephalitis: a zoonosis following aberrant measles. Lancet ii: 500–501, 1970

175 Bronisch, F. W.: Multiple Sklerose. 5 Fortbildungsvorträge, 3rd ed. Enke, Stuttgart 1975

176 Bronisch, F. W.: Die Reflexe und ihre Untersuchung in Klinik und Praxis, 5th ed. 1979

177 Broser, F.: Topische und klinische Diagnostik neurologischer Krankheiten. Urban und Schwarzenberg, München 1975

178 Broser, F. et al.: Chlorierte Acetylene als Ursache einer irreparablen Trigeminusstörung bei zwei Patienten. Dtsch. Z. Nervenheilk. 197: 163–170, 1970

179 Brown, E. L., E. G. Knox: Epidemiological

approach to Parkinson's disease. Lancet i: 974–976, 1972

180 Brown, K. W., E. Glen Sarah, T. White: Low serum iron status and akathisia. Lancet i: 1234–1236, 1987

181 Brown, M., A. K. Asbury: Diabetic neuropathy. Ann. Neurol. 15: 2–12, 1984

182 Brown, R. D., O. Wiebers, G. Forbes et al.: The natural history of unruptured intracranial arteriovenous malformations. J. Neurosurg. 68, 352–357, 1988

183 Brudny, J. et al.: Sensory feedback therapy as a modality of treatment in central nervous system disorders of voluntary movement. Neurology 24: 925–932, 1974

184 Brügger, A.: Die Erkrankungen des Bewegungsapparates und seines Nervensystems. Grundlagen und Differentialdiagnose. Ein interdisziplinäres Handbuch für die Praxis. Fischer, Stuttgart 1977

185 Bruguier, A., P. Texier, W. Sluzewski et al.: Les calcinoses des dermatomyositis infantiles: à propos de 10 cas. Helv. Paediat. Acta 39: 47–54, 1984

186 Brunner, G., G. Schnaberth: Epileptische Manifestationen bei Inselzelladenom. Nervenarzt 51: 630–632, 1980

187 Brunner, N. G. et al.: Corticosteroids in management of severe, generalized myasthenia gravis: effectiveness and comparison with corticotropin therapy. Neurology 22: 603–610, 1972

188 Brust, J. C. M.: Transient ischemic attacks: natural history and anticoagulation. Neurology 27: 701–707, 1977

189 Bruyn, G. W., P. J. Vinken: Handbook of Clinical Neurology. North-Holland, Amsterdam 1969 1982

190 Buchler, P., F. G. Kubina: Spontane (essentielle) Aliquorrhoe. Nervenarzt 52: 361–363, 1981

191 Buchs, S., P. Pfister: Die Letalität und die Gefährlichkeit von 14 eitrigen Meningitisarten in der Vor-Ampicillin- und in der Ampicillin-Aera. Schweiz. Med. Wschr. 114: 136–140, 1984

192 Buchtahl, F., F. Behse: Peroneal muscular atrophy (PMA) and related disorders. 1: clinical manifestations as related to biopsy findings, nerve conduction and electromyography. Brain 100: 41–66, 1977

193 Buck-Gramcko, D.: Ischämische Kontrakturen an Unterarm und Hand. Handchirurgie 6: 141–158, 1974

194 Bucknall, R. C. et al.: Myasthenia gravis associated with penicillamine treatment for rheumatoid arthritis. Brit. Med. J. i: 600–602, 1975

195 Budka, H. et al.: Adult adrenoleukodystrophy: spastic paraplegia associated with Addison's disease: adult variant of adreno-leukodystrophy. J. Neurol. 213: 237–250, 1976

196 Buge, A. et al.: Encéphalopathies myocloniques par les sels de bismuth: six cas observés

lors de traitements oraux au long cours. Nouv. Presse Méd. 3: 2315–2320, 1974

197 Bühlmann, A. A.: Dekompressionskrankheit des Rückenmarks. Resultate der Früh- und Spätbehandlung. Schweiz. Med. Wschr. 115, 796–800, 1985

198 Bulens, C. et al.: Benign intracranial hypertension. J. Neurol. Sci. 40: 147–157, 1979

199 Burke, D. et al.: The action of a GABA derivative in human spasticity. J. Neurol. Sci. 14: 199–208, 1971

200 Burns, R. et al.: Reversible encephalopathy possibly associated with bismuth subgallate ingestion. Brit. Med. J. i: 220–223, 1974

201 Busis, S. N.: Vertigo in children. Pediat. Ann. 5: 15–22, 1976

202 Busse, O., D. Stolke, B. U. Seidel: Die postoperative Discitis intervertebralis lumbalis. Nervenarzt 47: 604–608, 1976

203 Busse, O., T. Grumme, A. L. Agnoli: Abszeßbildung nach zerebraler Massenblutung und ischämischem Infarkt. Akt. Neurol. 8: 69–72, 1981

204 Caflisch, U., O. Tönz, U. B. Schaad et al.: Die Zecken-Meningoradikulitis – eine Spirochätose. Schweiz. Med. Wschr. 114: 630–634, 1984

205 Calne, D. B.: Parkinsonism: Physiology, Pharmacology and Treatment. Arnold, London 1970

206 Calne, D. B.: Therapeutics in Neurology. Blackwell, Oxford 1975

207 Calne, D. B. et al.: Treatment of parkinsonism with bromocriptine. Lancet ii: 1355–1356, 1974

208 Cambier, J., M. Masson, P. Delaporte: Le syndrome de contracture abdomino-crurale au cours de la maladie d'Addison. Presse Méd. 78: 2281–2282, 1970

209 Cameron, M. M.: Chronic subdural haematoma: a review of 114 cases. J. Neurol. Neurosurg. Psychiat. 41: 834–839, 1978

210 Campbell, J. N., D. M. Long: Peripheral nerve stimulation in the treatment of intractable pain. J. Neurosurg. 45: 692–699, 1976

211 The Canadian Cooperative Study Group: A randomized trial of aspirin and sulfinpyrazone in threatened stroke. New Engl. J. Med. 299: 53–59, 1978

212 Caplan, L. R., C. Schoene: Clinical features of subcortical arteriosclerotic encephalopathy (Binswanger disease). Neurology 28: 1206–1215, 1978

213 Capute, A. J. et al.: Primitive Reflex Profile. Monographs in Developmental Pediatrics, vol. I. University Park Press, Baltimore 1978

214 Carlier, G., M. Reznik, G. Franck et al.: Etude anatomo-clinique d'une forme infantile de la maladie de Huntington. Acta Neurol. Belg. 74: 36–63, 1974

215 Carpenter, S. et al.: The ultrastructural characteristics of the abnormal cytosomes in Batten-Kufs' disease. Brain 100: 137–156, 1977

216 Cartlidge, N. E. F. et al.: Carotid and vertebral-basilar transient cerebral ischemic attacks: a community study. Mayo Clin. Proc. 52: 117–120, 1977

217 Casaer, P., M. Azou: Flunarizine in alternating hemiplegia in childhood. Lancet ii: 579, 1984

218 Cassel, G. H., B. C. Cole: Mycoplasmas as agents of human disease. New Engl. J. Med. 304: 80–89, 1981

219 Castaigne, P. et al.: La maladie de Marchiafava-Bignami: étude anatomoclinique de dix observations. Rev. Neurol. 125: 179–196, 1971

220 Castaigne, P. et al.: Atrophie optique posthémorragique. Presse Méd. 5: 1631–1633, 1976

221 Castaigne, P., P. Brunet, J. J. Hauw, J. M. Léger: Système nerveux periphérique et panartérite noueuse: revue de 27 cas. Rev. Neurol. 140: 343–352, 1984

222 Castaigne, P., R. Escourolle, F. Chain et al.: Sclérose concentrique de Balo. Rev. Neurol. 140: 479–487, 1984

223 Cavanagh, N. P. C., A. Eames, R. J. Galvin et al.: Hereditary sensory neuropathy with spastic paraplegia. Brain 102: 79–94, 1979

224 Caveness, W. F. et al.: The nature of posttraumatic epilepsy. J. Neurosurg. 50: 545–553, 1979

225 Celesia, G. G., R. F. Daly: Visual electroencephalographic computer analysis (VECA): a new electrophysiologic test for the diagnosis of optic nerve lesions. Neurology 27: 637–641, 1977

226 Chapoy, P., C. Angelini, S. Cederbaum: Déficit systémique en carnitine: place dans le syndrome de Reye. Nouv. Presse Méd. 10: 499–502, 1981

227 Charron, L. et al.: Sensory neuropathy associated with primary biliary cirrhosis. Arch. Neurol. 37: 84–87, 1980

228 Chatrian, G. E. et al.: Congenital insensitivity at noxious stimuli. Arch. Neurol. 32: 141–145, 1975

229 Chaves-Carballo, E. et al.: Encephalopathy and fatty infiltration of the viscera (Reye-Johnson syndrome): A 17-year experience. Mayo Clin. Proc. 50: 209–215, 1975

230 Chemnitz, G.: Erhöhte Kreatinkinase-Aktivität. Dtsch. Med. Wschr. 109: 1172–1173, 1984

231 Cherington, M.: Botulism: 10-year experience. Arch. Neurol. (Chic.) 30: 432–437, 1974

232 Cherington, M., S. Ginsburg: Wound botulism. Arch. Surg. 110: 436–438, 1975

233 Cheson, B. D., A. Z. Bluming, J. Alroy: Cogan's syndrome: a systemic vasculitis. Amer. J. Med. 60: 549–555, 1976

234 Chester, E. M. et al.: Hypertensive encephalopathy: a clinicopathologic study of 20 cases. Neurology 28: 928–939, 1978

235 Chiappa, K. H., C. Yiannikas: Evoked potentials in clinical medicine. Raven Press, New York 1983

236 Ch'ien, L. T., R. M. Boehm, H. Robinson et al.: Characteristic early electroencephalographic changes in herpes simplex encephalitis: clinical and virologic studies. Arch. Neurol. 34: 361–364, 1977

237 Chokroverty, S., F. A. Rubino: "Pure" motor hemiplegia. J. Neurol. Neurosurg. Psychiat. 38: 896–899, 1975

238 Chokroverty, S. et al.: Pure motor hemiplegia due to pyramidal infarction. Arch. Neurol. 32: 647–648, 1975

239 Chokroverty, S. et al.: The syndrome of diabetic amyotrophy. Ann. Neurol. 2: 181–194, 1977

240 Christie, R., C. Bay, I. A. Kaufman: Lesch-Nyhan disease: clinical experience with 19 patients. Develop. Med. Child Neurol. 24: 293–306, 1982

241 Churcher, M. D.: Algodystrophy after aortic bifurcation surgery. Lancet ii: 131–133, 1984

242 Chusid, J. G.: Correlative Neuroanatomy and Functional Neurology, 18th ed. Lange, Los Altos, California 1982

243 Clair, F., S. Caillat, J. C. Soufir et al.: Syndrome myasthénique induit par la D,L-carnitins chez un hémodialysé chronique. Presse Méd. 13: 1154–1155, 1984

244 Clarke, C. R. A., M. J. G. Harrison: Neurological manifestations of Paget's disease. J. Neurol. Sci. 38: 171–178, 1978

245 Coers, C., N. Telerman-Toppet, J. Durdu: Neurogenic benign fasciculations, pseudomyotonia and pseudotetany. Arch. Neurol. 38: 282–287, 1981

246 Cohn, D. F., M. Streifler, E. Schujman: Das motorische Neuron im chronischen Lathyrismus. Nervenarzt 48: 127–129, 1977

247 Cohn, D. F., E. Avrahami: Intraventricular haemorrhage, CT and arteriographic findings in thirty-five patients. J. Neurol. 230: 137–140, 1983

248 Cole, M. et al.: Experimental ammonia encephalopathy in the primate. Arch. Neurol. 26: 130–136, 1972

249 Collins, R. C. et al.: Neurologic manifestations of intravascular coagulation in patients with cancer: a clinicopathologic analysis of 12 cases. Neurology 25: 795–806, 1975

250 Compston, D. A. S. et al.: Factors influencing the risk of multiple slerosis developing in patients with optic neuritis. Brain 101: 495–511, 1978

251 Confavreux, C.: Sclérose en plaques: conceptions étiopathogéniques actuelles. Presse Méd. 13: 1889–1894, 1984

252 Cook, S. D., P. C. Dowling: The role of autoantibody and immune complexes in the pathogenesis of Guillain-Barré syndrome. Ann. Neurol. 9 (Suppl.): 70–79, 1981

253 Cooper, P. R.: Head Injury. Williams and Wilkins, Baltimore 1982

254 Corbett, J. J., P. J. Savino, H. S. Thompson et al.: Visual loss in pseudotumor cerebri: follow-up of 57 patients from five to 41 years and a profile of 14 patients with permanent severe visual loss. Arch. Neurol. 39: 461–474, 1982

255 Couch, J. R., S. A. Weiss: Gliomatosis cerebri: report of four cases and review of the literature. Neurology 24: 504–511, 1974

256 Cos-Klazinga, M., L. J. Endtz: Peripheral nerve involvement in pernicious anaemia. J. Neurol. Sci. 45: 367–371, 1980

257 Crawford, P. M., C. R. Wet, D. W. Chadwick et al.: Arteriovenous malformations of the brain: natural history in unoperated patients. J. Neurol. Neurosurg. Psychiat. 49: 1–10, 1986

258 Crews, J. et al.: Muscle pathology of myotonia congenita. J. Neurol. Sci. 28: 449–457, 1976

259 Critchley, E.: Clinical manifestations of essential tremor. J. Neurol. Neurosurg. Psychiat. 35: 365–372, 1972

260 Crockard, H. A. et al.: Hydrocephalus as a cause of dementia: evaluation by computerised tomography and intracranial pressure monitoring. J. Neurol. Neurosurg. Psychiat. 40: 736–740, 1977

261 Crocker, J. F. S. et al.: Insecticide and viral interaction as a cause of fatty visceral changes and encephalopathy in the mouse. Lancet ii: 22–24, 1974

262 Cruz Martinez, A., M. C. Perez Conde, M. T. Ferrer et al.: Neuromuscular disorders in a new toxic syndrome: electrophysiological study: a preliminary report. Muscle Nerve 7: 12–22, 1984

263 Cummings, J. L., J. W. Gittinger: Central dazzle: a thalamic syndrome? Arch. Neurol. 38: 372–374, 1981

264 Currie, S., J. N. Walton: Immunosuppressive therapy in polymyositis. J. Neurol. Neurosurg. Psychiat. 34: 447–452, 1971

265 Dalakas, M. C., W. K. Engel: Polyneuropathy with monoclonal gammopathy: studies of 11 patients. Ann. Neurol. 1: 45–52, 1981

266 Dalakas, M. C., W. K. Engel: Chronic relapsing (dysimmune) polyneuropathy: pathogenesis and treatment. Ann. Neurol. 9 (Suppl.): 134–143, 1981

267 Dalakas, M. C., H. Teräväinen, W. K. Engel: Tremor as a feature of chronic relapsing and dysgammaglobulinemic polyneuropathies: incidence and management. Arch. Neurol. 41: 711–714, 1984

268 Dalakas, M. C., G. Elder, M. Hallet et al.: A long-term follow-up study of patients with postpoliomyelitis neuromuscular symptoms. New Engl. J. Med. 314: 959–963, 1986

269 Danilowicz, D., M. Tutkowski, D. Myung, D. Schively: Echocardiography in Duchenne dystrophy. Muscle Nerve 3: 298–303, 1980

270 Danks, D. M. et al.: Menke's kinky hair syndrome: an inherited defect in copper absorption with widespread effects. Pediatrics 50: 188–201, 1972

271 DaSilva, J. A. G., C. E. G. DaSilva: Postoperative Komplikationen bei 126 Fällen basilärer Impressionen und Arnold-Chiarischer Mißbildung. Neurochirurgia 24: 153–157, 1981

272 Dastur, D. K., D. K. Manghani, B. O. Osuntokun et al.: Neuromuscular and related changes in malnutrition. J. Neurol. Sci. 55: 207–230, 1982

273 Daun, H., G. Hartwich: Die Vincristin-Polyneuritis. Fortschr. Neurol. Psychiat. 39: 151–165, 1971

274 David, D. J., D. E. Poswillo, D. Simpson: The Craniosynostoses. Springer, Berlin 1982

275 Davis, C. H., V. M. Joglekar: Cerebellar astrocytomas in children and young adults. J. Neurol. Neurosurg. Psychiat. 44: 820–828, 1981

276 Davis, L. E., D. B. Drachman: Myeloma neuropathy. Arch. Neurol. 27: 507–511, 1972

277 Davis, L. E., J. C. Standefer, M. Kornfeld: Acute thallium poisoning: toxicological and morphological studies of the nervous system. Ann. Neurol. 1: 38–44, 1981

278 Davis, P. H., C. Bergeron, D. R. McLachlan: Atypical presentation of progressive supranuclear palsy. Ann. Neurol. 17: 337–343, 1985

279 Dawson, D. M., M. Hallett, L. H. Millender: Entrapment Neuropathies. Little, Brown and Company, Boston 1983

280 de Anquin, C. E.: Spina bifida occulta with engagement of the fifth lumbar spinous process: a cause of low back pain and sciatica. J. Bone Jt. Surg. 41 B: 486–490, 1959

281 De Bono, D. P., C. P. Warlow: Potential sources of emboli in patients with presumed transient cerebral or retinal ischaemia. Lancet i: 343–345, 1981

282 De Bray, J. M., J. Emile, M. Basle et al.: Chorée fibrillaire de Morvan. Rev. Neurol. 135: 827–833, 1979

283 Debrunner, A. M.: Orthopädie. Die Störungen des Bewegungsapparates in Klinik und Praxis. Huber, Bern 1983

284 De Jong, R. N.: The Neurologic Examination, 3rd ed. Hoeber Medical Division, London 1967

285 Delaney, P.: Gouty neuropathy. Arch. Neurol. 40: 823–824, 1983

286 Dement, W. C., M. Carskadon, R. Ley: The prevalence of narcolepsy II. Sleep Res. 2: 147, 1973

287 Derome, P. J., A. Visot: La dysplasie fibreuse crânienne (fibrous dysplasia of the skull). Neuro-chirurgie 29, Suppl. 1, 1983

288 Deruty, R. et al.: Tentatives de revascularisation cérébrale par anastomose extra-intracranienne dans certaines ischémies. Neuro-chirurgie 20: 345–368, 1974

289 Desai, B. T., J. R. Porter, J. K. Penry: Psychogenic seizures: a study of 42 attacks in 6 patients, with intensive monitoring. Arch. Neurol. 39: 202–209, 1982

290   De Smet, Y., M. Ruberg, M. Serdarn et al.: Confusion dementia and anticholinergics in Parkinson's disease. J. Neurol. Neurosurg. Psychiat. 45: 1161–1164, 1982

291   Detels, R., V. A. Clark, N. Valdiviezo et al.: Factors associated with a rapid course of multiple sclerosis. Arch. Neurol. 39: 337–341, 1982

292   Devoize, J. D., F. Rigal, A. Eschalier, A. d'Ambrosio: Aspects cliniques et pharmacologiques de l'effet antalgique des antidépresseurs tricycliques. Presse Méd. 13: 2806–2809, 1984

293   Devoize, J. L., J. Rouanet, P. Cellerier et al.: Paralysie bénigne des quatre derniers nerfs crâniens. Presse Méd. 14: 1328–1330, 1985

294   DeWitt, L. D., F. S. Buonanno, J. P. Kistler et al.: Central pontine myelinolysis: demonstration by nuclear magnetic resonance. Neurology 34: 570–576, 1984

295   Diaz Espejo, C. E., F. V. Chaves, B. S. Ramis: Chronic intracranial hypertension secondary to neurobrucellosis. J. Neurol. 234, 59–61, 1987

296   DiDonato, St., D. Pelucchetti, M. Rimoldi et al.: Systemic carnitine deficiency: clinical, biochemical and morphological cure with L-carnitine. Neurology 34: 157–162, 1984

297   Di Lorenzo, N., A. Fortuna, B. Guidetti: Craniovertebral junction malformations. J. Neursurg. 57: 603–608, 1982

298   Diethelm, U., M. Cadalbert, A. Huggler: Zur transitorischen Algodystrophie der Hüfte. Schweiz. Med. Wschr. 110: 1159–1163, 1980

299   Digre, K. B., M. W. Varner, J. J. Corbett: Pseudotumor cerebri and pregnancy. Neurology 34: 721–729, 1984

300   Dix, M. R. et al.: Progressive supranuclear palsy (the Steele-Richardson-Olszewski syndrome). A report of 9 cases with particular reference to the mechanism of the oculomotor disorder. J. Neurol. Sci. 13: 237–256, 1971

301   Dobyns, W. B., N. P. Goldstein, H. Gordon: Clinical spectrum of Wilson's disease (Hepatolenticular degeneration). Mayo Clin. Proc. 54: 35–42, 1979

302   Donaldson, I. M., J. Cuningham: Persisting neurologic sequelae of lithium carbonate therapy. Arch. Neurol. 40: 747–751, 1983

303   Donaldson, I. M., E. A. Espiner: Disseminated lupus erythematosus presenting as chorea gravidarum. Arch. Neurol. (Chic.) 25: 240–244, 1971

304   Donat, J. R., R. Auger: Familial periodic ataxia. Arch. Neurol. (Chic.) 36: 568–569, 1979

305   Donnan, G. A., F. W. Sharbrough, J. P. Whisnant: Carotid occlusive disease: effect of bright light on visual evoked response. Arch. Neurol. 39: 687–689, 1982

306   Doose, H., E. Völzke: Petit mal status in early childhood and dementia. Neuropädiatrie 10: 10–14, 1979

307   Dorndorf, W.: Schlaganfälle (Klinik und Therapie), 2nd ed. Thieme, Stuttgart 1983

308   Dowling, P. C., S. D. Cook: Role of infection in Guillain-Barré Syndrome: laboratory confirmation of herpes virus in 41 cases. Ann. Neurol. 9 (Suppl.): 44–55, 1981

309   Dowling, P. et al.: Cytomegalovirus complement fixation antibody in Guillain-Barré syndrome. Neurology 27: 1153–1156, 1977

310   Doyle, F. H., J. M. Pennock, J. S. Orr et al.: Imaging of the brain by nuclear magnetic resonance. Lancet ii: 53–57, 1981

311   Doyle, P. W., G. Gibson, C. L. Dolman: Herpes zoster ophthalmicus with contralateral hemiplegia: identification of cause. Ann. Neurol. 14: 84–85, 1983

312   Drachman, D. B. et al.: Prednisone in Duchenne muscular dystrophy. Lancet ii: 1409–1412, 1974

313   Drachman, D. B. et al.: Experimental arthrogryposis caused by viral myopathy. Arch. Neurol. 33: 362–367, 1976

314   Dravet, C., B. B. Dalla, E. Mesdjian et al.: Dyskinésies paroxystiques au cours de traitements par la diphenylhydantoine. Rev. Neurol. 136: 1–14, 1980

315   Drury, I., J. P. Whisnant, W. M. Garraway: Primary intracerebral hemorrhage: impact of CT on incidence. Neurology 34: 653–657, 1984

316   Dumermuth, G.: Elektroencephalographie im Kindesalter. Einführung und Atlas, 3rd ed. Thieme, Stuttgart 1976

317   Dvorak, J., F. von Orelli: Wie häufig sind Komplikationen nach Manipulationen der Halswirbelsäule? Praxis 71: 64–69, 1982

318   Dyck, P. J. et al.: Histologic and lipid studies of sural nerves in inherited hypertrophic neuropathy: preliminary report of a lipid abnormality in nerve and liver in Déjerine-Sottas disease. Mayo Clin. Proc. 45: 286–327, 1970

319   Dyck, P. J. et al.: Chronic inflammatory polyradiculoneuropathy. Mayo Clin. Proc. 50: 621–637, 1975

320   Dyck, P. J., P. C. O'Brien, K. F. Oviatt et al.: Prednisone improves chronic inflammatory demyelinating polyradiculoneuropathy more than no treatment. Ann. Neurol. 11: 136–141, 1982

321   Dyck, P. J., P. A. Low, J. C. Stevens: Burning feet as the only manifestation of dominantly inherited sensory neuropathy. Mayo Clin. Proc. 58: 426–429, 1983

322   Dyck, P. J., P. K. Thomas, E. H. Lambert, R. Bunge: Peripheral Neuropathy, vol. II, 2nd ed. Saunders, Philadelphia 1984

323   Dyken, P., O. Kolar: Dancing eyes, dancing feet: infantile polymyocoinia. Brain 91: 305–320, 1968

324   Dyken, P. P., A. Swift, R. H. DuRant: Long-term follow-up of patients with subacute sclerosing panencephalitis treated with Inosiplex. Ann. Neurol. 11: 359–365, 1982

325   Eames, R. A., L. S. Lange: Clinical and pathological study of ischaemic neuropathy. J. Neurol. Neurosurg. Psychiat. 30: 215–266, 1967

326 Earnest, M. P.: Neurologic Emergencies. Churchill Livingstone, Edinburgh 1983

327 Easton, J. D., D. G. Sherman: Somatic anxiety attacks and propranolol. Arch. Neurol. 33: 689–691, 1976

328 Ebeling, U., H. J. Reulen: Der laterale lumbale Bandscheibenvorfall. Nervenarzt 54: 521–524, 1983

329 Ebstein, R. P. et al.: A familial study in serum dopamine-beta-hydroxylase levels in torsion dystonia. Neurology 24: 684–687, 1974

330 EC/IC Bypass Study Group: Failure of extracranial-intracranial arterial bypass to reduce the risk of ischemic stroke. New Engl. J. Med. 313: 1191–1223, 1985

331 Edwards, P. D. et al.: Chorea, polycythaemia and cyanotic heart disease. J. Neurol. Neurosurg. Psychiat. 39: 729–739, 1975

332 Eggers, C., J. Hamer: Hydrosyringomyelia in childhood: clinical aspects, pathogenesis and therapy. Neuropädiatrie 10: 87–99, 1979

333 Eisenstein, S.: Injection for disc prolapse – whatever happened to chymopapain? S. Afr. Med. J. 66: 201–203, 1984

334 Ell, J. J., D. Uttley, J. R. Silver: Acute myelopathy in association with heroin addiction. J. Neurol. Neurosurg. Psychiat. 44: 448–450, 1981

335 Ell, J., D. Prasher, P. Rudge: Neuro-otological abnormalities in Friedreich's ataxia. J. Neurol. Neurosurg. Psychiat. 47: 26–32, 1984

336 Elsberg, Ch. A., F. Kennedy: A peculiar and undescribed disease of the roots of the cauda equina. J. Nerv. Ment. Dis. 40: 787, 1913

337 Engel, A. G.: Myasthenia gravis and myasthenic syndromes. Ann. Neurol. 16: 519–534, 1984

338 Engel, A. G., R. G. Siekert: Lipid storage myopathy responsive to prednisone. Arch. Neurol. (Chic.) 27: 174–181, 1972

339 Engel, A. G. et al.: Carnitine deficiency: clinical, morphological, and biochemical observations in a fatal case. J. Neurol. Neurosurg. Psychiat. 40: 313–322, 1977

340 Engel, W. K. et al.: Myasthenia gravis. Ann. Intern. Med. 81: 225–246, 1974

341 Engel, W. K., P. van den Bergh, V. Askanas: Subcutaneous thyrotropin-releasing hormone seems ready for wider trials in treating lower motor neuron-produced weakness and spasticity. Ann. Neurol. 16: 109–110, 1984

342 Espir, M. L. E., P. Millac: Treatment of paroxysmal disorders in multiple sclerosis with carbamazepine (Tegretol). J. Neurol. Neurosurg. Psychiat. 33: 528–531, 1970

343 Esses, S. I., W. J. Peters: Electrical burns: pathophysiology and complications. Canad. J. Surg. 24: 11–14, 1981

344 Esslen, E., U. Fisch: Zur Lokalisation der Nervenschädigung bei der idiopathischen Fazialisparese und zur Frage der Dekompression. Schweiz. Med. Wschr. 101: 386–387, 1971

345 Evans, D. E. et al.: Cardiac arrhythmias resulting from experimental head injury. J. Neurosurg. 45: 609–616, 1976

346 Evarts, E. V., H. T. Teräväinen, D. E. Beuchert, D. B. Calne: Pathophysiology of motor performance in Parkinson's disease. In: Dopaminergic Ergot Derivatives and Motor Functions, ed. by K. Fuxe, D. G. Calne. Pergamon Press, Oxford 1979, 45–59

347 Everet, D., G. Lawrenson, ed.: Tinnitus. Ciba Foundation symposium, 85. Pitman Books, London 1981

348 Faden, A.: Neurological sequelae of malignant external otitis. Arch. Neurol. 32: 204–205, 1976

349 Fager, C. A.: Results of adequate posterior decompression in the relief of spondylotic cervical myelopathy. J. Neurosurg. 38: 684–692, 1973

350 Fahn, S., S. B. Bressman: Should levodopa therapy for parkinsonism be started early or late? Evidence against early treatment. Canad. J. Neurol. Sci. 11: 200–206, 1984

351 Fambrough, D. M. et al.: Neuromuscular junction in myasthenia gravis: decreased acetylcholine receptors. Science 182: 293–295, 1973

352 Farrel, D. A.: Trigeminal neuropathy in progressive systemic sclerosis. Amer. J. Med. 73: 57–62, 1982

353 Feibel, J. H., J. F. Campa: Thyrotoxic neuropathy (Basedow's paraplegia). J. Neurol. Neurosurg. Psychiat. 39: 491–497, 1976

354 Feinsod, M., W. F. Hoyt: Subclinical optic neuropathy in multiple sclerosis: how early VER components reflect axon loss and conduction defects in optic pathways. J. Neurol. Neurosurg. Psychiat. 38: 1109–1114, 1975

355 Feinsod, M. et al.: Visually evoked response: use in neurologic evaluation of posttraumatic subjective visual complaints. Arch. Ophthal. 94: 237–240, 1976

356 Feldman, R. G., C. E. Pippenger: The relation of anticonvulsant drug levels to complete seizure control. J. Clin. Pharmacol. 16: 51–59, 1976

357 Feldman, Y. M., J. A. Nikitas: Syphilis serology today. Arch. Derm. 116: 84–89, 1980

358 Feldmeyer, J. J., J. Bogousslavsky, F. Regli: Asterixis uni- ou bilatéral en cas de lésion thalamique ou pariétale: un trouble moteur afférentiel? Schweiz. Med. Wschr. 114: 167–171, 1984

359 Ferell, M. R., G. Smallberg, L. D. Lewis et al.: A benign motor neuron disorder: delayed cramps and fasciculation after poliomyelitis or myelitis. Ann. Neurol. 11: 423–427, 1982

360 Fidler, S. M. et al.: Choreoathetosis as a manifestation of thyrotoxicosis. Neurology 21: 55–57, 1971

361 Fields, W. S.: Selection of stroke patients for vascular surgery. Z. Ges. Neurol. Psychiat. 201: 95–96, 1972

362 Finelli, P. F. et al.: Whipple's disease with

predominantly neuroophthalmic manifestations. Ann. Neurol. 1: 247–252, 1977

363 Finelli, P. F. et al.: Adult celiac disease presenting as cerebellar syndrome. Neurology 30: 245–249, 1980

364 Fisch, U., E. Esslen: Total intratemporal exposure of the facial nerve: pathologic findings in Bell's palsy. Arch. Otolaryng. 95: 335–341, 1972

365 Fischbeck, K. H., R. B. Layzer: Paroxysmal choreoathetosis associated with thyrotoxicosis. Ann. Neurol. 6: 453–454, 1979

366 Fischbeck, K. H., R. P. Simon: Neurological manifestations of accidental hypothermia. Ann. Neurol. 10: 384–387, 1981

367 Fischer, K. C., R. J. Schwartzman: Oral corticosteroids in the treatment of ocular myasthenia gravis. Neurology 24: 795–798, 1974

368 Fischer, P. A., W. Enzensberger: Neurological complications in AIDS. J. Neurol. 324: 269–279, 1987

369 Fisher, C. M.: An unusual variant of acute idiopathic polyneuritis (syndrome of ophthalmoplegia, ataxia and areflexia). New Engl. J. Med. 255: 57–65, 1956

370 Fisher, C. M.: Binswanger's encephalopathy: a review. J. Neurol. (in press)

371 Fisher, M., R. Long Randall, D. A. Drachmann: Hand muscle atrophy in multiple sclerosis. Arch. Neurol. 40: 811–815, 1983

372 Fleischer, K.: Geschmacksverlust nach Tonsillektomie. Dtsch. Med. Wschr. 106: 1274–1275, 1981

373 Flügel, K. A.: Transitorische globale Amnesie – ein paroxysmales amnestisches Syndrom. Fortschr. Neurol. Psychiat. 43: 471–485, 1975

374 Foley, K., J. B. Posner: Does pseudotumor cerebri cause the empty sella syndrome? Neurology 25: 565–569, 1975

375 Foltz, E., J. D. Loeser: Craniosynostosis. J. Neurosurg. 43: 48–57, 1975

376 Fontana, A. et al.: IgA deficiency, epilepsy and hydantoin medication. Lancet ii: 228–231, 1976

377 Ford, F. R.: Diseases of the nervous system. In: Infancy, Childhood and Adolescence, 6th ed. Thomas, Springfield/Ill. 1973

378 Forfar, J. C., G. J. Brown, R. E. Cull: Proximal myopathy during beta-blockade. Brit. Med. J. ii: 1331–1332, 1979

379 Fragerberg, S. E.: Diabetic neuropathy: a clinical and histological study on the significance of vascular affections. Acta Med. Scand. 164, Suppl. 345: 1–80, 1959

380 Frank, G.: Amnestische Episoden. Springer, Berlin 1981

381 Frank, Y., R. E. Kravath, K. Inoue et al.: Sleep apnea and hypoventilation syndrome associated with acquired nonprogressive dysautonomia: clinical and pathological studies in a child. Ann. Neurol. 1: 18–27, 1981

382 Fraser, J. G., P. C. Harborow: Labyrinthine window rupture. J. Laryng. 89: 1–7, 1975

383 Freemon, F.: Akinetic mutism and bilateral anterior cerebral artery occlusion. J. Neurol. Neurosurg. Psychiat. 34: 693–698, 1971

384 Freund, H.-J., K. Kendel: Vincristin zur Behandlung der Spastik. Dtsch. Med. Wschr. 96: 1155–1159, 1971

385 Frick, M., H. Rösler, M. Mumenthaler, K. Steinsiepe: Der prognostische Wert des Radiozisternogramms für die Shuntoperation beim Hydrocephalus communicans internus. Fortschr. Röntgenstr. 121: 634–643, 1974

386 Friede, R. L.: Alexander disease and related conditions. In: Developmental Neuropathology. Springer, Berlin 1975, pp. 458–464

387 Friedhoff, A. J., T. N. Chase: Advances in Neurology, vol. XXXV. Raven Press, New York 1982

388 Friedman, E. et al.: Menkes disease: neurophysiological aspects. J. Neurol. Neurosurg. Psychiat. 41: 505–510, 1978

389 Friedman, G., S. Harrison: Mucocoele of the sphenoidal sinus as a cause of recurrent oculomotor nerve palsy. J. Neurol. Neurosurg. Psychiat. 33: 172–179, 1970

390 Fromm, G. H., C. F. Terrence, A. S. Chattha: Baclofen in the treatment of trigeminal neuralgia: double-blind study and long-term follow-up. Ann. Neurol. 15: 240–244, 1984

391 Fromm, G. H., C. F. Terrence, J. C. Maroon: Trigeminal neuralgia: current concepts regarding etiology and pathogenesis. Arch. Neurol. 41: 1204–1207, 1984

392 Fujii, N., T. Tabira, H. Shibasaki et al.: Acute autonomic and sensory neuropathy associated with elevated Epstein-Barr virus antibody titer. J. Neurol. Neurosurg. Psychiat. 45: 656–657, 1982

393 Fulpius, B. W.: Characterization, isolation and purification of cholinergic receptors. In: Motor Innervation of Muscle, ed. by S. Thesleff. Academic Press, New York 1976, p. 1

394 Gadoth, N., R. Dagan, U. Sandbank et al.: Permanent tetraplegia as a consequence of tetanus neonatorum. J. Neurol. Sci. 51: 273–278, 1981

395 Galbraith, J. G., V. W. Barr: Epidural abscess and subdural empyema. Advanc. Neurol. 6: 257–267, 1974

396 Galvin, R. J. et al.: A possible means of monitoring the progress of demyelination in multiple sclerosis: effect of body temperature on visual perception of double light flashes. J. Neurol. Neurosurg. Psychiat. 39: 861–865, 1976

397 Gamstorp, I.: Intermittierende Muskellähmungen und Kaliumstoffwechsel. Nervenarzt 43: 1–8, 1972

398 Gandolfi, A., D. Horoupian, I. Rapin et al.: Deafness in Cockayne's syndrome: morphological, morphometric and quantitative study of the auditory pathway. Ann. Neurol. 15: 135-143, 1984

399 Gänshirt, H · Der Hirnkreislauf. Physiologie, Pathologie, Klinik. Thieme, Stuttgart 1972

400 Gänshirt, H., R. Keuler: Intracerebrale Blutungen. Nervenarzt 51: 201-206, 1980

401 Garcia, C. A., R. H. Fleming: Reversible corticospinal tract disease due to hyperthyroidism. Arch. Neurol. 34: 647-648, 1977

402 Gardner, W. J.: Hydrodynamic mechanism of syringomyelia: its relationship to myelocele. J. Neurol. Neurosurg. Psychiat. 28: 247-259, 1965

403 Gardner, W. J. et al.: Terminal ventriculostomy for syringomyelia. J. Neurosurg. 46: 609-617, 1977

404 Gardner-Thorpe, C., S. Benjamin: Peripheral neuropathy after disulfiram administration. J. Neurol. Neurosurg. Psychiat. 34: 253-259, 1971

405 Gastaut, J. L., B. Michel: La neuropathie mentonnière. Presse Méd. 13: 1071-1074, 1984

406 Geisler, L. S.: Das Pickwick-Syndrom. Dtsch. Med. Wschr. 96: 212-216, 1971

407 Gendelman, H. E., J. S. Wolinsky, R. T. Johnson, N. J. Pressman: Measles encephalomyelitis: lack of evidence of viral invasion of the central nervous system and quantitative study of the nature of demyelination. Ann. Neurol. 15: 353-360, 1984

408 Gentilini, M., E. DeRenzi, G. Crisi: Bilateral paramedian thalamic artery infarcts: report of eight cases. J. Neurol. Neurosurg. Psychiat. 50: 900-909, 1987

409 Geraghty, J. J., J. Jankovic, W. J. Zetusky: Association between essential tremor and Parkinson's disease. Ann. Neurol. 17: 329-333, 1985

410 Gerstenbrand, F.: Das traumatische apallische Syndrom. Springer, Wien 1967

411 Gerster, J. C., S. Guggi, H. Perroud, R. Bovet: Lyme arthritis appearing outside the United States: a case report from Switzerland. Brit. Med. J. 283: 951-952, 1981

412 Gettelfinger, D. M., E. Kokmen: Superior sagittal sinus thrombosis. Arch. Neurol. 34: 2-6, 1977

413 Gibbels, E.: Tabellarische Anleitung zur Differentialdiagnose der Polyneuropathien. Fortschr. Neurol. Psychiat. 48: 31-66, 1980

414 Gibbels, E., G. Schliep: Fragen der Ätiologie, Pathogenese, Syndromgenese und Therapie bei der diabetischen Polyneuropathie. Dargestellt aufgrund des neueren Schrifttums und einer Analyse von 120 eigenen Fällen. Fortschr. Neurol. Psychiat. 39: 579-629, 1971

415 Gill, G. V., D. R. Bell: Persisting nutritional neuropathy amongst former war prisoners. J. Neurol. Neurosurg. Psychiat. 45: 861-865, 1982

416 Gilles de la Tourette, G.: Etude sur une affection nerveuse, caracterisée par de l'incoordination motrice, accompagnée d'echolalie et de coprolalie. Arch. Neurol. (Paris) 9: 19-42, 158-200, 1885

417 Gilsanz, V. et al.: Controlled trial of glycerol versus dexamethasone in the treatment of cerebral oedema in acute cerebral infarction. Lancet i: 1049-1051, 1975

418 Girard, P. L., M. Dumas, R. Escourolle et al.: Angéite granulomateuse à cellules géantes du système nerveux central. Rev. Neurol. 132: 369-382, 1976

419 Giuffré, R., P. Curatolo: Cranial dermal sinuses in childhood and adolescence. Neurochirurgia 21: 72-75, 1978

420 Gjorup Lone: Obstetrical lesion of the brachial plexus. Acta Neurol. Scand. 42: Suppl. 18, 1966

421 Glaser, M. A.: Atypical neuralgia, so called: a critical analysis of one hundred and fortythree cases. Arch. Neurol. Psychiat. 20: 537-558, 1928

422 Godwin-Austen, R. B., J. Smith: Comparison of the effects of bromocriptine and levodopa in Parkinson's disease. J. Neurol. Neurosurg. Psychiat. 40: 479-482, 1977

423 Goldhammer, Y., J. L. Smith: Acquired intermittent Brown's syndrome. Neurology 24: 666-668, 1974

424 Goldschmidt, B. et al.: Mycoplasma antibody in Guillain-Barré syndrome and other neurological disorders. Ann. Neurol. 7: 108-112, 1980

425 Gomez Manuel, R.: Tuberous sclerosis. Raven Press, New York 1979

426 Gonsette, R. E. et al.: Intensive immunosuppression with cyclophosphamide in multiple sclerosis. J. Neurol. 214: 173-181, 1977

427 Gonyea, E. F.: The spectrum of primary blastomycotic meningitis: a review of central nervous system blastomycosis. Ann. Neurol. 3: 26-39, 1978

428 Goodman, J. M., W. L. Zink, D. F. Cooper: Hemilingual paralysis caused by spontaneous carotid artery dissection. Arch. Neurol. 40: 653-654, 1983

429 Gordon, R. M., A. Silverstein: Neurologic manifestations in progressive systemic sclerosis. Arch. Neurol. 22: 126-134, 1970

430 Gorelick, P. B., M. Rosenberg, R. J. Pagano: Enhanced ptosis in myasthenia gravis. Arch. Neurol. 38: 351, 1981

431 Gottstein, U., I. Sedlmeyer, A. Heuss: Behandlung der akuten zerebralen Mangeldurchblutung mit niedermolekularem Dextran. Therapie-Ergebnisse einer retrospektiven Studie. Dtsch. Med. Wschr. 101: 223-227, 1976

432 Gottwald, W.: Melkersson-Rosenthal-Syndrom. Fortschr. Med. 99: 249-252, 1981

433 Gourie-Devi, M., T. S. Suresh, S. K. Shankar: Monomelic amyotrophy. Arch. Neurol. 388-394, 1984

434 Grandas, F., J. Elston, N. Quinn et al.: Blepharospasm: a review of 264 patients. J. Neurol. Neurosurg. Psychiat. 51: 767-772, 1988

435 Greenberg, J. O. et al.: Idiopathic normal pressure hydrocephalus: a report of 73 patients. J. Neurol. Neurosurg. Psychiat. 40: 336–341, 1977

436 Greenfield, J. G.: Greenfield's Neuropathology, 4th ed., ed. by J. H. Adams, J. A. N. Corsellis, L. W. Duchen. Arnold, London 1984

437 Griggs, R. C., R. T. Moxley, R. A. Lafrance, J. McQuillen: Hereditary paroxysmal ataxia: response to acetazolamide. Neurology 28: 1259–1264, 1978

438 Grisold, W., B. Mamoli: The syndrome of continuous muscle fibre activity following gold therapy. J. Neurol. 231: 244–249, 1984

439 Grob, U., E. Ketz: Posttraumatische Epilepsie nach Schädelimpressionsbrüchen. Schweiz. Med. Wschr. 104: 209–212, 1974

440 Grobe, T., D. Raithel, M. Klupp, A. Schröder: Hämodynamische Wirksamkeit von Karotisstenosen und Langzeitverlauf nach Karotisoperation. Fortschr. Neurol. Psychiat. 52: 6–10, 1984

441 Groothuis, D. R., S. Schulman, R. Wollman et al.: Demyelinating radiculopathy in the Kearns-Sayre Syndrome: a clinicopathological study. Ann. Neurol. 8: 373–380, 1980

442 Grote, W.: Neurochirurgie. Thieme, Stuttgart 1975

443 Gschwandtner, W. R., H. Münzberger: Lipoatrophia semicircularis. Ein Beitrag zu bandförmig-circulären Atrophien des subcutanen Fettgewebes im Extremitätenbereich. Hautarzt 25: 222–227, 1974

444 Guggenheim, M. A., S. P. Ringel: Progressive neuromuscular disease in children with chronic cholestasis and vitamin E deficiency: diagnosis and treatment with alpha tocopherol. Pediatrics 1: 51–58, 1982

445 Guidetti, B., F. M. Gagliardi: Epidermoid and dermoid cysts: clinical evaluation and late surgical results. J. Neurosurg. 47: 12–18, 1977

446 Guillain, G. et al.: Sur un syndrome de radiculo-névrite avec hyperalbuminose du liquide céphalo-rachidien sans réaction cellulaire. Bull. Soc. Méd. Hôp. Paris 40: 1462–1470, 1916

447 Guilleminault, C., W. C. Dement: 235 cases of excessive daytime sleepiness: diagnosis and tentative classification. J. Neurol. Sci. 31: 13–27, 1977

448 Guiloff, R. J., P. K. Thomas, M. Contreras et al.: Linkage of autosomal dominant type I hereditary motor and sensory neuropathy to the Duffy locus on chromosome 1. J. Neurol. Neurosurg. Psychiat. 45: 669–674, 1982

449 Gumbinas, M. et al.: Progressive spastic paraparesis and adrenal insufficiency. Arch. Neurol. 33: 678–680, 1976

450 Gunby, P.: Chymopapain: tropical tree to surgical suite. J. Amer. Med. Ass. 249: 1115–1123, 1983

451 Gurney, M. E., A. C. Belton, N. Cashman, J. P. Antel: Inhibition of terminal axonal sprouting by serum from patients with amyotrophic lateral sclerosis. New Engl. J. Med. 311: 933–939, 1984

452 Gusella, J. F. et al.: A polymorphic DNA marker genetically linked to Huntington's disease. Nature 206: 234–238, 1983

453 Guthkelch, A. N.: Diastematomyelia with median septum. Brain 97: 729–742, 1974

454 Gutzwiller, F., P. J. Grob, I. Boppart, P. Marguerat: Früherfassung kindlicher Mißbildungen des Rückenmarkes und des Gehirns: Das AFP-Screening – Ergebnisse einer Studie bei 16000 schwangeren Frauen in der Schweiz. Schweiz. Ärzteztg. 66: 274–283, 1985

455 Hackett, E. R. et al.: Optic neuritis in systemic lupus erythematosus. Arch. Neurol. 31: 9–11, 1974

456 Haerer, A. R., W. A. Dallas, B. S. Schoenberg: Prevalence of essential tremor: results from the Copiah county study. Arch. Neurol. 39: 750–751, 1982

457 Hagberg, B., J. Aicardi, K. Dias, O. Ramos: A progressive syndrome of autism, dementia, ataxie and loss of purposeful hand use in girls: Rett's syndrome: report of 35 cases. Ann. Neurol. 14: 471–479, 1983

458 Hagedorn, H.-J.: Syphilisantikörper im Liquor cerebrospinalis und ihre diagnostische Bedeutung. Dtsch. Med. Wschr. 105: 155–161, 1980

459 Hagel, K., H. Freytag, H. Kindt: Das Kleine-Levin-Critchley Syndrom. Ein Beitrag zu seiner differentialdiagnostischen Klärung. Fortschr. Neurol. Psychiat. 48: 267–278, 1980

460 Hageman, G., J. Willemse: Arthrogryposis multiplex congenita. Neuropediatrics 14: 6–11, 1983

461 Hallen, O. et al.: Neurologische Erkrankungen bei chronischem Alkoholismus. Nervenarzt 42: 57–65, 1971

462 Hallenbeck, J. M. et al. Mechanisms underlying spinal cord damage in decompression sickness. Neurology 25: 308–316, 1975

463 Haller, J. S., J. A. Fabara: Tick paralysis: case report with emphasis on neurological toxicity. Amer. J. Dis. Child. 124: 915–917, 1972

464 Halliday, A. M., E. Halliday: Cortical evoked potentials in patients with benign essential myoclonus and progressive myoclonic epilepsy. Electroenceph. Clin. Neurophysiol. 29: 106–107, 1970

465 Halliday, A. M. et al.: Visual evoked response in diagnosis of multiple sclerosis. Brit. Med. J. 4: 661–664, 1973

466 Hallpike, J. F., C. W. M. Adams, W. W. Tourtellotte: Multiple Sclerosis: Pathology, Diagnosis and Management. Chapman and Hall, London 1983

467 Halpert, J., P. Larroque, J. Heyraud, J.-L. Lesbordes: Encéphalopathie aiguë hypercalcémique iatrogène. Nouv. Presse Méd. 35: 3152, 1978

468 Hamburger, F. A., F. Hollwich: Augenmuskellähmungen, 2nd ed. Enke, Stuttgart 1977
469 Hamel, E. et al.: Cervial myelopathy. Neurosurg. Rev. 1: 101-110, 1978
470 Hammar, C.-H., F. Regli: Zerebellare Ataxie infolge Hypothyreose beim Erwachsenen. Dtsch. Med. Wschr. 100: 1504-1506, 1975
471 Hancock, D. O.: A study of 49 patients with acute spinal extradural abscess. Paraplegia 10: 285-288, 1973
472 Hansen, K., H. Schliack: Segmentale Innervation. Ihre Bedeutung für Klinik und Praxis, 2nd ed. Thieme, Stuttgart 1962
473 Hanson, P. A., R. Chodos: Hemiparetic seizures. Neurology 28: 920-923, 1978
474 Hara, M., K. Takeuchi: A temporal study of survival of patients with pontine gliomas. J. Neurol. 216: 189-196, 1977
475 Harada, H., S. Nishikawa, K. Takahashi: Epidemiology of Parkinson's disease in a Japanese city. Arch. Neurol. 40: 151-154, 1983
476 Harding, A. E.: Idiopathic late onset cerebellar ataxie. J. Neurol. Sci. 51: 259-271, 1981
477 Harding, A. E.: Hereditary "pure" spastic paraplegia: a clinical and genetic study of 22 families. J. Neurol. Neurosurg. Psychiat. 44: 871-883, 1981
478 Harding, A. E.: Friedreich's ataxia: a clinical and genetic study of 90 families with an analysis of early diagnosis criteria and intrafamilial clustering of clinical features. Brain 104: 589-620, 1981
479 Harding, A. E.: Classification of the hereditary ataxias and paraplegias. Lancet i: 1151-1155, 1983
480 Harding, A. E., P. K. Thomas: Autosomal recessive forms of hereditary motor and sensory neuropathy. J. Neurol. Neurosurg. Psychiat. 43: 669-678, 1980
481 Harding, A. E., P. K. Thomas: The clinical features of hereditary motor and sensory neuropathy types I and II. Brain 103: 259-280, 1980
482 Harding, A. E., P. K. Thomas: Peroneal muscular atrophy with pyramidal features. J. Neurol. Neurosurg. Psychiat. 47: 168-172, 1984
483 Hardy, A. G., A. B. Rossier: Spinal Cord Injuries. Thieme, Stuttgart 1975
484 Harik, S. I., M. J. Post: Computer tomography in Wilson disease. Neurology 31: 107-110, 1981
485 Harper, C.: Wernicke's encephalopathy: a more common disease than realised. J. Neurol. Neurosurg. Psychiat. 42: 226-231, 1979
486 Harrington, D. O.: The Visual Fields: A Textbook and Atlas of Clinical Perimetry, 3rd ed. Mosby, Saint Louis 1971
487 Harrison, M. S., C. Ozsahinoglu: Positional vertigo: aetiology and clinical significance. Brain 95: 369-372, 1972
488 Hartmann, A., E. Alberti: Differentiation of communicating hydrocephalus and presenile

dementia by continuous recording of cerebrospinal fluid pressure. J. Neurol. Neurosurg. Psychiat. 40: 630-640, 1977
489 Hartmann, A., P. Berlit, D. Olbert, H. Krastel: Neurologische Komplikationen bei Morbus Behçet. Akt. Neurol. 9: 78-82, 1982
490 Hase, U., H.-J. Reulen: Läsionen des Plexus brachialis. de Gruyter, Berlin 1985
491 Hassan, I.: Cauda equina syndrome in ankylosing spondylitis: a report of six cases. J. Neurol. Neurosurg. Psychiat. 39: 1172-1177, 1976
492 Haymaker, W., J. W. Kernohan: The Landry-Guillain-Barré syndrome. Medicine (Baltimore) 28: 59-141, 1949
493 Haymaker, W., B. Woodhall: Peripheral Nerve Injuries, 2nd ed. Saunders, Philadelphia 1959
494 Haynes, F., M. I. Kaiser-Kupper, P. Mason et al.: Cogan syndrome: studies in thirteen patients, long-term follow-up, and a review of the literature. Medicine (Baltimore) 59: 426-441, 1980
495 Heimann, H., D. Naumann: Alkohol und Nervensystem. Therapiewoche 31: 4706-4710, 1981
496 Heiser, J. C., R. B. Rutherford, S. P. Riagel: Thymectomy for myasthenia gravis: a changing perspective. Arch. Surg. 117: 533-537, 1982
497 Henkin, R. I.: Syndrome of acute zinc loss. Cerebellar dysfunction, mental changes, anorexia, and taste and smell dysfunction. Arch. Neurol. 32: 745-751, 1975
498 Hennerici, M., W. Rautenberg, S. Mohr: Stroke risk from symptomless extracranial arterial disease. Lancet ii, 1180-1183, 1982
499 Henriksson, K. G., P. Sandstedt: Polymyositis — treatment and prognosis: a study of 107 patients. Acta Neurol. Scand. 65: 280-300, 1982
500 Henson, R. A., H. Ulrich: Cancer and the Nervous System: the Neurological Manifestation of Systemic Malignant Disease. Blackwell, Oxford 1982
501 Herberhold, C.: Störungen des Riechsinnes. Dtsch. Ärztebl. 75: 2901-2907, 1978
502 Herold, S., R von Kummer, C Jaeger: Follow-up of spontaneous intracerebral haemorrhage by computed tomography. J. Neurol. 228: 267-276, 1982
503 Hertel, G. et al.: Die Syringomyelie. Klinische Verlaufsbeobachtungen bei 323 Patienten. Nervenarzt 44: 1-13, 1973
504 Hertel, G., H.-G. Mertens, K. Ricker, K. Schimrigk: Myasthenia gravis und andere Störungen der neuromuskulären Synapse. Thieme, Stuttgart 1977
505 Herzberg, L., E. Bayliss: Spinal-cord syndrome due to non-compressive Paget's disease of bone: a spinal-artery steal phenomenon reversible with calcitonin. Lancet ii: 13-15, 1980
506 Hess, C. W., C. Scharfetter, M. Mumen-

thaler: Klinik der Narkolepsie-Kataplexie-Syndrome. Nervenarzt 55. 391–401, 1984

507 Hess, K.: Lage- und Lagerungsnystagmus aus neurologischer Sicht. Akt. Neurol. 10: 113–117, 1983

508 Heyck, H.: Der Kopfschmerz. Differentialdiagnostik und Therapie für die Praxis, 5th ed. Thieme, Stuttgart 1982

509 Heyman, A. et al.: Risk of stroke in asymptomatic persons with cervical arterial bruits. New Engl. J. Med. 297: 838–841, 1980

510 Heyman, A., W. E. Wilkinson, B. J. Hurwitz, C. S. Haynes: Risk of ischemic heart disease in patients with TIA. Neurology 34: 626–630, 1984

511 Hilal, S. K., J. W. Jichelsen: Therapeutic percutaneous embolization for extraaxial vascular lesions of the head, neck, and spine. J. Neurosurg. 43: 275–287, 1975

512 Hilt, D. C., D. Buchholz, A. Krumholz et al.: Herpes zoster ophthalmicus and delayed contralateral hemiparesis caused by cerebral angiitis: diagnosis and management approaches. Ann. Neurol. 14: 543–553, 1983

513 Hilton-Jones, D., J. R. Ponsford, N. Graham: Transient visual obscurations, without papilloedema. J. Neurol. Neurosurg. Psychiat. 45: 832–834, 1982

514 Hindfelt, B., O. Nilsson: The prognosis of ischemic stroke in young adults. Acta Neurol. Scand. 55: 123–130, 1977

515 Hoes, M. J. A. J. M., G. W. Bruyn, G. J. Velevoye: The Tolosa-Hunt syndrome - literature review: 7 new cases and a hypothesis. Cephalalgia 1: 181–184, 1981

516 Holman, R. R., V. Mayon-White, C. Orde-Peckar et al.: Prevention of deterioration of renal and sensory-nerve function by more intensive management of insulin-dependent diabetic patients. Lancet i: 204–208, 1983

517 Holmes, G. L., B. A. Shaywitz: Strumpell's pure familial spastic paraplegia: case study and review of the literature. J. Neurol. Neurosurg. Psychiat. 40: 1003–1008, 1977

518 Hoogenraad, T. U., C. J. van der Hamer, J. van Hattum: Effective treatment of Wilson's disease with oral zinc sulphate: two case reports. Brit. Med. J. 289: 273–276, 1984

519 Hopf, H. C., A. Struppler: Elektromyographie. Lehrbuch und Atlas. Thieme, Stuttgart 1974

520 Hopkins, A. P., P. K. P. Narvey: Chronic benign lymphocytic meningitis. J. Neurol. Sci. 18: 443–453, 1973

521 Hopmann, G., H. Wanke: Höchstdosierte Atropinbehandlung bei schwerer Alkylphosphatvergiftung. Dtsch. Med. Wschr. 99: 2106–2108, 1974

522 Hormes, J. T., C. M. Filley, N. L. Rosenberg: Neurologic sequelae of chronic solvent vapor abuse. Neurology 36: 698–702, 1986

523 Hoskins, B. et al.: Hyperkalemic periodic paralysis: effects of potassium, exercise glucose, and acetazolamide on blood chemistry. Arch. Neurol. 32: 519–523, 1975

524 Hösli, P. et al.: Hair-roots in screening and diagnosis of Tay-Sachs disease. Lancet i: 285–287, 1977

525 Hossain, M.: Neurological and psychiatric manifestations in idiopathic hypoparathyroidism: response to treatment. J. Neurol. Neurosurg. Psychiat. 33: 153–156, 1970

526 Houdart, R. et al.: La chirurgie d'urgence dans les traumatismes vertébromédullaires fermés. Nouv. Presse Méd. 2: 2331–2334, 1973

527 Hougaard, K. et al.: Regional cerebral blood flow in focal cortical epilepsy. Arch. Neurol. 33: 527–535, 1976

528 Houston, C. S., J. Dickinson: Cerebral form of high-altitude illness. Lancet ii: 758–761, 1975

529 Hoyt, W. F., J. R. Keane: Superior oblique myokymia: report and discussion on five cases of benign intermittent uniocular microtremor. Arch. Ophthal. 84: 461–467, 1970

530 Huber, A.: Eye Symptoms in Brain Tumors, 3rd ed. Mosby, St. Louis 1976

531 Huber, A., M. Meyer: Anwendung von Botulintoxin in der Ophthalmologie. Klin. Mbl. Augenheilk. 188: 89–94, 1986

532 Hudgins, W. R.: The predictive value of myelography in the diagnosis of ruptured lumbar discs. J. Neurosurg. 32: 152–162, 1970

533 Hudgson, P., J. N. Walton: Polymyositis and other inflammatory myopathies. In: Handbook of Clinical Neurology, vol. 41, ed. by P. S. Vinken, G. W. Bruyn. North Holland, Amsterdam 1979, pp. 51–93

534 Hudson, A. J. et al.: The muscular painfasciculation syndrome. Neurology 28: 1105–1109, 1978

535 Hughes, R. A. C., M. Kadlubowski, A. Hufschmidt: Treatment of acute inflammatory polyneuropathy. Ann. Neurol. 9 (Suppl.): 125–133, 1981

536 Huhn, A.: Die Thrombosen der intrakraniellen Venen und Sinus. Schattauer, Stuttgart 1965

537 Huhn, A., L. Daniels: Die Syntropie von Encephalomyelitis disseminata und Trigeminusneuralgie. Fortschr. Neurol. Psychiat. 41: 477–496, 1973

538 Hunt, W. E.: Tolosa-Hunt syndrome: one cause of painful ophthalmoplegia. J. Neurosurg. 44: 544–549, 1976

539 Huracek, J., K. Zuppinger, K. Karbowski: Epileptische Manifestationen bei Typ-1-Diabetes. Schweiz. Rundsch. Med. Praxis 73: 753–757, 1984

540 Hutchinson, W. M.: Acute optic neuritis and the prognosis for multiple sclerosis. J. Neurol. Neurosurg. Psychiat. 39: 283–289, 1976

541 Iannaccone, S. T. et al.: Familial progressive external ophthalmoplegia and ragged-red fibers. Neurology 24: 1033–1038, 1974

542 Illis, L. S., F. M. Taylor: Neurological and electroencephalographic sequelae of tetanus. Lancet i: 826–830, 1971

543 Innes, S. G. B.: Encephalomyelitis resembling benign myalgic encephalomyelitis. Lancet i: 969–971, 1970

544 Iqbal, A., J. J.-F. Oger, B. G. W. Arnason: Cell-mediated immunity in idiopathic polyneuritis. Ann. Neurol. 9 (Suppl.) 65–69, 1981

545 Isaacs, H., J. J. A. Heffron: The syndrome of continuous muscle-fibre activity cured: further studies. J. Neurol. Neurosurg. Psychiat. 37: 1231–1235, 1974

546 Iwakuma, T., A. Matsumoto, N. Nakamura: Hemifacial spasm: comparison of three different operative procedures in 110 patients. J. Neurosurg. 57: 753–756, 1982

547 Jabre, J. F., R. W. Bryan: Bent-knee pulling in the diagnosis of upper lumbar root lesions. Arch. Neurol. 39: 669–670, 1982

548 Jacobs, L. et al.: The lesions producing paralysis of downward but not upward gaze. Arch. Neurol. 28: 319–323, 1973

549 Jacobson, D. M., C. F. Terrence, O. M. Reinmuth: The neurologic manifestations of fat embolism. Neurology 36: 847–851, 1986

550 Jacobson, R. I.: More "goggle headache": supraorbital neuralgia. New Engl. J. Med. 308: 1363, 1983

551 Jaffe, H. W., K. Choi, P. A. Thomas et al.: National case-control study of Kaposi's sarcoma and pneumocystis carinii pneumonia in homosexual men, 1: epidemiologic results. Ann. Intern. Med. 99: 145–151, 1983

552 Jane, J. A., M. D. Neal, F. Kassell: The natural history of aneurysms and arteriovenous malformations. J. Neurosurg. 62: 321–323, 1985

553 Jankovic, J., J. Ford: Blepharospasm and orofacial-cervical dystonia: clinical and pharmacological findings in 100 patients. Ann. Neurol. 31: 402–411, 1983

554 Jannetta, P. J.: Observations on the etiology of trigeminal neuralgia, hemifacial spasm, acoustic nerve dysfunction and glossopharyngeal neuralgia: definitive microsurgical treatment and results in 117 patients. Neurochirurgia 20: 145–154, 1977

555 Janz, D.: Die Epilepsien. Spezielle Pathologie und Therapie, 2nd ed. Thieme, Stuttgart 1969

556 Janz, D.: Über das Risiko von Mißbildungen und Entwicklungsstörungen bei Kindern von Eltern mit Epilepsie. Nervenarzt 50: 555–562, 1979

557 Janz, D.: Epidemiologie und Klassifikation von Epilepsien und epileptischen Anfällen. Akt. Neurol. 6: 189–196, 1979

558 Jatzkewitz, H.: Zerebrale Sphingolipidosen als angeborene Stoffwechselstörungen. Dtsch. Med. Wschr. 95: 131–139, 1970

559 Jefferson, A., J. Clark: Treatment of benign intracranial hypertension by dehydrating agents with particular reference to the measurement of the blind spot area as a means of recording improvement. J. Neurol. Neurosurg. Psychiat. 39: 627–639, 1976

560 Jellinger, K.: Durchblutungsstörungen des Rückenmarks. Nervenarzt 43: 549–556, 1972

561 Jellinger, K., K. W. Sturm: Delayed radiation myelopathy in man: report of twelve necropsy cases. J. Neurol. Sci. 14: 389–408, 1971

562 Jemsek, J., S. B. Greenberg, L. Taber et al.: Herpes zoster-associated encephalitis: clinicopathologic report of 12 cases and review of the literature. Medicine (Baltimore) 62: 81–97, 1983

563 Jenkyn, L. R. et al.: The nuchocephalic reflex. J. Neurol. Neurosurg. Psychiat. 38: 561–566, 1975

564 Jennett, B.: Early traumatic epilepsy: incidence and significance after nonmissile injuries. Arch. Neurol. 30: 394–398, 1974

565 Jenzer, G.: Epilepsie und Schwangerschaft. Praxis 67: 848–853, 1978

566 Jenzer, G. et al.: Autonomic dysfunction in botulism B: a clinical report. Neurology 25: 150–153, 1975

567 Jenzer, G., L. Fierz: Visible "angular pulse" with internal carotid occlusion. J. Neurol. 214: 151–153, 1977

568 Jerusalem, F.: Hypotheses and recent findings concerning aetiology and pathogenesis of the muscular dystrophies. J. Neurol. 213: 155–162, 1976

569 Jerusalem, F.: Muskelerkrankungen. Thieme, Stuttgart 1979

570 Jerusalem, F., P. Imbach: Granulomatöse Myositis und Muskelsarkoidose. Klinische und bioptisch-histologische Diagnose. Dtsch. Med. Wschr. 95: 2184–2190, 1970

571 Jestico, J. V., P. D. M. Ellis: Changes in nystagmus on raising body temperature in clinically suspected and proved multiple sclerosis. Brit. Med. J. ii: 970–972, 1976

572 Johnson, C. C., T. Kuwabara: Oculopharyngeal muscular dystrophy. Amer. J. Ophthal. 77: 872–879, 1974

573 Johnson, K. P., B. J. Nelson: Multiple sclerosis: diagnostic usefulness of cerebrospinal fluid. Ann. Neurol. 2: 425–431, 1977

574 Johnson, P. C. et al.: Paraneoplastic vasculitis of nerve: a remote effect of cancer. Ann. Neurol. 5: 437–444, 1979

575 Johnson, R. T.: Current Therapy in Neurologic Disease. 1985–1986. Decker, Philadelphia 1985

576 Johnson, W. G., S. Fahn: Treatment of vascular hemiballism and hemichorea. Neurology 27: 634–636, 1977

577 Johnson, W. G., H. J. Wigger, H. R. Karp et

al.: Juvenile spinal muscular atrophy: a new hexosaminidase deficiency phenotype. Ann. Neurol.
11: 11-16, 1982
578 Jones, A. M., J. Biller, A. R. Cowley et al.:
Extracranial carotid artery arterisclerosis: diagnosis with continuous-wave Doppler and real-
time ultrasound studies. Arch. Neurol. 39:
393-394, 1982
579 Jones, D. A.: Volkmann's ischemia. Surg.
Clin. N. Amer. 50: 329-342, 1970
580 Jones, M. W., J. C. E. Kaufmann: Vertebrobasilar artery insufficiency in rheumatoid atlantoaxial subluxation. J. Neurol. Neurosurg.
Psychiat. 39: 122-128, 1976
581 Jörg, J., W. Daust, R. Körfer: Neue
Aspekte zur Zusammenhangsfrage kardialer und
spinaler Kreislaufstörungen. Nervenarzt 47:
112-117, 1976
582 Kaell, A. T., M. Shetty, B. C. P. Lee: The di-
versity of neurologic events in systemic lupus
erythematosus: prospective clinical and computed tomographic classification of 82 events in 71
patients. Arch. Neurol 43: 273-276, 1986
583 Kaeser, H. E.: Behandlung der Polyneuritiden. Dtsch. Med. Wschr. 96: 1442-1443, 1971
584 Kaeser, H. E.: Zur Frage der Behandlung
der chronisch-progredienten Strahlenmyelopa-
thie. Dtsch. Med. Wschr. 105: 446-447, 1980
585 Kaeser, H. E.: Drug-induced myasthenic
syndromes. Acta Neurol. Scand. 70, Suppl. 100:
39-45, 1984
586 Kaeser, H. E., R. Wüthrich: Zur Frage der
Neurotoxizität der Oxychinoline. Dtsch. Med.
Wschr. 95: 1685-1688, 1970
587 Kaeser, H. E., R. Dietrich, R. Kocher:
Zerebrospinale Toxoplasmose. Aktuelles zum
Erregernachweis, der Klinik und Therapie.
Schweiz. Med. Wschr. 107: 1482-1487, 1977
588 Kales, A. et al.: Successful treatment of
narcolepsy with propranolol: a case report.
Arch. Neurol. 36: 650-651, 1979
589 Kales, A., R. J. Cadieux, C. R. Soldatos et
al.: Narcolepsy - Cataplexy. Arch. Neurol. 39:
164-168, 1982
590 Kanchandani, R., J. G. Howe: Lhermitte's
sign in multiple sclerosis: a clinical survey and
review of the literature. J. Neurol. Neurosurg.
Psychiat. 45: 308-312, 1982
591 Kaneko, M. et al.: Early surgical treatment
for hypertensive intracerebral hemorrhage. J.
Neurosurg. 46: 579-583, 1977
592 Kapoor, W. N., M. Karpf, Y. Maher et al.:
Syncope of unknown origin: the need for a more
costeffective approach to its diagnostic evaluation. J. Amer. Med. Ass. 247: 2687-2691, 1982
593 Kapoor, W. N., M. Karpf, S. Wieand et al.:
A prospective evaluation and follow-up of patients with syncope. New Engl. J. Med. 309:
197-204, 1983
594 Karbowski, K.: Nomenklaturwandel in der
Epileptologie. Nutzen oder Schaden? Nervenarzt 52: 17-18, 1981

595 Karbowski, K.: Der Schwindel aus inter-
disziplinärer Sicht. Springer, Berlin 1981
596 Karbowski, K.: Epileptische Anfälle,
Phänomenologie, Differentialdiagnose und
Therapie. Springer, Heidelberg 1985
597 Karbowski, K. et al.: Electroencephalographic aspects of Lennox syndrome. Europ.
Neurol. 4: 301-311, 1970
598 Kark, P. R. et al.: Physostigmine in familial
ataxias. Neurology 27: 70-72, 1977
599 Kark, R. A. P., M. Rodriguez-Budelli: Pyruvate dehydrogenase deficiency in spinocerebellar degenerations. Neurology 29: 126-131, 1979
600 Karp, H. R. et al.: Transient cerebral ischemia: prevalence and prognosis in a biracial rural
community. J. Amer. Med. Ass. 225: 125-128,
1973
601 Karyofilis, A. et al.: Heredopathia atactica
polyneuritiformis. Fortschr. Neurol. Psychiat. 38:
321-330, 1970
602 Kaufman, M. D., L. C. Hopkins, B. J. Hurwitz: Progressive sensory neuropathy in patients
without carcinoma: a disorder with distinctive
clinical and electrophysiological findings. Ann.
Neurol. 9: 237-242, 1981
603 Kawakami, Y., K. Tabuchi, R. Ohnishi et
al.: Primary central nervous system lymphoma. J.
Neurosurg. 62: 522-527, 1985
604 Keane, J. R.: Bilateral sixth nerve palsy:
analysis of 125 cases. Arch. Neurol. 33: 681-683,
1976
605 Keane, J. R.: Tonic pupils with acute ophthalmoplegic polyneuritis. Ann. Neurol. 2:
393-396, 1977
606 Keane, J. R.: Acute bilateral ophthalmoplegia: 60 cases. Neurology 36: 279-281, 1986
607 Keesey, J., F. Naiem, J. Lindstrom et al.:
Acetylcholine receptor antibody titer and
HLA-B8 antigen in myasthenia gravis. Arch.
Neurol. 39: 73-77, 1982
608 Kellaway, P. et al.: Precise characterization
and quantification of infantile spasms. Ann.
Neurol. 6: 214-218, 1979
609 Keller, H., C. G. Baumgartner: Doppler-Ul-
traschallsonogfaphie: eine nicht-belastende Un-
tersuchungsmethode zur Diagnose und Thera-
piekontrolle von Karotisstenosen. Schweiz. Med.
Wschr. 104: 1281-1291, 1974
610 Keller, H., A. Müller, W. Meier et al.:
Transorale Doppler-Sonographie unter Schleim-
hautanästhesie zur Beurteilung der Strömungs-
verhältnisse in den Aa. vertebrales (Vertebralis-
Doppler). Dtsch. Med. Wschr. 100: 943-946,
1975
611 Kelly, J. J. et al.: The natural history of peripheral neuropathy in primary systemic amyloidosis. Ann. Neurol. 6: 1-7, 1979
612 Kelly, J. J., Jr., R. A. Kyle, J. M. Miles et al.:
The spectrum of peripheral neuropathy in myeloma. Neurology 31: 24-31, 1981
613 Kern, S., K. Hess, H. Schiller: Katamnesen

ungeklärter Trigeminus-Neuropathien. Schweiz. Arch. Neurol. Neurochir. Psychiat. 130: 13-24, 1982

614 Kerschensteiner, M., K. Poeck, W. Huber et al.: Die Untersuchung auf Aphasie. Akt. Neurol. 2: 151-157, 1975

615 Kesselring, J.: Neurologic manifestations in acquired immune deficiency syndrome (AIDS). Dtsch. Med. Wschr. 111: 1068-1073, 1986

616 Kessler, J. T.: Congenital narrowing of the cervical spinal canal. J. Neurol. Neurosurg. Psychiat. 38: 1218-1224, 1975

617 Khaleeli, A., R. D. Levy, R. Edwards et al.: The neuromuscular features of acromegaly: a clinical and pathological study. J. Neurol. Neurosurg. Psychiat. 47: 1009-1015, 1984

618 Kim, R. C., H. R. Smith, M. L. Henbest et al.: Nonhemorrhagic venous infarction of the spinal cord. Ann. Neurol. 15: 379-385, 1984

619 Kim, R. C., H. R. Smith, M. L. Henbest, B. H. Choi: Nonhemorrhagic venous infarction of the spinal cord. Ann. Neurol. 15: 379-385, 1984

620 Kirschbaum, W. R.: Jakob-Creutzfeld disease. Elsevier, Amsterdam 1968

621 Kiwak, K. J., M. J. Deray, W. D. Shields: Torticollis in three children with syringomyelia and spinal cord tumor. Neurology 33: 946-948, 1983

622 Klapatek, J.: Extrapyramidaler Tremor und Vitamin B6 in hohen Dosen: eine therapeutische Anmerkung. Nervenarzt 41: 251-255, 1970

623 Klawans, H. L., J. L. Topel: Parkinsonism as a falling sickness. J. Amer. Med. Ass. 230: 1555-1557, 1974

624 Knight, A. H., E. G. Rhind: Epilepsy and pregnancy: a study of 153 pregnancies in 59 patients. Epilepsia 16: 99-110, 1975

625 Kocen, R. S., P. K. Thomas: Peripheral nerve involvement in Fabry's disease. Arch. Neurol. 22: 81-88, 1970

626 Koch, G.: Microcephalie. Exogen bedingte und erbliche Formen. Dtsch. Ärztebl. 71: 3313-3322, 1974

627 Kocher, P., M.-E. Linder, D. Stula: Primäre Hirntumoren in einer psychiatrischen Klinik. Der informierte Arzt 5: 43-44, 1984

628 Köhler, H., E. Uehlinger, J. Kutzner et al.: Sterno-kosto-klavikuläre Hyperostose. Ein bisher nicht beschriebenes Krankheitsbild. Dtsch. Med. Wschr. 100: 1519-1523, 1975

629 Kokmen, E.: Dementia - Alzheimer type. Mayo Clin. Proc. 59: 35-42, 1984

630 Kolenda, K.-D.: Geschmacksstörungen und Leberparenchymschäden bei der Behandlung mit Thiamazol. Dtsch. Med. Wschr. 101: 84-86, 1976

631 Kollegger, H., R. Schmoliner, P. Dal-Bianco: Der Mitralklappenprolaps als Risikofaktor für den juvenilen Insult. Nervenarzt 59: 629-635, 1988

632 Kölmel, H. W. et al.: Meningosis leucaemica des Erwachsenen. Klinik, Liquorcytologie, Therapie. Nervenarzt 44: 527-536, 1973

633 Kölmel, H. W., G. Beck-Mannagetta: Intrakranielle Drucksteigerung und Stauungspapille bei Polyradikulitis. Nervenarzt 52: 460-463, 1981

634 Komàr, J., M. Szegavari: Der peripher-neurologische Hintergrund des Schreibkrampfes: mittlere N. medianus-Läsion. Nervenarzt 54: 322-325, 1983

635 Komàr, J., B. Varga: Syndrome of the rectus abdominis muscle: a peripheral neurological condition causing abdominal diagnostic problems. J. Neurol. 210: 121-125, 1975

636 Kömpf, D.: Der benigne pseudovestibuläre Kleinhirninsult. Nervenarzt 57: 163-166, 1986

637 Kondo, K., Y. Kuriowa: A case control study of Creutzfeldt-Jakob disease: association with physical injuries. Ann. Neurol. 11: 377-381, 1982

638 Kondo, K. et al.: Parkinson's disease. Genetic analysis and evidence of a multifactorial etiology. Mayo Clin. Proc. 48: 465-475, 1973

639 Kopell, H. P., W. A. L. Thompson: Peripheral Entrapment Neuropathies. Williams and Wilkins, Baltimore 1963

640 Koprowski, H., V. ter Meulen: Multiple sclerosis and parainfluenza 1 virus: history of the isolation of the virus and expression of phenotypic differences between the isolated virus and Sendai virus. J. Neurol. 208: 175-190, 1975

641 Korczyn, A.: Bell's palsy and diabetes mellitus. Lancet i: 108-109, 1971

642 Kori, S. H., K. M. Foley, J. B. Posner: Brachial plexus lesions in patients with cancer: 100 cases. Neurology 31: 45-50, 1981

643 Kozin, F. et al.: Neuro-Behçet disease: two cases and neuroradiologic findings. Neurology 27: 1148-1152, 1977

644 Krägeloh, I., J. Aicardi: Alternating hemiplegia in infants: report of five cases. Develop. Med. Child. Neurol. 22: 784-791, 1980

645 Krayenbühl, H., G. Yasargil: Zerebrale Angiographie für Klinik und Praxis, ed. P. Huber, 3rd ed. Thieme, Stuttgart 1979

646 Kristoferitsch, W., G. Spiel, P. Wessely: Zur Meningopolyneuritis (Garin-Bujadoux, Bannwarth). Klinik und Laborbefunde. Nervenarzt 54: 640-646, 1983

647 Krüger, G.: Wismut-Enzephalopathie. Fortschr. Neurol. Psychiat. 52: 24-31, 1984

648 Krüger, K. W.: Lupus erythematodes und Zentralnervensystem. Nervenarzt 55: 165-172, 1984

649 Kruglak, L., I. Nathan, A. D. Korczyn et al.: Platelet aggregability, disaggregability and serotonin uptake in migraine. Cephalalgia 4: 221-225, 1984

650 Krumholz, A., E. Niedermeyer: Psychogenic seizures: a clinical study with follow-up data. Neurology 33: 498–502, 1983

651 Kudrow, L.: Cluster headache: mechanisms and management. Oxford University Press, London 1980

652 Kugelberg, E., L. Welander: Heredofamilial juvenile muscular atrophy simulating muscular dystrophy. Arch. Neurol. Psychiat. 75: 500–509, 1956

653 Kuhl, W.: Vestibulär-zerebrale Synkopen. Dtsch. Med. Wschr. 105: 41–42, 1980

654 Kunze, K., R. Gothe: Neurophysiological investigations in tick paralysis. 4th International Congress of Electromyography, Brussels 12.–15. 9. 1971, Abstracts pp. 86–87

655 Kuritzky, A., R. Hering, G. Goldhammer, M. Bechar: Clonidine treatment in paroxysmal localized hyperhidrosis. Arch. Neurol. 41: 1210–1211, 1984

656 Kurland, L. T., J. G. Kurtze, I. D. Goldberg: Epidemiology of Neurologic and Sense Organ Disorders. Harvard University Press, Cambridge, MA 1973

657 Kurtzke, J. F.: The current neurologic burden of illness and injury in the United States. Neurology 32, 1207–1214, 1982

658 Kurtzke, J. F.: Rating neurologic impairment in multiple sclerosis: an expanded disability status scale (EDSS). Neurology 33: 1444–1452, 1983

659 Kurtzke, J. F., K. Hyllested: Multiple sclerosis in the Faroe Islands, 1: clinical and epidemiological features. Ann. Neurol. 5: 6–21, 1979

660 Kurtzke, J. F., G. W. Beebe, B. Nagler et al.: Studies on the natural history of multiple sclerosis, 5: long-term survival in young men. Arch. Neurol. 22: 215–225, 1970

661 Kurtzke, J. F., G. W. Beebe, B. Nagler et al.: Studies on the natural history of multiple sclerosis, 6: clinical and laboratory findings at first diagnosis. Acta Neurol. Scand. 48: 19–46, 1972

662 Kutt, H.: Interactions of antiepileptic drugs. Epilepsia 16: 393–402, 1975

663 Kyllermann, M., G. Steen: Intermittently progressive dyskinetic syndrome in glutaric aciduria. Neuropädiatrie 8: 397–404, 1977

664 Labauge, R., M. Boukocza, J. Zinzner et al.: Hématomes spontanés du cervelet: vingt-huit observations personnelles. Rev. Neurol. 139: 193–204, 1983

665 Labauge, R., M. Boukocza, M. Pages et al.: Occlusion de l'artère vertébrale. Rev. Neurol. 143: 6–7, 490–509, 1987

666 Lackner, K., R. Janson, T. Franken et al.: Digitale Subtraktionsangiographie (DAS). Dtsch. Med. Wschr. 108: 350–355, 1983

667 Ladurner, G., E. Jeindl, G. Schneider: Die Beziehung zwischen multiplen Infarkten und vaskulärer (Multiinfarkt-)Demenz. Fortschr. Neurol. Psychiat. 51: 124–127, 1983

668 Lamoureux, G. et al.: Cerebrospinal fluid proteins in multiple sclerosis. Neurology 25: 537–546, 1975

669 Lance, J. W.: Headaches related to sexual activity. J. Neurol. Neurosurg. Psychiat. 39: 1226–1230, 1976

670 Lance, J. W.: Mechanism and Management of Headache, 4th ed. Butterworths, London 1982

671 Landrieu, P., J. Selva, F. Alvarez et al.: Peripheral nerve involvement in children with chronic cholestasis and vitamin E deficiency: a clinical, electrophysiological and morphological study. Neuropediatrics 16: 194–201, 1985

672 Lane, R. J. M., P. A. Routledge: Drug-induced neurological disorders. Drugs 26: 124–247, 1983

673 Lang, B., J. Newsom-Davis, D. Wra, D. Vincent: Autoimmune etiology for myasthenic Eaton-Lambert syndrome. Lancet ii: 224–226, 1981

674 Langohr, H. D., M. Stöhr, F. Petruch: An open and double-blind cross-over study of the efficacy of clomipramine (Anafranil) in patients with painful mono- und polyneuropathies. Europ. Neurol. 21: 309–317, 1982

675 Laplane, D., V. Meininger, J. Bancaud et al.: Contribution à l'étude anatomo-clinique des phénomenes d'évitement. Rev. Neurol. 135: 775–787, 1979

676 Laplane, D., M. Baulac, D. Widlöcher, B. Dubois: Pure psychic akinesia with bilateral lesions of basal ganglia. J. Neurol. Neurosurg. Psychiat. 47: 377–385, 1984

677 Lapresle, J., R. Metreau: Atteintes trigéminales révélatrices d'une syringomyélie et d'une malformation de la charnière occipito-vertébrale. Nouv. Presse Méd. 7: 103–104, 1978

678 Lapresle, J., G. Said: Ophtalmoplégie douloureuse, alternante et récidivante. Rev. Neurol. 131: 583–588, 1975

679 Lapresle, J., I. Fernandez-Machola, P. Lasjaunias: L'atteinte trigéminale sensitive au cours de la paralysie faciale périphérique essentielle. Nouv. Presse Méd. 9: 291–293, 1980

680 Lascelles, R. G. et al.: Infectious mononucleosis presenting as acute cerebellar syndrome. Lancet ii: 707–709, 1973

681 Lascelles, R. G. et al.: The thoracic outlet syndrome. Brain 100: 601–612, 1977

682 Layzer, R. B.: Myeloneuropathy after prolonged exposure to nitrous oxide. Lancet ii, 1227–1230, 1978

683 Lazaro, R. P., H. S. Kirshner: Proximal muscle weakness in uremia. Arch. Neurol. 37: 555–558, 1980

684 Lazaro, R. P. et al.: Congenital muscular dystrophy: case reports and reappraisal. Muscle Nerve 2: 349–355, 1979

685 Le Beau, J. et al.: Sur le prognostic des abcès du cerveau. Neuro-chirurgie 18: 181–188, 1972

686 Lechtenberg, R., A. Shulmann: The neurologic implications of tinnitus. Arch. Neurol. 41: 718–721, 1984

687 Lecuire, J. et al.: A propos de 641 interventions pour névralgies sciatiques par hernies discales: étude statistique des résultats par ordinateur. Neuro-chirurgie 19: 501–512, 1973

688 Lederman, R. J., C. E. Henry: Progressive dialysis encephalopathy. Ann. Neurol. 4: 199–204, 1978

689 Lee, M. C. et al.: Superficial temporal to middle cerebral artery anastomosis. Arch. Neurol. 36: 1–4, 1979

690 Lees, A. J., M. Robertson, M. R. Trimble et al.: A clinical study of Gilles de la Tourette syndrome in the United Kingdom. J. Neurol. Neurosurg. Psychiat. 47: 1–8, 1984

691 Léger, J. M., S. Dancea, P. Brunet, J. J. Hauw: Polyneuropathie au cours d'un traitement par le carbimazole. Rev. Neurol. 140: 652–656, 1984

692 Leibel, R. L., V. E. Shih, S. I. Goodman et al.: Glutaric acidemia: a metabolic disorder causing progressive choreoathetosis. Neurology 30: 1163–1168, 1980

693 Leibowitz, S., R. A. C. Hughes: Immunology of the Nervous System. Arnold, London 1983

694 Lenard, H. G., D. Kettler: Malignant hyperpyrexia and myopathy. Neuropädiatrie 6: 7–12, 1975

695 Leon-Sotomayor, L. A.: Cardiac migraine: report of twelve cases. Angiology 25: 161–171, 1974

696 Lesoine, W.: Das stylo-kerato-hyoidale Syndrom. Dtsch. Ärztebl. 38: 2381–2386, 1976

697 Levin, B., J. B. Posner: Swallow syncope: report of a case and review of the literature. Neurology 22: 1086–1093, 1972

698 Levine, D. P., C. B. Lauter, A. M. Lerner: Simultaneous serum and CSF antibodies in herpes simplex virus encephalitis. J. Amer. Med. Ass. 240: 356–360, 1978

699 Levy, N. L. et al.: A blood test for multiple sclerosis based on the adherence of lymphocytes to measles-infected cells. New Engl. J. Med. 294: 1423–1427, 1976

700 Lewis, R. A., A. J. Summer, M. J. Brown et al.: Multifocal demyelinating neuropathy with persistent conduction block. Neurology 32: 958–964, 1982

701 Leys, D., F. Lesoin, A. Destee et al.: Les épidurites aiguës à germes banals: vingt-trois observations. Presse Méd. 13: 597–599, 1984

702 Lhermitte, F., R. Marteau, E. Roullet, H. de Saxcé: Traitement prolongé de la sclérose en plaques par l'azathioprine à doses moyennes: bilan de quinze années d'expérience. Rev. Neurol. 140: 553–558, 1984

703 Lieberman, A. et al.: The antiparkinsonian efficacy of bromocriptine. Neurology 26: 405–408, 1976

704 Lieberman, A. et al.: Dementia in Parkinson disease. Ann. Neurol. 6: 355–359, 1979

705 Lincoln, N. B., G. P. Mulley, A. C. Jones et al.: Effectiveness of speech therapy for aphasic stroke patients: a randomised controlled trial. Lancet i: 1197–1200, 1984

706 Lindegaard, K.-F., S. J. Mork, G. E. Eide: Statistical analysis of clinicopathological features, radiotherapy, and survival in 170 cases of oligodendroglioma. J. Neurosurg. 67: 224–230, 1987

707 Lindsay, J., C. Pimstedt, P. Richards: Long-term outcome in children with temporal lobe seizures, 5: indications and contraindications for neurosurgery. Develop. Med. Child Neurol. 26: 25–32, 1984

708 Lindstrom, J. M. et al.: Antibody to acetylcholine receptor in myasthenia gravis. Neurology 26: 1054–1059, 1976

709 Link, H. et al.: Immunoglobulin abnormalities and measles antibody response in chronic myelopathy. Arch. Neurol. 33: 26–32, 1976

710 Lipinski, C. G.: Die benigne Epilepsie im Kindesalter mit Rolando-Sharp-Wave-Fokus. Nervenarzt 51: 579–581, 1980

711 Little, J. R., C. S. MacCarty: Colloid cysts of the third ventricle. J. Neurosurg. 39: 230–235, 1974

712 Livingston, S.: Comprehensive Management of Epilepsy in Infancy, Childhood and Adolescence. Thomas, Springfield/Ill. 1972

713 Lockman, L. A. et al.: Relief of pain of Fabry's disease by diphenylhydantoin. Neurology 23: 871–875, 1973

714 Loewenfeld, I. E., H. S. Thompson: Mechanism of tonic pupil. Ann. Neurol. 10: 275–276, 1981

715 Löffel, N. B. et al.: The Landry-Guillain-Barré syndrome: complications, prognosis and natural history in 123 cases. J. Neurol. Sci. 33: 71–79, 1977

716 Logue, V.: Angiomas of the spinal cord: review of the pathogenesis, clinical features and results of surgery. J. Neurol. Neurosurg. Psychiat. 42: 1–11, 1979

717 Loiseau, P., J. M. Orgogozo: An unrecognised syndrome of benign focal epileptic seizures in teenagers. Lancet II: 1070–1071, 1978

718 Loiseau, P., P. Henry, P. Jallon et al.: Encéphalopathies myocloniques iatrogènes aux sels de Bismuth. J. Neurol. Sci. 27: 133–143, 1976

719 Loiseau, P., A. Brachet-Liermain, M. Legroux et al.: Intérêt du dosage des anticonvulsivants dans le traitement des épilepsies. Nouv. Presse Méd. 6: 813–817, 1977

720 Loizou, L. A., B. E. Kendall, J. Marshall: Subcortical arteriosclerotic encephalopathy: a clinical and radiological investigation. J. Neurol. Neurosurg. Psychiat. 44: 294–304, 1981

721 Lott, I. T., T. Coulombe, R. V. Di Paolo: Vitamin B 6-Dependent seizures: pathology and

chemical findings in brain. Neurology 28: 47–54, 1978

722 Low, P. A. et al.: The sympathetic nervous system in alcoholic neuropathy: a clinical and pathological study. Brain 98: 357–364, 1975

723 Low, P. A. et al.: The splanchnic autonomic outflow in Shy-Drager syndrome and idiopathic orthostatic hypotension. Ann. Neurol. 4: 511–514, 1978

724 Ludin, H.-P.: Electromyography in Practice. Thieme, Stuttgart 1980

725 Ludin, H. P.: Das Parkinson-Syndrom. Sandoz, Basel 1984

726 Ludin, H. P.: Das Parkinsonsyndrom. Kohlhammer, Stuttgart 1988

727 Ludin, H. P.: Der Tremor. Klinik und Therapie. Therap. Umschau 45: 19–23, 1988

728 Ludin, H. P., F. Bass-Verrey: Study of deterioration in long-term treatment of parkinsonism with L-Dopa plus decarboxylase inhibitor. J. Neur. Transm. 38: 249–258, 1976

729 Ludin, H. P., W. Tackmann: Sensory Neurography. Thieme, Stuttgart 1981

730 Ludin, H. P., W. Tackmann: Polyneuropathien. Thieme, Stuttgart 1984

731 Luessenhop, A. J., L. Rosa: Cerebral arteriovenous malformations: indications for and results of surgery and the role of intravascular techniques. J. Neurosurg. 60: 14–22, 1984

732 Lütschg, J. et al.: The syndrome of "continuous muscle fibre activity". Arch. Neurol. 35: 198–205, 1978

733 Lyons, J. C., L. F. A. Peterson: The snapping iliopsoas tendon. Mayo Clin. Proc. 59: 327–329, 1984

734 Macris, S. G.: Methylphenidate of hiccups. Anesthesiology 34: 200–201, 1971

735 McAlpine, D. et al.: Multiple Sclerosis: a Reappraisal, 2nd ed. Livingstone, Edinburgh 1972

736 McCloskey, J. R., S. M. K. Chung: Quadriceps contracture as a result of multiple intramuscular injection. Amer. J. Dis. Child. 131: 416–417, 1977

737 McCormick, D. P.: Herpes-simplex virus as cause of Bell's palsy. Lancet i: 937–939, 1972

738 McCormick, G. F., C.-S. Zee, J. Heiden: Cysticercosis cerebri: review of 127 cases. Arch. Neurol. 39: 534–539, 1982

739 McFarland, H. R. et al.: Papulosis atrophicans maligna (Köhlmeier-Degos disease): a disseminated occlusive vasculopathy. Ann. Neurol. 3: 388–392, 1978

740 McFarlin, D. E., H. F. McFarland: Multiple sclerosis. New Engl. J. Med. 307: 1183–1188; 1246–1251, 1982

741 McFarlin, D. A., J. O. Susac: Hoquet diabolique: intractable hiccups as a manifestation of multiple sclerosis. Neurology 29: 797–801, 1979

742 McLeod, J. G.: Electrophysiological studies in the Guillain-Barré syndrome. Arch. Neurol. 9 (Suppl.): 20–27, 1981

743 McLeod, J. G. et al.: Acute idiopathic polyneuritis. J. Neurol. Sci. 27: 145–162, 1976

744 McNamara, J. O. et al.: The value of carotid endarterectomy in treating transient cerebral ischemia of the posterior circulation. Neurology 27: 682–684, 1977

745 Madersbacher, H.: Zur Diagnostik neurogener Blasenentleerungsstörungen. Urologe A 13: 276–280, 1974

746 Maeder, R. P., M. Mumenthaler, H. Markwalder: Symptomatische zervikale Syringomyelie. Dtsch. Med. Wschr. 95: 164–168, 1970

747 Maendly, R., M. Mumenthaler, J. M. Martinez-Lage: Die Erythroprosopalgie. Übersicht mit Einschluß 224 eigener Beobachtungen. Dtsch. Med. Wschr. 107: 186–191, 1982

748 Mager, J.: Klinik des Opsoklonus. Nervenarzt 47: 29–33, 1976

749 Magnaes, B.: Communicating hydrocephalus in adults. Diagnostic tests and results of treatment with medium pressure shunts. Neurology 28: 478–484, 1978

750 Magnaes, B.: Cerebrospinal fluid hydromechanics in adult patients with benign noncommunicating hydrocephalus: one-hour test shunting and balanced cerebrospinal fluid infusion test to select patients for intracranial bypass operation. Neurosurgery 11: 769–775, 1982

751 Maia, M: Sjögren-Larsson syndrome in two sibs with peripheral nerve involvement and albuminaemia. J. Neurol. Neurosurg. Psychiat. 37: 1306–1315, 1974

752 Maigne, R. et al.: Lombalgies basses d'origine dorso-lombaire: traitement chirurgical par excision des capsules articulaires postérieures. Nouv. Presse Méd. 7: 565–568, 1978

753 Malin, J. P., E. Stark, U. Wurster: Borreliose-Radikulitis der Cauda equina. Aktuelle Neurologie (in press)

754 Malouf, R., J. C. M. Brust: Hypoglycemia: Causes, neurological manifestations, and outcome. Ann. Neurol. 17: 421–430, 1985

755 Mamoli, B., H. P. Ludin: Electrophysiological investigations in a case of cephalic tetanus. J. Neurol. 214: 251–255, 1977

756 Mamoli, B. et al.: Recurrent Bell's palsy: etiology, frequency, prognosis. J. Neurol. 216: 119–125, 1977

757 Mancall, E. L. et al.: Hypertrophic branchial myopathy: idiopathic enlargement of the masticatory muscles as a neglected myopathic disorder. Neurology 24: 1166–1170, 1974

758 Manz, F.: Konservative Behandlung des leichten Karpaltunnelsyndroms. Infiltration des Karpalkanals mit Corticoid-Kristallsuspension (Celestan R. Depot). Nervenarzt 45: 387–388, 1974

759 Marcea, J. T.: Das Raeder-Syndrom. Nervenarzt 50: 563–569, 1979

760 Marchac, D., D. Renier: Craniofacial surgery for craniosynostosis: Little, Brown, Boston 1983

761 Mariani, C. et al.: Bilateral perisylvian softenings: bilateral anterior opercular syndrome (Foix-Chavany-Marie syndrome). J. Neurol. 223: 269–284, 1980

762 Markakis, E., R. Heyer, L. Stoeppler, H. Werry: Die Aplasie der perisylvischen Region. Neurochirurgia 22: 211–220, 1979

763 Markand, O. N., B. P. Garg, D. D. Weaver: Familial startle disease (hyperexplexia): electrophysiologic studies. Arch. Neurol. 41: 71–74, 1984

764 Markham, C. H., S. G. Diamond: Evidence to support early levodopa therapy in Parkinson disease. Neurology 31: 125–131, 1981

765 Marsden, C. D.: Blepharospasm-oromandibular dystonia syndrome (Brueghel's syndrome): a variant of adult-onset torsion dystonia? J. Neurol. Neurosurg. Psychiat. 39: 1204–1209, 1976

766 Marsden, C. D., S. Fahn: Movement Disorders. Butterworth, London 1982

767 Marsden, C. D., M. J. G. Harrison: Idiopathic torsion dystonia (dystonia musculorum deformans): a review of forty-two patients. Brain 97: 793–810, 1974

768 Marshall, J.: The Management of Cerebrovascular Disease, 3rd ed. Churchill, London 1976

769 Martin, J. R.: Herpes simplex virus type 1 and 2 and multiple sclerosis. Lancet ii: 777–781, 1981

770 Masdeu, J. C., F. A. Rubino: Management of lobar intracerebral hemorrhage: medical or surgical. Neurology 34: 381–383, 1984

771 Masters, C. L., J. O. Harris, D. C. Gajdusek et al.: Creutzfeldt-Jakob disease: patterns of worldwide occurrence and the significance of familial and sporadic cases. Ann. Neurol. 5: 177–188, 1979

772 Masucci, E. F., J. F. Kurtzke, N. Saini: Myorhythmia: a widespread movement disorder: clinicopathological correlations. Brain 107: 53–79, 1984

773 Masui, Y., T. Mozai, K. Kakehi: Functional and morphometric study of the liver in motor neuron disease. J. Neurol. 232: 15–19, 1985

774 Mathey, D., R. Montz, P. Hanrath et al.: Kurzfristige regionale Myokardischämie und ihre Folgen bei Prinzmetal-Angina-pectoris. Dtsch. Med. Wschr. 103: 969–971, 1978

775 Mathis, J., C. W. Hess: Das Schlaf-Apnoe-Syndrom. Schweiz. Rundsch. Med. Prax. 77: 908–919, 1988

776 Matsumoto, A., K. Watanabe, T. Negoro et al.: Long-term prognosis after infantile spasms: a statistical study of prognostic factors in 200 cases. Develop. Med. Child Neurol. 23: 51–65, 1981

777 Matthes, A.: Epilepsie. Diagnostik und Therapie für Klinik und Praxis, 3rd ed. Thieme, Stuttgart 1977; 4th ed. 1984

778 Matthews, W. B.: Paroxysmal symptoms in MS. J. Neurol. Neurosurg. Psychiat. 38: 617–623, 1975

779 Matthews, W. B., M. Esiri: The migrant sensory neuritis of Wartenberg. J. Neurol. Neurosurg. Psychiat. 46: 1–4, 1983

780 Mattle, H.: Neurologische Manifestationen der gestörten Osmolalität. Schweiz. Med. Wschr. 115: 882–889, 1985

781 Maxion, H. et al.: Der Spasmus facialis – Klinischer Bericht über 25 Patienten. Nervenarzt 42: 590–595, 1971

782 May, W. E.: Nutritional sensory neuronopathy: an emerging new syndrome. Arch. Neurol. 41: 559–560, 1984

783 Meador, K. J., T. R. Swift: Tinnitus from intracranial hypertension. Neurology 34: 1258–1261, 1984

784 Mechelse, K. et al.: Bell's palsy: prognostic criteria and evaluation of surgical decompression. Lancet ii: 57–59, 1971

785 Medina, J. L., S. Diamond: The clinical link between migraine and cluster headaches. Arch. Neurol. 34: 470–472, 1977

786 Meek, D., L. S. Wolfe, E. Andermann, F. Andermann: Juvenile progressive dystonia: a new phenotype of GM2 gangliosidosis. Ann. Neurol. 15: 348–352, 1984

787 Mehta, A. J., S. S. Seshia: Orbicularis oculi reflex in brain death. J. Neurol. Neurosurg. Psychiat. 39: 784–787, 1976

788 Meienberg, O.: Störungen der Pupillenmotorik. Akt. Neurol. 5: 245–252, 1978

789 Meienberg, O.: Sparing of the temporal crescent in homonymous hemianopsia and its significance for visual orientation. Neuro-Ophthalm. 2: 129–134, 1981

790 Meienberg, O.: Lesion site in Fisher's syndrome. Arch. Neurol. 41: 250–251, 1984

791 Meienberg, O., K. Karbowski: Die Epilepsia partialis continua Kozevnikov. Zur Klinik und Pathophysiologie. Dtsch. Med. Wschr. 102: 781–784, 1977

792 Meienberg, O., G. Kommerell: Die Pupillenprüfung mit dem "swinging flashlight-Test". Alternierende tangentiale Belichtung der Augen zur Erfassung geringgradiger Opticusläsionen. Nervenarzt 49: 197–200, 1978

793 Meienberg, O., E. Ryffel: Supranuclear eye movement disorders in Fisher's syndrome of ophthalmoplegia, ataxia and areflexia. Arch. Neurol. 40: 402–405, 1983

794 Meier, C.: Polyneuropathy in paraproteinaemia. J. Neurol. 232: 204–214, 1985

795 Meier, C., H. P. Ludin, A. Bischoff: Polyneuropathien bei Hypothyreose. Akt. Neurol 8: 114–118, 1981

796 Meier, C., C. Moll: Hereditary neuropathy with liability to pressure palsies: report of two families and review of the literature. J. Neurol. 228: 73–95, 1982

797   Meier, C., W. Tackmann: Die hereditären motorisch-sensiblen Neuropathien. Fortschr. Neurol. Psychiat. 50: 349–365, 1982

798   Meier, C., H. P. Ludin, M. Mumenthaler: Die vaskulitische Ischiasneuritis. Nervenarzt 53: 196–199, 1982

799   Meier, C., M. Vandevelde, A. Steck, A. Zurbriggen: Demyelinating polyneuropathy associated with monoclonal IgM-paraproteinaemia. J. Neurol. Sci. 63: 353–367, 1983

800   Melamed, N., S. Satya-Murti: Cerebellar hemorrhage: a review and reappraisal of benign cases. Arch. Neurol. 41: 425–428, 1984

801   Mertens, H. G.: Störungen des Stoffwechsels, bei welchen Muskelsymptome im Vordergrund stehen. Periodische Lähmungen bei Dyskaliämien. In: Innere Medizin in Praxis und Klinik, 3rd ed., vol. 2, ed. H. Hornbostel, W. Kaufmann, W. Siegenthaler. Thieme, Stuttgart 1985

802   Mertin, J., M. Kremer, S. C. Knight et al.: Double-blind controlled trial of immunosuppression in the treatment of multiple sclerosis. Final report. Lancet ii: 351–354, 1982

803   Merx, W., S. Effert, P. Hanrath et al.: Hyperaktiver Carotissinusreflex. Diagnostischer Wert und Prognose im höheren Lebensalter. Dtsch. Med. Wschr. 106: 135–140, 1981

804   Messert, B., W. W. Orrison, M. J. Hawkins, C. E. Quaglieri: Central pontine myelinolysis. Considerations on etiology, diagnosis and treatment. Neurology 29: 147–160, 1979

805   Messiha, F. S., A. D. Kenny: Parkinson's disease: neurophysiological, clinical and related aspects. Plenum Press, New York 1977

806   Metha, D., R. Khatib, S. Patel: Carcinoma of the breast and meningioma: association and management. Cancer 51: 1937–1940, 1983

807   Metzger, J., A. Buge, G. Rancurel et al.: Aspects tomodensitométriques de trois observations d'encéphalopathies bismuthiques aiguës. Rev. Neurol. 134: 619–624, 1978

808   Meyer-Rienecker, H. J., B. Hitzschke: Lymphocytic meningoradiculitis (Bannwarth's syndrome). In: Handbook of Clinical Neurology, vol. 34/2, ed. by P. J. Vinken, G. W. Bruyn. North-Holland, Amsterdam 1978, pp. 571–586

809   Michel, D., M. Tommasi, B. Laurent et al.: Dégénérescence striato-nigrique: à propos de deux observations anatomo-cliniques. Rev. Neurol. 132: 3–22, 1976

810   Michel, E. M., B. T. Troost: Palinopsia: cerebral localization with computed tomography. Neurology 30: 887–889, 1980

811   Miller, D. H., P. Rudge, G. Johnson et al.: Serial gadolinium enhanced magnetic resonance imaging in multiple sclerosis. Brain 111: 927–939, 1988

812   Miller, F., H. Korsvik: Baclofen in the treatment of stiff-man syndrome. Ann. Neurol. 9: 511–512, 1981

813   Millikan, C. H.: Cerebral vasospasm and ruptured intracranial aneurysm. Arch. Neurol. 32: 433–449, 1975

814   Mimaki, T., N. Itoh, J. Abe et al.: Neurological manifestations in xeroderma pigmentosum. Ann. Neurol. 20: 70–75, 1986

815   Minder-von Goumoëns, I.: Polycythaemie, Polyglobulie und neurologische Symptome. Praxis 60: 423–429, 1971

816   Mitsumoto, H., A. J. Wilbourn, S. H. Subramony: Generalized myokymia and gold therapie. Arch. Neurol. 39: 449–450, 1982

817   Mizuno, T., Y. Yugari: Prophylactic effect of L-5-hydroxytryptophan on self-mutilation in the Lesch-Nyhan syndrome. Neuropädiatrie 6: 13–23, 1975

818   Moeschlin, S.: Klinik und Therapie der Vergiftungen, 7th ed. Thieme, Stuttgart 1986

819   Moeschlin, S.: Therapie-Fibel der inneren Medizin für Klinik und Praxis, 6th ed. Thieme, Stuttgart 1982

820   Mokri, B., D. G. Piepgrad, O. Wayne Houser: Traumatic dissections of the extracranial internal carotid artery. J. Neurosurg. 68: 189–197, 1988

821   Mokri, B., T. M. Sundt, O. W. Houser: Spontaneous internal carotid dissection, hemicrania and Horner's syndrome. Arch. Neurol. 36: 677–680, 1979

822   Mollaret, P.: La méningite endothélio (?) - leucocytaire multirécurrente bénigne. Rev. Neurol. 133: 225–244, 1977

823   Monnier, V. M., B. W. Fulpius: A radioimmunoassay for the quantitative evaluation of antihuman acetylcholine receptor antibodies in myasthenia gravis. Clin. Exp. Immunol. 29: 16–22, 1977

824   Montagna, P., F. Cirignotta, T. Sacquegna et al.: "Painful legs and moving toes" associated with polyneuropathy. J. Neurol. Neurosurg. Psychiat. 46: 399–403, 1983

825   Montero, C. G., A. J. Martinez: Neuropathology of heart transplantation: 23 cases. Neurology 36: 1149, 1986

826   Morariu, M. A.: Progressive supranuclear palsy and normal pressure hydrocephalus. Neurology 29: 1544–1546, 1979

827   Moretti, G., P. Caffarra, M. Parma: Transient topographical amnesia. Ital. J. Neurol. Sci. 4: 361, 1983

828   Morris, H. H. et al.: Neuroleptic malignant syndrome. Arch. Neurol. 37: 462–463, 1980

829   Moser, H.: Klinik der Muskelkrankheiten. In: Innere Medizin in Praxis und Klinik, 3rd ed., vol. 2, ed. H. Hornbostel, W. Kaufmann, W. Siegenthaler. Thieme, Stuttgart 1985, pp. 88–89

830   Moser, H., A. E. H. Emery: The manifesting carrier in Duchenne muscular dystrophy. Clin. Genet. 5: 271–284, 1974

831   Moser, H. W., A. E. Moser, I. Singh, B. P. O'Neill: Adrenoleukodystrophy: survey of

303 cases: biochemistry, diagnosis and therapy. Ann. Neurol. 16: 628–641, 1984

832 Moshell, A. N. et al.: Radiosensitivity in Huntington's disease: implications for pathogenesis and presymptomatic diagnosis. Lancet i: 9–11, 1980

833 Mottiert, D., G. Bergeret, M. F. Perreaut et al.: Myopathie thyroïdienne chronique simulant une sclérose laterale amyotrophique. Presse Méd. 10: 1655, 1981

834 Mouret, J., P. Sanchez, J. Taillard: Treatment of narcolepsy with L-tyrosine. Lancet ii: 1458–1459, 1988

835 Moutsopoulos, H. M., B. L. Webber, N. A. Pavlidis: Diffuse fasciitis with eosinophilia: a clinicopathologic study. Am. J. Med. 68: 701–709, 1980

836 Muenter, M. D.: Should levodopa therapy be started early or late? Canad. J. Neurol. Sci. 11: 195–199, 1984

837 Mulder, D. W.: The Diagnosis and Treatment of Amyotrophic Lateral Sclerosis. Mifflin, Boston 1980

838 Mulder, D. W., F. M. Howard: Patient resistance and prognosis in amyotrophic lateral sclerosis. Mayo Clin. Proc. 51: 537–541, 1976

839 Müller, W.: Die Lyme Arthritis. Erythemamigrans-Arthritis. Schweiz. Med. Wschr. 114: 265–269, 1984

840 Müller-Jensen, A.: Einseitige und seitenwechselnde Ophthalmoplegia interna bei seitenwechselnder Hemikranie. Nervenarzt 46: 97–99, 1975

841 Mumenthaler, M.: Myopathy in neuropathy. In: Muscle Diseases. Excerpta Medica International Congress Series No. 199. Excerpta Medica, Amsterdam 1970, pp. 585–598

842 Mumenthaler, M.: Giant-cell arteritis: cranial arteritis, polymyalgia rheumatica. J. Neurol. 218: 219–236, 1978

843 Mumenthaler, M.: Der Schulter-Arm-Schmerz, 2nd ed. Huber, Bern 1982

844 Mumenthaler, M.: Die besonderen neurologischen Nystagmusformen. Akt. Neurol. 10: 128–131, 1983

845 Mumenthaler, M.: Synkopen und Sturzanfälle. Thieme, Stuttgart 1984

846 Mumenthaler, M.: Neuropathies due to physical agents. In: Handbook of Clinical Neurology, ed. by P. J. Vinken, G. W. Bruyn. North-Holland, Amsterdam 1985

847 Mumenthaler, M.: Didaktischer Atlas der klinischen Neurologie, 2nd ed. Springer, Berlin 1986

848 Mumenthaler, M.: Neurologische Differentialdiagnostik. Syndrome und Leitsymptome, 3rd ed. Thieme, Stuttgart 1988

849 Mumenthaler, M., C. Probst: Das Querschnittssyndrom mit schlaffer Paraplegie. Beitrag zu den vasculären Rückenmarksläsionen anhand von 12 eigenen Beobachtungen. Z. ges. Neurol. Psychiat. 201: 6–23, 1972

850 Mumenthaler, M., J. Lütschg: Die Myasthenia gravis pseudoparalytica. Diagnostische und therapeutische Aspekte anhand von 60 eigenen Beobachtungen. Schweiz. Arch. Neurol. Neurochir. Psychiat. 118: 23–56, 1976

851 Mumenthaler, M., H. Schliack: Läsionen peripherer Nerven. Diagnostik und Therapie, 5th ed. Thieme, Stuttgart 1987

852 Mumenthaler, M., T. Treig: Amnestische Episoden. Analyse von 111 eigenen Beobachtungen. Schweiz. Med. Wschr. 114, 1163–1170, 1984

853 Mumenthaler, M. et al.: Transient global amnesia after clioquinol: five personal observations from outside Japan. J. Neurol. Neurosurg. Psychiat. 42: 1084–1090, 1979

854 Mumenthaler, Manuela, M. Mumenthaler, C. Meier: Amnestische Episoden. In: Status psychomotoricus und seine Differentialdiagnose, ed. K. Karbowski. Huber, Bern 1980

855 Munsat, T. L., J. N. Walton: Prednisone in Duchenne muscular dystrophy. Lancet i: 276–277, 1975

856 Munsat, T. L. et al.: Serum enzyme alterations in neuromuscular disorders. J. Amer. Med. Ass. 226: 1536–1543, 1973

857 Münzenberg, K. J.: Schmerzen im Bein. Edition Medizin, Weinheim 1982

858 Müri, R. M.: The clinical spectrum of internuclear ophthalmoplegia in multiple sclerosis. Diss., Bern 1984

859 Murphy, M. J., L. W. Lyon, J. W. Taylor: Subacute arsenic neuropathy: clinical and electrophysiological observations. J. Neurol. Neurosurg. Psychiat. 44: 896–900, 1981

860 Myers, R. H., D. Boldman, E. D. Bird et al.: Maternal transmission in Huntington's disease. Lancet i: 208–210, 1983

861 Myllylä, V. V., A. Saarinen, P. Ylöstalo, E. Hokkanen: Efficacy of small doses of bromocriptine in Parkinson's disease. Curr. Ther. Res. 33: 144–149, 1983

862 Nadeau, S. E., J. D. Trobe: Pupil sparing in oculomotor pasly: a brief review. Ann. Neurol. 13: 143–148, 1983

863 Nadel, A. M., W. P. Wilson: Dialysis encephalopathy: a possible seizure disorder. Neurology 26: 1130–1134, 1976

864 Nadjmi, M., U. Piepgras, H. Vogelsang: Kranielle Computertomographie. Thieme, Stuttgart 1981

865 Nagao, H., K. Kida, H. Matsuda et al.: Alexander disease: clinical, electrodiagnostic and radiographic studies. Neuropediatrics 12: 22–32, 1981

866 Nakae, K. et al.: Relation between subacute myelo-optic neuropathy (SMON) and clioquinol: nationwide survey. Lancet i: 171–173, 1973

867 Nakamura, Y., Y. K. Inoue: Pathogenicity of virus associated with subacute myelo-opticoneuropathy. Lancet i: 223–226, 1972

868 Nakano, K. K. et al.: The cervical myelopathy associated with rheumatoid arthritis: analysis of 32 patients, with 2 postmortem cases. Ann. Neurol. 3: 144–151, 1978

869 Namba, T. et al.: Idiopathic giant cell polymyositis: report of a case and review of the syndrome. Arch. Neurol. 31: 27–30, 1974

870 Narins, R. G., E. R. Jones, M. C. Stom et al.: Diagnostic strategies in disorders of fluid, electrolyte and acid-base homeostasis. Amer. J. Med. 72: 496–520, 1982

871 Nass, R., A. Chutorian: Dysaesthesias and dysautonomia: a self-limited syndrome of painful dysaesthesias and autonomic dysfunction in childhood. J. Neurol. Neurosurg. Psychiat. 45: 162–165, 1982

872 Nathan, P. W.: Painful legs and moving toes: evidence on the site of the lesion. J. Neurol. Neurosurg. Psychiat. 41: 934–939, 1978

873 Nausieda, P. A. et al.: Chorea induced by oral contraceptives. Neurology 29: 1605–1609, 1979

874 Nee, L. E. et al.: Gilles de la Tourette syndrome: clinical and family study of 50 cases. Ann. Neurol. 7: 41–49, 1980

875 Nelson, K. B., G. D. Eng: Congenital hypoplasia of the depressor anguli oris muscle: differentiation from congenital facial palsy. J. Pediat. 81: 16–20, 1972

876 Nelson, K. B., J. H. Ellenberg: Predictors of epilepsy in children who have experienced febrile seizures. New Engl. J. Med. 295: 1029–1033, 1976

877 Neundörfer, B.: Differentialtypologie der Polyneuritiden und Polyneuropathien. Schriftenreihe Neurologie, vol. 11. Springer, Berlin 1973

878 Neundörfer, B., H. Kuhn: Roussy-Lévy-Syndrom. Nervenarzt 47: 153–156, 1976

879 Nevsimalova-Bruhova, S., B. Roth: Heredofamilial aspects of narcolepsy and hypersomnia. Schweiz. Arch. Neurol. Neurochir. Psychiat. 110: 45–54, 1972

880 Newman, R. P., W. R. Kinkel: Paroxysmal choreoathetosis due to hypoglycemia. Arch. Neurol. 41: 341–342, 1984

881 Newsom-Davis, J., N. M. F. Murray: Plasma exchange and immunosuppressive drug treatment in the Lambert-Eaton myasthenic syndrome. Neurology 34: 480–485, 1984

882 Niedermeyer, E.: Epilepsy Guide: Diagnosis and Treatment of Epileptic Seizure Disorders. Urban and Schwarzenberg, München 1983

883 Nishioka, H., C. Torner, C. J. Graf et al.: Cooperative study of intracranial aneurysms and subarachnoid hemorrhage: a long-term prognostic study: ruptured intracranial aneurysms managed conservatively. Arch. Neurol. 41: 1142–1146, 1984

884 Nishioka, H., C. Torner, C. J. Graf et al.: Cooperative study of intracranial aneurysms and subarachnoid hemorrhage: a long-term prognostic study: subarachnoid hemorrhage of undetermined etiology. Arch. Neurol. 41: 1147–1151, 1984

885 Nordgren, R. E. et al.: Seven cases of cerebromedullospinal disconnection: the locked-in syndrome. Neurology 21: 1140–1148, 1971

886 Norris, F. H., Jr.: The remote effects of cancer on the nervous system. Z. Ges. Neurol. Psychiat. 201: 201–210, 1972

887 Noseworthy, J., D. Paty, T. Wonnacott et al.: Multiple sclerosis after age 50. Neurology 33: 1537–1544, 1983

888 Notter, O.: Das Tolosa-Hunt Syndrom. Fortschr. Neurol. Psychiat. 44: 429–440, 1977

889 Nukada, H., M. Pollock, S. Allpress: Experimental cold injury to peripheral nerve. Brain 104: 779–811, 1981

890 Nutt, J. G., J. P. Hammerstad: Blepharospasm and oromandibular dystonia (Meige's syndrome) in sisters. Ann. Neurol. 9: 189–191, 1981

891 Nyland, H., R. Matre, S. Mork: Immunological characterization of sural nerve biopsies from patients with Guillain-Barré syndrome. Ann. Neurol. 9 (Supp.), 80–86, 1981

892 O'Brien, T. A., P. S. Harper: Course prognosis and complications of childhood-onset myotonic dystrophy. Dev. Med. Child. Neurol. 26: 62–67, 1984

893 O'Neill, B. P.: Passive ocular proptosis. J. Neurol. Neurosurg. Psychiat. 40: 1198–1202, 1977

894 O'Sullivan, D. J. et al.: Multiple progressive intracranial arterial occlusing (moyamoya disease). J. Neurol. Neurosurg. Psychiat. 40: 853–860, 1977

895 Obeso, J. A., J. F. Marti-Masso, W. Astudillo et al.: Treatment of hemiballism with reserpine. Ann. Neurol. 4: 581, 1978

896 Oh, S. J.: Subacute demyelinating polyneuropathy responding to corticosteroid treatment. Arch. Neurol. 35: 509–516, 1978

897 Ohta, T. et al.: Sinus pericranii. J. Neurosurg. 42: 704–712, 1975

898 Okada, F. et al.: Two cases of acute pandysautonomia. Arch. Neurol. 32: 146–151, 1975

899 Olanow, C. W., J. M. R. Lande, A. D. Roses: Thymectomy in late-onset myasthenia gravis. Arch. Neurol. 39: 82–83, 1982

900 Olson, W. et al.: Oculocraniosomatic neuromuscular disease with "ragged-red" fibers. Histochemical and ultrastructural changes in limb muscles of a group of patients with idiopathic progressive external ophthalmoplegia. Arch. Neurol. 26: 193–211, 1972

901 Omasitis, M., M. Brainin: Zur primär chronischen Neurobrucellose. Fortschr. Neurol. Psychiat. 55: 291–293, 1987

902 O'Neill, J. H., K. R. Mills, N. M. F. Murray: McArdle's sign in multiple sclerosis. J. Neurol. Neurosurg. Psychiatry 50: 1691–1693, 1987

903 O'Neill, J. H., N. M. F. Murray, J. Newsom-Davis: The Lambert-Eaton myasthenic syndrome (a review of 50 cases). Brain 111: 577–596, 1988

904 Oosterhuis, H. J. G. H.: Myasthenia gravis. In: Clinical Neurology and Neurosurgery Monographs. Churchill Livingstone, Edinburgh 1984

905 Orfei, R., O. Meienberg: Carotidynia: report of eight cases and prospective evaluation of therapy. J. Neurol. 230: 65–72, 1983

906 Österman, P. O., C. E. Westerberg: Paroxysmal attacks in MS. Brain 98: 189–202, 1975

907 Ott, K. M. et al.: Cerebellar hemorrhage: diagnosis and treatment: a review of 56 cases. Arch. Neurol. 31: 160–167, 1974

908 Ouvrier, R. A.: Progressive dystonia with marked diurnal fluctuation. Ann. Neurol. 4: 412–417, 1978

909 Ouvrier, R. A., J. G. McLeod, G. J. Morgan et al.: Hereditary motor and sensory neuropathy of neuronal type with onset in early childhood. J. Neurol. Sci. 51: 181–197, 1981

910 Palliyath, S., C. A. Garcia: Multifocal interstitial myositis associated with localized lipoatrophy: a benign course. Arch. Neurol. 39: 722–724, 1982

911 Pamphlett, R., R. Mackenzie: Severe peripheral neuropathy due to lithium intoxication. J. Neurol. Neurosurg. Psychiat. 45: 656–661, 1982

912 Pampiglione, G. E., E. J. Moynahan: The tuberous sclerosis syndrome: clinical and EEG studies in 100 children. J. Neurol. Neurosurg. Psychiat. 39: 666–673, 1976

913 Pampus, I., I. Seidenfaden: Die posttraumatische Epilepsie. Fortschr. Neurol. Psychiat. 42: 329–384, 1974

914 Panayiotopoulos, C. P., S. Scarpalezos: Dystrophia myotonica: peripheral nerve involvement and pathogenetic implications. J. Neurol. Sci. 27: 1–16, 1976

915 Park, T. S., H. J. Hoffmann, E. B. Hendrick et al.: Medulloblastoma: clinical presentation and management. J. Neurosurg. 58: 543–552, 1983

916 Parkes, J. D. et al.: Controlled trial of amantadine hydrochloride in Parkinson's disease. Lancet I: 259–262, 1970

917 Parkin, P. J., R. Hierons, W. I. McDonald: Bilateral optic neuritis: a long-term follow-up. Brain 107: 951–964, 1984

918 Parry, G. J., S. Clarke: Multifocal acquired demyelinating neuropathy masquerading as motor neuron disease. Muscle Nerve 11: 103–107, 1988

919 Pasternak, J. F., J. Hageman, M. A. Adams et al.: Exchange transfusion in neonatal myasthenia. J. Pediat. 99: 644–646, 1981

920 Patten, B. M., M. Pages: Severe neurological disease associated with hyperparathyreoidism. Ann. Neurol. 15: 453–456, 1984

921 Patten, B. M. et al.: Multiple sclerosis associated with defects in neuromuscular transmission. J. Neurol. Neurosurg. Psychiat. 35: 385–394, 1972

922 Paul, K. S., R. N. Lye, F. A. Strang, J. Dutton: Arnold Chiari malformation. J. Neurosurg. 58: 183–187, 1983

923 Paulson, G. W.: Benign essential tremor in childhood: symptoms, pathogenesis, treatment. Clin. Pediat. 15: 67–75, 1976

924 Payk, T. R.: Psychopathologische Besonderheiten bei Kranken mit Encephalomyelitis disseminata ("Multiple Sklerose"). Nervenarzt 44: 378–380, 1973

925 Pearn, J.: Neuromuscular paralysis caused by tick envenomation. J. Neurol. Sci. 34: 37–42, 1977

926 Pearn, J. H. et al.: A clinical and genetic study of spinal muscular atrophy of adult onset. Brain 101: 591–606, 1978

927 Pearson, J.: Familial dysautonomia. J. Auton. Nerv. Syst. 1: 119–126, 1979

928 Pedersen, E.: Epidemic vertigo: clinical picture, epidemiology and relation to encephalitis. Brain 82: 566–580, 1959

929 Peele, T. L.: The Neuroanatomic Basis for Clinical Neurology, 3rd ed. McGraw-Hill, New York 1977

930 Peiffer, J. et al.: Alcohol embryo and fetopathy. J. Neurol. 41: 125–137, 1979

931 Pena, S. D. J.: Giant axonal neuropathy: an inborn error of organization of intermediate filaments. Muscle Nerve 5: 166–172, 1982

932 Penn, A. S. et al.: Muscular dystrophy in young girls. Neurology 20: 247–259, 1970

933 Pépin, B., J. Frenay, B. Goldstein et al.: Syndrome syringomyélique après méningite tuberculeuse (à propos de quatre observations). Rev. Neurol. 133: 697–708, 1977

934 Perentes, E., F. Donati: La méningo-encéphalite herpétique. Rev. Méd. Suisse Rom. 101: 713–728, 1981

935 Perret, E.: Gehirn und Verhalten. Neuropsychologie des Menschen. Huber, Bern 1973

936 Perret, G., H. Nishioka: Report on the cooperative study of intracranial aneurysms and subarachnoid hemorrhage, section 6: arteriovenous malformations: an analysis of 545 cases of craniocerebral arteriovenous malformations and fistulae reported to the cooperative study. J. Neurosurg. 25: 467–490, 1966

937 Perry, T. L. et al.: Hereditary mental depression and parkinsonism with taurine deficiency. Arch. Neurol. 32: 108–113, 1975

938 Pestel, M.: Sclérose en plaques et assurance-vie. Nouv. Presse Méd. 5: 1071–1073, 1976

939 Peters, B. H. et al.: Neurologic and psychologic manifestations of decompression illness in divers. Neurology 27: 125–127, 1977

940 Petitti, D. B., J. Wingerd: Use of oral contraceptives, cigarette smoking and risk of subarachnoid hemorrhage. Lancet ii: 234–235, 1978

941 Pettigrew, L. C., J. P. Glass, M. Maor, J. Zornoza: Diagnosis and treatment of lumbosacral plexopathies in patients with cancer. Arch. Neurol. 41: 1282–1285, 1984
942 Pfaltz, C. R.: Schwindel aus hals-nasen-ohrenärztlicher Sicht. Ther. Umsch. 41: 689–693, 1984
943 Pfeiffer, J.: Stoffwechselkrankheiten des Gehirns. Dtsch. Ärztebl. 45: 2931–2942, 1972
944 Pfeiffer, R. A., H. Bauer, C. Petersen: Das Syndrom von Schwartz-Jampel (Myotonia chondrodystrophica). Helv. Paediat. Acta 32: 251–261, 1977
945 Pfister, H. W., K. Einhäupl, V. Preac-Mursic et al.: The spirochetal etiology of lymphocytic meningoradiculitis of Bannwarth (Bannwarth's syndrome). J. Neurol. 231: 141–144, 1984
946 Philipp, M., N. Seyfeddinipur, A. Marneros et al.: Epileptische Anfälle beim Delirium tremens. Nervenarzt 47: 192–197, 1976
947 Philippon, J. et al.: Résultats de la dérivation du liquide céphalorachidien dans l'hydrocéphalie à pression normale de l'adulte. Rev. Neurol. 130: 333–342, 1974
948 Pickett, J. B. E. et al.: Neuromuscular complications of acromegaly. Neurology 25: 638–645, 1975
949 Pilz, H.: Clinical, morphological and biochemical aspects of sphingolipidoses. Neuropädiatrie 1: 383–427, 1970
950 Pilz, H. et al.: Neurologische Symptome bei Fabryscher Krankheit. Angiokeratoma corporis diffusum. Z. Ges. Neurol. Psychiat. 202: 307–322, 1972
951 Pirovino, M., J. Meier, M. Meyer et al.: Malignes Neuroleptika-Syndrom. Dtsch. Med. Wschr. 109: 378–381, 1984
952 Piscol, K.: Die Durchblutung des Rückenmarkes und ihre klinische Relevanz. Schriftenreihe Neurologie, vol. 13. Springer, Berlin 1972
953 Plaitakis, A., J. T. Caroscio: Abnormal glutamate metabolism in amyotrophic lateral sclerosis. Ann. Neurol. 22: 575–579, 1987
954 Plaitakis, A. et al.: Glutamate dehydrogenase deficiency in three patients with spinocerebellar syndrome. Ann. Neurol. 7: 297–303, 1980
955 Plaitakis, A., S. Berl, M. D. Yahr: Neurological disorders associated with deficience of glutamate dehydrogenase. Ann. Neurol. 15: 144–153, 1984
956 Plaitakis, A., J. Smith, J. Mandeli et al.: Pilot trial of branched-chain aminoacids in amyotrophic lateral sclerosis. Lancet i: 1015–1018, 1988
957 Pleet, A. B., E. W. Massey: Notalgia paresthetica. Neurology 28: 1310–1313, 1978
958 Plum, F., J. B. Posner: The Diagnosis of Stupor and Coma, 3rd ed. Davis, Philadelphia 1980
959 Poeck, K.: Die Differentialdiagnose Migraine accompagnée und sensible Jackson-Anfälle. Dtsch. Med. Wschr. 97: 637–641, 1972

960 Poeck, K.: Neuropsychologische Symptome ohne eigenständige Bedeutung. Akt. Neurol. 2: 199–208, 1975
961 Poeck, K.: Studies on language comprehension in hemispherectomy, split brain and aphasic patients: a possible contribution to the knowledge of the psychological mechanisms of speech comprehension. Experimental Brain Research Supplementum II: Hearing Mechanisms and Speech. Springer, Berlin 1979
962 Poeck, K.: Klinische Neuropsychologie. Thieme, Stuttgart 1982
963 Poeck, K.: Neurologie. Ein Lehrbuch für Studierende und Ärzte, 6th ed. Springer, Berlin 1982
964 Pongratz, D., H. Kötzner, G. Hübner et al.: Adulte Form des Mangels an saurer Maltase unter dem Bild einer progressiven spinalen Muskelatrophie. Dtsch. Med. Wschr. 109: 537–541, 1984
965 Pönkä, A.: The occurrence and clinical picture of serologically verified Mycoplasma pneumoniae infections with emphasis on central nervous system, cardiac and joint manifestations. Ann. Clin. Res. 11: Suppl. 24, 1–60, 1979
966 Porter, J., H. Jick: Drug-induced anaphylaxis, convulsions, deafness and extrapyramidal symptoms. Lancet i: 587–588, 1977
967 Poser, S., W. Poser: Toxische Wirkungen von Arzneimitteln auf das Zentralnervensystem. Nervenarzt 54: 615–623, 1983
968 Posner, J., N. L. Chernick: Intracranial metastases from systemic cancer. Advanc. Neurol. 19: 579–592, 1978
969 Powell, H. C., M. Rodriguez, R. A. C. Hughes: Microangiopathy of vasa nervorum in dysglobulinemic neuropathy. Ann. Neurol. 15: 386–394, 1984
970 Price, R. W., J. B. Posner: Chronic paroxysmal hemicrania: a disabling headache syndrome responding to indomethacin. Ann. Neurol. 3: 183–184, 1978
971 Prill, A., E. Volles: Zentralnervöse Manifestationen der akuten und chronischen Niereninsuffizienz. Dtsch. Med. Wschr. 97: 1953–1957, 1972
972 Prineas, J. W.: Pathology of the Guillain-Barré syndrome. Ann. Neurol. 9 (Suppl.): 6–19, 1981
973 Puvanendran, K. et al.: Delayed facial palsy after head injury. J. Neurol. Neurosurg. Psychiat. 40: 342–350, 1977
974 Quandt, J., H. Sommer: Neurologie. Grundlagen und Klinik, 2nd ed. VEB Thieme, Leipzig 1983
975 Rabe, F.: Isolierte Ageusie. Ein neues Symptom als Nebenwirkung von Medikamenten. Nervenarzt 41: 23–27, 1970
976 Radanov, B.: Schwindel mit dem Schwindel? Psychiatrische Aspekte. Ther. Umsch. 41: 715–719, 1984

977 Radü, E. W., V. Skorpil, H. E. Kaeser: Facial myokymia. Europ. Neurol. 13: 499–512, 1975

978 Raman, P. T., G. M. Taori: Prognostic significance of electrodiagnostic studies in the Guillain-Barré syndrome. J. Neurol. Neurosurg. Psychiat. 39: 163–170, 1976

979 Raskin, N. H., S. Prusiner: Carotidynia. Neurology 27: 43–46, 1977

980 Rau, H. et al.: Hydrocephalus communicans. Beitrag zur Klinik der ätiologisch ungeklärten Liquorzirkulationsstörungen. J. Neurol. 207: 279–287, 1974

981 Rebollo, M., J. F. Val, F. Garijo et al.: Livedo reticularis and cerebrovascular lesions (Sneddon's syndrome). Brain 106: 965–979, 1983

982 Rechthand, E., D. R. Cornblath, B. J. Stern, J. O. Meyerhoff: Chronic demyelinating polyneuropathy in systemic lupus erythematosus. Neurology 34: 1375–1377, 1984

983 Refsum, S.: Heredopathia atactica polyneuritiformis: phytanic acid storage disease (Refsum's disease) with particular reference to therapeutic and pathogenetic aspects. In: The Nervous System, vol. 2, ed. by D. B. Tower. The Clinical Neurosciences. Raven Press, New York 1975, pp. 229–234

984 Regli, F.: Die flüchtigen ischämischen zerebralen Attacken. Natürlicher Verlauf und Pathogenese. Dtsch. Med. Wschr. 96: 525–530, 1971

985 Regli, F. et al.: Der see-saw-Nystagmus. Nervenarzt 42: 316–319, 1971

986 Reik, L., A. C. Steere, N. H. Bartenhaben et al.: Neurologic abnormalities of Lyme disease. Medicine (Baltimore) 58: 281–294, 1979

987 Reisner, T., E. Maida: Computerized tomography in multiple sclerosis. Arch. Neurol. 37: 475–477, 1980

988 Reker, U., H. Rudert: Akute isolierte Vestibularisstörung. HNO 25: 122–126, 1977

989 Remillard, G. et al.: Facial asymmetry in patients with temporal lobe epilepsy. Neurology 27: 109–114, 1977

990 Reulecke, M., M. Dumas, C. Meier: Specific antibody activity against neuroendocrine tissue in a case of POEMS syndrome with IgG gammopathy. Neurology 38: 614–616, 1988

991 Reulen, J. P. H., E. A. C. M. Sander, L. A. H. Hogenhuis: Eye movement disorders in multiple sclerosis and optic neuritis. Brain 106: 121–140, 1983

992 Riccardi, V. M., J. J. Mulvihill: Neurofibromatosis: genetics, cell biology and biochemistry. Advances in Neurology, vol. 2. Raven Press, New York 1981

993 Rice, G. P. A. et al.: Familial stroke syndrome associated with mitral valve prolapse. Ann. Neurol. 7: 130–134, 1980

994 Richards, P., H. Shawdon, R. Illingworth: Operative findings on microsurgical exploration of the cerebello-pontine angle in trigeminal neuralgia. J. Neurol. Neurosurg. Psychiat. 46: 1098–1101, 1983

995 Richter, H. R.: Einklemmungsneuropathien der Rami dorsales als Ursache von akuten und chronischen Rückenschmerzen. Ther. Umsch. 34: 435–438, 1977

996 Ridley, A.: The neuropathy of acute intermittent porphyria. Quarterly J. Med., n. s. 38: 307–333, 1969

997 Rieben, F. W.: Hustensynkope. Dtsch. Med. Wschr. 105: 360–362, 1980

998 Riikonen, R.: A long-term follow-up study of 214 children with the syndrome of infantile spasms. Neuropediatrics 13: 14–23, 1982

999 Riley, C. M.: Familial dysautonomia. Advanc. Pediat. 9: 157–190, 1957

1000 Ring, J. et al.: Intensive immunosuppression in the treatment of multiple sclerosis. Lancet ii: 1093–1096, 1974

1001 Ritter, G., S. Poser: Epilepsie und multiple Sklerose. Münch. Med. Wschr. 116: 1983–1986, 1974

1002 Robbins, J. H., K. H. Kraemer, M. A. Lutzner et al.: Xeroderma pigmentosum: an inherited disease with sun sensitivity, multiple cutaneous neoplasms and abnormal DNA repair. Ann. Intern. Med. 80: 221–248, 1974

1003 Robert, F., M. Mumenthaler: Kriterien des Hirntodes. Schweiz. Med. Wschr. 107: 335–341, 1977

1004 Robertson, D. M., D. H. Mellor: Asymmetrical palatal paresis in childhood: a transient cranial mononeuropathy? Develop. Med. Child Neurol. 24: 842–849, 1982

1005 Robertson, W. C., Jr., D. B. Clark, W. R. Markesbery: Review of 38 cases of subacute sclerosing panencephalitis: effect of amantadine on the natural course of the disease. Ann. Neurol. 8: 422–425, 1980

1006 Rohmer, F.: Les méningoradiculites: données cliniques, électromyographiques et étiologiques à propos de 36 observations: limites nosologiques. Rev. Neurol. 130: 415–431, 1974

1007 Rollinson, R. D., B. S. Gilligan: Postanoxic action myoclonus (Lange-Adams syndrome) responding to Valproate. Arch. Neurol. 36: 44–45, 1979

1008 Roman, G. et al.: Neurological manifestations of hereditary hemorrhagic teleangiectasia (Rendu-Osler-Weber disease): report of 2 cases and review of the literature. Ann. Neurol. 4: 130–144, 1978

1009 Rompf, G.: Zum elektiven Befall des Zentralnervensystems durch Lupus erythematodes. Fortschr. Neurol. Psychiat. 39: 229–245, 1971

1010 Romy, M. et al.: De la fréquence des anévrismes artériels intracranies et de leur rupture, d'après une serie d'autopsie de routine. Neuro-chirurgie 19: 611–626, 1973

1011 Roos, R. P., M. V. Viola, R. Wollmann:
Amyotropic lateral sclerosis with antecedent
poliomyelitis. Arch. Neurol. 37: 312–313, 1980
1012 Ropper, A. H., D. C. Poskanzer: The
prognosis of acute and subacute transverse myelopathy based on early signs and symptoms.
Ann. Neurol. 4: 51–59, 1978
1013 Ropper, A. H., B. T. Shahani: Pain in
Guillain-Barré syndrome. Arch. Neurol. 41:
511–514, 1984
1014 Rosen, J. A.: Prolonged azathioprine
treatment of nonremitting multiple sclerosis. J.
Neurol. Neurosurg. Psychiat. 42: 338–344, 1979
1015 Rosenberg, R. N.: The Treatment of Neurological Disease. SP Medical Books, New York
1979
1016 Rosenberg, R. N.: Biochemical genetics
of neurologic disease. New Engl. J. Med. 305:
1181–1193, 1981
1017 Rosenberger, K.: Vaskuläre Polyneuropathien bei primär chronischer Polyarthritis.
Fortschr. Neurol. Psychiat. 45: 536–544, 1977
1018 Rosenhamer, H. J., B. P. Silfverskiöld:
Slow tremor and delayed brainstem auditory
evoked responses in alcoholics. Arch. Neurol.
37: 293–296, 1980
1019 Rosenstock, H. A. et al.: Chronic man-
ganism. Neurologic and laboratory studies during treatment with levodopa. J. Amer. Med. Ass.
217: 1354–1358, 1971
1020 Rosman, N. P.: The cerebral defect and
myopathy in Duchenne muscular dystrophy: a
comparative clinicopathological study. Neurology 20: 329–335, 1970
1021 Rossi, L. N. et al.: Guillain-Barré syndrome in children with special reference to the
natural history of 38 personal cases. Neuropediatrics 7: 42–51, 1976
1022 Rossi, L. N., M. Mumenthaler, F. Vasella:
Complicated migraine (migraine accompagnée)
in children. Neuropädiatrie 11: 27–35, 1980
1023 Rossi, L. N., F. Vasella, M. Mumenthaler:
Obstetrical lesions of the brachial plexus: natural
history in 34 personal cases. Europ. Neurol. 21:
1–7, 1982
1024 Rossi, L. N., F. Vasella, M. Mumenthaler
et al.: Benign migraine-like syndrome with CSF
pleocytosis in children. Develop. Med. Child
Neurol. 1985
1025 Roth, G., J. Rohr, M. R. Magistris et al.:
Motor neuropathy with proximal multifocal persistent conduction block, fasciculations and
myokymia. Eur. Neurol. 25: 416–423, 1986
1026 Rothrock, J. F., P. C. Johnson, S. M. Rothrock, R. Merkley: Fulminant polyneuritis after
overdose of disulfiram and ethanol. Neurology
34: 357–359, 1984
1027 Rott, H.-D., D. Mulz: Muskeldystrophie
Duchenne: Konduktorinnenerfassung mit Ul-
traschall. Dtsch. Med. Wschr. 107: 1678–1681,
1982

1028 Rougemont, D., M. G. Bousser, B. Wechs-
ler et al.: Manifestations neurologiques de la
maladie de Behçet (vingt-quatre observations).
Rev. Neurol. 138: 493–505, 1982
1029 Rouhani, F.: Artérite temporale giganto-
cellulaire à vitesse de sédimentation basse.
Schweiz. Med. Wschr. 114: 54–56, 1984
1030 Rosseaux, P., M. H. Bernard, B. Scher-
pereel et al.: Thrombose des sinus veineux intra-
craniens. Neuro-chirurgie 24: 197–203, 1978
1031 Rowland, L. P.: Advances in Neurology,
vol. 36: Human Motor Neuron Disease. Raven
Press, New York 1982
1032 Rowland, L. P.: Looking for the cause of
amyotrophic lateral sclerosis. New Engl. J. Med.
311: 979–981, 1984
1033 Rowland, L. P.: Merritt's Textbook of
Neurology, 7th ed. Lea and Febiger, Philadelphia 1984
1034 Rowland, L. P., R. Defendini, W. Sherman
et al.: Macroglobulinemia with peripheral neuropathy simulating motor neuron disease. Ann.
Neurol. 11: 532–536, 1982
1035 Rubenstein, A. E., S. F. Wainapel: Acute
hypokalemic moypathy in alcoholism: a clinical
entity. Arch. Neurol. 34: 553–555, 1977
1036 Ruel, M., Y. Keravel, B. Mignot et al.: Les
cavernomes cérébraux: une malformation vascu-
laire rare. Presse Méd. 15: 1029–1032, 1986
1037 Rushton, J. G., J. C. Stevens, R. H. Miller:
Glossopharyngeal (vasoglossopharyngeal) neuralgia. Arch. Neurol. 38: 201–205, 1981
1038 Russell, D. S., L. J. Rubinstein: Pathology
of Tumours of the Nervous System, 4th ed. Arnold, London 1977
1039 Russell, J. A., M. D. M. Shaw: Chronic
abscess of the brain stem. J. Neurol. Neurosurg.
Psychiat. 40: 625–629, 1977
1040 Russell, W. R.: The Traumatic Amnesias.
Oxford University Press, Oxford 1971
1041 Rüther, E. et al.: Zur Symptomatologie
des narkoleptischen Syndroms. Nervenarzt 43:
640–643, 1972
1042 Ryan, M. S., T. K. F. Taylor: Acute spinal
cord compression in Scheuermann's disease. J.
Bone Jt. Surg. 64: 409–412, 1982
1043 Saadi, A. A., M. Palutke, G. K. Kumar:
Chromosome abnormality in ataxia teleangiectasia. Hum. Genet. 55, 23–29, 1980
1044 Sabouraud, O., J. Oger, F. Darcel,
M. Madigand: Immunosuppression au long
cours dans la sclérose en plaques: évaluation des
traitements commencés avant 1972. Rev. Neurol.
140: 125–130, 1984
1045 Sabra, A. F., M. Hallett, L. Sudarsky,
W. Mullally: Treatment of action tremor in multiple sclerosis with isoniazid. Neurology 32: 913,
1982
1046 Sackellares, J. C., T. R. Swift: Shoulder
enlargement as the presenting sign in syringomyelia. J. Amer. Med. Ass. 236: 2878–2879, 1979

1047 Saenz-Lope, E., F. J. Herranz, J. C. Masdeu: Startle epilepsy: a clinical study. Ann. Neurol. 16: 78–81, 1984

1048 Saffer, D. et al.: Carbohydrate metabolism in motor neurone disease. J. Neurol. Neurosurg. Psychiat. 40: 533–537, 1977

1049 Sagar, H. J., C. P. Warlow, P. W. E. Sheldon, M. M. Esiri: Multiple sclerosis with clinical and radiological features of cerebral tumour. J. Neurol. Neurosurg. Psychiat. 45: 802–808, 1982

1050 Sage, J. I., R. L. Van Uitert, F. E. Lepore: Alcoholic myelopathy without substantial liver disease: a syndrome of progressive dorsal and lateral column dysfunction. Arch. Neurol. 41: 999–1001, 1984

1051 Said, G.: Les dystonies. Nouv. Presse Méd. 1: 527–532, 1972

1052 Sakai, T., S. Mawatari, H. Iwashita et al.: Choreoacanthocytosis: clues to clinical diagnosis. Arch. Neurol. 38: 335–338, 1981

1053 Salazar, O. M., H. Castro-Vita, P. van-Houtte et al.: Improved survival in cases of intracranial ependymoma after radiation therapy: late report and recommendations. J. Neurosurg. 59: 652–659, 1983

1054 Salisachs, P.: Charcot-Marie-Tooth disease associated with "essential tremor": report of 7 cases and a review of the literature. J. Neurol. Sci. 28: 17–40, 1976

1055 Salloum, A., M. Lobel, J. Reiher: Accès céphalalgiques simulant une hémorragie méningée. Rev. Neurol. 133: 131–138, 1977

1056 Sambrook, M. A. et al.: Myasthenia gravis: clinical and histological features in relation to thymectomy. J. Neurol. Neurosurg. Psychiat. 39: 38–43, 1976

1057 Samii, M., P. J. Jannetta: The Cranial Nerves. Springer, Berlin 1981

1058 Sanchez, J. E., V. F. Lopez: Sex-linked sudanophilic leukodystrophy with adrenocortical atrophy (so-called Schilder's disease): report of a case and review of the literature. Neurology 26: 261–269, 1976

1059 Sandok, B. A. et al.: Guidelines for the management of transient ischemic attacks. Mayo Clin. Proc. 53: 665–674, 1978

1060 Satran, R.: Déjerine-Sottas disease revisited. Arch. Neurol. 37: 67–68, 1980

1061 Satya-Murti, S., L. Howard, G. Kohel: The spectrum of neurologic disorder from vitamin E deficiency. Neurology 36: 917–921, 1986

1062 Sawaya, R., R. I. McLauren: Dandy-Walker syndrome. J. Neurosurg. 55: 89–98, 1981

1063 Sayk, J., F.-M. Loebe: Therapie neurologischer Erkrankungen, 2nd ed. VEB Fischer, Jena 1974

1064 Scarlato, G. et al.: Quantitative EMG and histological carrier detection of Duchenne muscular dystrophy. J. Neurol. 216: 235–249, 1977

1065 Schadé, J. P., D. H. Ford: Basic Neurology, 2nd ed. Elsevier, Amsterdam 1975

1066 Scharf, D.: Neurocysticercosis: two hundred thirty-eight cases from a California hospital. Arch. Neurol. 45: 777–780, 1988

1067 Schaumburg, H. H., P. S. Spencer, P. K. Thomas: Disorders of Peripheral Nerves. Davis, Philadelphia 1983

1068 Scheid, W.: Lehrbuch der Neurologie, 5th ed. Thieme, Stuttgart 1983

1069 Scherer, H.: Das Gleichgewicht. Praktische Gleichgewichtsdiagnostik, Teil 1. Springer, Berlin 1984

1070 Schiff, H. B., M. P. Alexander, A. Naeser, A. M. Galaburda: Aphemia: clinical-anatomic correlations. Arch. Neurol. 40: 720–727, 1983

1071 Schiffman, S. S.: Taste and smell in disease. New Engl. J. Med. 308: 1275–1279 and 1337–1343, 1983

1072 Schiffter, R.: Die internukleären Ophthalmoplegien. Nervenarzt 46: 116–127, 1975

1073 Schiffter, R., H. Schliack: Über ein charakteristisches neurologisches Syndrom bei Ischämien in der Arteria-carotis-interna-/-cerebri-media-Strombahn. (Ergebnisse von Schweiß-sekretionstest nach Schlaganfällen). Fortschr. Neurol. Psychiat. 42: 555–562, 1974

1074 Schilt, U.: Der virologische Untersuchungsgang. Ther. Umsch. 37: 891–899, 1980

1075 Schlegel, U.: Neurosarkoidose. Diagnostik und Therapie. Fortschr. Neurol. Psychiat. 55: 1–15, 1987

1076 Schlenska, G. K.: Zur Symptomatik, Diagnostik und Therapie der zentralnervösen Erwachsenen-Toxoplasmose. Fortschr. Neurol. Psychiat. 46: 287–294, 1978

1077 Schliack, H.: Zur Therapie der idiopathischen Fazialislähmung. Dtsch. Ärztebl. 70: 562–565, 1973

1078 Schliack, H.: Ninhydrin-Schweißtest nach Moberg. Dtsch. Med. Wschr. 101: 1336, 1976

1079 Schliack, H., R. Schiffter: Umschriebene Störungen der Schweißsekretion als diagnostisches Kriterium. Med. Welt 22: 1421–1425, 1971

1080 Schliep, G., U. Ritter: Klinik der Syringomyelie. Fortschr. Neurol. Psychiat. 39: 53–82, 1971

1081 Schmidley, J. W., R. P. Simon: Postictal Pleocytosis. Ann. Neurol. 9: 81–83, 1981

1082 Schmidt, D., G. Kommerell: Lidretraktion bei chronisch progressiver okulärer Muskeldystrophie (v. Graefe). Klin. Mbl. Augenheilk. 167: 314–317, 1975

1083 Schmidt, D.: Behandlung der Epilepsie. Medikamentös, psychosozial, operativ, 2nd ed. Thieme, Stuttgart 1984

1084 Schmidt, R., R. Ackermann: Durch Zecken übertragene Meningo-Polyneuritis (Garin-Bujadoux, Bannwarth). Erythema-Chronicum-migrans-Krankheit des Nervensystems. Fortschr. Neurol. Psychiat. 53: 145–153, 1985

1085 Schmidt, R. T. et al.: A pharmacologic

study of the stiff-man syndrome. Neurology 25: 622-626, 1975

1086 Schneider, E., P. A. Fischer, P. Jacobi, A. Grotz: Exogene Psychosen beim Parkinsonsyndrom. Fortschr. Neurol. Psychiat. 52: 207-214, 1984

1087 Schneider, H. et al.: The Lennox syndrome: a clinical study of 40 children. Europ. Neurol. 4: 289-300, 1970

1088 Schonberger, L. B., E. S. Hurwitz, P. Katona et al.: Guillain-Barré syndrome: its epidemiology and associations with influenza vaccination. Ann. Neurol. 9 (Suppl.): 31-38, 1981

1089 Schott, G. D.: Painful legs and moving toes: the role of trauma. J. Neurol. Neurosurg. Psychiat. 44: 344-346, 1981

1090 Schulte, F. J.: Intracranial tumors in childhood - concepts of treatment and prognosis. Neuropediatrics 15: 3-12, 1984

1091 Schulte, F. J., M. Vollrath: Treatment of haemophilus influenzae meningitis. Neuropädiatrie 5: 349-352, 1974

1092 Schulte-Sasse, U., H. J. Eberlein: Maligne Hyperthermie - eine jetzt beherrschbare, potentiell letale Narkosekomplikation. Dtsch. Med. Wschr. 106: 1405-1408, 1981

1093 Schwarz, J. et al.: Außenrotation des Beines bei gesunden und hemiparetischen Probanden. Z. Ges. Neurol. Psychiat. 207: 327-334, 1974

1094 Scot, A. B., R. A. Kennedy, H. A. Stubbs: Botulinum A toxin as a treatment for blepharospasm. Arch. Ophthalm. 103: 347-350, 1985

1095 Scrimgeour, E. M., D. C. Gajdusek: Involvement of the central nervous system in Schistosoma Mansoni and S. Haematobium infection: a review. Brain 108: 1023-1038, 1985

1096 Segawa, M., A. Hosaka, F. Miyagawa: Hereditary progressive dystonia with marked diurnal fluctuation. Advanc. Neurol. 14: 215-233, 1976

1097 Seiler, R.: Die Kombinationstherapie der undifferenzierten supratentoriellen Astrozytome. Schweiz. Med. Wschr. 107: 836-840, 1977

1098 Seitz, D., H. C. Hopf, R. W. C. Janzen et al.: Penicillamin-induzierte Myasthenie bei chronischer Polyarthritis. Dtsch. Med. Wschr. 101: 1153-1158, 1976

1099 Selhorst, J. B. et al.: Diphenylhydantoin-induced cerebellar degeneration. Arch. Neurol. 27: 453-456, 1972

1100 Shapiro, S. et al.: Anticonvulsants and parenteral epilepsy in the development of birth defects. Lancet i: 272-275, 1976

1101 Sharf, B., E. Bental: Pancreatic encephalopathy. J. Neurol. Neurosurg. Psychiat. 34: 357-361, 1971

1102 Sharp, G. C. et al.: Mixed connective tissue disease: an apparently distinct rheumatic disease syndrome associated with a specific antibody to an extractable nuclear antigen (ENA). Amer. J. Med. 52: 148-159, 1972

1103 Shaw, M. D. M., J. A. Russell: Cerebellar abscess: a review of 47 cases. J. Neurol. Neurosurg. Psychiat. 38: 429-435, 1975

1104 Shaw, P. J., D. Bates, N. E. F. Dartlidge et al.: Neurological complications of coronary artery bypass graft surgery: six month follow-up study. Brit. Med. J. 293: 165-167, 1986

1105 Sheehy, M. P., C. D. Marsden: Writer's cramp - a focal dystonia. Brain 105: 461-480, 1982

1106 Shephard, R. H.: Prognosis of spontaneous (non-traumatic) subarachnoid haemorrhage of unknown cause: a personal series 1958-1980. Lancet i: 777-779, 1984

1107 Shuman, R. M. et al.: The biology of childhood ependymomas. Arch. Neurol. 32: 731-739, 1975

1108 Shy, G. M., G. A. Drager: A neurological syndrome associated with orthostatic hypotension. Arch. Neurol. 2: 511-527, 1960

1109 Sima, A. A. F., D. M. Robertson: Involvement of peripheral nerve and muscle in Fabry's disease. Arch. Neurol. 35: 291-301, 1978

1110 Simard, J. M., F. Garcia-Bengochea, W. E. Ballinger et al.: Cavernous angioma: a review of 126 collected and 12 new clinical cases. Neurosurgery 18: 162-172, 1986

1111 Simpson, J.: Listeria monocytogenes meningitis: an opportunistic infection. J. Neurol. Neurosurg. Psychiat. 34: 657-663, 1971

1112 Singer, W. D.: Transient Gilles de la Tourette syndrome after chronic neuroleptic withdrawal. Develop. Med. Child Neurol. 4: 518-530, 1981

1113 Singhal, B. S., D. K. Dastur: Eales' disease with neurological involvement, part 1: clinical features in 9 patients. J. Neurol. Sci. 27: 313-321, 1976

1114 Sipe, J. C.: Leigh's syndrome: the adult form of subacute necrotizing encephalomyelopathy with predilection for the brainstem. Neurology 23: 1030-1038, 1973

1115 Sköldenberg, B., M. Forsgren, K. Alestig et al.: Acyclovir versus vidarabine in herpes simplex encephalitis: randomised multicentre study in consecutive swedish patients. Lancet ii: 707-711, 1984

1116 Skouteli, H., V. Dubowitz: Fasciculation of the eyelids: an additional clue to clinical diagnosis in spinal muscular atrophy. Neuropediatrics 15: 145-146, 1984

1117 Smith, R. R., S. C. Boone, R. W. Crowell et al.: Stroke and the extracranial vessels. Raven Press, New York 1984

1118 Snider, W. D., D. M. Simpson, S. Nielsen et al.: Neurological complications of acquired immune deficiency syndrome: analysis of 50 patients. Ann. Neurol. 14: 403-418, 1983

1119 Snow, R. M., W. W. Dismukes: Cryptococcal meningitis. Arch. Intern. Med. 135: 1155, 1975

1120 Snyder, B. D. et al.: Neurological status and prognosis after cardiopulmonary arrest: a retrospective study. Neurology 27: 807–811, 1977

1121 So, E. L., J. F. Toole, P. Dalal, D. M. Moody: Cephalic fibromuscular dysplasia in 32 patients: clinical findings and radiologic features. Arch. Neurol. 38: 619–622, 1981

1122 Sobue, I. et al.: Myeloneuropathy with abdominal disorders in Japan: a clinical study of 752 cases. Neurology 21: 168–173, 1971

1123 Sobue, I. et al.: Myeloneuropathy with abdominal disorders in Japan: neuropathology findings in seven autopsied cases. Neurology 22: 1034–1039, 1972

1124 Soffer, D. et al.: Paroxysmal choreoathetosis as a presenting symptom in idiopathic hypoparathyroidism. J. Neurol. Neurosurg. Psychiat. 40: 692–694, 1977

1125 Soffer, D., H. W. Grotzky, I. Rapin, K. Suzuki: Cockayne syndrome: unusual neuropathological findings and review of the literature. Ann. Neurol. 6: 340–348, 1979

1126 Sokol, R. J.: Alcohol and abnormal outcomes of pregnancy. Amer. J. Med. Ass. 125: 143 148, 1981

1127 Solingen, L. D. et al.: Subclinical eye movement disorders in patients with multiple sclerosis. Neurology 27: 614–619, 1977

1128 Soliven, B. C., D. J. Lange, A. S. Penn: Seronegative myasthenia gravis. Neurology 38: 514–516, 1988

1129 Solomon, G. E., M. Engel, H. L. Hecht, A. R. Rapoport: Progressive dyskinesia due to internal cerebral vein thrombosis. Neurology 32: 769–772, 1982

1130 Soloway, S. S., J. C. Moench: Progressive and treatable cerebellar ataxia in macroglobulinemia. Neurology 30: 536–538, 1980

1131 Sorensen, S. C., R. T. Eagan, M. Scott: Meningeal carcinomatosis in patients with primary breast or lung cancer. Mayo Clin. Proc. 59: 91–94, 1984

1132 Soyka, D.: Kopfschmerz. Medizin, Basel 1984

1133 Sparacio, R. R. et al.: Hypernatremia and chorea: a report of two cases. Neurology 26: 46–50, 1976

1134 Spatz, R.: Klassifikation epileptischer Anfälle. Münchn. Med. Wschr. 124: 689–690, 1982

1135 Spector, G. J. et al.: Neurologic manifestations of glomus tumors in the head and neck. Arch. Neurol. 33: 270–274, 1976

1136 Spector, R. H. et al.: Edrophonium infrared optokinetic nystagmography in the diagnosis of myasthenia gravis. Neurology 25: 317–321, 1975

1137 Spector, R. H. et al.: Phenytoin-induced ophthalmoplegia. Neurology 26: 1031–1034, 1976

1138 Spiess, H.: Schädigungen am peripheren Nervensystem durch ionisierende Strahlen. Monographien aus dem Gesamtgebiet der Neurologie. Springer, Berlin 1972

1139 Spillane, J. D. et al.: Painful legs and moving toes. Brain 94: 541–556, 1971

1140 Spillane, J. D., H. Urich: Trigeminal neuropathy with nasal ulceration: report of two cases and one necropsy. J. Neurol. Neurosurg. Psychiat. 39: 105–113, 1976

1141 Staehelin Jensen, T.: Transient global amnesia in childhood. Develop. Med. Child Neurol. 22: 654–667, 1980

1142 Staehelin Jensen, T., B. de Fine Olivarius: Transient global amnesia – its clinical and pathophysiological basis and prognosis. Acta Neurol. Scand. 63: 220–230, 1981

1143 Stahl, S. M., P. A. Berger: Bromocriptine in dystonia. Lancet ii: 745, 1981

1144 Stalberg, E. et al.: Neuromuscular transmission in myasthenia gravis studied with single fibre electromyography. J. Neurol. Neurosurg. Psychiat. 37: 540–547, 1974

1145 Stamm, T., D. Lubach: Livedo racemosa generalisata und zerebrale Durchblutungsstörungen. Akt. Neurol. 8: 59–61, 1981

1146 Stark, J. R., R. A. Henson, S. J. W. Evans: Spinal metastases: a retrospective survey from a general hospital. Brain 105: 189–213, 1982

1147 Starosta-Rubinstein, S., A. B. Young, K. Kluin: Clinical assessment of 31 patients with Wilson's disease: correlations with structural changes on magnetic resonance imaging. Arch. Neurol. 44: 365–370, 1987

1148 Steck, A. J., C. Meier, M. Vandevelde, F. Regli: Polyneuropathies et gammapathies: une forme avec anticorps anti-glycoproteine MAG. Rev. Neurol. 140: 28 36, 1984

1149 Steck, A. J., N. Murray, J. C. Justafre et al.: Passive transfer studies in demyelinating neuropathy with IgM monoclonal antibodies to myelin associated glycoprotein. J. Neurol. Neurosurg. Psychiat. 48: 927–929, 1985

1150 Steele, J. C., A. Vasuvat: Recurrent multiple cranial nerve palsies: a distinctive syndrome of cranial polyneuropathy. J. Neurol. Neurosurg. Psychiat. 33: 828 832, 1970

1151 Steele, J. C. et al.: Progressive supranuclear palsy. Arch. Neurol. 10: 333–359, 1964

1152 Steere, A. C., S. E. Malawista, J.-H. Newman et al.: Antibiotic therapy in Lyme disease. Ann. Intern. Med. 93: 1–8, 1980

1153 Stefan, H., D.-K. Böker, J. Müller, F. Gullotta: Glykogenose Typ II (Morbus Pompe) als Myopathie des Erwachsenen. Dtsch. Med. Wschr. 102: 1512–1514, 1977

1154 Steiger, H.-J.: Zur Behandlung der traumatischen Karotisdissektion. Neurochirurgia 31: 128–133, 1988

1155 Steiger, H.-J., R. V. Markwalder, H.-J. Reulen: Das zerebrale Kavernom als Ursache von rezidivierenden Hirnblutungen und epileptischen Anfällen. Schweiz. Med. Wschr. 118: 471–477, 1988

1156 Stein, S. C., T. W. Langfitt: Normal-pressure hydrocephalus: predicting the results of cerebrospinal fluid shunting. J. Neurosurg. 41: 463–470, 1974

1157 Stephenson, J. B. P.: Reflex anoxic seizures ("white breath-holding"): non-epileptic vagal attacks. Arch. Dis. Childh. 53: 193–200, 1978

1158 Sterman, A. A. et al.: The acute sensory neuronopathy syndrome: a distinct clinical entity. Ann. Neurol. 7: 354–358, 1980

1159 Stern, B. J., A. Krumholz, C. Johns et al.: Sarcoidosis and its neurological manifestations. Arch. Neurol. 42: 909–917, 1985

1160 Stevens, D. L., W. B. Matthews: Cryptogenic drop-attacks: an affliction of women. Brit. Med. J. I: 439–442, 1973

1161 Stober, T., K. Schimrigk, S. Dietzsch, T. Thielen: Intrathecal thyrotropin-releasing hormone therapy of amyotrophic lateral sclerosis. J. Neurol. 232: 13–14, 1985

1162 Stöhr, M.: Iatrogene Nervenläsionen. Thieme, Stuttgart 1980

1163 Stöhr, M., J. Dichgans, H. C. Diener, U. W. Buettner: Evozierte Potentiale. Springer, Berlin 1982

1164 Störtebecker, P.: Motor Neuron Disorder: Deficiency of Arterial Blood Supply to Spinal Cord and Brain Stem. Störtebecker Foundation for Research, Stockholm 1983

1165 Streib, E. W., A. D. Rothner: Eaton-Lambert myasthenic syndrome: long-term treatment of three patients with Prednisone. Ann. Neurol. 10: 448–453, 1981

1166 Stucki, P., W. Hadorn: Lehrbuch der Therapie, 7th ed. Huber, Bern 1983

1167 Sturm, W., W. Hartje, V. J. Kitteringham et al.: Die psychologische Diagnose allgemeiner hirnorganischer Leistungsstörungen. Akt. Neurol. 2: 141–150, 1975

1168 Suchenwirth, R.: Gibt es ein Syndrom der Arteria sulcocommissuralis? Nervenarzt 44: 604–605, 1973

1169 Suchenwirth, R. M. A.: Beitrag zum Problem Morbus Behçet und Nervensystem. 10jährige Verlaufsbeobachtung mit Schwangerschaft. Fortschr. Neurol. Psychiat. 52: 41–47, 1984

1170 Sunderland, S.: Nerves and Nerve Injuries, 2nd ed. Churchill Livingstone, Edinburgh 1978

1171 Supino, V. et al.: Toxic encephalopathy due to ingestion of bismuth salts: clinical and EEG studies of 45 patients. J. Neurol. Neurosurg. Psychiat. 40: 748–752, 1977

1172 Susac, J. O. et al.: Superior oblique myokymia. Arch. Neurol. 29: 432–434, 1973

1173 Sutcher, H. D. et al.: Orofacial dyskinesia: a dental dimension. J. Amer. Med. Ass. 216: 1459–1463, 1970

1174 Suter, C. C., B. F. Westmoreland, F. W. Sharbrough, R. C. Hermann, Jr.: Electroencephalographic abnormalities in interferon encephalopathy: a preliminary report. Mayo Clin. Proc. 59: 847–850, 1984

1175 Sutherland, J. M. et al.: The Epilepsies: Modern Diagnosis and Treatment, 2nd ed. Churchill Livingstone, Edinburgh 1974

1176 Swank, R. L.: Multiple sclerosis: twenty years on low fat diet. Arch. Neurol. 23: 460–474, 1970

1177 Swanson, J. W., J. J. Kelly, Jr., W. M. McConahey: Neurologic aspects of thyroid dysfunction. Mayo Clin. Proc. 56: 504–512, 1981

1178 Swash, M. et al.: Treatment of involuntary movement disorders with tetrabenazine. J. Neurol. Neurosurg. Psychiat. 35: 186–191, 1972

1179 Sweet, W. H., J. G. Wespsic: Controlled thermocoagulation of trigeminal ganglion and rootlets for differential destruction of pain fibers. J. Neurosurg. 40: 143–146, 1974

1180 Syndyk, R., M. J. W. Brennan: "Lhermitte's sign" as a presenting symptom of subacute combined degeneration of the cord. Ann. Neurol. 13: 215–216, 1983

1181 Tabira, T., H. Shibasaki, Y. Kuroiwa: Reflex sympathetic dystrophy (causalgia) treatment with guanethidine. Arch. Neurol. 40: 430–432, 1983

1182 Taddei, I. M., H.-P. Ludin: Der essentielle Tremor: Eine katamnestische Untersuchung. Schweiz. Arch. Neurol. Neurochir. Psychiat. 139: 33–46, 1988

1183 Tahmoush, A. J. et al.: Hartnup disease: clinical, pathological and biochemical observations. Arch. Neurol. 33: 797–807, 1976

1184 Takamori, M. et al.: Myasthenic syndromes in hypothyroidism: electrophysiological study of neuromuscular transmission and muscle contraction in two patients. Arch. Neurol. 26: 326–335, 1972

1185 Tal, Y. et al.: Dandy-Walker syndrome: analysis of 21 cases. Develop. Med. Child Neurol. 22: 189–201, 1980

1186 Tanaka, H. et al.: Cardiac involvement in the Kugelberg-Welander syndrome. Amer. J. Cardiol. 38: 528–532, 1976

1187 Tator, C. H., K. Meguro, D. W. Rowed: Favorable results with syringosubarachnoid shunts for treatment of syringomyelia. J. Neurosurg. 56: 517–523, 1982

1188 Tenny, R. T., E. R. Laws, B. R. Younge, J. A. Rush: The neurosurgical management of optic glioma: results in 104 patients. J. Neurosurg. 57: 452–458, 1982

1189 Teräväinen, H. et al.: Effect of propranolol on essential tremor. Neurology 26: 27–30, 1976

1190 Terrence, C. F. et al.: Unexpected, unexplained death in epileptic patients. Neurology 25: 594–598, 1975

1191 Terry, R. D., R. Katzmann: Senile dementia of the Alzheimer type. Ann. Neurol. 14: 497–506, 1983

1192 Teuscher, U., O. Meienberg: Ischemic oculomotor nerve palsy. J. Neurol. 232: 144–149, 1985

1193 Teychenne, P. F., D. Bergsrud, A. Racy, B. Vern: Low dose bromocriptine therapy in Parkinson's disease. Res. Clin. Forums 3: 37–48, 1981

1194 Thaler, M. M. et al.: Reye's syndrome due to a novel protein-tolerant variant of ornithine-transcarbamylase deficiency. Lancet ii: 438–440, 1974

1195 Thomalske, G. et al.: Zur chirurgischen Behandlung der cervicalen Myelopathie. Nervenarzt 43: 520–524, 1972

1196 Thomas, J. E. et al.: Epilepsia partialis continua: a review of 32 cases. Arch. Neurol. 34: 266–275, 1977

1197 Thomas, P. K., H. H. Schaumburg, P. S. Spencer et al.: Central distal axonopathy syndromes: newly recognized models of naturally occuring human degenerative disease. Ann. Neurol. 15: 313–315, 1984

1198 Thompson, B. M., J. J. Corbett, L. B. Kline, H. S. Thompson: Pseudo-Horner's syndrome. Arch. Neurol. 39: 108–111, 1982

1199 Tobin, W. D., D. D. Layton: The diagnosis and natural history of spinal cord arteriovenous malformations. Mayo Clin. Proc. 51: 637–646, 1976

1200 Todorov, A. B.: Clinical Neurology: the Resident's Guide. Thieme-Stratton, New York 1983

1201 Toglia, J. U.: Acute flexion-extension injury of the neck: electronystagmographic study of 309 patients. Neurology 26: 808–814, 1976

1202 Tomashefsky, A. F. et al.: Acute autonomic neuropathy. Neurology 22: 251–255, 1972

1203 Toole, J. F. et al.: Transient ischemic attacks: a prospective study of 225 patients. Neurology 28: 746–753, 1978

1204 Toole, J. F., H. J. M. Barnett, V. Hachinski et al.: Cerebrovascular Disorders, 3rd ed. Raven Press, New York 1984

1205 Tosi, C., F. Regli, J. Wenk: Die Creutzfeldt-Jakob'sche Krankheit. Klinische, epidemiologische, pathogenetische und ätiologische Gesichtspunkte. Fortschr. Neurol. Psychiat. 48: 353–384, 1980

1206 Toyka, K. V. et al.: Myasthenia gravis. New Engl. J. Med. 296: 125–131, 1977

1207 Traub, R., D. C. Gajdusek, C. J. Gibbs: Transmissible virus dementia: the relation of transmissible spongiform encephalopathy to Creutzfeld-Jakob disease. In: Aging and Dementia, ed. by W. L. Smith, M. Kinsbowne. New York 1977

1208 Trend, P. S., C. M. Wiles, G. T. Spencer et al.: Acid maltase deficiency in adults: diagnosis and management in five cases. Brain 108: 845–860, 1985

1209 Trouillas, P., G. Aimard: Le syndrome prémonitoire de l'hémorrhagie méningée. Nouv. Presse Méd. 1: 2235–2236, 1972

1210 Tuck, R. R., J. G. McLeod: Autonomic dysfunction in Guillain-Barré syndrome. J. Neurol. Neurosurg. Psychiat. 44: 983–990, 1981

1211 Twomey, J. A., M. L. E. Espir: Paroxysmal symptoms as the first manifestations of multiple sclerosis. J. Neurol. Neurosurg. Psychiat. 43: 296–304, 1980

1212 Ucar, S. et al.: Increased intracranial pressure associated with spinal cord tumours. Neurochirurgia 19: 265–268, 1976

1213 Ueno, T., N. Takahata: Chronic brainstem encephalitis with mental symptoms and ataxia. J. Neurol. Neurosurg. Psychiat. 41: 516–524, 1978

1214 Uldry, P. A., F. Regli, A. Uske: Ramollissements cérébelleux. Presentation clinique et évaluation en tomodensitométrie cérébrale. Schweiz. Med. Wschr. 116: 34–41, 1986

1215 Ullrich, J.: Das Fisher-Syndrom. Zur Symptomatik und Nosologie einer Sonderform der Polyradiculoneuritis. Nervenarzt 46: 417–421, 1975

1216 Ulrich, J.: Die cerebralen Entmarkungskrankheiten im Kindesalter. Diffuse Hirnsklerosen. Schriftenreihe Neurologie, vol. 6. Springer, Berlin 1971

1217 Ulrich, J.: Grundriß der Neuropathologie. Springer, Berlin 1975

1218 Ungar-Sargon, J. Y., R. E. Lovelace, J. C. M. Brust: Spastic paraplegia-paraparesis. J. Neurol. Sci. 46: 1–12, 1980

1219 Utterback, R. A. et al.: Pancreatic function in amyotrophic lateral sclerosis. J. Neurol. Neurosurg. Psychiat. 33: 544–547, 1970

1220 Vahar-Matiar, H. et al.: Zur ektodermalen Dysplasie Typ Bloch-Sulzberger sc. Incontinentia pigmenti. Nervenarzt 45: 88–93, 1974

1221 Valli, G., S. Barbieri, S. Cappa et al.: Syndromes of abnormal muscular activity: overlap between continuous muscle fibre activity and the stiff man syndrome. J. Neurol. Neurosurg. Psychiat. 46: 241–247, 1983

1222 Valli, G., S. Barbieri, P. Sergi et al.: Evidence of motor neuron involvement in chronic respiratory insufficiency. J. Neurol. 47: 1117–1121, 1984

1223 Valpey, R. et al.: Acute and chronic progressive encephalopathy due to gasoline sniffing. Neurology 28: 507–510, 1978

1224 Van den Bergh, R.: Neurochirurgische Behandlung der Syringomyelie. In: Spinale raumfordernde Prozesse, ed. W. Schiefer, H. Wieck. Perimed, Erlangen 1976, pp. 333–338

1225 Van der Ark, G. D.: Cardiovascular changes with acute subdural hematoma. Surg. Neurol. 3: 305–308, 1975

1226 van Staveren, G., R. M. Kosanin:

Anesthesia in myotonic dystrophy. Rev. Anesthesiol. 10: 26-27, 1983

1227 Van Woert, M., V. H. Sethy: Therapy of intention myoclonus with L-5-hydroxytryptophan and a peripheral decarboxylase inhibitor, MK 486. Neurology 25: 135-140, 1975

1228 Van Zandycke, M., J.-J. Martin, L. Vande Gaer, P. van den Heyning: Facial myokymia in the Guillain-Barré syndrome: a clinicopathologic study. Neurology 32: 744-748, 1982

1229 Vanasse, M. et al.: Shuddering attacks in children: an early clinical manifestation of essential tremor. Neurology 26: 1027-1030, 1976

1230 Vassella, F.: Benigne Epilepsien beim Kind und beim Jugendlichen. Praxis 68: 691-695, 1979

1231 Vassella, F., J. Lütschg, M. Mumenthaler: Cogan's congenital ocular motor apraxia in two successive generations. Develop. Med. Child Neurol. 14: 788-796, 1972

1232 Vermeulen, M., K. W. Lindsay, G. D. Murray et al.: Antifibrinolytic treatment in subarachnoid hemorrhage. New Engl. J. Med. 311: 432-437, 1984

1233 Vlahovitch, B., J. M. Fuentes, Y. Coucair et al.: Valeur pronostique indissociable des fonctions spinothalamique et corticospinale dans les traumatismes médullaires graves. Neuro-chirurgie 23: 55-72, 1977

1234 Vom Brocke, I., F. Regli: Die idiopathische Trigeminusneuropathie. Schweiz. Med. Wschr. 104: 1029-1031, 1974

1235 Von Torklus, D.: Zervikaler Schwindel. Orthop. Prax. 14: 167-172, 1978

1236 von Wartburg, J.-P., R. Bühler: Alcoholism and aldehydism: new biomedical concepts. Lab. Invest. 50: 5-15, 1984

1237 Vroom, F. Q., M. Greer: Mercury vapour intoxication. Brain 95: 305-318, 1972

1238 Wadia, R. S. et al.: Neurological manifestations of organophosphorous insecticide poisoning. J. Neurol. Neurosurg. Psychiat. 37: 841-847, 1974

1239 Wahle, H.: Behandlung und Rehabilitation bei Patienten mit Querschnittslähmungen. In: Klinik der Gegenwart, vol. 1, ed. H. E. Bock, W. Gerok, F. Harmann. Urban and Schwarzenberg, München 1977, pp. 161-182

1240 Walker, J. E., J. D. Cook, P. Harrison, P. Stastny: HLA and the response of lymphocytes to viral antigens in patients with multiple sclerosis. Hum. Immunol. 4: 71-78, 1982

1241 Wall, M., H. S. Wray: The one-and-a-half syndrome - a unilateral disorder of the pontine tegmentum: a study of 20 cases and review of the literature. Neurology 33: 971-980, 1983

1242 Wallace, D. C.: A new manifestation of Leber's disease and a new explanation for the agency responsible for its unusual pattern of inheritance. Brain 93: 121-132, 1970

1243 Walls, T. J., R. A. Jones, N. E. F. Cartlidge,

M. Saunders: Alexander's disease with Rosenthal fibre formation in an adult. J. Neurol. Neurosurg. Psychiat. 47: 399-403, 1984

1244 Walser, H., H. Mattle, H. M. Keller: Komabeurteilung mit Hilfe evozierter Hirnpotentiale. Schweiz. Med. Wschr. 113: 1757-1765, 1983

1245 Walsh, F. B., W. F. Hoyt: Clinical Neuro-Ophthalmology, 4th ed. Williams and Wilkins, Baltimore 1982

1246 Walsh, J.: The neuropathy of multiple myeloma: an electrophysiologic and histologic study. Arch. Neurol. 25: 404-414, 1971

1247 Walton, J. N.: Disorders of Voluntary Muscle, 5th ed. Churchill Livingstone, Edinburgh 1988

1248 Waespe, W., J. Hayek, W. Wichmann et al.: Die olivo-ponto-zerebelläre Atrophie als wichtige Differentialdiagnose ataktischer Gangstörungen beim älteren Patienten. Schweiz. Med. Wschr. 118: 1032-1038, 1988

1249 Wassmann, H., K. H. Holbach, A. P. Bonatelli et al.: Stenose des Spinalkanals bei Chondrodystrophie. Nervenarzt 48: 342-344, 1977

1250 Waters, W. E., P. J. O'Connor: Prevalence of migraine. J. Neurol. Neurosurg. Psychiat. 38: 613-616, 1975

1251 Webster, D. D.: Critical analysis of the disability in Parkinson's disease. Mod. Treatm. 5: 257-282, 1968

1252 Weder, B., M. Mumenthaler: Neurolues in einer Schweizerischen Neurologischen Universitätsklinik. Nervenarzt 54: 633-639, 1983

1253 Weder, B., O. Meienberg, E. Wildi, C. Meier: Neurological disorder of vitamin E deficiency in acquired intestinal malabsorption. Neurology 34: 1561-1565, 1984

1254 Weidmann, P.: Die orthostatische Hypotonie. Schweiz. Med. Wschr. 114: 246-260, 1984

1255 Weiner, L. P.: Possible role of androgen receptors in amyotrophic lateral sclerosis: hypothesis A. Arch. Neurol. 37: 129-131, 1980

1256 Weingeist, T. A., E. J. Goldman, J. C. Folk et al.: Terson's syndrome. Ophthalmology 93: 1435-1442, 1986

1257 Weisberg, L.: Multiple spontaneous intracerebral hematomas: clinical and computed tomographic correlations. Neurology 7: 897-900, 1981

1258 Weisberg, L. A. et al.: Empty sella syndrome as complication of benign intracranial hypertension. J. Neurosurg. 43: 177-180, 1975

1259 Weiss, M., M. Schmid, T. Hess et al.: Extrapulmonale Komplikationen der Mycoplasma pneumoniae-Infektion. Dtsch. Med. Wschr. 112: 1896-1901, 1987

1260 Wende, S., B. Ludwig, T. Kishikawa et al.: The value of CT in diagnosis and prognosis of different inborn neurodegenerative disorders in childhood. J. Neurol. 231: 57-70, 1984

1261 Werlin, S. L., B. J. D'Souza, W. J. Hogan et al.: Sandifer syndrome: an unappreciated clinical entity. Develop. Med. Child Neurol. 22: 374–378, 1980

1262 West, T., R. J. Davies, R. E. Kelly: Horner's syndrome and headache due to carotid artery disease. Brit. Med. J. 1: 818–820, 1976

1263 Westmoreland, F. et al.: Alpha-coma: electroencephalographic, clinical, pathologic and etiologic correlations. Arch. Neurol. 32: 713–718, 1975

1264 Wheeler, S. D., J. Ochoa: Poliomyelitis-like syndrome associated with asthma: a case report and review of the literature. Arch. Neurol. 37: 52–53, 1980

1265 Whisnant, J. P. et al.: The effect of anticoagulant therapy on the prognosis of patients with transient cerebral ischemic attacks in a community: Rochester, Minnesota, 1955 through 1969. Mayo Clin. Proc. 48: 844–848, 1973

1266 Whitaker, J. N. et al.: Hereditary sensory neuropathy: association with increased synthesis of immunoglobulin A. Arch. Neurol. 30: 359–371, 1974

1267 White, K. T., T. R. Fleming, E. R. Laws: Single metastasis to the brain. Mayo Clin. Proc. 56: 424–428, 1981

1268 Whiteley, A. M. et al.: Progressive encephalomyelitis with rigidity – its relation to "subacute myoclonic spinal neuronitis" and to the "stiff man syndrome". Brain 99: 27–42, 1976

1269 Whitley, R. J.: Adenine arabinoside therapy of biopsy-proved herpes simplex encephalitis. New Engl. J. Med. 297: 289–294, 1977

1270 Whitley, R. J., S.-J. Soong, M. S. Hirsch et al.: Herpes simplex encephalitis: vidarabine therapy and diagnostic problems. New Engl. J. Med. 304: 313–318, 1981

1271 Wiebers, D. O. et al.: The ophthalmologic manifestations of Wilson's disease. Mayo Clin. Proc. 52: 409–416, 1977

1272 Wiebers, D. O., W. N. Folger, G. S. Forbes et al.: Ophthalmodynamometry and ocular pneumoplethysmography for detection of carotid occlusive disease. Arch. Neurol. 39: 690–691, 1982

1273 Wiederholt, W. C.: Therapy for Neurologic Disorders, Wiley, New York 1982

1274 Wiederholt, W. C., R. G. Siekert: Neurological manifestations of sarcoidosis. Neurology 15: 1147–1154, 1965

1275 Wieser, H. G., C. Probst, G. Costabile: Das gekreuzte Lasègue'sche Zeichen. Schweiz. Arch. Neurol. Neurochir. Psychiat. 116: 315–324, 1975

1276 Wiesner, H., M. Mumenthaler: Schleuderverletzungen der Halswirbelsäule. Eine katamnestische Studie. Arch. Orthop. Unfall-Chir. 81: 13–36, 1975

1277 Williams, F. J. B., J. M. Walshe: Wilson's disease: an analysis of the cranial computerized tomographic appearances found in 60 patients and the changes in response to treatment with chelating agents. Brain 104: 735–752, 1981

1278 Willner, J. P., G. A. Graboski, R. E. Gordon et al.: Chronic GM_2 gangliosidosis masquerading as atypical Friedreich ataxia: clinical, morphologic and biochemical studies of nine cases. Neurology 7: 787–798, 1981

1279 Wills, M. R., J. Savory: Aluminium poisoning: dialysis encephalopathy, osteomalacia and anaemia. Lancet ii: 29–33, 1983

1280 Willvonseder, R. et al.: A hereditary disorder with dementia, spastic dysarthria, vertical eye movement paresis, gait disturbance, splenomegaly and abnormal copper metabolism. Neurology 23: 1039–1049, 1973

1281 Windorfer, A., Jr., W. Sauer: Drug interactions during anticonvulsant therapy in childhood: diphenylhydantoin, primidone, phenobarbitone, clonazepam, nitrazepam, carbamazepine and dipropylacetate. Neuropädiatrie 8: 29–41, 1977

1282 Winkelmann, W.: L-Dopa-Langzeitbehandlung einer Torsionsdystonie. J. Neurol. 208: 319–323, 1975

1283 Winn, H. R. et al.: The long-term prognosis in untreated cerebral aneurysms, 1: the incidence of late hemorrhage in cerebral aneurysm: a 10-year evaluation of 364 patients. Ann. Neurol. 1: 358–370, 1977

1284 Wisniewski, H. M., A. B. Keith: Chronic relapsing experimental allergic encephalomyelitis: an experimental model of multiple sclerosis. Ann. Neurol. 1: 144–148, 1977

1285 Wisniewski, K., M. Dambska, J. H. Sher, Q. Quazi: A clinical neuropathological study of the fetal alcohol syndrome. Neuropediatrics 14: 197–201, 1983

1286 Wolf, P.: Nomenklatur und Klassifikation epileptischer Anfälle und Syndrome. Nervenarzt 50: 547–554, 1979

1287 Wolf, P.: Familiäre episodische Ataxie. Nervenarzt 51: 355–358, 1980

1288 Wolf, P., H. Assmus: Paroxysmale Dysarthrie und Ataxie. Ein pathognomonisches Anfallssyndrom bei multipler Sklerose. J. Neurol. 208, 27–38, 1974

1289 Wolf, P. A. et al.: Epidemiologic assessment of chronic atrial fibrillation and risk of stroke: the Framingham study. Neurology 28: 973–977, 1978

1290 Wolf, S. M. et al.: Treatment of Bell palsy with prednisone: a prospective, randomized study. Neurology 28: 158–161, 1978

1291 Wolff, H. G.: Headache and Other Head Pain, 3rd ed. Oxford University Press, Oxford 1972

1292 Wolfgram, F., L. Myers: Amyotrophic lateral sclerosis: effect of serum on anterior horn cells in tissue culture. Science 179: 579–580, 1973

1293 Wolstenholme, G. E. W., M. O'Connor: Alzheimer's Disease and Related Conditions. Ciba Foundation Symposium, London. Churchill, London 1970

1294 Wood, J. H. et al.: Normal-pressure hydrocephalus: diagnosis and patient selection for
shunt surgery. Neurology 24: 517-526, 1974

1295 Wright, J. T.: Slipping-rib syndrome: Lancet ii: 632, 1980

1296 Wrobel, C. J., E. H. Oldfield, G. DiChiro
et al.: Myelopathy due to intracranial dural arteriovenous fistulas draining intrathecally into spinal medullary veins: report of three cases. J.
Neurosurg. 69: 934-939, 1988

1297 Yahr, M. D., A. T. Frontera: Acute autonomic neuropathy, its occurrence in infectious
mononucleosis. Arch. Neurol. 32: 132-133, 1975

1298 Yahr, M. D. et al.: Autopsy findings in
parkinsonism following treatment with levodopa. Neurology Suppl. 22, Nr. 5, part 2: 56-71,
1972

1299 Yamamoto, I., M. Matsumae, A. Ikeda:
Thoracic spinal stenosis: experience with seven
cases. J. Neurosurg. 68: 37-40, 1988

1300 Yasargil, M. G.: Microneurosurgery,
vol. 1: Microsurgical Anatomy of the Basal Cisterns and Vessels of the Brain. Thieme, Stuttgart
1984

1301 Yasargil, M. G.: Microneurosurgery,
vol. 2: Clinical Considerations, Surgery of the Intracranial Aneurysms and Results. Thieme, Stuttgart 1984

1302 Yasargil, M. G. et al.: Hydrocephalus following spontaneous subarachnoid hemorrhage:
clinical features and treatment. J. Neurosurg. 39:
474-479, 1973

1303 Yase, Y.: The pathogenesis of amyotrophic lateral sclerosis. Lancet i: 292-296,
1972

1304 Yiannikas, C., J. G. McLeod, J. C. Walsh:
Peripheral neuropathy associated with polycythemia vera. Neurology 33: 139-143, 1983

1305 Young, A. C. et al.: Mental change as an
early feature of multiple sclerosis. J. Neurol.
Neurosurg. Psychiat. 39: 1008-1013, 1976

1306 Young, I. R., A. S. Hall, C. A. Pallis et al.:
Nuclear magnetic resonance imaging of the
brain in multiple sclerosis. Lancet ii: 1063-1066,
1981

1307 Young, R. R. et al.: Pure pan-dysauto-
nomia with recovery: description and discussion
of diagnostic criteria. Brain 98: 613-636, 1975

1308 Younger, D. S., S. Chou, A. P. Hays et al.:
Primary lateral sclerosis: a clinical diagnosis
reemerges. Arch. Neurol. 45: 1304-1307, 1988

1309 Zahn, J. R.: Incidence and characteristics
of voluntary nystagmus. J. Neurol. Neurosurg.
Psychiat. 41: 617-623, 1978

1310 Zeh, W.: Progressive Paralyse. Verlaufs-
und Korrelationsstudien. Thieme, Stuttgart 1984

1311 Ziegler, D. K.: Prolonged relief of dystonic movements with diazepam. Neurology 31:
1457-1458, 1981

1312 Ziegler, D. K., S. Batnitzky: Coccygody-
nia caused by perineural cyst. Neurology 34:
829-830, 1984

1313 Ziegler, D. K. et al.: Correlation of bruits
over the carotid artery with angiographically
demonstrated lesions. Neurology 21: 860-865,
1971

1314 Zschocke, St.: Pathogenese epileptischer
Reaktionen beim arteriovenösen Angiom des
Gehirns. Beitrag zur Frage epileptischer Reak-
tionen bei zerebralen Durchblutungsstörungen.
Fortschr. Neurol. Psychiat. 42: 433-453, 1974

1315 Zülch, K. J.: Brain Tumors: their Biology
and Pathology, 2nd English ed. [based on 4th
German ed.] Springer, New York 1965

1316 Zülch, K. J.: Trigiminal paresthesias in
cervical 5/6 disk involvement. In: The Cranial
Nerves, ed. M. Samii, P. J. Jannetta, Springer,
Berlin 1981, pp. 359-360

Subject Index

Bold-faced page numbers refer to illustrations.

notes